Nephrology

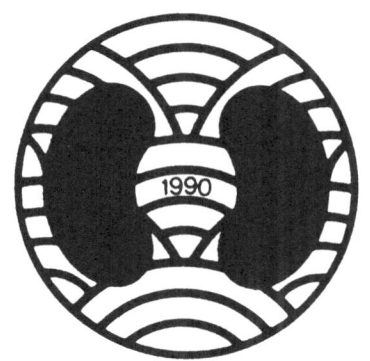

Nephrology VOLUME II

PROCEEDINGS OF THE
XITH INTERNATIONAL CONGRESS OF NEPHROLOGY

Editor
Michinobu Hatano

Associate Editors
Nishio Honda · Hyoe Ishikawa · Kenkichi Koiso
Kiyoshi Kurokawa · Tadao Niijima
Nobuhiro Sugino · Susumu Takahashi

With 239 Figures

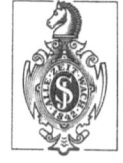

Springer Japan KK

Editor

Michinobu Hatano, m.d., Professor of Medicine, Director, Department of Internal Medicine, Nihon University School of Medicine, Tokyo, Japan

Associate Editors

Nishio Honda, Tokyo Senbai Hospital, Tokyo
Hyoe Ishikawa, Nara Medical University, Nara
Kenkichi Koiso, The University of Tsukuba, Ibaraki
Kiyoshi Kurokawa, University of Tokyo, Tokyo
Tadao Niijima, Tokyo Seamen's Medical College, Tokyo
Nobuhiro Sugino, Tokyo Women's Medical College, Tokyo
Susumu Takahashi, Nihon University, Tokyo

ISBN 978-3-540-70074-6

Library of Congress Cataloging-in-Publication Data
International Congress on Nephrology (11th: 1990: Tokyo, Japan); Nephrology: proceedings of the XIth International Congress of Nephrology/editors, Michinobu Hatano: associate editors, Nishio Honda...[et al.].
p. cm. Congress held in Tokyo, Japan, July 15-20, 1990. Includes bibliographical references. Includes index.
ISBN 978-3-540-70074-6   ISBN 978-3-662-35158-1 (eBook)
DOI 10.1007/978-3-662-35158-1
1. Kidneys – Diseases – Congresses.
2. Nephrology – Congresses. 3. Kidney Diseases – congresses. 4. Nephrology – congresses. I. Hatano, Michinobu, 1926- . II. Honda, Nishio. III. Title. [DNLM: WJ 300 I59n 1990]. RC902.A2I56 1990. 616.6'1 –dc20. DNLM/DLC. for Library of Congress 91-4651

© Springer Japan 1991

Originally published by Springer-Verlag Tokyo Berlin Heidelberg New York in 1991
Softcover reprint of the hardcover 1st edition 1991

Typesetting: Publishers Service of Montana, Bozeman, Montana

Foreword

The proceedings of the XIth International Congress of Nephrology held in Tokyo in 1990, form the most international and complete document of the present state of basic and clinical science in nephrology. In addition, they document the progress made in this field during the 3 years since the London Congress. The result is nothing short of impressive. The material presented by the invited lecturers and the participants of the symposia all show a remarkable pattern; not only the "height" of the science, but also the depth of the specialized knowledge, both prerequisites of excellency in science, which do not necessarily imply narrowness of outlook. On the contrary, this written document of the Tokyo Congress is a witness to the enormous progress made over the last few years in communication between basic scientists and clinical scientists.

The International Society of Nephrology is a fine example of how fruitful and productive this interaction can be, if it is conducted with the desire to understand each other. The members of the Scientific Program Committee of the Tokyo Congress are to be congratulated, not only for a thoughtful and well designed program, but also for carefully selecting those speakers who, besides their own contribution to nephrological science, also have the talent of being able to communicate with a large, international audience. In particular, I would like to express my deep appreciation to the editors of the Proceedings for their commitment and industriousness which made it possible for this publication to appear so soon after the Congress.

Since the first Congress of the International Society of Nephrology in Evian in 1960, nephrologists have witnessed a phenomenal increase in knowledge, a progress which still continues and will do so in the future. The present proceedings are a snapshot of this process. The counterpoint to the intellectual challenge of acquiring deeper understanding is the duty and promise to utilize that understanding for the benefit of our patients.

KLAUS THURAU, M.D.
President,
International Society of Nephrology
(1987–1990)

Preface

The XIth International Congress of Nephrology was held in Tokyo, Japan from July 15–20, 1990.

Since the first congress in Evian, France in 1960, this is the first time that this prestigious congress has been held in Asia. Therefore, enthusiastic expectations were held by nephrologists not only in Japan but also throughout the world.

In organizing the congress under the estimable guidance of Prof. Klaus Thurau, President of the International Society of Nephrology, the ISN Executive Committee and the International Advisory Committee, Prof. Michinobu Hatano, Chairman of the local organizing committee as well as the organizing committee made every effort to make the congress a success.

Over three thousand participants from 71 countries attended the congress. These included 1,470 participants from Japan, 472 from the United States, 150 from France, and 128 from Italy. We were particularly pleased to welcome eight representatives from Czechoslavakia as well as an increased participation from other eastern European countries, the Soviet Union, and China. Forty-nine delegates from Taiwan were also in attendance.

The opening ceremony was held at the New Takanawa Prince Hotel in the presence of the Crown Prince, whose address noted that progress in nephrology would contribute greatly to the welfare of patients worldwide.

The scientific program consisted of 15 state-of-the-art lectures, 36 symposia, 11 workshops, 256 oral and 1,778 poster presentations. Following the advice of the ISN Executive Committee, the Scientific Program Committee encouraged the presentation of clinical and research papers at the same time in each session. This ensured that throughout the scientific program, discussions were constructive, and this helped to make the congress both stimulating and fruitful.

A total of 12 ISN satellite symposia, 4 overseas and 8 in Japan, were also held. The specific topics discussed at each symposium, combined with sightseeing tours at each site, contributed greatly to exchanges of both friendship and information.

Finally, we would like to express our sincere thanks and appreciation to the ISN Committee and all the participants of the congress.

KENZO OSHIMA, M.D.
President

YAWARA YOSHITOSHI,
M.D.
Vice-President

YASUSHI UEDA, M.D.
Vice-President

HIROSHI ABE, M.D.
Vice-President

XIth International Congress of Nephrology

ORGANIZED BY: The Organizing Committee of the XIth International
                          Congress of Nephrology

UNDER THE AUSPICES OF: International Society of Nephrology

SPONSORED BY: Japanese Society of Nephrology
                          The Kidney Foundation, Japan

IN COOPERATION WITH: The Japanese Association of Medical Science
                          Japan Medical Association
                          The Japanese Urological Association
                          The Japan Society for Transplantation
                          Japanese Society for Artificial Organs
                          Japanese Society for Dialysis Therapy
                          The Japanese Society of Pediatric Nephrology
                          Japan Incorporated Medical Association for Dialysis

SUPPORTED BY: Ministry of Education, Science and Culture
                          Ministry of Health and Welfare
                          Science Council of Japan
                          Tokyo Metropolitan Government

The International Society of Nephrology

MANAGEMENT COMMITTEE

XIth International Congress Officers

President	Kenzo Oshima
Vice Presidents	Yawara Yoshitoshi
	Yasushi Ueda
	Hiroshi Abe

Organizing Committee

Chairman	Michinobu Hatano
Secretary-General	Susumu Takahashi

Members

Yoshio Aso	Tadashi Miyahara
Toshiyuki Furukawa	Toshihiko Nagasawa
Kohei Hara	Mitsuharu Narita
Nishio Honda	Hiromi Nihira
Takeshi Hoshi	Tadao Niijima
Kazunari Iidaka	Teruo Omae
Hyoe Ishikawa	Zensuke Ota
Chuichi Kawai	Fuminori Sakai
Teruo Kitagawa	Takao Sonoda
Kenkichi Koiso	Nobuhiro Sugino
Kiyoshi Kurokawa	Shizuo Tojo
Sunao Maki	

SCIENTIFIC PROGRAM COMMITTEE

Chairmen — Nobuhiro Sugino
Nishio Honda

Executive Secretary — Kiyoshi Kurokawa

Members

Akitoshi Ando	Koichi Matsumoto
Kikuo Arakawa	Toshihiko Nagasawa
Masaaki Arakawa	Mitsumasa Nagase
Hitoshi Endou	Yasushi Nakamoto
Mamoru Fujimoto	Hiroshi Nihei
Gerhard Giebisch	Michio Odaka
Takashi Harada	Hiroyuki Ohi
Eiji Higashihara	Yoshimasa Orita
Kazunari Iidaka	Kazuo Ota
Masashi Imai	Hideto Sakai
Hiroshi Kida	Osamu Sakai
Hikaru Koide	Tadasu Sakai
Kenkichi Koiso	Takao Saruta
Shozo Koshikawa	Hidekazu Shigematsu
Akio Koyama	Kenjiro Yamamoto
Kenji Maeda	Nobuyuki Yoshizawa
Sunao Maki	

FUND RAISING COMMITTEE

Chairmen — Tadao Niijima
Hyoe Ishikawa

Members

Keishi Abe	Joichi Kumazawa
Yoshio Aso	Yuji Nagura
Tohru Azuma	Zensuke Ota
Kohei Hara	Tsutomu Sanaka
Yoshihei Hirasawa	Takao Sonoda
Hiroshi Kida	Naohiko Ueda

FINANCE COMMITTEE

Chairman — Kenkichi Koiso

Members

Hiroshi Kawamura	Gengo Osawa

Contents of Volume II

Symposia

Cytokines, Mitogens and Their Receptors on Glomerular Cells

Frontiers of Research on Natriuretic Peptides

Glomerular Cells and Extracellular Matrix

Renal Tubular Acidosis

Endothelin and the Kidney

Transplantation

Cystic Diseases of the Kidney

Continuous Ambulatory Peritoneal Dialysis (CAPD)

Autacoids and the Kidney

Ion Channels of the Kidney

Contents of Volume I

State of the Art Lectures

Symposia

Cyclosporine Nephrotoxicity: From Experimental Animal to Clinical Practice

Cell Volume Regulation in Health and Disease

Mechanisms of Renal Cell Injury of Acute Renal Failure

List of Contributors

For contributors' addresses see chapter opening pages

List of Contributors

Renal Growth Factors

Chair: F. Gary Toback (USA)
Harry R. Jacobson (USA)

Expression of Growth-Related Genes in Human Fetal Kidney

Paul R. Goodyer[1], Jehane Fata[1], Lois Mulligan[2],
Cynthia G. Goodyer[3], Harvey Guyda[3], and Daniel Fischer[4]

SUMMARY. In early to midgestational human fetal life, branches of the ureteric bud begin to induce successive generations of nephrons from undifferentiated metanephric mesenchyme. Development of each evolving nephron is highly dependent on brisk, organized cell division. In order to identify molecular mechanisms potentially involved in fetal kidney growth, we screened a panel of fetal and adult kidneys for expression of 22 growth-related genes. Among the seven genes selectively expressed in fetal kidney, IGF-II, N-myc, and c-erbA have been investigated elsewhere. The "anti-oncogene", p53, and the homeobox gene, HHO.c13, are most likely involved in restriction of growth rather than in mitogenic events. The expression of epidermal growth factor (EGF) receptor in fetal kidney suggests a role for this pathway as an arbiter of rapid cell division. Using specific radioimmunoassays, we demonstrated that transforming growth factor (TGF)-Alpha peptide, but not EGF, was present in extracts of midgestation fetal kidney and amniotic fluid. Using the polymerase chain reaction, we identified TGF-Alpha messenger RNA (mRNA) in fetal kidney, indicating endogenous production of the peptide.

Introduction

Between the fifth and sixth weeks of human fetal life, undifferentiated metanephric mesenchyme is contacted by the ureteric bud (an outpouching of the Wolffian duct)

---

[1]Division of Pediatric Nephrology, McGill University-Montreal Children's Hospital Research Institute, Montreal, Quebec H3H 1P3, Canada
[2]Ludwig Cancer Institute, Royal Victoria Hospital, McGill University, Montreal, Quebec H3H 1P3, Canada
[3]Division of Pediatric Endocrinology, McGill University-Montreal Children's Hospital Research Institute, Montreal, Quebec H3K 1P3, Canada
[4]Nephrology Resident, Royal Victoria Hospital, McGill University, Montreal, Quebec H3H 1P3, Canada

resulting in induction of the first generation of nephrons [1]. Prior to induction, the metanephric tissue consists of loosely organized vimentin-positive cells proliferating in an extracellular matrix of fibronectin and collagens type I and III. As in the cells in Wilm's tumors, messenger RNA (mRNA) for insulin-like growth factor II is abundant [2]. Histologic observations indicate that clusters of metanephric cells condense at the point of contact with individual branches of the ureteric bud and then vesiculate to form S-shaped tubular structures [3]. The cells become polarized through laminin-mediated attachment to newly formed basement membrane, changes in cytoskeletal components, and increased lateral adhesion [1,4,5]. Recent work by Hastie et al. indicates that the committed cells of the emerging renal vesicle exhibit intense expression of the Wilm's tumor gene [3].

Induction of metanephric mesenchyme causes a shift in cellular phenotype, but it also initiates a phase of rapid cell division. It is intriguing to note that IGF-II mRNA is most intense in the undifferentiated cells of the metanephric mesenchyme rather than in the rapidly proliferating cells of the evolving nephron [6]. Little is known about the mitogenic signals which direct this proliferation, but it is clear that local regulatory events are involved. The nephron develops a primitive glomerulus at its proximal end through ingrowth of capillaries; fusion with the ureteric bud at its distal end achieves continuity with the bladder. Over the course of fetal life, successive branches of the ureteric bud penetrate nests of metanephric mesenchyme at the outer rim of the developing organ; tiers of newly formed units are layered upon deeper zones of the more advanced nephrons already producing fetal urine. By thirty-five weeks of gestation the ureteric bud stops dividing and the metanephric blastema involutes as the final generation of nephrons is formed.

In order to characterize the molecular mechanisms potentially responsible for the rapid growth of evolving nephrons, we probed a panel of human adult and fetal kidney RNAs with 23 known protooncogene probes. Among those genes expressed at especially high levels in fetal tissue was the EGF receptor. Further studies support the view that transforming growth factor-alpha (TGF-Alpha) is the most likely physiologic ligand for the EGF receptor in fetal kidney.

Materials and Methods

For Northern analyses, frozen tissues were pulverized on dry ice; total RNA was prepared by the guanidinium/cesium chloride gradient method [7]. For gene expression screening, 30 μg of total RNA was separated on 1% agarose/formaldehyde gels and was transferred to Hybond-N membranes (Amersham) using 20X SSC. The Northern blots were hybridized for 36 hours to [32P]-labelled probes (random oligonucleotide priming) in 50% formamide 40mM Na_2HPO_4 (pH=6.7), 5X SSC, 0.05% SDS, 0.02% PVP, 0.02% Ficoll, and 0.02% bovine serum albumin at 42°C. For detailed analysis of the EGF receptor, nitrocellulose Northern blots were hybridized overnight (55% deionized formamide, 5X SSC, 1X Denhardt's solution, 50 mM Na_2HPO_4, and 10% dextran sulfate at 42°C) to a [32-P]-labelled complementary DNA (cDNA) probe for the human EGF receptor (ATCC). The blots were washed and submitted to autoradiography.

For assay of transforming growth factor-alpha (TGF-Alpha), frozen kidney was pulverized on dry ice and homogenized in 5 volumes of buffer containing 20mM

TRIS (ph 7.4), 0.25M sucrose, 1mM phenylmethylsulfonylfluoride, and 0.1%
Triton-X 100. TGF-Alpha was measured in amniotic fluid and tissue extracts in triplicate with the Biotope TGF-Alpha RIA kit (Biotope, Redmond, Washington) as previously described [8]. The kit utilizes antiserum raised against synthetic TGF-Alpha
peptide (17 residues, 34–50) and gives linear displacement for human TGF-Alpha
standard between 0.5–5 pmoles/ml, but does not recognize human EGF. Half-
maximal competition is at 1.4 nM TGF-Alpha. Serial dilutions of kidney extracts or
amniotic fluid samples produced displacement of TGF-Alpha tracer parallel to the
standard curve; Triton X-100 buffer gave no displacement in the assay.

For assay of human EGF, tissues were prepared as above. EGF was measured by
radioimmunoassay as described previously [9]. The antiserum used was raised in
rabbits against recombinant human EGF (Amgen); it detects human EGF but not rat
EGF or TGF-Alpha from either species. Half maximal competition is 0.3 nM.

Specific high-affinity EGF binding was performed as previously described [10].
Frozen tissues were homogenized in 5 volumes of buffer containing 20 mM TRIS
(pH 7.4) and 0.25M sucrose. The homogenate was centrifuged twice at 500Xg, and
the supernatant respun at 20,000Xg for 20 minutes to obtain a membrane pellet.
Human EGF was iodinated by the chloramine T method and incubated (50000
CPM/assay) with 200–300 µg kidney membrane protein, or 100 µg placental membrane protein in 500 µl final volume of 25mM TRIS (pH 7.4)/10mM magnesium
chloride buffer containing 1 mg/ml bovine serum albumin and 1 mg/ml bacitracin at
4°C. for 18 hours. Specific binding was estimated by comparing the fraction of total
tracer bound in the presence or in the absence of excess unlabelled EGF (500ng/ml).

Results

Gene Expression in Fetal and Adult Kidney

The expression profile of 23 genes suspected of involvement in regulation of cell
growth was assessed by Northern analysis, using a panel of total RNA samples
(30 µg per lane) from human fetal ($n=11$) and adult kidneys ($n=4$). Fetal foot length
was used to determine fetal age; the fetal samples ranged from 14–24 weeks gestation
at 410 day intervals. For simplicity, semi-quantitative estimates of signal intensity
for each gene were assigned to early (14–20 weeks) and mid (21–24 weeks) gestation
fetal kidney samples and to the adult panel.

Of the 22 genes studied, 5 (NGF, IGF1, IL-2, c-abl, and L-myc) were undetectable by Northern analysis in any of the fetal or adult kidney samples. Transcripts for
10 of the 22 genes (c-myc, c-raf, neu, TGF-B1, met, yes, sis, RB1, K-ras, H-ras) were
detected in all samples, but the level of gene expression was equivalent in the early
fetal, mid-fetal, and adult kidney groups. The expression pattern for the remaining
7 genes is summarized in Table 1. In each case, transcript was detected in fetal kidney
but was much reduced or absent in adult kidney.

EGF Receptor

Among the genes selectively expressed in fetal kidney, the EGF receptor was chosen
for further analysis. We noted that primary transcripts for the EGF receptor (9.4 and

Table 1. Summary of expression pattern for 7 of 22 genes studied

Gene	Gestational age 10–14 weeks	Fetal kidney 14–20 weeks	Adult kidney
IGF-II	+++	+++	−
EGF Receptor	+	+	−
N-myc	++	++	−
N-ras	++	+	+
c-erbA	++	++	±
HHO.c13	+	+	−
p53	++	+	±

5.6 kb) in fetal kidney RNA co-migrated with transcripts in mid-gestational human placenta but were absent in adult kidney; no unusual transcripts were seen. Specific high-affinity EGF binding in membrane fractions of fetal kidney was 2–5 times higher than in adult kidney, but was less than in mid-gestation placenta (Table 2).

TGF-Alpha and EGF

If the EGF receptor is to initiate mitogenic signals in fetal kidney, it must be activated by an appropriate ligand. Levels of TGF-Alpha and EGF peptides were assayed in detergent extracts of fetal kidney and amniotic fluid. As seen in Table 2, TGF-Alpha was detectable, by RIA, in fetal kidneys of 11–15 weeks gestation. In one pair of kidneys obtained at 7–8 weeks gestation, the level was significantly lower. TGF-Alpha was also present in all amniotic fluid samples tested (13–39 weeks gestation, $n=20$) (Table 3). Primer oligonucleotides, prepared from the published sequence for human TGF-Alpha, were used to convert TGF-Alpha mRNA in human fetal kidney total RNA to cDNA, using the reverse transcriptase reaction; this was followed by 25 cycles of PCR amplification. PCR products were dotted on nitrocellulose and identified with a cDNA probe for human TGF-Alpha. Significant TGF-Alpha expression was identified in all fetal kidneys (13–19 weeks gestation) tested ($n=7$).

Midgestational kidney extracts were also assessed for EGF content. In three fetal kidney samples, EGF was undetectable (lower limit of assay = 0.1 pmoles/ml). By contrast the extract from the normal kidney of an adult was 6 pmol/g. Significant levels of EGF in amniotic fluid were undetectable before 30 weeks gestation, when they began to rise (Table 3). At term, amniotic fluid EGF was still only 4% of the

Table 2. EGF binding, TGF-Alpha, and EGF in human fetal kidney

	Fetal	Adult
% EGF binding/200 µg protein	1.1 ± 0.1 (n=9)	0.3 (n=2)
pmoles TGF-Alpha/g wet weight	42.1 ± 1.4 (n=7)	ND
pmoles EGF/g wet weight	0.0 (n=3)	6.0 (n=3)

Table 3. TGF-Alpha and EGF in human amniotic fluid

Gestational age	TGF-Alpha (nM)	EGF (nM)
15–20 weeks (n = 5)	4.0 ± 0.3	< 0.05
20–25 weeks (n = 5)	6.1 ± 0.4	< 0.05
25–30 weeks (n = 3)	4.6 ± 0.5	< 0.05
30–35 weeks (n = 2)	2.5	< 0.05
35–40 weeks (n = 5)	3.9 ± 0.2	0.12 ± 0.04

level of TGF-Alpha. Although PCR amplification was not performed, EGF mRNA was identified in adult, but not in fetal kidney, by Northern analysis.

Discussion

In this report, we examined the expression profile of a panel of growth-related genes in human fetal kidney, in order to identify some which may be of particular importance to kidney development. As reported by others, we noted increased expression of IGF-II, N-myc, N-ras, and c-erbA (thyroxine receptor) in fetal kidney. The possible roles of these genes in kidney development have recently been reviewed [1]. The characteristics of the "anti-oncogene", p53, and the human homeobox gene, HHO.C13, suggest that their expression in human fetal kidney may be related to restrictions of cell division rather than to their acting as mitogenic signals. However, the increase in EGF receptor mRNA and the increase in EGF binding in midgestational renal tissue, compared to levels in the adult tissue, suggests that this receptor may be among the important mediators of rapid fetal kidney growth. Renal cells are known to proliferate in response to EGF in vitro [11].

Some controversy remains about whether fetal kidney can produce a physiologic ligand for the EGF receptor. Several groups have reported an EGF-like peptide in fetal kidneys of sheep and mice [12–14]; others have reported TGF-Alpha mRNA in fetal mouse [15], and in adult human [16] kidneys by Northern blotting. On the other hand, Han was unable to identify TGF-Alpha mRNA in fetal rat kidney [17] and Mydlo found none in normal adult human kidney by Northern blotting [18]. Using specific radioimmunoassays, we have demonstrated the presence of TGF-Alpha peptide, but not EGF, in extracts of human kidney and in amniotic fluid from early to mid-gestation. Using PCR amplification, we were able to demonstrate the presence of TGF-Alpha mRNA in fetal kidney, indicating endogenous synthesis there. We cannot rule out small quantities of renal EGF synthesis during fetal life, but the relative amounts of TGF-Alpha and EGF in amniotic fluid suggest that the former is the dominant physiologic EGF receptor ligand.

It is certain that the interaction between paracrine growth factors and critical nuclear transcription factors during renal development is extremely complex. Signals directing cell division must be exerted under tight spatial and temporal restrictions relevant to differentiation of the renal tubule. Nevertheless, efforts to identify the key molecular mechanisms involved in normal development are likely to shed light on the repair of renal injury in later life.

References

1. Bacallao R, Fine LG (1989) Molecular events in the organization of renal tubular epithelium: from nephrogenesis to regeneration. Am J Physiol 257:F913–F924
2. Paik S, Rosen N, Jung W, You JM, Lippman ME, et al. (1989) Expression of insulin-like growth factor II in RNA in fetal kidney and Wilm's tumor. Lab Invest 61:522–526
3. Hastie N, Pelletier J, et al. (to be published) Expression of a candidate Wilm's Tumour gene in human fetal tissues and Wilm's tumour. Nature
4. Ekblom M, Klein G, Mugrauer G, Fecker L, Deutzmann R, Trumph R, Ekblom P (1990) Transient and locally restricted expression of laminin A-chain in RNA by developing epithelial cells during kidney organogenesis. Cell 60:337–346
5. Klein G, Langegger M, Gordis C, Ekblom P (1988) Neural adhesion molecules during embryonic induction and development of the kidney. Develop 102:749–761
6. Han VKM, D'Ercole AJ, Lund PK (1987) Cellular localization of somatomedin (insulin-like growth factor) messenger RNA in the human fetus. Science 236:193–196
7. Goodyer PR, Langshur S, Fata J (1990) Renal synthesis of epidermal growth factor is unchanged by vitamin D deficiency. Can J Physiol Pharmacol 68:733–736
8. Goodyer PR, Fata J, Goodyer CG (to be published) Transforming growth factor-alpha and the ontogeny of epidermal growth factor receptors in rat kidney
9. Goodyer PR (1990) Excretion of epidermal growth factor-like material in acute Henoch-Schonlein purpura nephritis. Pediatr Nephrol 4:101–104
10. Goodyer PR, Fata J, Goodyer CG, Mulligan L, Guyda H (to be published) Transforming growth factor-alpha and epidermal growth factor receptor in human fetal kidney
11. Goodyer PR, Kachra Z, Bell C, Rozen R (1988) Renal tubular cells are potential targets for epidermal growth factor. Am J Physiol 255:F1191–F1196
12. Nexo E, Hollenberg MD, Figuerou A, Pratt RM (1980) Detection of epidermal growth factor-urogastrone and its receptor during fetal mouse development. Proc Natl Acad Sci (USA) 77:2782–2785
13. Freemark M, Comer M (1987) Epidermal growth factor (EGF)-like transforming growth factor (TGF) activity and EGF receptors in ovine fetal tissues: possible role for TGF in ovine fetal development. Pediatr Res 22:609–615
14. Twardzik Dr, Ranchalis JR, Todaro GJ (1982) Mouse embryos contain growth factors related to those from tumour cells. Cancer Res 42:590–593
15. Derynck R, Jarett JA, Chen EY, et al. (1985) Human transforming growth factor-beta complementary DNA sequence and expression in normal and transformed cells. Nature 316:701–705
16. Gomella LG, Sargent ER, Wade TP, Anglard P, Linehan WM, Kasid A (1989) Expression of transforming growth factor-alpha in normal human adult kidney and enhanced expression of transforming growth factors alpha and beta1 in renal cell carcinoma. Cancer Res 49:6972–6975
17. Han VKM, Hunter E III, Pratt RM, Zendegin JG, Lee DC (1987) Expression of rat transforming growth factor alpha in RNA during development occurs predominantly in the maternal decidua. Mol Cell Biol 7:2335–2343
18. Mydlo JH, Michaeli J, Cordon-Cardo C, Goldenberg AS, Heston WDW, Fair WR (1989) Expression of transforming growth factor alpha and epidermal growth factor receptor messenger RNA in neoplastic and nonneoplastic human kidney tissue. Cancer Res 49:3407–3411

Growth Hormone, Insulin-Like Growth Factor I, and Kidney

MARC R. HAMMERMAN and STEVEN B. MILLER

SUMMARY. Insulin-like growth factor I (IGF I) exerts a variety of actions on kidney. To shed light upon its role in regulation of renal function and renal growth we have characterized its cellular biology in two parts of the nephron, proximal tubule and collecting duct. Receptors for IGF I are present in the basolateral membrane of the renal proximal tubular cell, but not in collecting duct. The peptide IGF I enhances gluconeogenesis in proximal tubule. IGF I is produced in collecting duct. Gene expression for IGF I in collecting duct is stimulated by both normal and supraphysiological levels of growth hormone (GH). Levels of IGF I in collecting duct are elevated in the setting of compensatory renal hypertrophy. IGF I of collecting duct origin could act as a paracrine growth factor in other portions of the nephron. IGF I may be causative of renal hypertrophy that occurs in the settings of hypersomatotropism and unilateral nephrectomy (compensatory hypertrophy).

Introduction

Insulin-like growth factor I (IGF I) is the predominant growth hormone (GH)-responsive IGF. It is present in circulation, where it can interact, as an endocrine hormone, with receptors present on the plasma membranes of a variety of cells. In addition, it is produced locally within a number of GH-sensitive tissues, where it acts as an autocrine or paracrine growth factor [1]. Kidney is a site of IGF I synthesis [2].

Receptors for IGF I have been described in renal glomerulus and proximal tubule [3,4]. IGF I is known to exert several actions on kidney. Administration of this peptide to rats [5] and humans [6] increases glomerular filtration rate and renal plasma flow. In addition, IGF I increases kidney size when infused directly into rats [7]. States of GH excess (hypersomatotropic states) are characterized by elevations of cir-

Renal and Endocrine Divisions, Departments of Internal Medicine and Cell Biology and Physiology, Washington University School of Medicine, St. Louis, MO 63110, USA

culating IGF I and are accompanied by hypertrophy of the renal glomerulus and proximal tubule [8]. Indeed, many actions of GH on renal size and kidney function appear to be mediated indirectly through stimulation of the synthesis and release of insulin-like growth factor I (IGF I).

In order to gain an understanding of the cellular biological mechanisms by which GH and IGF I regulate renal growth, renal metabolism, and renal function, we have characterized binding of, signal-transduction by, and metabolic actions of IGF I in proximal tubule, and IGF I gene expression in collecting duct. Our findings have shed new light on the GH-IGF I axis within the kidney.

Materials and Methods

The methodology used to generate data presented in this manuscript has been detailed elsewhere. Methods include measurement of ^{125}I-IGF I binding by rapid centrifugation and covalent crosslinking techniques [4], phosphorylation of canine renal proximal tubular basolateral membranes [9], measurement of gluconeogenesis in suspensions of canine renal proximal tubular segments [10], measurement of IGF I mRNA using a solution-hybridization, nuclease-protection assay [11], and measurement of IGF I of collecting duct origin using high performance liquid chromatography and radioimmunoassay [12]. A probe derived from a subclone of rat IGF I exon 3 was provided by Dr. Peter Rotwein, Washington University, St. Louis Mo. Recombinant bovine GH (bGH) was the gift of Monsanto Chemical Co., St. Louis Mo. Recombinant human IGF I (hIGF I) was purchased from Amgen Biologicals, Thousand Oaks CA.

Results

Renal Proximal Tubule

Receptors for IGF I are distributed asymmetrically in the plasma membrane of the renal proximal tubular cell, being localized predominantly on the basolateral side [4] (Fig. 1). In isolated proximal tubular basolateral membranes IGF I-stimulated phosphorylation of the beta subunit of its receptor can be demonstrated (Fig. 2), consistent with signal transduction being effected via this mechanism in proximal tubule, as it is in other IGF I-sensitive tissues [9]. In isolated proximal tubular segments IGF I stimulates gluconeogenesis (Fig. 3).

Renal Collecting Duct

Kidney is a site of GH-stimulated IGF I production [2]. We and other groups of investigators have shown that collecting duct is the site of IGF I synthesis within rat kidney [11–13]. IGF I has been localized to collecting duct by immunohistochemistry; IGF I mRNA is co-localized to this portion of the nephron [11] (Fig. 4). Administration of recombinant bovine GH (bGH) to normal [14] or hypophysectomized [11,15] rats results in enhanced immunostainable IGF I in collecting duct, as well as increased levels of IGF I mRNA.

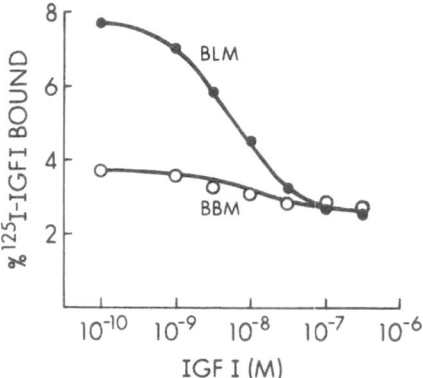

Fig. 1. Binding of ^{125}hI-IGF I to canine renal proximal tubular basolateral (*BLM*) and brush border membranes (*BBM*). Binding is expressed as % ^{125}I-IGF I bound

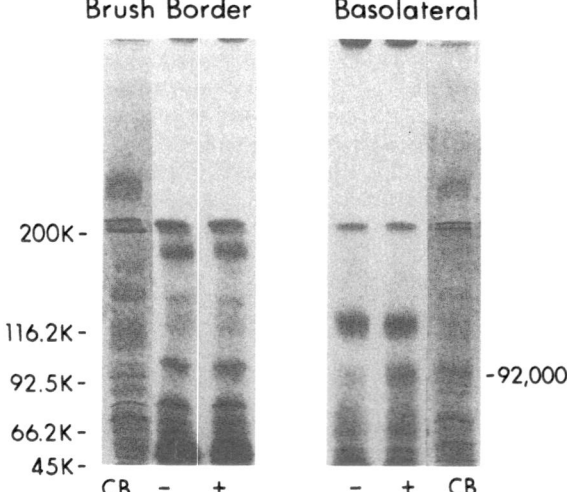

Fig. 2. IGF I-stimulated phosphorylation of canine renal proximal tubular brush border and basolateral membranes. Shown are Coomassie blue stained SDS-polyacrylamide gels (*CB*) and autoradiograms originating from proximal tubular brush border and basolateral membranes incubated without (-) or with (+) 10^{-6} M hIGF I prior to phosphorylation. Several M_r markers are shown. IGF I-stimulated phosphorylation of a 92000 M_r protein is demonstrable in basolateral membranes, but not in brush border membranes. (From [9] with permission)

Fig. 3. Stimulation of glucose production from gluconeogenic substrates by varying concentrations of hIGF I in suspensions of canine renal proximal tubular segments. (From [10] with permission)

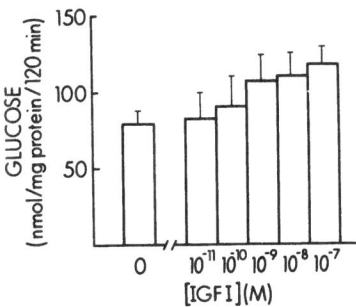

Incubation of collecting ducts isolated from rat kidney with bGH results in elevated levels of total IGF I extractable from total suspensions (cells plus media). In addition, GH enhances levels of IGF I present in extracellular suspending media [12] (Fig. 5). Prior to measurement by radioimmunoassay, IGF I of collecting duct origin (cdIGF I) is separated from IGF binding activity, using high performance liquid chromatography. It co-elutes with recombinant human ^{125}I-IGF I [12]. IGF I of collecting duct origin inhibits binding of ^{125}I-IGF I to the 135000 M_r alpha subunit of its receptor in canine proximal tubular basolateral membranes, identically to authentic human IGF I (hIGF I) (Fig. 6). Incubation of isolated collecting ducts with bGH elevates levels of IGF I mRNA in vitro (Fig. 7) [12]. These findings demonstrate that GH enhances IGF I gene expression via a direct action on renal collecting ducts.

Discussion

The Renal GH-IGF I Axis

The studies detailed above establish the potential for a GH-IGF I axis within kidney [16]. IGF I produced in isolated rat renal collecting ducts is released into extracellular

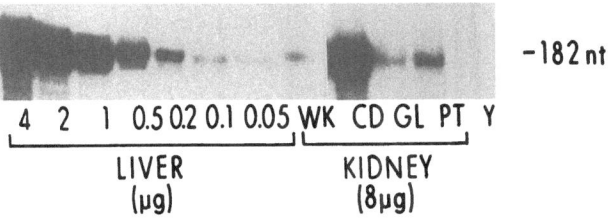

Fig. 4. Levels of IGF I mRNA in kidney. Shown is an autoradiogram depicting the results of a solution-hybridization nuclease-protection experiment using a ^{32}P-labeled rat IGF I exon 3 antisense probe (protected fragment = 182 nucleotides). Illustrated are protected RNA fragments from rat liver and from whole kidneys (*WK*), collecting duct (*CD*), glomeruli (*GL*), proximal tubule (*PT*), or yeast tRNA (*Y*). (Reproduced from the *Journal of Cell Biology* [11] by copyright permission of the Rockefeller University Press)

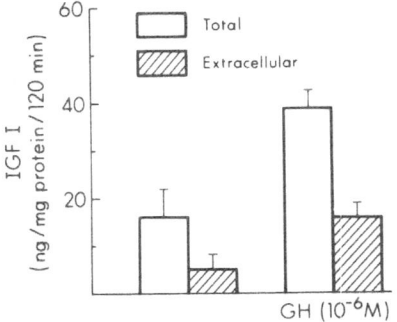

Fig. 5. Levels of immunoreactive IGF I present in whole collecting duct suspensions (*total*) and in extracellular media of the suspensions. Data are expressed ± SE of 3 experiments

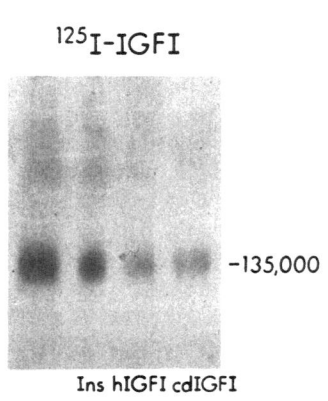

Fig. 6. Crosslinking of ^{125}I-hIGF I to canine renal proximal tubular basolateral membranes in the absence or presence of 2×10^{-8} M insulin (*Ins*), hIGF I or IGF I of collecting duct origin (*cdIGF I*). (From [12] with permission)

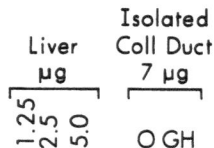

Fig. 7. Levels of IGF I mRNA in isolated rat renal collecting duct incubated with (*GH*) or without (*0*) 10^{-6} M bGH for 2 h. Shown is an autoradiogram depicting the results of a solution-hybridization nuclease-protection experiment conducted as described in Fig. 4. (From [12] with permission)

media. This is likely to reflect peptide secretion into renal tissue in vivo. Although IGF I can be detected in urine, its concentration is small (approximately 10^{-11} M) [17]. This suggests that IGF I is not secreted into the collecting duct lumen, but rather, exits from collecting duct across the basolateral membrane. Receptors for IGF I are not present in collecting duct [15]. Therefore IGF I produced there must act at other sites in kidney at which receptors are present, such as glomerulus and proximal tubule, where IGF I could function as a paracrine growth factor. IGF I produced in cortical collecting duct is located immediately adjacent to the basolateral membrane of the renal proximal tubular cell where IGF I receptors are present. IGF I produced in medullary collecting duct could reach the renal cortex via the ascending vasa recta, the walls of which are extensively fenestrated like those of renal capillaries. Indeed, segments of proximal tubule and other tubular structures in the outer stripe of medulla receive their blood supply from these vessels [16].

A role for renal IGF I as causative of the glomerular and proximal tubular hypertrophy that occurs in hypersomatotropic states and in compensatory renal hypertrophy is suggested by observations from several laboratories. First, IGF I may be the major stimulus for renal cellular growth in hypersomatotropic states such as acromegaly [8], since GH administered in vivo, or added to collecting ducts in vitro, enhances IGF I gene expression. Second, IGF I could function as a hypertrophic stimulus in compensatory renal hypertrophy. We [15] and other investigators [18,19] have demonstrated enhanced IGF I expression within kidney in the setting of compensatory growth.

Our knowledge of the GH-IGF I axis within kidney is incomplete. A number of important issues remain to be addressed. First, it is likely that factors in addition to GH affect IGF I gene expression in collecting duct. This is illustrated by the fact that the increase in renal IGF I that accompanies compensatory hypertrophy occurs in the hypopituitary state [18]. Second, the nature of feedback-loops for GH and IGF I in kidney is undefined. Third, sites of action for GH and IGF I, in addition to those that have been characterized, may exist along the nephron. In addition, interactions may occur between GH, IGF I, and other polypeptide growth factors within renal tissue. Future investigations will shed light on these and other important questions regarding the GH-IGF I axis in kidney.

Acknowledgments. We acknowledge the typing skills of Ms. Lynn Wesselmann. Contributions to the work upon which much of this review is based were made by Dr. Peter Bechtel, University of Illinois, Champaign-Urbana Ill.; Dr. James R. Gavin III, Oklahoma City Okla.; and Dr Jonathan Bortz, Dr. Rosemary Lajara, Dr. Peter Rotwein, Ms. Virginia Hansen, and Ms. Sharon Rogers, Washington University, St. Louis Mo. M.R. Hammerman was supported by N.I.H. grants DK-27600 and DK-09976 and by Grant 186270 from the Juvenile Diabetes Foundation. S. Miller was supported by N.I.H. training grant DK-07126.

References

1. Daughaday WH (1989) Growth hormone, normal synthesis, secretion, control, and mechanism of action. In: DeGroot LJ (ed) Endocrinology, vol 1. Saunders, Philadelphia, pp 318–329

2. D'Ercole JA, Stiles AD, Underwood LE (1984) Tissue concentrations of somatomedin C: further evidence for multiple sites of synthesis and paracrine or autocrine mechanisms of action. Proc Natl Acad Sci USA 81:935–939

3. Pillion DJ, Haskell JF, Meezen E (1988) Distinct receptors for insulin-like growth factor I in rat renal glomeruli and tubules. Am J Physiol 255:E504–E512

4. Hammerman MR, Rogers SA (1987) Distribution of IGF receptors in the plasma membrane of proximal tubular cells. Am J Physiol 253:F841–F847

5. Hirschberg R, Kopple JD (1989) Evidence that insulin-like growth factor I increases renal plasma flow and glomerular filtration rate in fasted rats. J Clin Invest 83:3267–3330

6. Guler HP, Schmid C, Zapf J, Froesch ER (1989) Effects of recombinant insulin-like growth factor I on insulin secretion and renal function in normal human subjects. Proc Natl Acad Sci USA 86:2868–2872

7. Guler HP, Zapf J, Schweiller E, Froesch ER (1988) Recombinant human insulin-like growth factor I stimulates growth and has distinct effects on organ size in hypophysectomized rats. Proc Natl Acad Sci USA 85:4889–4893

8. Gershberg H, Heinemann O, Stumpf HH (1957) Renal function studies and autopsy report in a patient with gigantism and acromegaly. J Clin Endocrinol Metab 17:377–385

9. Hammerman MR, Gavin JR III (1986) Binding of IGF I and IGF I-stimulated phosphorylation in canine renal basolateral membranes. Am J Physiol 251:E32–E41

10. Rogers SA, Karl IE, Hammerman MR (1989) Growth hormone directly stimulates gluconeogenesis in canine renal proximal tubule. Am J Physiol 257:E751–E756

11. Bortz JD, Rotwein P, DeVol D, Bechtel PJ, Hansen V, Hammerman MR (1988) Focal expression of insulin-like growth factor I in rat kidney collecting duct. J Cell Biol 107:811–819

12. Rogers SA, Miller SB, Hammerman MR (1990) Growth hormone stimulates IGF I gene expression in isolated rat renal collecting duct. Am J Physiol 259:F474–F479

13. Hansson HA, Nilsson A, Isgaard J, Billig H, Isaksson O, Skottner A, Andersson IK, Rozel B (1988) Immunohistochemical localization of insulin-like growth factor I in the adult rat. Histochemistry 89:403–410

14. Miller SB, Rotwein P, Bortz JD, Bechtel PJ, Hansen VA, Rogers SA, Hammerman, MR (1990) Renal expression of IGF I in hypersomatotropic states. Am J Physiol 259:F251–F257

15. Lajara R, Rotwein P, Bortz JD, Hansen VA, Sadow JL, Betts CR (1989) Dual regulation of insulin-like growth factor I expression during renal hypertrophy. Am J Physiol 257:F252–F261

16. Hammerman MR (1989) The growth hormone-insulin-like growth factor axis in kidney (editorial review). Am J Physiol 257:F503–F514

17. Hizuka N, Takano K, Tanaka I, Asakawa K, Miyakawa M, Horikawa R, Shizume K (1987) Demonstration of insulin-like growth factor I in human urine. J Clin Endocrinol Metab 64:1309–1312

18. Stiles AD, Sosenko RS, D'Ercole AJ, Smith BT (1985) Relation of kidney tissue somatomedin-C/insulin-like growth factor I to postnephrectomy renal growth in the rat. Endocrinology 117:2397–2401

19. Andersson GL, Skottner A, Jennische E (1988) Immunocytochemical and biochemical localization of insulin-like growth factor I in the kidney of rats before and after uninephrectomy. Acta Endocrinol (Copenh) 119:555–560

Epidermal Growth Factor and the Kidney

Raymond C. Harris[1]

Epidermal growth factor (EGF), a 53 amino acid polypeptide, with a molecular weight of 6045, is derived by proteolytic processing from a precursor (prepro-EGF) of 1207 amino acids in humans or 1217 amino acids in rodents [1,2]. PreproEGF is a membrane-spanning protein that contains a hydrophobic domain adjacent to the EGF moiety. EGF was originally isolated as the factor that stimulates precocious tooth eruption and eyelid opening in newborn mice; subsequently, it has been found to produce a wide variety of effects both in vitro and in vivo, including proliferation of cultured cells, acceleration of lung maturation, corneal healing, and inhibition of gastric acid secretion [1].

EGF binds to a 170 kilodalton plasma membrane receptor that contains intrinsic tyrosine kinase activity [2]. Binding of EGF to its receptor stimulates receptor autophosphorylation, as well as tyrosine phosphorylation of a number of other cellular proteins. Specific high affinity EGF receptors have been detected in cultured cells of epithelial, mesenchymal and endothelial origin. Receptors have also been detected in a variety of tissues, including kidney [3], breast [4], liver [5], and intestine [6]. EGF has been demonstrated to promote hyperplasia and maturation of the cells in the gastrointestinal epithelium [7], pancreas, and liver [8]. In addition to inhibition of gastric acid secretion, EGF also preserves the integrity of the intestinal epithelium and reduces ulceration [9]. Addition of EGF to cultured cells stimulates a number of intracellular responses including increased Na^+/H^+ antiport activity [10], activation of glycolysis [1], increased DNA, RNA, protein, and hyaluronic acid synthesis [1] and increased glucosamine incorporation in glycosaminoglycans [11].

In 1978, Delarco and Todaro described a peptide, released by retrovirally transformed fibroblasts, that bound to EGF receptors and promoted anchorage independent growth of normal rat kidney (NRK) cells in soft agar [12]. They termed this growth factor, transforming growth factor alpha (TGF-α). TFG-α possesses both structural and functional homology with EGF. Both TFG-α and EGF bind with simi-

---

[1]Vanderbilt University School of Medicine, Nashville, TN 37232, USA

lar affinity to the same receptor, and TFG-α binding will activate EGF receptor tyrosine kinase activity. Such observations raise the obvious possibility that "EGF receptors" may actually be targets for TFG-α and that EGF is one, possibly specialized, member of the family of TGF-α peptides. In many biological systems, the effects elicited by EGF and TGF-α are very similar, while in others, TGF-α appears quantitatively more potent than EGF.

Originally, EGF was detected in mouse submaxillary gland, the most abundant source of production in the rodent. Although levels of EGF are high in saliva, circulating blood levels are low [1]. Furthermore, in humans, EGF concentrations are much higher in serum than in plasma, and EGF in blood is not freely circulating but is associated with platelets [14]. Subsequent to its discovery in saliva, EGF has also been noted to be present in high (nanogram concentrations) in milk, urine, secretions of Brunner's glands [15], and in prostatic secretions [16]. Immunohistochemical localization in rodents has shown EGF to be present in submaxillary glands, exocrine glands of the gastrointestinal tract, and serous acini of the nasal cavity, as well as in kidney, further indicating the possible exocrine role for this peptide [17]. Urinary EGF, or urogastrone, is present in high concentrations in urine [18]. In humans, urinary EGF concentrations are 50–70 ng/mg creatinine.

A number of studies have indicated a renal source of urinary EGF. Urinary EGF/creatinine ratios are greater than one. Intravenously injected ^{125}I EGF is not detected in urine [19]. Following sialoadenctomy and duodenectomy, urinary EGF levels were unchanged [20], but following unilateral nephrectomy, urinary EGF levels fell to 50% of control, and did not increase over the subsequent 14 days [20,21]. In humans, urinary EGF levels have been demonstrated to be decreased in chronic renal failure of multiple etiologies [22]. In addition, in experimental renal failure induced by cis platinum [23] or ischemia [24], urinary EGF levels decreased markedly. However, Nielsen et al. have recently found that in isolated rabbit proximal tubules only 4% of filtered EGF is reabsorbed (compared to 73% for insulin) [25]. These authors also detected a small amount of apical secretion of EGF after presentation of EGF to proximal tubular basolateral membrane and suggested the possibility that a component of urinary EGF may originate from blood.

High concentrations of prepro-EGF mRNA have been found in the kidney [26]. In situ hybridization localization of prepro-EGF indicates the site of renal synthesis to be the thick ascending limb of Henle (TALH) and early distal convoluted tubule (DCT) [26]. Immunocytochemical and immunoelectron microscopic localization of EGF and preproEGF to cortical thick ascending limb and early distal convoluted tubule has been demonstrated. No staining of macula densa was observed [27,28].

The predicted structure of preproEGF suggests that it is a membrane protein, with an extracellular EGF moiety (amino acids 977-1029). The immunocytochemical identification of preproEGF in the TALH and DCT indicates that the protein is predominantly, if not exclusively, found anchored in the apical membrane [28]. This polarized distribution suggests that renal preproEGF may be acted upon by proteases in the tubular fluid and/or apical membrane and the derived EGF is released directly into the urine. The protease(s) responsible for processing of renal preproEGF have not been characterized. Arginine esterase, the protease responsible for cleaving submaxillary preproEGF, is not found in the kidney or in urine [29]. It has been suggested that the renal kallikrein or related enzymes may be responsible for cleavage of the precursor [30]. In addition to EGF, the EGF precursor contains other sequences homologous to EGF, as well as sequences homologous to atrial natriuretic factor precursor. Whether these sequences are processed to biologically active peptides is not known.

Processing of preproEGF may not be necessary for biological activity. Fibroblasts transfected with human preproEGF cDNA produce and secrete intact preproEGF, which binds to EGF receptors, activates EGF receptor tyrosine kinase and induces mitogenesis [31]. Since preproEGF appears to be an intrinsic membrane protein, and since it possesses homology to the low-density lipoprotein receptor, it has also been suggested that preproEGF may itself serve as a receptor for a yet unidentified ligand, but confirming evidence for this hypothesis has not been forthcoming.

The regulation of synthesis and release of renal EGF is not well understood. Unlike serum EGF, urinary EGF concentrations are higher in females than in males, and, unlike results in submaxillary gland, androgen administration to female mice increases neither preproEGF mRNA expression in the kidney nor urinary EGF levels [32]. In fact, estrogen administration increases urinary EGF levels in males [33]. Although human urinary EGF levels are not affected by menstrual cycle or oral contraceptives, pregnancy does induce a doubling of urinary EGF, with a peak at 20 weeks [34]. Chronic thyroxine and growth hormone administration also increase urinary EGF levels [35]. Evidence to date suggests that β-adrenergic stimulation increases, and β-adrenergic blockade decreases, urinary EGF levels, in contrast to salivary gland release, which is stimulated by a-adrenergic agonists [36].

In rat, EGF immunoreactivity in the kidney does not appear until after birth [37], although in human fetuses, EGF immunoreactivity is present from half-term onwards. Matilla et al. found that urinary EGF in humans was low at birth, rose progressively, peaked at two years of postnatal life (235 ng/mg creatinine), gradually fell to age 16 (30–60 ng/mg creatinine), and then remained stable until age 55, when it began to decline [38]. Urinary EGF levels are greater in term than in premature infants [39]. In contrast, in the rat embryo, TGF-α is present at days 8–10 but is not detectable near term (day 18) [40] . Similarly, fetal sheep kidney possesses high TGF-α activity [41], suggesting a role for this peptide in fetal renal development. Thus, it is likely that TGF-α is the physiologic ligand for the EGF receptors that have been detected in fetal kidney.

The physiologic roles of EGF produced in the kidney are not yet well understood. EGF may serve as a cytoprotective agent of the distal nephron, ureters, and bladder. It is of interest that EGF is produced in the TALH, a nephron segment just proximal to the nephron segments in which urinary acidification is accomplished; the collecting duct, ureters, and bladder are exposed to urine pH of as low as 4.5, as well as to a hypertonic mileau. There is evidence suggesting a role for EGF in modulation of growth and function of these distal structures. Specific, high affinity receptors have been demonstrated in microdissected cortical collecting ducts [42], cultured papillary collecting duct cells, and freshly isolated suspensions of papillary collecting ducts [43]. In isolated perfused cortical collecting ducts, EGF inhibits hydroosmotic conductivity [44], electrogenic Na reabsorption [45], and K secretion [46]. EGF has been shown to be mitogenic for cultured rabbit thick ascending limb and cortical collecting duct cells [47], cultured rat papillary collecting duct cells [43], and cultured bladder epithelial cells [48].

In addition to its mitogenic effects upon cultured papillary collecting duct cells, EGF increases arachidonate release and prostaglandin production in these cells [43].

The latter is of especial interest, since renal medullary prostaglandins have been implicated in solute and fluid reabsorption in this segment. Medullary interstitial cells, thought to be an important site of medullary arachidonate metabolism, also possess specific EGF receptors, and EGF is a potent mitogen for these cells [44]. In addition, EGF stimulates arachidonate release and prostaglandin production in MDCK cells, a cell line with many characterictics of distal nephron [45].

EGF is a potent mitogen for cultured rabbit [46] and rat [47] proximal tubule cells, as well as LLC-PKl cells, a cell line with many characteristics of proximal tubule [48]. In cultured rabbit proximal tubule cells, EGF also stimulates protein synthesis and S6 kinase activity [49]. In freshly isolated rat proximal tubule segments, EGF inhibits both basal and angiotensin-stimulated gluconeogenesis [50] and stimulates hexose monophosphate shunt activity [47] and protein synthesis [49].

Therefore, in cultured cells and isolated tubule segments, a number of potential tubular effects for EGF have been proposed. The unanswered question remains whether the EGF synthesized and secreted by the kidney serves a paracrine function in the kidney and/or in the lower urinary tract. As mentioned above, immuno-histochemical studies localize preproEGF to the apical membrane of the thick ascending limb and distal convoluted tubule. However, studies to date suggest that EGF receptors are on basolateral membranes of polarized epithelia in the kidney. High affinity EGF binding was localized exclusively to basolateral membranes of proximal tubule of rat [50], rabbit [51], and mouse [52]. That the basolateral EGF binding represented binding to functional receptors was indicated by demonstration of EGF-mediated tyrosine kinase activity that was also localized to basolateral membranes [50]. Furthermore, all of the above-mentioned modulatory effects of EGF upon isolated perfused cortical collecting duct are induced only by administration of EGF to the basolateral membrane.

In spite of the apparent apical localization of preproEGF, it is possible that basolateral secretion of EGF does occur, thereby allowing access to receptors on adjacent tubules (which might include both proximal tubules as well as more distal tubule segments, given the topology of the cortex). Alternatively, EGF may be secreted into the lumen and then transcytosed in more distal nephron segments to the basolateral surface. In this regard, EGF is transcytosed from lumen to blood in the ileum of suckling mice [53]. However, in MDCK cells [54], transcytosis of EGF occurs only in the direction of basolateral to apical membrane.

It is also possible that under normal circumstances, the EGF produced in the kidney does not interact with EGF receptors in the kidney or the distal uroepithelium. However, following injury, either localized or general, intercellular tight junctions would be disrupted and EGF could traverse to the basolateral surfaces and interact with the EGF receptors located there. A potential role for EGF, in repair of renal tubules following injury, is suggested by the observations of the mitogenic effects of EGF on cells cultured from various tubule segments and by the indication that EGF serves to inhibit differentiated tubule functions (gluconeogenesis, salt and water reabsorption) either directly or through generation of prostaglandins. Since disruption of tight junctions (as well as loss of cell polarity) may occur following non-fatal cell injury, EGF may serve to inhibit the normal functioning of injured cells, thereby allowing repair and regeneration. A similar function for EGF in the bladder is suggested by the demonstration that only cells in the basal layer express EGF receptors [55].

These cells would not be exposed to urinary EGF unless there were injury and disruption of the superficial mucosa.

That EGF or TGF-α may play an important role in repair of renal injury is further suggested by recent studies of experimental tubular injury. In rat, following 50 minutes of unilateral renal ischemia induced by renal artery clamping, ^{125}I EGF binding increased, with the greatest relative increases seen in the cortex [24]. The increased binding was detectable at 24 hours following ischemia, and no change was noted in the contralateral, non-ischemic kidney. Similar findings have been reported in rabbit kidney following ischemia [56], and in rat kidney following folic acid administration [57]. Following ischemic renal injury in the rat, subcutaneous injection of EGF significantly accelerates ^{3}H thymidine incorporation and recovery of tubular function [58].

Although EGF and/or TGF-α may be important mediators of renal regeneration following acute tubular necrosis, EGF produced by the thick ascending limb/distal convoluted tubule is likely not involved. Following either cis-platinum renal toxicity [23] or ischemic tubular necrosis [24], both preproEGF mRNA levels and urinary EGF levels decrease and remain significantly depressed for up to 7 days. Whether this decrease in renal EGF production is a nonspecific result of cellular damage or whether it is a specific response to injury that is linked to the upregulation of receptors and increased sensitivity to EGF, remains to be determined. That renal EGF production decreased as a result of renal tubular damage was further suggested by the finding that in a series of patients with a variety of chronic renal diseases, urinary EGF excretion was depressed, and the relative decrease correlated with the decrease in renal function [22].

In contrast to renal regeneration, there is little current evidence suggesting a role for EGF in the mediation of compensatory hypertrophy. In cultured proximal tubule cells, the cells that undergo the greatest compensatory hypertrophy in vivo, EGF is a mitogenic rather than a hypertrophic agent. Following uninephrectomy, EGF receptors have been reported either to be unchanged [57], or to decrease slightly [59]. As previously mentioned, following unilateral nephrectomy, urinary EGF levels decrease by 50% and do not increase over the subsequent 14 days. However, immunolocalization studies indicate that EGF expression may be increased at 7, but not at 2 days, after contralateral nephrectomy [60]. Thus, the increases in expression of both EGF and insulin-like growth factor (IGF)-1 are not seen early after contralateral nephrectomy, during the period of greatest hypertrophy. Whether this late increase in growth factor expression serves a physiologic function in the growth process or is a response to the hypertrophy is unclear. A preliminary report by Uchida et al. has also suggested a role for serum EGF in renal hypertrophy. They found that sialoadenectomy inhibited compensatory hypertrophy following contralateral nephrectomy in mice, and that exogenous EGF administration overcame this inhibition [61].

In either streotpzotocin-induced or autoimmune diabetes mellitus, urinary EGF levels increase 4–9-fold, with partial normalization following insulin therapy [62]. Of interest, in mice with either streptozotocin-induced or genetic diabetes, submaxillary but not renal preproEGF mRNA expression was drastically reduced, with normalization following insulin therapy [63]. No role in either the hypertrophy or the glomerular pathology of diabetes has yet been attributed to EGF.

Preliminary evidence does suggest there may be a possible role for EGF/TGF-α in the mediation of the epithelial proliferation seen in cystic renal disease. In

C57BL/6J-cpk mice, which manifest an inheritable autosomal recessive form of polycystic kidney disease, with cystic dilatatior. of the collecting duct, no renal preproEGF mRNA could be detected [64]. Furthermore, although submaxillary preproEGF mRNA was present in these animals, testosterone did not stimulate expression, suggesting the possibility of a systemic disorder in regulation of EGF production. Of interest, cyst fluid from these animals has been reported to contain high concentrations of EGF (60 ng/ml). Cyst fluid from humans with adult polycystic kidney disease has EGF concentrations higher than plasma but lower than urine (0.5 ng/ml) [65]. Whether EGF contributes to cyst development and/or growth in vivo, as has been recently suggested in a murine metanephric culture system [66], will have to be determined in further studies.

EGF and/or TGF-α may also be involved in modulation of glomerular hemodynamics, either under physiologic conditions or following inflammatory injury. Intrarenal infusion of EGF into rats [67] or sheep [68] produced decreases in renal blood flow and GFR. Micropuncture studies in rat indicated that EGF induced both afferent and efferent arteriolar vasoconstriction, as well as a profound fall in K_f [67]. That the fall in K_f was secondary to mesangial cell contraction was further suggested by identification of specific high-affinity EGF receptors on cultured rat mesangial cells, and demonstration that EGF stimulated Na^+/H^+ exchange and contraction of these cells [67]. In cultured mesangial cells, EGF has been demonstrated to activate phospholipase A_2 activity [69], to release arachidonic acid, and to increase prostaglandin production in synergism with phorbol esters or vasopressin [70]. Furthermore, following irreversible cyclooxygenase inactivation by aspirin, EGF stimulated synthesis of new cyclooxygenase in mesangial cells [71]. Therefore, it is possible that EGF or TGF-α may modulate glomerular prostaglandin production.

Recent studies have suggested a role for both cyclooxygenase and non-cyclooxygenase arachidonate metabolites in the mediation of EGF's renal hemodynamic effects [72]. In the presence of cyclooxygenase inhibition by ibuprofen, the vasoconstrictive effects of EGF were abolished. Instead, intrarenal EGF infusion led to both systemic and renal microcirculatory vasodilation. This vasodilatory effect was also suggested to be mediated by non-cyclooxygenase arachidonate metabolites, because pretreatment with the competitive inhibitor of arachidonate release, 5,8,11,14-eicosatetraynoic acid (ETYA), abolished the vasodilation. In the face of complete inhibition of arachdionate release, EGF was found to again induce mild vasoconstriction. That the non-cyclooxygenase arachidonate metabolites mediating the vasodilation were generated from metabolism by cytochrome P450 was suggested by studies demonstrating that ketoconazole, a relatively selective inhibitor of renal P450, also inhibited the above-described EGF-induced vasodilation. EGF-induced stimulation of P450 arachidonate metabolite production was suggested by the demonstration that in suspensions of isolated rat proximal tubules, EGF administration led to a 100% increase in endogenous epoxyeicosatrienoic acids (EETs) within 5 minutes [73].

Although circulating EGF levels in most mammals are low, platelets are known to contain EGF[14], as well as TGF-α [74]. In addition, activated macrophages synthesize and secrete TGF-α [75,76]. Therefore, during inflammatory injury, local glomerular concentrations of EGF and TGF-α may be high and play a role in mediating both acute alterations in renal hemodynamics and subsequent mesangial proliferation. The recent observations that transmembrane prepro TGF-α can bind to EGF receptors and stimulate acute signal transduction events without proteolytic cleavage and secretion [77,78] also raises the possibility that infiltrating cells could alter glomerular function even in the absence of peptide release. Mroczkowski et al. have also found that preproEGF expressed in a recombinant system does not require proteolytic processing in order to bind to EGF receptors and activate tyrosine kinase activity [31].

Although EGF and TGF-α modulate acute renal hemodynamic events and stimulate proliferation of mesangial cells in culture, studies of collagen production by cultured rat mesangial cells suggest that EGF does not promote increased mesangial matrix production, since EGF actually inhibits both basal [79] and retinoic acid-stimulated [80] production of collagen in mesangial cells. Stimulation of wound healing by epidermal growth factor is due to its stimulation of fibroblast proliferation, rather than stimulation of collagen production per se [81]. Since EGF and TGF-α are both potent mitogens for NRK cells, a fibroblast cell line derived from rat kidney, it is possible that under pathophysiologic conditions these peptides might also stimulate proliferation of renal fibroblasts in vivo and thereby increase cortical or medullary scarring.

In summary, the kidney is one of the major sites for EGF synthesis and urinary EGF levels are high. The expression of preproEGF mRNA and immunoreactive preproEGF and EGF are localized to the cells of the TALH and early DCT. A diverse number of potential responses to EGF and/or TGF-α have recently been described, including modulation of glomerular hemodynamics, renal metabolism, tubular transport functions, and eicosanoid synthesis. In addition, these growth factors have been shown to be potent mitogens in vitro for a variety of cell types in the kidney and they may play an important role in renal embryogenesis and repair following injury.

References

1. Carpenter G, Cohen S (1979) Epidermal growth factor. Annu Rev Biochem 48:193
2. Carpenter G (1987) Receptors for epidermal growth factor and other polypeptide mitogens. Annu Rev Biochem 56:881
3. Cohen S, Fava RA, Sawyer ST (1982) Purification and characterization of epidermal growth factor receptor/protein kinase from normal mouse liver. Proc Natl Acad Sci USA 79:6237
4. Taketani Y, Oka T (1983) Epidermal growth factor stimulates cell proliferation and inhibits functional differentiation of mouse mammary gland cells in culture. Endocrinology 133:871
5. Chabot JG, Walker P, Pelletier G (1986) Distribution of epidermal growth factor binding sites in the adult rat liver. Am J Physiol 250:G760
6. Scheving LA, Shiurba RA, Nguyen TD, Gray Gary M (1989) Epidermal growth factor receptor of the intestinal enterocyte. Localization to laterobasal but not brush border membrane. J Biol Chem 264:1735
7. Deminski AB, Johnson LR (1985) Effect of EGF on development of rat gastric mucosa. Endocrinology 116:90
8. Deminski A, Gregory H, Kontrutek S, Polanski M (1982) Trophic action of EGF on the pancreas and gastroduodenal mucosa in rats. J Physiol 325:35
9. Konturek SJ (1988) Role of epidermal growth factor in gastroprotection and ulcer healing. Scand J Gastroenterol 23:129

10. Moolenaar WH, Yarden Y, deLaat SW, Schlessinger J (1982) Epidermal growth factor induces electrically silent Na$^+$ influx in human fibroblasts. J Biol Chem 275:8502

11. Lembach K (1977) Enhanced synthesis and extracellular accumulation of hyaluronic acid during stimulation of quiescent human fibroblasts by mouse epidermal growth factor. J Cell Physiol 89:277

12. DeLarco J, Todaro GJ (1978) Growth factors from murine sarcoma virus-transformed cells. Proc Natl Acad Sci USA 75:4001

13. Derynck R (1986) Transforming growth factor-a: Structure and biological activities. J Cell Biochem 32:293

14. Oka T, Orth DN (1983) Human plasma epidermal growth factor/β urogastrone is associated with blood platelets. J Clin Invest 72:249

15. Joh T, Itoh M, Katsumi K, Yokoyama Y, Takeuchi T, Kato T, Wada Y, Tanaka R (1986) Physiological concentrations of human epidermal growth factor in biological fluids: use of a sensitive enzyme immunoassay. Clin Chim Acta 158:81

16. Gregory H, Willshire IR, Kavanagh JP, Blacklock NJ, Chowdury S, Richards RC (1986) Urogastrone-epidermal growth factor concentrations in prostatic fluid of normal individuals and patients with benign prostatic hypertrophy. Clin Sci 70:359

17. Poulsen SS, Nexo E, Skov Olsen P, Hess J, Kirkegaard P (1986) Immunohistochemical localization of epidermal growth factor in rat and man. Histochemistry 85:389

18. Gregory H (1975) The isolation and structure of urogastrone and its relationship to epidermal growth factor. Nature 257:325

19. Kasselberg AG, Orth DN, Gray ME, Stahlman MT (1985) Immunocytochemical localization of human growth factor/urogastrone in several human tissues. J Histochem Cytochem 33:315

20. Skov Olsen P, Nexo E, Poulsen S, Hansen HF, Kirkegaard P (1984) Renal origin of rat urinary epidermal growth factor. Regul Pept 10:37

21. Harris RC, Gung A, Orth DN, Badr KF (1988) Effect of dietary protein and uninephrectomy on urinary epidermal growth factor excretion. FASEB J 2:1305A

22. Mattila A-L, Pasternack A, Viinikka L, Perheentupa J (1986) Subnormal concentrations of urinary epidermal growth factor in patients with kidney disease. J Clin Endocrinol Metab 62:1180

23. Safirstein R, Zelent AZ, Price PM (1989) Reduced renal prepro-epidermal growth factor mRNA and decreased EGF excretion in ARF. Kidney Int. 36:810

24. Safirstein R, Price PM, Saggi SJ, Harris RC (1990) Changes in gene expression after temporary renal ischemia. Kidney Int 37:1515

25. Nielsen S, Nexo E, Christensen EI (1989) Absorption of epidermal growth factor and insulin in rabbit renal proximal tubules. Am J Physiol 256:E55

26. Rall LB, Scott J, Bell GI, Crawford RJ, Penshcow JD, Niall HD, Coghlan JP (1985) Mouse prepro-epidermal growth factor synthesis by the kidney and other tissues. Nature 313:228

27. Salido EC, Barajas L, Lechago J, Laborde NP, Fisher DA (1986) Immunocytochemical localization of epidermal growth factor in mouse kidney. J Histochem Cytochem 34:1155

28. Salido EC, Yen PH, Shapiro LJ, Fisher DA, Barajas L (1989) In situ hybridization of prepro-epidermal growth factor mRNA in the mouse kidney. Am J Physiol F632

29. Drinkwater CC, Evans BA, Richards RI (1987) Mouse glandular kallikrein genes: identification and characterization of the genes encoding the epidermal growth factor binding proteins. Biochemistry 26:6750

30. Drinkwater CC, Evans BA, Richards RI (1988) Kallikreins, kinins and growth factor biosynthesis. Trends Biochem Sci 13:169

31. Mroczkowski B, Reich M, Chen K, Bell GI, Cohen S (1989) Recombinant human epidermal growth factor precursor is a glycosylated membrane protein with biological activity. Mol Cell Biol 9:2771

32. Perheentupa J, Lakshmanan J, Fisher DA (1985) Urine and kidney epidermal growth factor: ontogeny and sex difference in the mouse. Pediatr Res 19:428
33. Hoffmann GE, Rao CV, Brown MJ, Murray LF, Schultz GS, Siddiqi TA (1988) Epidermal growth factor in urine of nonpregnant women throughout pregnancy and at delivery. J Clin Endocrinol Metab 66:119
35. Mattila A-L, Perheentupa J, Salmi J, Miinikka L (1987) Human epidermal growth factor concentrations in urine, but not in saliva and serum, depend on thyroid state. Life Sci 41:2739
36. Olsen PS, Kirkegaard P, Poulsen SS, Nexo E (1985) Adrenergic effects on renal secretion of epidermal growth factor in the rat. Regul Pep 11:17
37. Raaberg L, Nexo E, Mikkelsen JD, Poulsen SS (1988) Immunohistochemical localisation and developmental aspects of epidermal growth factor in the rat. Histochemistry 89:351
38. Mattila A-L, Perheentupa J, Pesonen K, Viinikka L (1985) Epidermal growth factor in human urine from birth to puberty. J Clin Endocrinol Metab 61:997
39. Evans NJ, Rutter N, Gregory H (1986) Urinary excretion of epidermal growth factor in the newborn. Early Hum Dev 14:277
40. Lee DC, Rochford R, Todaro G, Villarreal LP (1985) Development expression of rat transforming growth factor alpha mRNA. Mol Cell Biol 5:3644
41. Freemark M, Comer M (1987) Epidermal growth factor (EGF)-like transforming growth factor (TGF) activity and EGF receptors in ovine fetal tissues: possible role for TGF in ovine fetal development. Pediatr Res 22:609
42. Rehda R, Lopez C, Breyer JA, Jacobson HR, Breyer MD (1989) Mapping of 125-I epidermal growth factor binding sites along the rabbit nephron. Kidney Int 35:319A
43. Harris RC (1989) Response of rat inner medullary collecting duct to epidermal growth factor. Am J Physiol 256:F1117
44. Breyer MD, Jacobson HR, Breyer JA (1988) Epidermal growth factor inhibits the hydroosmotic effect of vasopressin in the isolated perfused rabbit cortical collecting tubule. J Clin Invest 82:1313
45. Vehaskari VM, Hering-Smith KS, Moskowitz DW, Wiener ID, Hamm LL (1989) Effect of epidermal growth factor on sodium transport in the cortical collecting tubule. Am J Physiol 256:F803
46. Muto S, Furuya H, Tabei K, Asano Y (1990) Effect of epidermal growth factor on potassium transport in the rabbit cortical collecting duct. Kidney Int 37:568A
47. Wilson PD, Horster MF (1983) Differential response to hormones of defined distal nephron epithelia in culture. Am J Physiol 13:C166
48. Nissenkorn I, Mickey D, Soloway M (1982) Effect of media and growth promoters on in vitro cultivation of normal murine urinary bladder epithelium. J Urol 128:176
44. Breyer J, Harris RC (1988) EGF binds to specific EGF receptors and stimulates mitogenesis in renal medullary interstitial cells. Kidney Int 33:255A
45. Levine L, Hassid A (1977) Epidermal growth factor stimulates prostaglandin biosynthesis by canine kidney (MDCK) cells. Biochem Biophys Res Commun 76:1181
46. Norman J, Badie-Dezfooly B, Nord EP, Kurtz I, Schlosser J, Chaudhari A, Fine LG (1989) EGF-induced mitogenesis in proximal tubular cells: potentiation by angiotensin II. Am J Physiol 253:F299
47. Stanton RC, Seifter JL (1988) Epidermal growth factor rapidly activates the hexose monophosphate shunt in kidney cells. Am J Physiol 253:C267
48. Mullin JM, McGinn MT (1988) Epidermal growth factor-induced mitogenesis in kidney epithelial cells (LLC-PK1). Cancer Res 48:4886
49. Harris RC (1990) S6 kinase activity increases in cultured proximal tubule cells with epidermal growth factor and insulin and in renal cortex after uninephrectomy. Kidney Int 37:195A

50. Harris RC, Daniel TO (1989) Epidermal growth factor binding, stimulation of phosphorylation and inhibition of gluconeogenesis in rat proximal tubule. J Cell Physiol 139:383

51. Sack E, Talor Z (1988) High affinity binding sites for epidermal growth factor in renal membranes. Biochem Biophys Res Commun 154:312

52. Goodyer P, Kachra Z, Bell C, Rozen R (1988) Renal tubular cells are potential targets for epidermal growth factor. Am J Physiol 255:F1191

53. Gonnelia PA, Siminoski K, Murphy RA, Neutra MR (1987) Transepithelial transport of epidermal growth factor by absorptive cells of suckling rat ileum. J Clin Invest 80:22

54. Maratos-Flier E, Kao C-Y, Verdin E, King GL (1987) Receptor-mediated vectorial transcytosis of epidermal growth factor by Madin-Darby Canine Kidney Cells. J Cell Biol 105:1595

55. Neal DE, Marsh C, Bennett MK, Abel PD, Hall RR, Sainsbury JR, Harris AL (1985) Epidermal growth factor receptors in human bladder cancer: comparison of invasive and superficial tumours. Lancet I:366

56. Tsau YK, Norman JT, Fine LG (1989) Epidermal growth factor enhances renal regeneration and accelerates recovery from ischemic acute renal failure. Kidney Int 35:420A

57. Behrens MT, Corbin AL, Hise MK (1989) Epidermal growth factor receptor regulation in the rat kidney: two models of renal growth. Am J Physiol 257:F1059

58. Humes HD, Cieslinski DA, Coimbra TM, Messana JM, Calvao C (1989) Epidermal growth factor enhances renal tubule cell regeneration and repair and accelerates the recovery of renal function in postischemic acute renal failure. J Clin Invest 84:1757

59. Sack E, Arruda JAL, Talor Z (1989) EGF binding is decreased in compensatory renal hypertrophy. Kidney Int 35:319A

60. Jennische E, Andersson G, Hansson HA (1987) Epidermal growth factor is expressed by cells in the distal tubules during postnephrectomy renal growth. Acta Physiol Scand 129:449

61. Uchida S, Tsutsumi O, Hise MK, Oka T (1988) Role of epidermal growth factor in compensatory renal hypertrophy in mice. Kidney Int 33:387A

62. Hwang DL, Lev-Ran A, Tay YC, Chen CR, Dev N (1989) Epidermal growth factor excretion and receptor binding in diabetic rats. Life Sci 44:407

63. Kasayama S, Ohba Y, Oka T (1989) Epidermal growth factor deficiency associated with diabetes mellitus. Proc Natl Acad Sci USA 86:7644

64. Gattone VH, Fu-wen N, Andrews GK, Klein RM, Calvet JP (1989) Reduced ontogenic expression of epidermal growth factor (EGF) in a murine model of renal cystic disease. Kidney Int 35:311A

65. Moskowitz DW, Bonar SL, Marcus MD, Clayman RV, Avner ED (1989) Epidermal growth factor content of human and mouse (cpk) renal cysts. Clin Res 37:497A

66. Avner ED, Sweeney WE (1990) Epidermal growth factor induces hyperplastic tubular cysts and increased Na-K ATPase activity in vitro. Kidney Int 37:190A

67. Harris RC, Hoover RL, Jacobson HR, Badr KF (1988) Evidence for glomerular actions of epidermal growth factor in the rat. J Clin Invest 82:1028

68. Scoggins BA, Butkus A, Coghlan JP, Fei D, McDougall JG, Niall HD, Walsh JR, Wang X (1984) In vivo cardiovascular, renal and endocrine effects of epidermal growth factor in sheep. In: Labrie T, Prouix L (eds) Endocrinology. Elsevier, p 573

69. Margolis BL, Holub BJ, Troyer DA, Skorecki KL (1988) Epidermal growth factor stimulates phospholipase A2 in vasopressin-treated rat glomerular mesangial cells. Biochem J 256:469

70. Margolis BL, Bonventre JV, Kremer SG, Kudlow JE, Skorecki KL (1988) Epidermal growth factor is synergistic with phorbol esters and vasopressin in stimulating arachidonate release and prostaglandin production in renal glomerular mesangial cells. Biochem J 249:587

71. Harris RC, Badr KF (1990) Recovery of prostaglandin synthesis in rat glomerular mesangial cells after aspirin inhibition: induction of cyclooxygenase activity by serum and epidermal growth factor. Prostaglandins 39:213

72. Harris RC, Munger KA, Badr KF, Takahashi K (1990) Mediation of renal vascular effects of epidermal growth factor by arachidonate metabolites. FASEB J 4:1654

73. Capdevila JH, Harris RC, Karara A, Dishman E (1989) Characterization of the arachidonic acid epoxygenase reaction present in isolated rat kidney proximal tubule cells. Kidney Int 35:290A

74. Assoain RK, Grotendorst GR, Miller DM, Sporn MB (1984) Cellular transformation by coordinated action of three peptide growth factors from human platelets. Nature 309:804

75. Madtes DK, Raines EW, Sakariassen KS, Assoain RK, Sporn MB, Bell GJ, Ross R (1988) Induction of transforming growth factor-α in activated human macrophages. Cell 53:285

76. Rappolee DA, Mark D, Banda MJ, Werb Z (1988) Wound macrophages express TGF-α and other growth factors in vivo: Analysis by mRNA phenotyping. Science 241:708

77. Brachman R, Lindquist PB, Nagashima M, Kohr W, Lipari T, Napier M, Derynck R (1989) Transmembrane TGF-α precursors activate EGF/TGF-α receptors. Cell 56:691

78. Song ST, Winchell LF, McCune BK, Earp HS, Teixido J, Massague J, Herman B, Lee DC (1989) The TGF-α precursor expressed on the cell surface binds to the TGF receptor on adjacent cells, leading to signal transduction. Cell 56:495

79. Hoover RL, Harris RC, Haralson MA (1989) Effects of epidermal growth factor on collagen biosynthesis in cultured rat kidney mesangial cells. Kidney Int 35:349A

80. Haralson MA, DiMari SJ, Hoover RL, Harris RC (1990) Epidermal growth factor suppresses collagen biosynthesis in retinoic acid-treated cultured rat kidney mesangial cells. Kidney Int 37:195A

81. Laato M, Kahari V-M, Niinikoski J, Vuorio E (1987) Epidermal growth factor increases collagen production in granulation tissue by stimulation of fibroblast proliferation and not by activation of procollagen genes. Biochem J 247:385

Determinants of Autocrine and Paracrine Growth Factor Release by Kidney Epithelial Cells

F. Gary Toback, Sreedharan Kartha, and Margaret M. Walsh-Reitz[1]

SUMMARY. During studies of mitogenic signal transduction mechanisms in nontransformed monkey kidney epithelial cells in culture, evidence for the release of autocrine and paracrine growth factors was obtained. Reduction of the K or Na concentration of the culture medium induced rapid release of novel growth-promoting activities, whereas addition of the mitogen, adenosine diphosphate, stimulated the appearance of a platelet-derived growth factor-like protein which could function in a paracrine manner. These cells constitutively release transforming growth factor β2, which acts as a negative autocrine growth factor. Thus, growth in culture appears to be regulated by the interplay of positive and negative autocrine growth factors and the responses of cell surface receptors and post-receptor events. Autocrine and paracrine growth factors released in response to alterations in the ionic and nutrient composition of the extracellular environment could play an important role in physiological and pathological states in the kidney.

Introduction

Few factors that regulate the growth of kidney epithelial cells have been defined. During the past decade, we have used a tissue culture model system to identify determinants of renal cell proliferation. Experiments were carried out using kidney epithelial cells of the nontransformed African green monkey (*Cercopithecus aethiops*) line, BSC-1. Although the growth of cells in culture may differ in certain respects from that in the intact organ, this approach eliminates many of the problems inherent in studies of growth in a tissue as complex as kidney. Studies were often carried out in quiescent, high-density cultures in order to simulate the low proliferative

[1]The University of Chicago, Department of Medicine, Chicago, IL 60637, USA

activity of kidney cells in vivo [1]. Under these conditions, the epithelial cell monolayer appears to form small domes (3 to 4 cells in size), which suggests that the cells carry out transepithelial transport.

Several determinants of growth regulation have been identified in BSC-1 cells [2]. These include growth factors and hormones in normal serum and their receptors on the cell surface, and low molecular weight nutrients. Specific growth-stimulatory molecules contained in serum include vasopressin, glucagon, and epidermal growth factor (EGF) [3]. The growth of BSC-1 cells in culture is also regulated by the cellular production of several inhibitors. These include lactate, ammonium ion, and a secreted protein which has an M_r of 25000 [4]. This inhibitor protein, which has been identified as transforming growth factor (TGF)-β2, is active at very low concentrations (1 ng/ml) on epithelial cells grown in culture, impedes exit of cells from the G_0/G_1 (resting) phase of the cell cycle, and can be overcome by the stimulatory action of serum or EGF [5]. We have reported that this protein appears to exert its growth inhibitory effect by interfering with cell Na flux [6]. Although the substratum upon which cells grow in culture is often considered a critical determinant of replication and differentiation [7], the contribution of collagen, fibronectin, and other extracellular factors to the growth of BSC-1 cells has not yet been defined in detail.

Growth Factors Isolated from Renal Tissue

While no growth factor specific to kidney has been described, several factors initially described in other types of cells have been identified in kidney tissue or have been shown to have actions on renal cells in culture. Growth factors isolated from kidney tissue include EGF, TGF-α and β, platelet-derived growth factor (PDGF), insulin-like growth factor (IGF)-I and II, acidic and basic fibroblast growth factor (FGF), and interleukin-1 [8]. EGF is found in abundance in urine and renal cyst fluid, and its precursor protein, preproEGF, is made by cells of the distal nephron in the mouse [9]. TGF-β1 has been isolated from bovine kidney, and TGF-β2 is an autocrine growth inhibitor for kidney epithelial cells in culture [6]. PDGF is produced by mesangial cells, stimulates mesangial cell contraction, and is an autocrine and paracrine mitogen for different types of renal cells [8]. IGF-I and II are probably synthesized in the kidney, although their physiologic functions in the organ are unknown. Both acidic and basic FGF are found in kidney and may play a role in angiogenesis during renal embryonic development [10].

The metabolism and excretion of growth factors in acute and chronic renal failure has not yet been studied in detail. Although most of the factors probably act locally, their presence has also been detected in the circulation and in urine. Some may be filtered at the glomerulus or may require intact tubular cells for degradation and might accumulate progressively in the extracellular fluid as glomerular and tubular function diminish. In this scenario, cells of the injured kidney could be exposed to abnormal concentrations of growth factors and thereby subjected to nonphysiologic growth-regulatory signals.

Initiation of DNA Synthesis and Multiplication is Induced in BSC-1 Cells Exposed to Altered Extracellular Concentrations of K or Na

Studies of renal epithelial cells in culture provided the first support for the hypothesis that cell proliferation can be induced by perturbations of the ionic environment. In 1980 it was shown that addition of NaCl to the culture medium of BSC-1 cells initiated DNA synthesis and induced cell multiplication in high-density, quiescent BSC-1 cells [1]. In 1983 a report from this laboratory demonstrated that BSC-1 cells exposed to a reduced concentration of K in the medium (control of 5.4 mM to 3.2 mM) exhibited accelerated growth analogous to that observed in kidneys of rats fed a K-deficient diet [11]. In addition, growth stimulation provoked by lowering the extracellular K concentration required a transient increase in intracellular Na content [12]. When this increment was prevented, low-K stimulation of cell multiplication was not observed. Since augmented influx of Na occurs during the onset of proliferation, one would expect that exposure of kidney cells to a reduced concentration of Na might inhibit mitogenesis. Contrary to this expectation, cell growth was stimulated when the concentration of the medium was reduced from 155 mM (control) to 130 mM [13]. It should be noted that the mitogenic effects in each condition cited above were shown not to be a consequence of increments or reductions in either the osmolality or the anion concentration of the culture medium. In summary, renal epithelial cells can respond to perturbations in the extracellular fluid concentration of K or Na by initiating DNA synthesis.

Reduced Extracellular Potassium Concentration Stimulates Growth of Renal Cells by an Autocrine Mechanism

More than fifty years ago, systemic K depletion, achieved experimentally by feeding rats a K-deficient diet, was found to induce kidney growth [14]. Sustained mild hypokalemia is associated with doubling of renal mass due to both hyperplasia and hypertrophy of kidney cells. An in vitro model to study this phenomenon became available when it was found that simply lowering the extracellular K concentration from 5.4 mM (control) to 3.2 mM in confluent cultures of BSC-1 cells induced accelerated growth [11]. Thus, these cells perceive a reduction in the K concentration of the medium as a mitogenic signal.

We tested the hypothesis that proliferation in response to low-K medium is mediated by release of a growth-promoting factor from the cells [15]. Low-K or control medium was conditioned by placing it on confluent cultures of BSC-1 cells. Growth-stimulating activity in low-K conditioned medium (CM) first appeared after 1 hour (Fig. 1, a) and was optimal when the K concentration during conditioning was 3.2 mM. Preliminary studies indicated that the growth factor(s) had an apparent M_r of 12000–30000, as determined by ultrafiltration and dialysis. The factor(s) is highly potent because it retains its stimulatory activity at dilutions greater than 1:1000. Its activity is destroyed by heating to 56°C for 30 minutes, but is stable at 4°C for at least 3 days. This activity differs from other previously described growth factors.

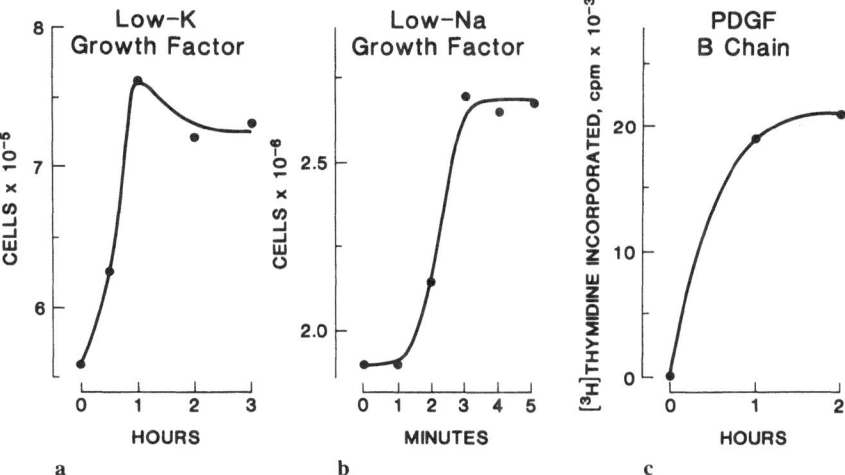

Fig. 1a-c. Release of autocrine and paracrine growth-promoting activities from BSC-1 cells exposed to low-K medium, low-Na medium, or adenosine diphosphate. **a** Appearance of growth-stimulating activity in low-K medium. Confluent, quiescent cultures of BSC-1 cells were exposed to medium containing 3.2 mM K and 0.01% calf serum for different periods of time and were collected. The K concentration of this low-K conditioned medium (*CM*) was adjusted to 5.4 mM by adding KCl. CM was filtered and its serum concentration was raised to 0.5%. Medium on fresh cultures was aspirated and replaced by the low-K CM. The effect of each medium on cell multiplication was assessed by counting the number of cells 3 days later. One hour of exposure of the cells to low-K CM was required to increase the growth-stimulating activity of this medium above that in control CM. **b** Appearance of growth-promoting activity in low-Na medium. At time 0, confluent cultures were exposed to low-Na medium (130 mM) containing 0.01% serum. At the times specified on the abscissa, the CM on the dish was collected. The Na concentration of this CM was adjusted to 155 mM by adding NaCl. CM was filtered and its serum concentration was raised to 0.5%. Medium on a fresh culture was aspirated and replaced by the low-Na CM. The number of cells per dish was counted 4 days later. Growth-promoting activity was maximal in low-Na CM after 3 minutes. **c** Release of PDGF-like mitogenic activity by ADP from high-density, quiescent cultures. BSC-1 cells were exposed to ADP for 1 or 2 hours, and CM was collected and assayed for its mitogenic activity in NRK fibroblasts. The stimulation of [³H]thymidine incorporation into DNA was inhibited 85% by human anti-PDGF IgG. After 1 hour of exposure to ADP, PDGF-like activity was about 10-fold greater than that measured in control CM. (Data adapted from [13,15,27])

The growth-promoting activity in low-K CM can be antagonized by the addition of purified TGF-β2, the autocrine inhibitor of BSC-1 cell growth.

This study indicated that stimulation of renal epithelial cell growth induced by lowering the extracellular K concentration is associated with the appearance of a mitogenic factor(s) in the medium, and provided the first evidence that cell growth induced by an alteration in the ion concentration of the extracellular fluid could be mediated by an autocrine mechanism.

Lowering Extracellular Sodium Concentration Induces Renal Cell Growth and Production of Growth Factors

Since augmented influx of Na ions probably occurs during the onset of proliferation in virtually all mammalian cells [16], one would expect to find that exposure of BSC-1 cells to medium containing a reduced concentration of Na would inhibit mitogenesis. Surprisingly, we found that cell multiplication was stimulated when the Na concentration of the medium was reduced from 155 mM (control) to 130 mM [13]. The capacity of low-Na medium to enhance cell proliferation depended upon the decreased Na concentration, as growth stimulation was equivalent whether equimolar amounts of choline chloride or equiosmolar amounts of sucrose were used to replace NaCl deleted from the medium.

After exposure of confluent cultures to low-Na medium (130 mM) for only 3–5 minutes (Fig. 1, b), the cells released two growth-stimulatory factors (apparent M_r 6200 and 9000). Release was not dependent upon new protein synthesis, since it occurred in the presence of cycloheximide. The activity in CM was stable at 56°C for 30 minutes and was retained after freezing for many weeks. Treatment with trypsin abolished the growth-promoting effect, whereas treatment with dithiothreitol did not, which suggests that the low-Na growth factors are proteins that have no accessible disulfide bonds required for activity. The growth response to a reduction in extracellular Na concentration appears to be cell-type specific, since low-Na medium does not stimulate proliferation of fibroblasts. Release of growth factor activity is also cell-type specific, as CM from fibroblasts exposed to a reduced extracellular Na concentration is not stimulatory for epithelial cells. The low-Na growth factors appear to be chemically and functionally different from other known growth factors.

Low-K and Low-Na Growth Factors

The observations summarized above indicate that exposure of kidney epithelial cells to low-K or low-Na medium results in the rapid appearance of growth-promoting activities in the extracellular fluid. These autocrine products appear to differ in that (a) the apparent M_r of the growth factor(s) in low-K CM is 12000–30000, whereas those in low-Na CM are 6200 and 9000, (b) the low-K factor(s) first appears in the medium after 60 minutes, whereas the low-Na factors are detected as early as 3 minutes, and (c) the growth-stimulating effect of low-K CM is destroyed by heating at 56°C for 30 minutes, whereas the low-Na activity is stable under this condition.

The liberation of active factors by renal epithelial cells in culture suggests that kidney cells may respond similarly in vivo. Thus, modest reductions in the extracellular concentration of K and Na may result in the rapid appearance of physiological mediators that could communicate information to other cells along the nephron. These factors might act as messengers between glomerular and tubular cells in different parts of the nephron, in response to changes in peritubular or luminal ion concentrations. Although the factors released in response to low-K and low-Na media induce proliferation in cell culture, their physiologic role may be different in the intact kidney. Since many mitogens stimulate fluxes of ions and nutrients [16,17], one possible role could be to modify epithelial transport in response to changes in the extracellular environment. Release of autocrine or paracrine factors with this property suggests a previously undisclosed mechanism for regulation of ion and nutrient transport in adjacent and nonadjacent epithelial cells. Additional studies will be required to determine whether these factors contribute to the control of kidney epithelial cell growth and/or transport in vivo.

Transforming Growth Factor β2 Is a Negative Autocrine Growth Factor for Kidney Cells

The autocrine release of growth-inhibitory activity was inferred from observations made on crowded cultures of BSC-1 cells by Holley and co-workers in 1978 [4]. They noted stimulation of [^{3}H]thymidine incorporation into DNA when CM containing serum was aspirated and replaced with fresh serum-free medium. As no serum growth factors were added to the cells, it appeared that DNA synthesis was initiated by removal of a cell-derived growth inhibitor. Subsequent purification of this inhibitor protein indicated that it could arrest sparse cultures of growing cells in the G_1 phase of the cell cycle, but proliferation resumed when it was removed [6]. This reversible effect on cell growth, and the low concentration required for inhibition, suggested a physiological role for the inhibitor in the control of proliferation. In 1984, this growth inhibitor was shown to be biologically and chemically similar to TGF-β [18]. The complete amino acid sequence of the BSC-1 cell growth inhibitor has been determined from the nucleotide sequence of the cDNA, and has been shown to correspond to that of TGF-β2 [5].

In primary cultures of rabbit proximal tubular cells, TGF-β2 appears to transform a mitogenic stimulus into a hypertrophic one [19], and suggests that this negative autocrine growth factor could play a regulatory role in compensatory renal growth after uninephrectomy. Perhaps release of this protein by kidney cells in vivo converts what might otherwise have been a largely hyperplastic response into one that is expressed by an increase in renal mass that is 75% cell hypertrophy and 25% proliferation [20].

Purine Nucleotides Are Potent Mitogens for Renal Epithelial Cells and Stimulate Proto-oncogene Expression

During the course of a study to define the role of cAMP in kidney epithelial cell growth, we observed that exogenous adenosine 5′-monophosphate (AMP), used as a control, acted as a powerful mitogen [21]. Each of the adenine nucleotides was able to stimulate DNA synthesis in confluent cultures of BSC-1 cells. ADP and AMP were more potent mitogens than ATP or adenosine, or guanine or inosine and their nucleotides. Furthermore, ADP stimulated DNA synthesis 3-fold more than any known growth-promoting agent for BSC-1 cells. Importantly, ADP and AMP were mitogenic under serum-free conditions, and their stimulatory effects were apparently not mediated by cAMP-dependent mechanisms. In addition, known metabolites such as adenosine, hypoxanthine, or inosine did not appear to mediate ADP or AMP stimulation of DNA synthesis, because they were not as potent when added to the culture medium. Autoradiography of [³H]thymidine-labeled cultures indicated that 6-fold more cells were synthesizing DNA. There was no detectable detachment of cells from the monolayer under these conditions. Finally, the mitogenic effect of ADP or AMP did not appear to be mediated through the adenosine receptor, because the predicted stimulation of DNA synthesis was observed in the presence of a large excess of theophylline or 5'-deoxy 5'-methylthioadenosine, which are potent adenosine receptor antagonists.

To explore the molecular mechanisms by which ADP exerts its mitogenic effect, we tested the hypothesis that stimulation of DNA synthesis in renal epithelial cells of the BSC-1 line is mediated by activation of proto-oncogenes. Transcripts of the c-Ha-*ras* proto-oncogene were identified in quiescent, high-density cells [22]. Addition of ADP to the culture medium stimulated expression by 4-fold. Maximal expression of c-*ras* was observed 12 hours following exposure to ADP, and preceded initiation of DNA synthesis. Expression of the c-*fos* and c-*myc* proto-oncogenes was not detected in unstimulated cells, but following exposure to ADP there was maximal accumulation of c-*fos* transcripts at 30 minutes and c-*myc* at 60 minutes.

We also evaluated the capacity of ADP to stimulate expression of the early growth response gene, Egr-1 [23]. ADP rapidly induced Egr-1 mRNA expression with a peak level about 10-fold higher than that attained for c-*fos*. Egr-1 mRNA induction occurred as early as 10 minutes following exposure of BSC-1 cells to ADP. This novel gene is also induced in serum-stimulated mouse fibroblasts, insulin-stimulated rat hepatoma cells, and phytohemagglutinin-stimulated human peripheral blood lymphocytes. Another early growth response gene, NAK1, the human homologue of mouse nur 77 and rat NGFI-B, also is induced by ADP [24]. NAK1 belongs to the superfamily of steroid and thyroid hormone and retinoic acid receptor genes. The expression of NAK1 is detected at 20 minutes, and is maximal after 1 hour of exposure to ADP. Genes which are activated rapidly and transiently are likely to be important in transduction of mitogenic signals and regulation of cell proliferation. The Egr-1 and NAK1 genes encode proteins with zinc-finger domains that could facilitate DNA binding [24,25]. These proteins are postulated to function as transcriptional regulators.

ADP stimulation of Egr-1, NAK1, and proto-oncogene expression occurred during the G_1 phase of the cell cycle because maximal expression of these transcripts was detected prior to the increment in DNA synthesis at 12–24 hours. These findings represent the first reported examples of enhanced expression of Egr-1, NAK1, c-*fos*, c-*myc*, c-Ha-*ras*, and transferrin receptor genes in stimulated, nontransformed epithelial cells.

Expression of 25 genes and proto-oncogenes, most of which contribute to growth control, were studied in BSC-1 cells in the absence and presence of ADP. The responses observed could be divided into four patterns, which are presented in Table 1; genes not constitutively expressed but induced by ADP, genes whose constitutive expression was enhanced or unaltered by the nucleotide, and genes that were neither constitutively expressed nor induced. It is possible that ADP represents a critical extracellular signal which activates genes such as Egr-1 and NAK1, which encode zinc-finger containing transcriptional regulatory proteins, and could in turn control induction of several other genes [24,25]. It is also of interest that ADP stimulates expression of the gene for TGF-β, which encodes a protein that inhibits growth of BSC-1 cells. Thus, ADP can mimic the action of a growth factor and stimulate

Table 1. Effect of ADP on gene expression in BSC-1 cells

Gene	Effect of ADP
Egr-1, NAK1, c-*fos*, c-*myc*	Expression induced
c-*Ha-ras*, c-*sis* (PDGF-B chain), TGF-β, transferrin receptor, fibronectin, plasminogen activator inhibitor	Constitutive expression enhanced
EGF receptor, β-actin, τ-actin, vimentin, cathepsin L, thymosin $β_{10}$	Constitutive expression unaltered by ADP
IGF-I, IGF-II, prepro EGF, TGF-α, PDGF receptor, PDGF-A chain, v-*src*, v-*fms*, v-*yes*	Genes not expressed or induced

expression of cell-cycle specific genes (Egr-1, NAK1, and proto-oncogenes), as well as the gene for TGF-β, whose expression could serve to limit cell proliferation by releasing a negative autocrine growth factor.

ADP Induces Release of PDGF-like Protein from Renal Epithelial Cells Which Could Act as a Paracrine Growth Factor

PDGF is produced by cells of mesodermal origin, such as fibroblasts and smooth muscle cells, and is released from platelets and macrophages during clotting and wound healing [26]. It is a mitogen for cells of mesenchymal origin, a chemoattractant for smooth muscle cells and monocytes, and a promoter of collagen, proteoglycan, and elastic fiber protein synthesis. PDGF is a dimeric glycoprotein of M_r 30000, comprised of A and/or B chains linked by disulfide bonds. It is most commonly found as a heterodimer (AB), although biologically active homodimers (AA and BB) have been described. The amino acid sequence of the B chain is nearly identical to the putative transforming protein of the simian sarcoma virus which is encoded by the v-*sis* oncogene; the cellular homologue is termed c-*sis*. Three classes of PDGF receptors have been defined, which are each comprised of two subunits located in the plasma membrane. During a study of ADP-induced gene expression, we showed that quiescent BSC-1 cells constitutively release PDGF-like activity [27]. The growth factor in BSC-1 CM was assayed for its mitogenic activity on NRK fibroblasts and its chemoattractant activity on bovine aortic smooth muscle cells. Both activities were found, and were blocked by human anti-PDGF IgG. The presence of a PDGF-like protein was unexpected because expression of PDGF was thought to be confined to cells of mesodermal origin [26]. The gene for the B chain of PDGF (c-*sis*) is constitutively expressed in these cells, whereas no PDGF A chain mRNA could be detected. Thus, the cells appear to synthesize and secrete a PDGF-like protein that is a BB homodimer. ADP increased by 3-fold the amounts of PDGF-B chain mRNA and secreted immunoreactive PDGF-like protein. Importantly, ADP rapidly induced release of PDGF-like activity, so that 1 hour after exposure of cells to the nucleotide, the amount of growth factor was increased by more than 10-fold (Fig. 1, c). TGF-β2 inhibited DNA synthesis in growing cultures and induced marked accumulation of c-*sis* RNA without a corresponding increase in released PDGF-like activity. Interestingly, BSC-1 cells do not exhibit a mitogenic response to authentic PDGF, nor do they express the gene encoding the PDGF receptor. These results imply that if PDGF-like protein is released by renal epithelial cells in vivo, it could

Table 2. Growth factors in renal physiology and pathology: possible roles

Embryonic growth and development of the kidney
Control of glomerular filtration and blood flow
Regulation of ionic and nutrient fluxes in tubular cells
Compensatory renal growth after uninephrectomy
Regeneration after acute renal failure
Proliferative glomerulonephritis
Cell proliferation in renal cystic diseases
Renal adenomas and adenocarcinomas

act by a paracrine mechanism to initiate proliferation of adjacent stromal (fibroblastic) and/or vascular (smooth muscle) cells within the organ.

Conclusions and Speculations

The studies described above indicate that brief alterations in the extracellular environment can signal release of physiological mediators from kidney epithelial cells of the BSC-1 line. The appearance of growth factors following reductions in the extracellular K or Na concentrations, within the physiological range, demonstrates the capacity of kidney cells to transduce changes in their ionic milieu into release of autocrine products. These growth factors could stimulate hypertrophic and/or proliferative cell growth, communicate information to other cells along the nephron, and/or facilitate adaptive changes in cell metabolism in response to the altered extracellular fluid composition. Thus, monkey renal epithelial cells can respond to extracellular ionic perturbations as do T-lymphocytes when presented with foreign antigens: they release polypeptide growth factors.

Infusion of adenine nucleotides can speed recovery of renal function and structure after ischemic, toxic, or obstructive injury [28]. The infused adenine nucleotides could exert their beneficial effects during renal regeneration by raising cell ATP content and thereby restoring the energy charge and metabolic integrity needed to carry out biosynthetic reactions [29,30]. The nucleotides could also stimulate DNA synthesis, and stimulate the release of growth-stimulating molecules which could accelerate the repair of sublethally-injured cells and the proliferation of new ones, thereby augmenting reepithelialization of the nephron. Provision of ADP stimulates release of PDGF-like protein by BSC-1 cells. If released from kidney cells in vivo, this growth factor could initiate proliferation of stromal and vascular cells by a paracrine mechanism at the site of renal injury. It should be noted that although BSC-1 cells are nontransformed they are immortal, so that their capacity to secrete growth factors in response to physiological signals may be one of the characteristics of their phenotype. Hence, caution should be used in extrapolating results obtained in these kidney epithelial cells in culture to renal tissue in vivo.

That autocrine and paracrine factors can be released by kidney cells in response to physiological and pathological signals suggests a previously unsuspected network of cell-to-cell communication within the organ. Growth factors may participate in many renal physiological and pathological processes, as suggested in Table 2. New research initiatives are needed to explore this heretofore unrecognized informational system, which, when defined in detail, could provide new insight into the normal regulation of renal function and the pathogenesis of kidney diseases.

Acknowledgments. Support for studies cited in the text was provided by National Institutes of Health Grants R01 DK39689, R01 DK18413, and R01 DK37227.

References

1. Toback FG (1980) Induction of growth in kidney epithelial cells in culture by Na⁺. Proc Natl Acad Sci USA 77:6654–6656
2. Holley RW, Armour R, Baldwin JH, Brown KD, Yeh Y-C (1977) Density-dependent regulation of growth of BSC-1 cells in cell culture: control of growth by serum factors. Proc Natl Acad Sci USA 74:5046–5050
3. Walsh-Reitz MM, Toback FG (1983) Vasopressin stimulates growth of renal epithelial cells in culture. Am J Physiol 245:C365–C370
4. Holley RW, Armour R, Baldwin JH (1978) Density-dependent regulation of growth of BSC-1 cells in cell culture: growth inhibitors formed by the cells. Proc Natl Acad Sci USA 75:1864–1866
5. Hanks SK, Armour R, Baldwin JH, Maldonado F, Spiess J, Holley RW (1988) Amino acid sequence of the BSC-1 cell growth inhibitor (polyergin) deduced from the nucleotide sequence of the cDNA. Proc Natl Acad Sci USA 85:79–82
6. Walsh-Reitz MM, Toback FG, Holley RW (1984) Cell growth and net Na⁺ flux are inhibited by a protein produced by kidney epithelial cells in culture. Proc Natl Acad Sci USA 81:793–796
7. Gospodarowicz D, Lepine J, Massoglia S, Wood I (1984) Comparison of the ability of basement membranes produced by corneal endothelial and mouse-derived endothelial PF-HR-9 cells to support the proliferation and differentiation of bovine kidney tubule epithelial cells in vitro. J Cell Biol 99:947–961
8. Mendley SR, Toback FG (1989) Autocrine and paracrine regulation of kidney epithelial cell growth. Annu Rev Physiol 51:33–50
9. Atkin BM, Franklin WA, Bell GI, Toback FG (1990) Macula densa cells of mouse kidney do not synthesize epidermal growth factor precursor mRNA. Nephron 54:313–317
10. Risau W, Ekblom P (1986) Production of a heparin-binding angiogenesis factor by the embryonic kidney. J Cell Biol 103:1101–1107
11. Walsh-Reitz MM, Toback FG (1983) Kidney epithelial cell growth is stimulated by lowering extracellular potassium concentration. Am J Physiol 244:C429–C432
12. Walsh-Reitz MM, Aithal HN, Toback FG (1984) Na regulates growth of kidney epithelial cells induced by lowering extracellular K concentration. Am J Physiol 247:C321–C326
13. Walsh-Reitz MM, Gluck SL, Waack S, Toback FG (1986) Lowering extracellular Na⁺ concentration releases autocrine growth factors from renal epithelial cells. Proc Natl Acad Sci USA 83:4764–4768
14. Schrader GA, Prickett CO, Salmon WD (1937) Symptomatology and pathology of potassium and magnesium deficiencies in the rat. J Nutr 14:85–110
15. Mordan LJ, Toback FG (1984) Growth of kidney epithelial cells in culture: evidence for autocrine control. Am J Physiol 246:C351–C354
16. Koch KS, Leffert HL (1979) Increased sodium ion influx is necessary to initiate rat hepatocyte proliferation. Cell 18:153–163
17. Weber MJ, Evans PK, Johnson MA, McNair TF, Nakamura KD, Salter DW (1984) Transport of potassium, amino acids, and glucose in cells transformed by Rous sarcoma virus. Fed Proc 43:107–112

18. Tucker RF, Shipley GD, Moses HL, Holley RW (1984) Growth inhibitor from BSC-1 cells closely related to platelet type β transforming growth factor. Science 226:705–707

19. Fine LG, Holley RW, Nasri H, Badie-Dezfooly B (1985) BSC-1 growth inhibitor transforms a mitogenic stimulus into a hypertrophic stimulus for renal proximal tubular cells: relationship to Na$^+$-H$^+$ antiport activity. Proc Natl Acad Sci USA 82:6163–6166

20. Johnson HA, Vera Roman JM (1966) Compensatory renal enlargement. Hypertrophy versus hyperplasia. Am J Pathol 49:1–13

21. Kartha S, Toback FG (1985) Purine nucleotides stimulate DNA synthesis in kidney epithelial cells in culture. Am J Physiol 249:F967–F972

22. Kartha S, Sukhatme VP, Toback FG (1987) ADP activates protooncogene expression in renal epithelial cells. Am J Physiol 252:F1175–F1179

23. Sukhatme VP, Kartha S, Toback FG, Taub R, Hoover RV, Tsai-Morris C-H (1987) A novel early growth response gene rapidly induced by fibroblast, epithelial cell and lymphocyte mitogens. Oncogene Res 1:343–355

24. Nakai A, Kartha S, Sakurai A, Toback FG, DeGroot LJ (1990) A human early response gene homologous to murine nur77 and rat NGFI-B, and related to the nuclear receptor superfamily. Mol Endocrinol 4:1438–1443

25. Sukhatme VP, Cao X, Chang LC, Tsai-Morris C-H, Stamenkovich D, Ferreira P, Cohen D, Edwards S, Shows T, Curran T, Le Beau M, Adamson E (1988) A zinc finger encoding gene coregulated with c-*fos* during growth, differentiation and after cellular depolarization. Cell 53:37–43

26. Deuel TF, Pierce GF, Hsiu-Jeng Y, Shawver LK, Milner PG, Kimura A (1987) Platelet-derived growth factors/*sis* in normal and neoplastic cell growth. J Cell Physiol [Suppl] 5:95–99

27. Kartha S, Bradham DM, Grotendorst GR, Toback FG (1988) Kidney epithelial cells express the c-*sis* proto-oncogene and secrete PDGF-like protein: evidence for a paracrine mechanism. Am J Physiol 255:F800–F806

28. Siegel NJ, Gaudio KM (1988) Amino acids and adenine nucleotides in acute renal failure. In: Brenner BM, Lazarus JM (eds) Acute renal failure, 2nd edn. Churchill Livingstone, New York, pp 857–873

29. Weinberg JM, Humes HD (1986) Increases of cell ATP produced by exogenous adenine nucleotides in isolated rabbit kidney tubules. Am J Physiol 250:F720–F733

30. Mandel LJ, Takano T, Soltoff SP, Murdaugh S (1988) Mechanisms whereby adenine nucleotides improve rabbit renal proximal function during and after anoxia. J Clin Invest 81:1255–1264

Diabetic Nephropathy, from Hyperfiltration and Microproteinuria to ESRD: Perspective of Intervention

Chair: Carl E. Mogensen (Denmark)
Masaaki Arakawa (Japan)

Renal Hypertrophy and Hyperfunction in Experimental Diabetes

ALLAN FLYVBJERG[1]

SUMMARY. Induction of experimental diabetes causes a rapid increase in renal size, accompanied by parallel increases in total kidney RNA and protein, demonstrable 48–72 h after injection of streptozotocin. Within four days of diabetes the total glomerular volume increases by 30%, while tubules, which constitute the greater part of the kidney, grow relatively more slowly. However, the renal growth is apparent before any measurable kidney hyperfiltration. The diabetic renal hypertrophy is preceded by a rise in renal tissue concentration of insulin-like growth factor I (IGF-I), which reaches a peak 24–48 h after induction of diabetes. Strict insulin treatment abolishes both kidney IGF-I accumulation and kidney growth. Administration of a long-acting somatostatin analogue (Octreotide) has an equally inhibitory effect on kidney IGF-I and growth and this without affecting the metabolic control. This finding supports the hypothesis that IGF-I accumulation is a prerequisite for initial renal growth. Furthermore, the renal IGF-I concentration is linearly dependent on the prevailing blood glucose levels, as has been shown for renal growth. The mechanisms responsible for kidney IGF-I accumulation are discussed, including a presentation of results for kidney IGF-I receptor number and affinity, as well as renal IGF-I mRNA levels during initial diabetic hypertrophy. These results thus indicate that IGF-I may contribute to early kidney growth in experimental diabetes and it is noteworthy that six months treatment with Octreotide in diabetic rats reduces both long-term renal hypertrophy and urinary albumin excretion without altering the metabolic status or renal function, suggesting that growth factors may be involved in long-term renal changes as well.

Introduction

Several lines of evidence indicate that renal hypertrophy and hyperfiltration are characteristic and early manifestations of human and experimental diabetes which

[1]Medical Department M, (Diabetes and Endocrinology), Aarhus Kommunehospital, DK-8000 Aarhus C, Denmark

may contribute to the later development of diabetic nephropathy [1]. The renal hypertrophy and hyperfunction persist even in long-term diabetes and it is obvious that an understanding of the genesis of initial renal growth may throw light upon the changes in the sequence of events that eventually lead to late diabetic nephropathy. Furthermore, it is to be expected that a deeper insight into these early cellular pathogenetic events in the diabetic kidney may allow the design of specific antagonists, possibly useful for therapeutic manipulation in the treatment of diabetic patients.

In this review, the current knowledge of kidney growth, as observed in experimental diabetes in rats, is summarized. Firstly, the phenomenon is described according to the classical biochemical, morphological and functional changes. Secondly, various studies are reviewed concerning possible mechanisms behind renal hypertrophy, with the focus on recent facets of evidence for the significance of growth factors from our laboratories.

Biochemical, Morphological and Functional Changes Associated with Renal Hypertrophy in Experimental Diabetes

Induction of experimental diabetes causes a rapid increase in renal size, regularly occurring 48–72 h after the injection of streptozotocin (i.e., about 36 h after the onset of glucosuria), that is not due to accumulation of water, since the total kidney protein content rises in parallel to wet kidney weight [2]. The initial diabetic kidney growth is due to both cellular hypertrophy and hyperplasia. The first sign of growth is an increase in total RNA as early as 24–36 h after the onset of glucosuria [2] and about the same time the cellular pools of RNA precursors and the incorporation of orotate into uridine triphosphate are increased [3]. Shortly thereafter, an increased protein/DNA ratio is seen, indicating cellular hypertrophy, while total DNA is unchanged for the first four days [2]. By means of thymidine incorporation techniques it has been shown that the hyperplastic response is primarily located in the proximal and distal tubules, with almost no hyperplasia in the glomeruli [4].

The morphological features of the hypertrophying diabetic kidney have been studied both by light and electron microscopy and have revealed a non-uniform growth in its early stages, presenting an anatomical glomerulo-tubular imbalance. Within four days of streptozotocin diabetes the total glomerular volume increases by 30%, while tubules, which constitute the greater part of the kidney, grow relatively more slowly [5]. Whether this glomerulo-tubular imbalance is also reflected functionally is not clear at present. However, after a few weeks of diabetes the ratio between glomerular and tubular size returns to almost non-diabetic levels [5].

Several studies have shown that kidney function is increased in animals with a moderate degree of hyperglycemia, whereas in severely diabetic rats glomerular filtration rate (GFR) is similar to that in non-diabetic controls [6], as it is true for the degree of renal hypertrophy [7]. However, the exact relationship between increased renal mass and hyperfunction is controversial and only recently have studies appeared on this topic. Most studies of early diabetic renal abnormalities have been cross-sectional and confined to a well established diabetic state, whereas studies of the initial dynamic phase, during which kidney growth and hyperfunction evolve, have been largely ignored. It seems evident, however, from a recent paper by Cortes et al. [8] on the temporal relationship of renal growth and kidney function, that renal growth is apparent before any measurable kidney hyperfunction. When GFR was expressed per unit kidney weight, there was a significant decrease 48 h after induction of diabetes, indicating that it is unlikely that initial renal metabolic changes and hypertrophy are initiated by increased function and exaggerated work load [8].

On the Pathogenesis of Early Diabetic Renal Hypertrophy and Hyperfunction: The Possible Role of Growth Factors

The term "growth factor" is used as a generic designation for any substance capable of inducing cellular proliferation and/or differentiation. Certain growth factors extend the known hormone cascade beginning with the hypothalamic releasing factors flowing through the pituitary trophic hormones to endocrine gland hormones released into the circulation, and culminating with peripheral tissue growth. Some growth factors, however, do not mediate their actions as hormones because their effects are directly promoted through local paracrine/autocrine mechanisms.

Several lines of evidence suggest that *growth hormone (GH)* modulates renal function and size. GH-deficient patients tend to have abnormally low renal plasma flow (RPF) and GFR, both of which normalize after GH administration [9]. Hirschberg et al. [10] recently demonstrated that a single intramuscular injection of GH did not affect RPF and GFR acutely, but that it increased both functions within 24 h in parallel with the rise in serum *insulin-like growth factor I (IGF-I)*. These findings indicate that GH increases RPF and GFR indirectly through the growth factor IGF-I.

Hirschberg and Kopple [11] infused IGF-I in fasted, anesthetized rats for 20 min and found rises in RPF and GFR and a fall in renal vascular resistance lasting for 2 h. The effects of IGF-I were blocked by simultaneous infusion of indomethacin, while no blocking effect was found with somatostatin infusion, suggesting a role for eicosanoids in the action of IGF-I on the kidney. These acute studies point at a direct effect of IGF-I on kidney function, independent of primary changes in kidney size. In addition, recent studies have shown that IGF-I administration induces kidney growth in GH (and IGF-I) deficient rats within some days [12]. Thus, it can be concluded that IGF-I administration acutely increases kidney function and after some days also induces renal growth in rodents.

Although the mechanism of renal hypertrophy and hyperfiltration, as seen in the early phase after clinical onset of diabetes and in experimental diabetes is unknown, recent studies have suggested that GH and IGF-I may be involved. The increased plasma GH concentration in patients with type 1 diabetes has been suggested as the cause of the increased RPF and GFR. Christiansen et al. [13] showed that when GH was given subcutaneously twice daily (2 and 4 IU) to well-controlled C-peptide negative diabetic patients for a week to induce plasma levels similar to those found in diabetic patients in average to very poor metabolic control, small but significant increases in RPF and GFR were found. Whether this effect is mediated through IGF-I is, however, unknown.

In contrast to the well-established paradox that hyperglycemia (poor metabolic control) does not suppress, but augments GH secretion in diabetic patients, recent studies have shown that GH secretion in the streptozotocin diabetic rat is inhibited rather than

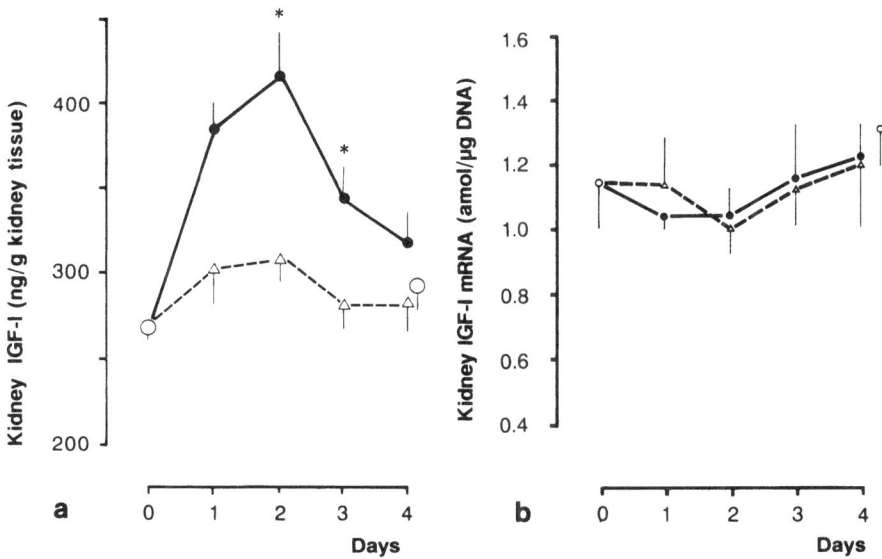

Fig. 1. Changes in **a** kidney insulin-like growth factor I (*IGF-I*) and **b** kidney IGF-I messenger RNA (*IGF-I mRNA*) in control (○), untreated diabetic (●——●), and insulin-treated diabetic rats (△---△) during the four days after induction of streptozotocin (*STZ*) diabetes. On day 0 STZ was injected i.v.; insulin treatment with a very long-acting, heat treated Ultralente Insulin was initiated after 18 h when all animals had blood glucose levels above 15 mmol/l. Insulin was given in an initial dose of 4–6 U, followed by 1–2 U daily thereafter depending on blood glucose values. Kidney IGF-I was measured by radioimmunoassay after previous extraction of the tissue in 1 mol/l acetic acid, while IGF-I mRNA was measured by solution-hybridization. *P < 0.05 between untreated and insulin-treated diabetic animals. Values are mean ± SEM, $n=6$ for kidney IGF-I values and $n=5$ for kidney IGF-I mRNA. (Reproduced from [17] with permission)

paradoxically stimulated [14]. This observation would, at first glance, along with the observation that short-term GH-treatment of diabetic rats has no effect on the degree of renal growth [15], preclude a causal role for GH in diabetic renal hypertrophy. Very recently, however, we found that diabetic dwarf rats with an isolated GH-deficiency (i.e. with normal secretion of the other pituitary hormones) underwent a slower and lesser degree of initial renal hypertrophy when compared to diabetic controls with intact pituitary. Thus, these findings seem to indicate that the *lack* of GH or some GH-dependent factors (e.g., IGF-I or IGF-I binding proteins) attenuates diabetic renal growth in rats (A. Flyvbjerg et al., unpublished results, 1990).

In line with this observation it is interesting that the initial renal hypertrophy is preceded by a rise in extractable renal tissue concentration of IGF-I, which reaches a peak 24–48 h after the induction of diabetes (Fig. 1a) and returns to basal levels after about 4 days, and thus precedes the first demonstrable increase in kidney RNA, protein [16,17], function [8], and size (Fig. 2). The kidney IGF-I accumulation pattern parallels that of labelled thymidine incorporation into renal tubules [4], being in good accordance with a mitogenic effect of IGF-I and thus precedes the pronounced

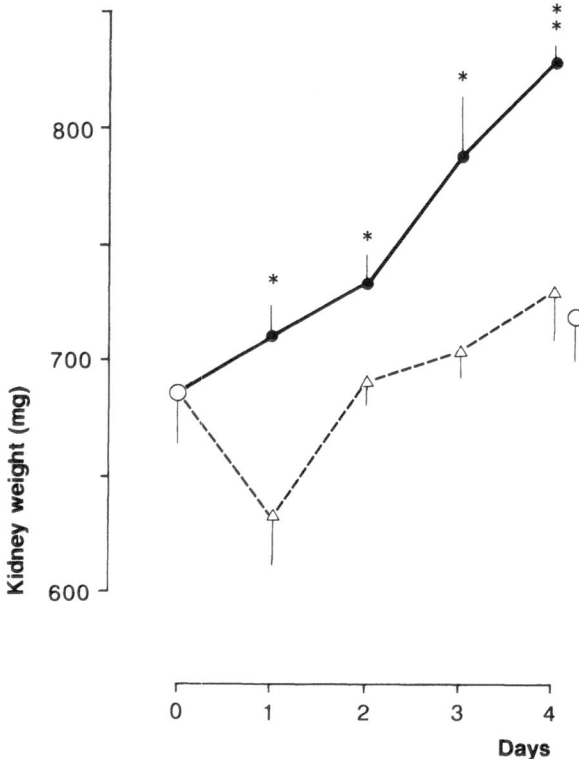

Fig. 2. Changes in kidney weight in streptozotocin-diabetic rats, untreated (●——●) and insulin-treated (△---△), over four days and in non-diabetic control rats on day 0 and 4 (0). Animals were treated as described in legend to Fig. 1. *P < 0.05, **P < 0.01 between untreated and insulin-treated diabetic animals. Values are given as mean ± SEM and every point represents 6 different animals. (Reproduced from [17] with permission)

hypertrophy of glomeruli [5]. Strict insulin treatment abolishes the increase in both kidney IGF-I and renal hypertrophy (Figs. 1a & 2), supporting the hypothesis of the involvement of this putative causal growth factor in renal hypertrophy and, furthermore, demonstrating that no toxic effect of streptozotocin is involved in the observed changes. Administration of a long-acting somatostatin analogue (Octreotide) has an equally inhibitory effect on kidney IGF-I accumulation and growth, and this without affecting the blood glucose levels, supporting the idea that renal IGF-I accumulation is a prerequisite for initial diabetic kidney growth [18]. It has previously been shown that diabetic kidney hypertrophy was linearly dependent on blood glucose levels one week after induction of diabetes [7]. Very recently it was shown that the degree of kidney IGF-I accumulation 48 h after injection with streptozotocin was directly proportional to the prevailing blood glucose in rats with graded severities of diabetes [19]. This adds weight to the hypothesis that renal IGF-I accumulation is promoted by the diabetic state in stimulating renal growth. The changes seen in kidney IGF-I and diabetic kidney growth have great similarities to those occurring in the remaining kidney after unilateral nephrectomy [16] and it is interesting therefore that induction of diabetes and unilateral nephrectomy combined in the same animal induce additive increase in both kidney IGF-I accumulation and renal enlargement [20].

It is still to be clarified how the increased IGF-I content arrives in the kidney, and thus whether it is due to increased uptake of circulating IGF-I or to increased local production. Traditionally, the liver has been considered to be the main site of IGF-I synthesis, mainly under the control of GH. However, the increase in kidney IGF-I after induction of moderate diabetes or after unilateral nephrectomy is accompanied by little or no change in hepatic or circulating levels of IGF-I [16–18]. Recent reports have shown the existence of distinct receptors for IGF-I in rat kidneys and we have recently shown that IGF-I receptor numbers and affinity in whole kidney homogenates, obtained from hypertrophying diabetic kidneys, are unchanged, suggesting that the increased kidney IGF-I concentration is not likely to be due to changes at receptor level [21]. Alternatively, sequestration of IGF-I within tubules and collecting ducts, or decreased breakdown of the peptide could be responsible for the IGF-I accumulation in the diabetic kidney.

By means of a sensitive solution-hybridization assay for the renal content of IGF-I messenger RNA (IGF-I mRNA), a marker of the cellular gene expression for IGF-I, changes in local kidney production of IGF-I were measured during the initial renal growth in diabetes (Fig. 1b). We found unaltered levels of IGF-I mRNA during the first four days after induction of diabetes, despite accumulation of IGF-I in the kidney (Fig. 1a); this thus seems to indicate that local production at transcriptional level is unchanged [17]. However, IGF-I accumulation in the diabetic kidney due to enhanced translatory regulation cannot be excluded, as has been suggested for IGF-I accumulation in unilateral nephrectomy [22].

The apparent dependence of diabetic renal hypertrophy on kidney IGF-I accumulation has been confirmed in a recent study [23], showing that renal hypertrophy in pre-pubertal rats is much slower than in post-pubertal, and that pre-pubertal rats have no significant increase in kidney IGF-I. This study was inspired by the fact that diabetic angiopathy takes a more benign course in pre-pubertal than in post-pubertal children. The reduced degree of renal hypertrophy in pre-pubertal animals seems to be independent of the presence of androgens, since castration does not attenuate the renotrophic activity of alloxan diabetes in mice [24].

Several observations on the streptozotocin rat model have suggested that increased intrarenal production of the vasodilating prostaglandins PGE_2 and PGI_2 may be involved in the early diabetic renal growth and hyperfiltration. Craven et al. [25] found that when indomethacin administration was begun concomitantly with induction of diabetes in rats, diabetic renal hypertrophy, hyperfiltration, and increased urinary prostaglandin excretion were all reduced, without affecting the metabolic state, when compared to untreated diabetic controls. By contrast, indomethacin treatment for three days in rats with diabetes which had lasted for four weeks, did not influence kidney size or function, indicating a possible role for prostaglandins in the very early renal changes in diabetic rats.

It may be hypothesized that blood glucose-dependent renal IGF-I accumulation, either directly or through eicosanoids, increases initial kidney growth and renal function. This is supported by the finding that indomethacin blocks both initial renal hypertrophy in experimental diabetes [25] and the IGF-I induced enhancement of renal function [11]. In addition, IGF-I is found to stimulate the synthesis of 6-keto PEG$_{1a}$ and PEG$_2$ in cultured rat liver cells [26].

Altogether our studies indicate that IGF-I may contribute to early kidney growth in experimental diabetes, although the precise cellular mechanisms are a matter of debate. The suggested hypothesis deals with the possible contribution of IGF-I, at a very early stage, to a sequence of events that may lead to late diabetic nephropathy. A considerable amount of further information is of course required to elucidate whether or not IGF-I and other growth factors are also directly involved in the further development of diabetic renal disease. It is, however, intriguing that six months treatment with a long-acting somatostatin analogue (Octreotide) had effects on long-term kidney changes in streptozotocin diabetic rats, by reducing both long-term renal hypertrophy and urinary albumin excretion [27]. These effects were seen without any drug effects on metabolic control (blood glucose, Hgb$_{Alc}$, 24h glucose output) or renal function in diabetic animals; thus indicating that chronic administration of a "growth factor inhibitor" reduces certain functional abnormalities regarded to be prognostic of late diabetic kidney disease.

Acknowledgments. This manuscript reflects the contribution of co-workers in our own laboratories (Jan Frystyk, Klavs W. Hansen, Sally M. Marshall, Kirsten Nyborg, Ida B. Sillesen, Ole Thorlacius-Ussing, Hans Ørskov and Ruth Østerby) and our colleagues at Linköping University, Sweden (Hans J. Arnqvist and Karin E. Bornfeldt). The studies were supported by grants from the Danish Diabetes Association.

References

1. Mogensen CE, Christensen CK (1984) Predicting diabetic nephropathy in insulin-dependent patients. N Engl J Med 311:89–93
2. Seyer-Hansen K (1983) Renal hypertrophy in experimental diabetes. Kidney Int 23:643–646
3. Cortes P, Lewin NW, Dumler F, Rubenstein AH, Verghese CP, Venkatachalam KK (1980) Uridine triphosphate and RNA synthesis during diabetes-induced kidney growth. Am J Physiol 238:E349–E357
4. Rasch R, Rytter-Nørgaard JO (1983) Renal enlargement: Comparative autoradiographic studies of ^{3}H-thymidine uptake in diabetic and uninephrectomized rats. Diabetologia 25:280–287
5. Seyer-Hansen K, Hansen J, Gundersen HJG (1980) Renal hypertrophy in experimental diabetes. A morphometric study. Diabetologia 18:501–505
6. Hostetter TH, Troy JL, Brenner BM (1981) Glomerular hemodynamics in experimental diabetes. Kidney Int 19:410–415
7. Seyer-Hansen K (1977) Renal hypertrophy in experimental diabetes: Relation to severity of diabetes. Diabetologia 13:141–143
8. Cortes P, Dumler F, Goldman J, Levin NW (1987) Relationship between renal function and metabolic alterations in early streptozocin-induced diabetes in rats. Diabetes 36:80–87
9. Falkheden T, Wickbom I (1965) Renal function and kidney size following hypophysectomy in man. Acta Endocrinol (Copenh) 48:348–354
10. Hirschberg R, Rabb H, Bergamo R, Kopple JD (1989) The delayed effect of growth hormone on renal function in humans. Kidney Int 35:865–870
11. Hirschberg R, Kopple JD (1989) Evidence that insulin-like growth factor I increases renal plasma flow and glomerular filtration rate in fasted rats. J Clin Invest 83:326–330

12. Guler HP, Zapf J, Scheiwiller E, Froesch ER (1988) Recombinant human insulin-like growth factor I stimulates growth and has distinct effects on organ size in hypophysectomized rats. Proc Natl Acad Sci USA 85:4889–4893

13. Christiansen JS, Gammelgaard J, Frandsen M, Ørskov H, Parving HH (1982) Kidney function and size in insulin dependent diabetics before and during growth hormone administration for one week. Diabetologia 22:333–337

14. Robinson ICAF, Clark RG, Carlsson LMS (1987) Insulin, IGF-I and growth in diabetic rats (letter). Nature 326:549

15. Seyer-Hansen K, Gundersen HJG, Østerby R (1981) Acute renal hypertrophy in experimental diabetes: Lack of effect of growth hormone administration. Diabetologia 21:373–375

16. Flyvbjerg A, Thorlacius-Ussing O, Naeraa R, Ingerslev J, Ørskov H (1988) Kidney tissue somatomedin C and initial renal growth in diabetic and uninephrectomized rats. Diabetologia 31:310–314

17. Flyvbjerg A, Bornfeldt KE, Marshall SM, Arnqvist HJ, Ørskov H (1990) Kidney IGF-I mRNA in initial renal hypertrophy in experimental diabetes in rats. Diabetologia 33:334–338

18. Flyvbjerg A, Frystyk J, Thorlacius-Ussing O, Ørskov H (1989) Somatostatin analogue administration prevents increase in kidney somatomedin C and initial renal growth in diabetic and uninephrectomized rats. Diabetologia 32:261–265

19. Flyvbjerg A, Ørskov H (1990) Kidney tissue insulin-like growth factor I and initial renal growth in diabetic rats: Relation to severity of diabetes. Acta Endocrinol (Copenh) 122:374–378

20. Flyvbjerg A, Frystyk J, Marshall SM (1990) Additive increase in kidney insulin-like growth factor I and initial renal enlargement in uninephrectomized-diabetic rats. Horm Metab Res 22:516–520

21. Marshall SM, Korsgaard L, Flyvbjerg A, Frystyk J, Ørskov H (1990) Renal insulin-like growth factor I binding in experimental diabetes (abstract). Diabetologia 33:A148

22. Lajara R, Rotwein P, Bortz JD, Hansen VA, Sadow JL, Betts CR, Rogers SA, Hammerman MR (1989) Dual regulation of insulin-like growth factor I expression during renal hypertrophy. Am J Physiol 257:F252–F261

23. Bach LA, Jerums G (1990) Effect of puberty on initial kidney growth and rise in kidney IGF-I in diabetic rats. Diabetes 39:557–562

24. Broulik PD, Schreiber V (1982) Effect of alloxan diabetes on kidney growth in intact and castrated mice. Acta Endocrinol (Copenh) 99:109–111

25. Craven PA, Caines MA, DeRubertis FR (1987) Sequential alterations in glomerular prostaglandin and thromboxane synthesis in diabetic rats: Relationship to the hyperfiltration of early diabetes. Metabolism 36:95–103

26. Levine L, Xiao D, Fujiki D (1986) Comparisons of polytoxin or 12-O-tetradecanoylphorbol-13-acetate and recombinant human insulin-like growth factor I or insulin synergistically stimulates prostaglandin production in cultured rat liver cells and squirrel monkey aorta smooth muscle cells. Prostaglandins 31:669–681

27. Flyvbjerg A, Marshall SM, Frystyk J, Hansen KW, Østerby R, Harris AG, Ørskov H (1990) Six months Sandostatin treatment in diabetic rats: Effects on kidney growth and urinary albumin excretion (abstract). Diabetologia 33:A65

Renal Pathology in Insulin Dependent (IDDM) and Noninsulin Dependent Diabetes Mellitus (NIDDM)

Pascale H. Lane, S. Michael Mauer[1], and Michael W. Steffes[2]

Summary. Much has been learned in the last decade regarding the pathology of the kidney in insulin-dependent diabetes mellitus (IDDM) and noninsulin-dependent diabetes mellitus (NIDDM). The major pathologic changes of diabetes include thickening of all renal extracellular basement membranes and mesangial matrix, and mesangial cell expansion. Although much less is known regarding renal pathology in NIDDM compared to IDDM, most proteinuric patients with NIDDM have typical diabetic nephropathy while approximately 25% have another form of renal disease. Two renal lesions appear critical in diabetic nephropathy. Mesangial expansion out of proportion to the size of the glomerulus is closely and inversely related to measures of peripheral capillary wall filtration surface; this expansion is also closely related to clinical features of proteinuria, hypertension, and declining glomerular filtration rate (GFR). Arteriolar hyalinosis is related to global glomerulosclerosis and both are correlated with the clinical features of nephropathy. Renal extracellular basement membrane and matrix expansion appears to be secondary to increased production or decreased turnover, or both, of normal structural constituents of the kidney. Microalbuminuria in the "predictive range" is frequently accompanied by rising blood pressure and/or falling GFR and is associated with well-established structural lesions. Thus, microalbuminuria is a marker of quite advanced diabetic nephropathology. Further natural history studies of variables which might influence the rate of development of the earlier lesions of diabetic nephropathy are critical to our understanding of this important disorder.

Introduction

Diabetic nephropathy represents the single most important cause of renal failure in adults in the Western world, causing 25% of all new cases of uremia [1]. The peak

[1]Department of Pediatrics and [2]Department of Laboratory Medicine and Pathology, University of Minnesota, Minneapolis, MN 55455, USA

incidence for the development of clinical renal disease occurs after about 16 years of diabetes but does not reach zero even after 40 years of insulin-dependent diabetes mellitus (IDDM) [2]. Overall, approximately 35%–45% of patients with longstanding IDDM will ultimately develop nephropathy, defined as dipstick-positive proteinuria, hypertension, and falling GFR [2]. It has been recently shown that it is the IDDM patients with nephropathy who manifest virtually all of the increased mortality associated with type I diabetes [2], while those who escape nephropathy have a mortality rate which is little different from that of the background population [2]. Although it is commonly thought that nephropathy is more common in IDDM patients [3] more recent studies of diabetic Pima Indians suggest that the cumulative risk of nephropathy in these NIDDM patients is at least as high as in IDDM patients [4]. Perhaps these younger NIDDM Pima patients live long enough to manifest diabetic nephropathy while older age NIDDM patients more frequently die of other causes before nephropathy becomes clinically apparent.

General Pathological Findings in Diabetic Nephropathy

The glomerulus seems to be normal at the onset of IDDM, as shown by the early pioneering work of Østerby [5] and confirmed by our studies of identical twins discordant for IDDM [6]. In the latter studies the nondiabetic twins, presumably identical to their IDDM twins but for the presence of diabetes, all had normal glomerular structure. This indicated that the diabetic state is a necessary prerequisite for diabetic glomerulopathy to be expressed. Osterby demonstrated that glomerular basement membrane (GBM) thickening can be detected two years after onset of IDDM; mesangial expansion can be quantitated after 5 years of diabetes [5]. Ultimately, in those developing serious renal disease, the dominant pathologic process becomes that of diffuse mesangial expansion [7–9]. The Kimmelstiel-Wilson nodular lesion is the most marked pathologic expression of diabetic mesangial expansion. While specific for diabetes, only a minority of patients progressing to overt diabetic nephropathy have nodular glomerulosclerosis [10].

Other lesions commonly seen in the kidney of patients with type I diabetes include hyaline degenerative changes in the afferent and efferent glomerular arterioles, and exudative hyaline lesions (fibrin cap) in the subendothelial space and under the parietal layer of the epithelium along Bowman's capsule (capsular drop) [10]. The hyaline lesions in the glomerular arterioles may be early changes in the kidney in IDDM and may be important in promoting glomerular scarring (R.D. Harris et al., unpublished data). Capillary loops may develop microaneurysms. These microaneurysms may be the forerunners of Kimmelstiel-Wilson nodules [11]. Epithelial and endothelial cell structure are generally well preserved until late in the course of nephropathy [12,13]. Interstitial fibrosis [14] and tubular changes may also be seen as the disease progresses [6,15,16].

Much less work has been done on the description of the pathology of the kidney in NIDDM compared to work done in IDDM. Schmitz et al. have performed light microscopy studies indicating that mesangial expansion occurs in NIDDM patients [17]. However, detailed electron microscopic morphometric studies in these patients are lacking. It is also important to note that more than 25% of NIDDM patients with proteinuria may have a renal disease other than diabetic nephropathy [18]; while in our experience this occurs in fewer than 5% of proteinuric IDDM patients (unpublished data). Thus, it is not safe to assume that NIDDM patients with clinical renal disease have this on the basis of diabetic nephropathology. Studies indicate that the direct relationships between glycemic control and the risk of diabetic nephropathy known to be present in IDDM [19] hold for NIDDM (FC Goetz, unpublished data). Thus, the severity of the lesions of diabetic nephropathy, assessed by light microscopy studies from kidneys obtained at autopsy in NIDDM patients, were closely predicted by the level of the blood sugar at the time of diagnosis, as well as by the summed glucose values obtained during glucose tolerance testing, in these NIDDM patients (GC Goetz, unpublished data).

Accurate stereologic techniques have allowed quantitation of the structural changes of diabetic nephropathy [20,21]. This has facilitated correlation of these changes with renal function.

Structural-Functional Relationships in Diabetic Nephropathy

Glomerular Basement Membrane

Measurements of GBM width, using the orthogonal intercept method [20], demonstrate thickening in almost all long-standing IDDM patients [5,7]. This thickening, measurable after two years of diabetes [5,22], is generally uniform both within and between glomeruli. The nature of this thickening is not completely understood, but it primarily involves the lamina densa. Immunofluorescent studies by Falk et al. [23] have shown increased staining for normal GBM and tubular basement membrane (TBM), and mesangial matrix constituents, suggesting that increased production or decreased turnover, or both, result in the accumulation of renal extracellular matrix materials. Also, there is increased localization of plasma proteins in GBM as well as in other renal extracellular membranes in diabetes, including the tubular basement membrane (TBM) and Bowman's capsule; this is detectable by immunofluorescence microscopy [24,25]. There is evidence suggesting that this increased localization is related to the charge of the circulating molecules, since anionic proteins bind preferentially [26]. However, this binding is relatively irreversible, requiring harsh treatment with collagenase or acids to release the bound protein, so charge alone is unlikely to explain the phenomenon [25].

The width of the GBM correlates poorly with mesangial volume fraction and with the functional parameters of glomerular filtration rate (GFR) and hypertension [7]. However, there is a weak correlation of GBM width with urinary albumin excretion (UAE). Increased GBM width is a sensitive marker of the diabetic state [5,10,22]. In seven pairs of identical twins discordant for IDDM, only diabetic twins showed GMB thickening, demonstrating that the diabetic state is a prerequisite for expression of this abnormality [6]. The width of the TBM is also increased in IDDM patients [6]. This latter fact suggests that pressure and flows in the glomerular capillaries, normally much higher than those present in other capillaries, are not prerequisites for the development of renal extracellular basement membrane thickening in IDDM.

Mesangium

Shortly after the onset of IDDM the fraction of the glomerular tuft occupied by mesangium is normal, with roughly equal proportions of cells and matrix. After two to three years, matrix begins to accumulate [13,27], and mesangial expansion, out of proportion to any increase in glomerular volume (increased mesangial volume fraction or VvMes), may become quite marked after many years of diabetes [7,28]. Approximately two-thirds of this mesangial expansion is due to matrix accumulation, and the mesangium contains increased amounts of the usual matrix antigens [23], including smooth muscle antigens [29]. One-third of this mesangial expansion is due to cellular expansion. It is unclear if mesangial cell number is increased in the later stages of diabetic nephropathy, although the total number of cell nuclei per glomerulus is increased [28].

Mesangial expansion demonstrates important correlations with renal function in diabetic nephropathy [7]. There is a strong inverse correlation between mesangial volume fraction and GFR. This probably results from the expanding mesangium compromising the structure of contiguous glomerular capillaries. Thus, fractional mesangial volume is precisely and inversely related to the peripheral capillary filtration surface density [7]. This suggests that as the relative volume of the glomerulus occupied by mesangium increases, the relative peripheral capillary wall available for filtration decreases. Stronger support of this concept comes from the work of Ellis et al. [30], which is confirmed by the work of Østerby et al. [31], who showed that filtration surface per glomerulus is directly related to GFR.

Virtually all patients with marked mesangial expansion (specifically, a mesangial volume fraction >37%) have had more than 400 mg of albumin in their urine per 24 hours; all patients in this earlier study had hypertension [7]. Thus, severe mesangial expansion is closely associated with all of the manifestations of overt nephropathy: decreased GFR, proteinuria, and hypertension. More recent studies (unpublished data) indicate that about 20% of patients with overt nephropathy and marked mesangial expansion do not have hypertension. Further, hypertension can occur in IDDM patients with lesser degrees of mesangial expansion. When hypertension is present in a patient with IDDM, this is almost always associated with increased UAE and well-established glomerular lesions. Thus, in our experience, hypertension, without other features of overt diabetic nephropathy, is distinctly uncommon in IDDM patients (unpublished data).

It is important to discuss the relationships of microalbuminuria to the structural lesions of diabetic nephropathy. Using mesangial expansion as the key structural parameter [8], it was found that patients with longstanding IDDM and entirely normal renal function, as indicated by normal UAE, GFR, and blood pressure, have mesangial volume fractions ranging from normal to levels bordering on those regularly associated with overt nephropathy [32]. Patients with microalbuminuria, normal GFR, and normal blood pressure (UAE usually <45 mg/24 hours or 30 µg/minute) have mesangial volume fractions completely overlapping with those whose renal function is entirely normal [32]. Those IDDM patients with microalbuminuria, hypertension, and/or decreased GFR (UAE usually >45 mg/24 hours) have more advanced mesangial expansion [32]. Thus, normal UAE does not preclude the presence of important lesions, while microalbuminuria does not necessarily predict structural abnormalities. However, if other manifestations of overt nephropathy are present, then micro-

albuminuria indicates more advanced structural injury. In other words, microalbuminuria in the range regularly "predictive" of the later development of proteinuria is,
in fact, a marker of well-established diabetic glomerulopathy.

Glomerular Arterioles

Hyaline changes, which can involve both the afferent and efferent glomerular arterioles, range in severity from the presence of small amounts of (PAS) positive translu-
cent material under the elastic membrane of the arterioles to virtually complete
replacement of the smooth muscle of the vessels by this material. Hyaline in these
vessel walls, along the parietal layer of Bowman's capsule (capsular drop), and in the
glomerular subendothelial space (fibrin cap) all appears to contain the same
materials; immunoglobulins, fibrinogen, and complement, as well as other plasma
proteins [37]. The pathogenesis of these lesions is unknown. We have recently found
that the more advanced glomerular arteriolar lesions, defined as complete replacement of smooth muscle cells by hyaline, are directly correlated with greater numbers
of globally sclerotic glomeruli [11]. This suggests that glomerular sclerosis in diabetic nephropathy may derive, in part, from vascular pathology. An additional
mechanism of glomerular sclerosis in diabetes may be extreme mesangial expansion
with consequent capillary closure [28].

Epithelial Cells

The epithelial cells in diabetic patients contain large numbers of mitochondria and
ribosomes, extensive endoplasmic reticula and prominent Golgi apparatuses, these
cells retain normal structure until overt proteinuria develops [12,13]. These findings
could reflect an increased GBM synthetic activity, biochemical evidence for which
has been presented [34]. Only in the later stages of diabetic nephropathy has measurable foot process expansion been observed [12], and we have also noted a parallel
loss in filtration slit length density [35]. These changes occur in association with
increased levels of UAE and suggest that these epithelial cell changes may be the consequence of the breakdown of the glomerular permselectivity barrier which develops
as the disease enters its terminal stages consequent to decreased available filtration
surface.

Endothelial Cells

Endothelial cell structure also appears to be well preserved in diabetic nephropathy
in man, although in advanced stages with capillary closure and massive mesangial
expansion, atrophic appearances have been described [36]. Scanning electron microscopy in alloxan diabetic rats has revealed subtle alterations in endothelial cell fenes-
trae [37]. To our knowledge, similar studies have not been reported in diabetic man.

Interstitium

Interstitial fibrosis is a concomitant of diabetic nephropathy. Bader et al. [14] have
shown that there is an inverse relationship between morphometric measures of the
severity of interstitial fibrosis and GFR. In our studies of structural-functional

relationships [7] we found that mesangial expansion and expansion of the inter-stitium were covariables predicting GFR, but that the correlation was stronger with measures of the mesangium; interstitial measures did not improve the correlation of mesangium with GFR. Interstitial fibrosis correlated with mesangial expansion. Thus, in our view, interstitial expansion correlates with glomerular function through correlations with mesangial changes, but the mesangial changes are more likely to be the major cause of the glomerular dysfunction. However, the interstitial fibrosis which develops in relation to nephron death may be important in contributing to the pathologic process which characterize the end stage kidney.

Tubules

The Armanni-Ebstein lesion represents the accumulation of PAS positive glycogen in the epithelial cells of the loop of Henle, and in the distal convoluted tubule and collecting duct; this lesion occurs as a concomitant of poor glycemic control [38]. The thick ascending limb of the loop of Henle shows the most pronounced lesions. This is the location of the macula densa, which demonstrates other structural abnormalities as well [38]. Spaces between the macula densa cells show altered size and geometry; the basal contact area between these cells and the juxtaglomerular apparatus is increased by 38% in diabetic animals compared to controls. This area of the nephron is important in regulating glomerular blood flow and GFR via tubuloglomerular feedback. Thus, these abnormalities may play a role in hyperfiltration and other alterations of renal function [38].

A layered thickening and splitting of the tubular basement membrane and Bowman's capsule has been described [15,16]. As noted above, we have found that increases in tubular basement membrane width paralleled those observed in GBM and mesangium [6].

Glomerular Structure and Loss of Renal Function

It is our hypothesis that decreasing filtration surface is "viewed" by the kidney as would be a decrease in renal mass. This pathologic change, we suggest, stimulates adaptive hemodynamic responses [39] and, perhaps, other forces [40,41], resulting in disruption of permselectivity and production of proteinuria and the development of hypertension. This hypothesis argues that once the lesions of diabetes produce clinically detectable renal dysfunction, then the forces propelling the kidney toward its ultimate destruction become largely independent of the diabetic state and become similar to those of advanced renal injury in general.

Filtration surface is ultimately determined by the filtration area per glomerulus and by the number of glomeruli. Filtration area per glomerulus is inversely proportional to the fractional mesangial volume [7,30]. As the mesangium expands and occupies a greater proportion of the glomerular tuft, the capillary volume must decrease unless accompanied by expansion of the entire glomerular volume. If accumulation of mesangial material exceeds the ability of the glomerulus to hypertrophy, the capillary loops will ultimately close, resulting in a completely obliterated glomerulus. Thus, mesangial expansion may decrease functioning filtration surface, both by decreasing the surface per glomerulus and by decreasing the number of functioning glomeruli.

Glomerular numbers may be decreased by other mechanisms as well. Horlych et al. [42] demonstrated a nonrandom distribution of sclerotic glomeruli in a plane perpendicular to the surface of the kidney and, therefore, along the course of the interlobular arteries. As already mentioned, advanced glomerular arteriolar lesions are correlated with global glomerular sclerosis. Thus, vascular lesions may lead to a loss of functioning glomeruli.

Overt diabetic nephropathy progresses inexorably to uremia. Evidence that this stage is associated with advanced structural lesions is neither surprising nor helpful. No functional tests prior to this stage accurately indicate the severity of the underlying renal pathology. In patients with normal albumin excretion or microalbuminuria without hypertension or reduced GFR, we found no correlations between GBM thickness, mesangial volume fraction, or peripheral capillary filtration surface density and levels of UAE [32]. In fact, it is our view that microalbuminuria gains in strength as a "predictor" or serious diabetic renal disease primarily when associated with hypertension and/or with early reduction in GFR, that is, as one manifestation of already established, albeit subtle, clinical diabetic nephropathy [6,32].

Conclusions

There have been substantial advances in our understanding of diabetic nephropathy through the study of renal structure and function in diabetic patients. It is becoming clearer that the important processes driving the kidney toward its functional demise are matrix accumulation, which occurs in the mesangium, in other renal extracellular membranes, and in the interstitium, and hyaline changes, which occur in the glomerular arterioles. It is also clear that functional studies are not indicative of underlying renal pathology, except relatively late in the pathologic evolution when glomerular injury is already quite far advanced. Only carefully designed, quantitative, prospective studies of renal pathology, beginning early in the course of type I diabetes, can further clarify the relationship of structure and function with a variety of risk factors in the nephropathy of IDDM and NIDDM patients.

Acknowledgments. Supported in part by NIH grants AM13083 and AM20742 and by the Juvenile Diabetes Foundation International.

References

1. Rao TKS, Hirsh S, Avram MM, et al. (1980) Prevalence of diabetic nephropathy in Brooklyn. In: Friedman EA, L'Esperance FA Jr (eds) Diabetic renal-retinal syndrome. Grune and Strattan, New York, pp 205–207
2. Christiansen JS, Anderson AR, Koch Anderson J, et al. (1985) The natural history of diabetic nephropathy. Diabetic Nephro 4:104–106
3. Herman WT, Teutsch SM (1986) Renal disorders associated with diabetes mellitus. In: Friedman EA, L'Esperance FA Jr (eds) Diabetic renal-retinal syndrome. Grune and Stratton, New York, pp 9–52

4. Knowler WC, Kungelman CL (1988) Population comparisons of the frequency of diabetic nephropathy. In: Mogensen CE (ed) The kidney and hypertension in diabetes mellitus. Martinus Nijhoff, Boston, pp 25–32

5. Østerby R (1975) Early phases in the development of diabetic glomerulosclerosis. Acta Med Scand 574(Suppl 1):1–80

6. Steffes MW, Sutherland DER, Goetz FC, Rich SS, Mauer SM (1985) Studies of kidney and muscle biopsy specimens from identical twins discordant for type I diabetes mellitus. N Engl J Med 312:1282–1287

7. Mauer SM, Steffes MW, Ellis EN, Sutherland DER, Brown DM, Goetz FC (1984) Structural-functional relationships in diabetic nephropathy. J Clin Invest 74:1143–1155

8. Steffes MW, Østerby R, Chavers B, Mauer SM (1989) Mesangial expansion as a central mechanism for loss of kidney function in diabetic patients. Diabetes 38:1077–1081

9. Gellmann DD, Pirani CL, Soothill JF, et al. (1959) Structure and function in diabetic nephropathy. The importance of diffuse glomerulosclerosis. Diabetes 8:251–256

10. Mauer SM, Steffes MW, Brown DM (1981) The kidney in diabetes. Am J Med 70:603–612

11. Saito Y, Kida H, Takeda S, et al. (1988) Mesangiolysis in diabetic glomeruli: Its role in the formation of nodular lesions. Kidney Int 34:389–396

12. Farquhar MG, Hopper J, Moon HD (1959) Diabetic glomerulosclerosis: Electron and light microscopic studies. Am J Pathol 35:721–753

13. Østerby R (1972) The number of glomerular cells and substructures in early juvenile diabetes. Acta Pathol Microbiol Immunol Scand [A] 80:785–800

14. Bader R, Bader H, Grund KE, et al. (1980) Structure and function of the kidney in diabetic glomerulosclerosis: Correlations between morphologic and functional parameters. Pathol Res Pract 167:204–216

15. Sabour MS, MacDonald MK, Robson JS (1962) An electron microscopic study of the human kidney in young diabetic patients with normal renal function. Diabetes 11:291–295

16. Churg J, Dachs S (1966) Diabetic renal disease: Arteriosclerosis and glomerulosclerosis. Pathol Annu 1:148–171

17. Schmitz A, Gundersen HJG, Østerby R (1988) Glomerular morphology by light microscopy in non-insulin dependent diabetes—lack of glomerular hypertrophy. Diabetes 37:38–43

18. Parving H-H, Gall M-A, Skott P, Jorgensen HE, Jorgensen F, Larsen S (1990) Prevalence and causes of albuminuria in non-insulin dependent diabetic (NIDDM) patients. Kidney Int 37:243A

19. Krolewski AS, Warram JH, Christlieb AR, Busick EJ, Kahn CR (1985) The changing natural history of diabetic nephropathy. Am J Med 78:785–794

20. Jensen EB, Gundersen HJG, Østerby R (1979) Determination of membrane thickness distribution from orthogonal intercepts. J Microsc 115:19–33

21. Weiber ER (1979) Stereological methods: Practical methods for biological morphometry. Academic, London

22. Østerby R (1972) Morphometric studies of the peripheral glomerular basement membrane in early juvenile diabetes. II. Development of initial basement membrane thickening. Diabetologia 8:84–92

23. Falk RJ, Scheinman JI, Mauer SM, Michael AF (1983) Polyantigenic expansion of basement membrane constituents in diabetic nephropathy. Diabetes 32:34–39

24. Miller K, Michael AF (1976) Immunopathology of renal extracellular membranes in diabetes mellitus. Specificity of tubular basement membrane immunofluorescence. Diabetes 25:701–708

25. Michael AF, Brown D (1981) Increased concentration of albumin in kidney basement membranes in diabetes mellitus. Diabetes 30:843–846

26. Melvin T, Kim Y, Michael AF (1984) Selective binding of IgG4 and other negatively charged plasma proteins in normal and diabetic human kidneys. Am J Pathol 115:443–446

27. Østerby R (1973) A quantitative electron microscopic study of mesangial regions in glomeruli from patients with short-term juvenile diabetes mellitus. Lab Invest 29:99–110
28. Gundersen HJG, Østerby R (1977) Glomerular size and structure in diabetes mellitus. II. Late abnormalities. Diabetologia 13:43–48
29. Scheinman JF, Fish AJ, Michael AF (1974) The immunohistopathology of glomerular antigens: The GBM, collagen, and actomyosin antigens in normal and diseased kidneys. J Clin Invest 54:1144–1154
30. Ellis EN, Steffes MW, Goetz FC, Sutherland DER, Mauer SM (1986) Glomerular filtration surface in type I diabetes mellitus. Kidney Int 29:889–894
31. Østerby R, Parving H-H, Nyberg G, et al. (1988) A strong correlation between glomerular filtration rate and filtration surface in diabetic nephropathy. Diabetologia 31:265–270
32. Chavers BM, Bilous RW, Ellis EN, Steffes MW, Mauer SM (1989) Glomerular lesions and urinary albumin excretion in type I diabetes without overt proteinuria. N Engl J Med 320:966–970
33. Burkholder PM (1965) Immunohistopathologic study of localized plasma protein and fixation guinea pig complement in renal lesions of diabetic glomerulosclerosis. Diabetes 14:755–770
34. Walker F (1972) The origin, turnover, and removal of glomerular basement membrane. J Pathol 110:233–244
35. Elllis EN, Steffes MW, Chavers BM, et al. (1986) Foot process width (FP) and filtration slit (FS) length in diabetes mellitus (DM) (abstract). Kidney Int 29:273
36. Huang TW (1980) The nature of the basal lamina alterations in human diabetic glomerulosclerosis. Am J Pathol 100:225–238
37. Evan AP, Luft FC (1980) Effect of alloxan-induced diabetes on the glomerular filtration barrier of the rat. Renal Physiol 3:257–264
38. Rasch R (1988) Nonglomerular lesions in the diabetic kidney. In: Davison AM (ed) Nephrology: Proceedings of the Xth international congress of nephrology. Bailliere Tindall, London, pp 744–757
39. Hostetter TH, Olson JL, Rennke HG, et al. (1981) Hyperfiltration in remnant nephrons: A potentially adverse response to renal ablation. Am J Physiol 241:F85–F93
40. Klahr S, Schreiner G, Ichikawa I (1988) The progression of renal disease. N Engl J Med 318:1657–1666
41. Keane WF, Kasiske BL, O'Donnell MP (1988) Lipids and progressive glomerulosclerosis. Am J Nephrol 8:261–271
42. Horlyck A, Gundersen HJG, Østerby R (1986) The cortical distribution pattern of diabetic glomerulopathy. Diabetologia 29:146–150

The Proteinuric Phase of Diabetic Nephrology

Timothy W. Meyer[1]

SUMMARY. In normal humans, very little protein is lost in the urine because the glomerular capillary wall imposes an efficient barrier to passage of macromolecules, excluding them from Bowman's space on the basis of both size and charge. Indeed, despite having an extraordinarily high permeability to water, the glomerular capillary wall, comprised of the fenestrated endothelial cells, basement membrane, and visceral epithelial cells with interdigitating podocytes, has a permeability to macromolecules which is among the lowest in the circulation. Leakiness of the glomerular capillary wall to proteins is the first sign of glomerular injury in diabetes and a reliable predictor of eventual renal failure in this disorder. Recent studies suggest, moreover, that antihypertensive therapies which reduce proteinuria will retard the progression of diabetic renal disease. This observation has provided a strong impetus to identify the mechanisms responsible for proteinuria in diabetic renal disease.

The Permeability of the Normal Glomerular Capillary Wall to Macromolecules

In order to discuss the mechanisms responsible for proteinuria in diabetic renal disease, it is necessary first to review current concepts of glomerular permeability to macromolecules. The principal basis on which the glomerular capillary wall excludes macromolecules from Bowman's space is *molecular size*. Molecules the size of inulin or smaller permeate the capillary wall as freely as water, but permeability decreases progressively with size for larger molecules, becoming very low as size nears that of serum albumin. Two methods have been employed to assess the size-selective properties of the glomerular capillary wall. The first method requires analysis of fluid samples collected from Bowman's space by micropuncture in

---

[1]Nephrology Division, Palo Alto Veterans Administration Medical Center, Palo Alto, CA 94304, USA

animals. The Bowman's space to plasma concentration ratio for a given protein then provides the fractional filtration or "sieving coefficient" (Θ) for that protein. The second method is based on measurement of the urinary clearance rates for intravenously infused test macromolecules [1]. This method avoids the difficulties encountered in analysis of small amounts of protein in tubule fluid samples, and can, moreover, be employed in human studies. The fractional clearance of a test macromolecule (M) is defined as the clearance of M divided by the glomerular filtration rate (GFR). When inulin is used to measure the GFR, the fractional clearance of a test macromolecule can be expressed as:

$$\text{Fractional clearance of M} = (U/P)_M/(U/P)_{In}$$

where $(U/P)_M$ and $(U/P)_{In}$ are the urine-to-plasma concentration ratios for the macromolecule M and for inulin. If, like inulin, the test macromolecule is neither reabsorbed nor secreted by the tubules, its fractional clearance will be equal to its fractional filtration by the glomerulus:

$$\text{Fractional clearance of M} = \Theta_M$$

The test substances most frequently employed to probe glomerular permeability to macromolecules have been the non-protein polymers dextran and polyvinylpyrrolidone [1]. These substances are available in a broad range of molecular sizes, appear not to be secreted or reabsorbed by renal tubules, and can be infused into humans. Results of studies in which dextran was used to assess the size-selectivity of the glomerular capillary wall are shown in Fig. 1. In these studies, dextran 40 was infused into 15 normal human volunteers [2,3]. Values for dextran fractional clearance (which are the same as values for the sieving coefficient, Θ) are plotted as a function of the Einstein-Stokes radii of the dextran molecules. A value of 1.0 on the y-axis represents equality of dextran and inulin clearances and indicates no measurable restriction to transport of dextran across the glomerular capillary wall when molecular radius is 20 Å or less. With increasing size, however, dextrans are progressively restricted, as indicated by a rapidly declining value for Θ. As indicated in Fig. 1, fractional clearances approach zero, indicating dextran impermeance in normal humans, when dextran radius exceeds 60 Å.

Theoretical studies employing mathematical models of solute transport through porous structures have shown that the size-selective properties of normal glomeruli, as exemplified in Fig. 1, can be accounted for by assuming that the glomerular capillary wall is permeated by numerous cylindrical pores with radius (r_o) ~ 55 Å [1–3]. It should be emphasized that structures of this size cannot be clearly distinguished even by the most sophisticated microscopic techniques, and that uniform cylindrical pores may not be a real feature of the glomerular capillary wall. Nevertheless, the assumption that the capillary wall is permeated by uniform pores accounts, with remarkable accuracy, for the dextran clearance profiles obtained in normal humans and animals. Theoretical analysis of dextran sieving curves based on this assumption thus provides a means to describe changes in glomerular size-selectivity associated with glomerular disease.

In addition to size, the glomerular capillary wall also excludes macromolecules from Bowman's space on the basis of *molecular charge*. The charge-selective proper-

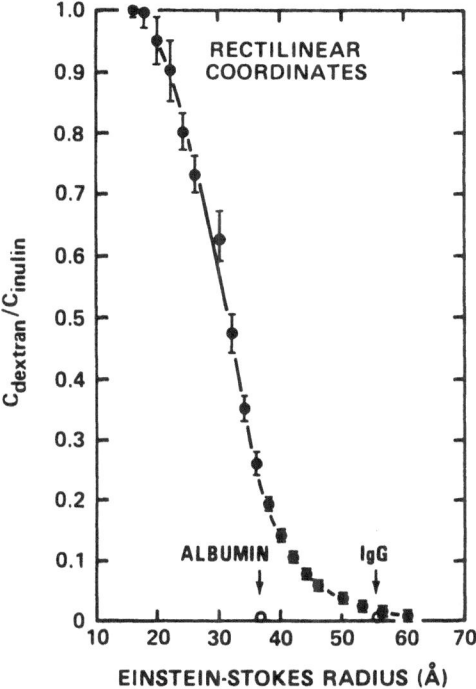

Fig. 1. The fractional dextran clearance profile of the normal glomerular capillary wall as determined in 15 healthy adult volunteers. Fractional dextran clearances are plotted as a function of the Einstein-Stokes radius of the dextran. The *vertical bars* represent 1 SEM. Data for albumin and IgG are illustrated for comparison. (Courtesy of B.D. Myers)

ties of the glomerular capillary wall have been most clearly demonstrated in animals, in which the clearances of charged and neutral test macromolecules can be directly compared. Bohrer et al. [4] showed that in normal rats the clearance of anionic dextran sulfate molecules is 10–50-fold lower than the clearance of neutral dextran molecules over the size range 26–42 Å. Further studies have shown that the capillary wall loses its ability to discriminate against anionic dextrans in rats with glomerular disease [5,6]. These results can be explained on the assumption that the normal glomerular capillary wall carries a fixed negative charge which is reduced by glomerular disease [7]. Presumably the glomerular capillary wall discriminates against anionic macromolecules in humans as it does it rats. Moreover, it is widely assumed that loss of capillary wall anionic charge contributes to proteinuria in human as well as in experimental glomerular disease. Because charged test macromolecules have not been available for human use, however, the contribution of reduced capillary wall charge to proteinuria in humans has not been quantified.

In addition to being determined by the intrinsic properties of the glomerular capillary wall, including size- and charge-selectivity, the glomerular filtration of macromolecules is determined by the *hemodynamic factors* which govern the GFR [2].

Thus proteinuria can be altered by hemodynamic events, such as changes in volume status or blood pressure, independent of any changes in capillary wall structure. The influence on macromolecule filtration of glomerular hemodynamic factors, which include the glomerular plasma flow rate, transcapillary hydraulic pressure, and the arterial plasma protein concentration, is complex and difficult to predict. In general, maneuvers which increase the filtration fraction while GFR remains constant may be expected to increase the glomerular filtration of macromolecules the size of albumin.

The Development of Proteinuria in Diabetic Renal Disease

Early "Functional" Proteinuria

During the first decade of diabetes, values for urinary albumin excretion rate (UAE) usually remain normal, averaging < 10 mg/day. There are, however, at least two circumstances in which transient increases in UAE may be observed in patients with early diabetes. First, elevation of UAE may be observed during episodes of poor metabolic control [8]. Values for UAE in this setting usually remain < 50 mg/day, but higher values have sometimes been recorded. Second, exercise may increase UAE to values as high as 500 mg/day in diabetic patients whose resting values for UAE are normal [9]. The mechanism(s) by which poor metabolic control and exercise increase filtration of albumin in diabetic patients have not been fully characterized. Poor metabolic control has been shown to increase the albumin excreting rate in patients with diabetes of only a few months duration, in whom defects in glomerular capillary wall structure presumably have not yet developed [8]. Albumin excretion rates are rapidly reduced following improvement in metabolic control and cessation of exercise, further suggesting that increased albumin filtration in these circumstances cannot be attributed to fixed defects in glomerular size- or charge-selectivity [8,9]. It thus seems likely that alterations in glomerular hemodynamic function cause transient increases in glomerular filtration of macromolecules early in the course of diabetes.

In patients with diabetes of several years duration, transient increases in UAE may result from the combination of altered glomerular hemodynamic function with early changes in glomerular capillary wall structure. In such patients, exercise may serve as a provocative test to reveal abnormalities in glomerular barrier function which are not apparent at rest [9]. It is not yet known, however, whether exercise-induced albuminuria, like resting "microalbuminuria," predicts development of clinical nephropathy in diabetes. At present, physicians should be aware of the effects of exercise and poor metabolic control on albumin filtration, chiefly in order to avoid over-interpretation of elevated values for UAE. As described by Viberti in this symposium, the diagnosis of "microalbuminuria" should be made only when urine specimens have been collected under well defined conditions, and should preferably be based on analysis of more than one urine sample.

Microalbuminuria

In clinical practice, the diagnosis of diabetic nephropathy has usually been established by the finding of "dipstick positive" proteinuria, representing an albumin excretion rate of approximately 500 mg/day. Recent studies, however, have emphasized the value of identifying patients with "microalbuminuria," usually defined as having albumin excretion rates in the range of 30–300 mg/day. Long term studies have shown that albumin excretion in such patients increases over several years to rates in excess of 500 mg/day. Development of this "clinical" level of albuminuria in turn reliably predicts the ultimate loss of kidney function in diabetic patients. The small defect in glomerular barrier function which causes "microalbuminuria" must therefore be regarded as the first sign of a pathological process which leads inexorably to renal failure.

The permselectivity defect(s) responsible for microalbuminuria have been difficult to identify because the macromolecule excretion rates, though abnormal, are still very low. It is important to note that excretion of proteins other than albumin is increased in patients with "microalbuminuria." Emphasis has been placed on albumin excretion because albumin is the predominant, and therefore the most easily measurable, protein in the urine as well as in the plasma. However, diabetic patients with values for UAE of 30–300 mg/day have been found also to exhibit increased excretion of IgG [10,11]. The finding of increased quantities of this large protein in the urine implies that a defect in glomerular size-selectivity contributes to proteinuria in patients with microalbuminuria. More rigorous proof that a defect in size selectivity contributes to early proteinuria in diabetes has been provided by a study showing that glomerular permeability to dextran molecules with radii of 50–60 Å is increased in type II diabetic patients with albumin excretion rates averaging <50 mg/day [12]. Given that a charge-selectivity defect accompanies the size-selectivity defect in diabetic patients with heavier proteinuria (see below), it seems likely that a charge-selectivity defect also accompanies the size-selectivity defect in diabetic patients with microalbuminuria. Attempts to identify a charge-selectivity defect early in the course of diabetic nephropathy, by comparing clearance values for IgG molecules with different isoelectric points, have yielded inconclusive results [11,13].

Clinical Proteinuria

The mechanisms responsible for proteinuria in diabetic patients with clinical nephropathy have been extensively investigated by Myers and coworkers [13–15]. These investigations have identified a size-selectivity defect, reflected by enhanced clearance of dextrans with radii of 50–60 Å, in diabetic patients with protein excretion which ranges from 300 mg/day to more than 10 g/day. To assess the magnitude of this size-selectivity defect, Myers and co-workers have employed a "heteroporous" model of the glomerular capillary wall [16]. The heteroporous model assumes that in injured, as in normal glomeruli, the major portion of the capillary wall is perforated by cylindrical pores of radius r_o. This model further assumes that a smaller portion of the capillary wall is permeated by "shunt" pores which are so large that they exhibit no size-selectivity. The portion of the capillary wall permeated by shunt pores denoted ω_o, as opposed to normal pores can be determined from dextran clearance profiles. Thus shunt parameter provides a quantitative measure of the magnitude of the size-selectivity defect in injured glomeruli.

Two important conclusions have so far emerged from the theoretical analysis of dextran clearance studies performed by Myers and co-workers in patients with diabetic renal disease [14,15]. First, these studies indicate that the magnitude of the "shunt" is sufficient to account for most of the protein excreted in the urine. Second, these studies have shown that the magnitude of the shunt increases as diabetic nephropathy advances. This latter finding has been most clearly demonstrated in a study in which dextran clearance studies were repeated at an interval of 24 months in ten patients with diabetic nephropathy [15]. During this interval, mean GFR decreased from 59 ± 9 to 34 ± 7 ml/min. Urinary excretion of albumin and IgG, however, did not change significantly. The finding that urinary protein excretion rates were maintained as the GFR fell clearly implies that fractional protein excretion rates increased over the course of the study. Dextran sieving studies revealed that this increase in fractional protein excretion was caused by a progressive impairment of glomerular size-selectivity, reflected by an increase in the shunt parameter ω_o as renal disease advanced. It should be noted that, in patients with other glomerular diseases, proteinuria may also remain at high levels as GFR declines. Experimental studies suggest that these findings may reflect aggravation of glomerular barrier injury, associated with hypertrophy of remnant glomeruli when nephrons are lost in the setting of established nephrosis [17].

The heteroporous model of glomerular injury used by Myers and co-workers, though it provides a useful index of impaired size-selectivity, clearly provides an incomplete description of glomerular permeability to macromolecules in diabetic renal disease. If circulating macromolecules escaped injured glomeruli exclusively through a non-discriminatory shunt, the glomerular clearances of various proteins would be equal. Multiple studies have shown, however, that values for the fractional clearance of albumin are several-fold greater than values for the fractional clearance of IgG in patients with diabetic nephropathy [10,11,14,15]. The most likely explanation for this finding is that impairment of glomerular charge-selectivity accompanies impairment of glomerular size-selectivity in diabetic renal disease, so that glomerular permeability to albumin is increased relatively more than glomerular permeability to IgG. Studies employing charged test macromolecules have shown that charge-selectivity defects almost invariably accompany size-selectivity defects in animals with heavy proteinuria.

The Relation of Proteinuria to Altered Glomerular Structure in Diabetes

The structural changes responsible for increased glomerular permeability to proteins in diabetes remain largely unidentified. Research in this area has been hampered by limited access to renal tissue in diabetic humans and by difficulties in creating suitable animal models of diabetic renal disease.

Early morphologic studies identified *thickening of the basement membrane* as a regular feature of diabetic glomerular injury, and it was natural to assume that increased permeability to macromolecules might be caused by this change in glomerular capillary wall structure. Recent studies have shown, however, that urine albumin excretion rates are not correlated with glomerular basement membrane thickness in diabetic patients [18,19]. Marked basement membrane thickening has been observed in patients who have been diabetic for less than ten years and who have had albumin excretion rates only slightly above normal [19].

While proteinuria in diabetic renal disease cannot be attributed to glomerular basement membrane thickening per se, it may well be caused by associated changes in *basement membrane composition*. It has been suggested that glycosylation of basement membrane constituents increases the permeability of the basement membrane to macromolecules. This attractive hypothesis remains to be tested experimentally. Increased permeability of the glomerular capillary wall has also been attributed to altered synthesis of various basement membrane constituents. To date, the most extensively investigated of these basement membrane constituents has been *heparan sulfate proteoglycan* (HSPG). Because HSPG is highly anionic, it has been widely assumed that distribution of this substance within the glomerular basement membrane is largely responsible for maintenance of glomerular charge-selectivity. Functional studies have suggested that HSPG is also necessary for the maintenance of glomerular size-selectivity [20]. A relation between basement membrane HSPG content and albumin excretion rate, however, has not yet been demonstrated in diabetic animals or humans.

In addition to changes in basement membrane structure, proteinuria in diabetic renal disease may be related to changes in *epithelial cell structure*. As in other glomerular diseases, proteinuria in diabetic renal disease is associated with broadening and retraction of epithelial cell foot processes. Recent morphometric studies have demonstrated early broadening of epithelial cell foot processes in diabetic patients with albumin excretion rates of <1 g/day [21,22]. It is not known whether this change in epithelial cell structure represents a cause or a consequence of increased glomerular permeability to macromolecules.

Maneuvers which Reduce Proteinuria in Diabetic Renal Disease

The observation that proteinuria precedes loss of renal function in diabetic patients has led naturally to the assumption that maneuvers which reduce proteinuria will retard the progression of diabetic renal disease. Extensive clinical trials are required to establish the validity of this hypothesis. As described by Mauer in this symposium, morphometric studies suggest that the reduction of the GFR in diabetic nephrology is caused by progressive expansion of the glomerular mesangium. Since the mechanisms responsible for mesangial expansion may differ from those responsible for glomerular barrier dysfunction, it is not certain that all maneuvers which reduce proteinuria will prevent reduction of the GFR in diabetic patients.

Among therapies examined to date, *antihypertensive agents* have proven most effective in reducing proteinuria in patients with diabetic renal disease. Moreover, antihypertensive agents have the same effect on glomerular barrier function. Overall, studies to date suggest that albumin excretion rates are comparably reduced by regimens including converting enzyme inhibitors and beta adrenergic receptor blockers, while variable effects on albumin excretion rates have been observed with calcium channel antagonists.

The mechanisms by which antihypertensive agents improve glomerular barrier function in diabetic renal disease have not been fully elucidated. It has frequently been suggested that antihypertensive agents improve glomerular barrier function by lowering glomerular transcapillary hydraulic pressure, ΔP. A recent modification of this "hemodynamic" hypothesis suggests that antihypertensive agents improve

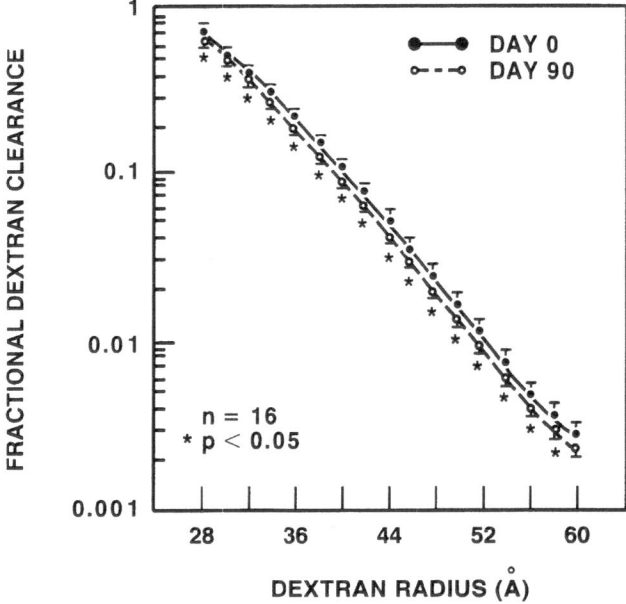

Fig. 2. The fractional dextran clearance profiles before (*day 0*) and after (*day 90*) converting enzyme inhibitor treatment in 16 diabetic patients with initial average proteinuria of 2.2 g/day. (From [26])

glomerular barrier function by reducing glomerular capillary wall tension, which is considered to be the product of ΔP and glomerular capillary radius. Studies in which converting enzyme inhibitor treatment was initiated at the outset of experimental diabetes are often cited in support of this hypothesis [25]. These studies have shown that continuous converting enzyme inhibitor treatment reduces ΔP and largely prevents development of albuminuria in diabetic rats. There is reason to question, however, whether lowering of capillary wall tension accounts for the beneficial effect of antihypertensive agents on glomerular barrier function in established diabetic nephropathy. A recent dextran clearance study suggests, alternatively, that converting enzyme inhibitor therapy may have a direct effect on glomerular capillary wall pore structure [26]. In this study, 16 diabetic patients with serum creatinine values < 2 mg/dl and proteinuria averaging 2.2 g/day were treated with a converting enzyme inhibitor for 90 days. Values for GFR remained stable during converting enzyme inhibitor treatment, while mean arterial pressure declined from 98 ± 3 to 92 ± 3 mmHg. As illustrated in Fig. 2, converting enzyme inhibitor treatment decreased fractional clearance values not only for large dextran molecules with radii of 50–60 Å, but also for dextran molecules with radii of 30–50 Å. This finding indicates that converting enzyme inhibitor therapy alters the structure of the capillary wall so as to shift the entire pore size distribution toward a lower value.

Other therapies which may reduce proteinuria in diabetic disease include *improved glycemic control* and *dietary protein restriction*. As described above, improved glycemic control has been shown to lower albumin excretion rates in patients with recent onset diabetes and poor initial glycemic control. The effect of rigorous glycemic control on albuminuria in patients with established diabetic renal disease is less well defined. Some, but not all, studies have shown that sustained normalization of blood glucose by insulin pump therapy reduces the albumin excretion rate in patients with microalbuminuria [27-29]. Viberti and coworkers [30] have shown, however, that long-term normalization of blood glucose neither reduces the protein excretion rate nor slows the progression of renal disease in diabetic patients with heavy proteinuria and reduction of the GFR. In contrast, dietary protein restriction has been shown to reduce the protein excretion rate in patients with established diabetic nephropathy [31].

Proteinuria in Type II Diabetes

Most of the studies described above have been performed in patients with type I diabetes. Available studies suggest, however, that the pattern of proteinuria is similar in type I and in type II diabetes [32-34]. One difference between the two conditions is that patients with type II diabetes may exhibit dipstick positive proteinuria at the time when diabetes is diagnosed [33,35,36]. Insulin resistance and hypertension may precipitate glomerular injury prior to development of overt hyperglycemia in these patients.

Acknowledgment. Supported by grants from the National Institutes of Health (DK35734) and the California Affiliate of the American Heart Association.

References

1. Deen WM, Bridges CR, Brenner BM (1983) Biophysical basis of glomerular permselectivity. J Membr Biol 71:1-10
2. Friedman S, Strober S, Field E, Silverman E, Myers BD (1984) Glomerular capillary wall function in human lupus nephritis. Am J Physiol 246 (Renal Fluid Electrolyte Physiol 15):F580-591
3. Shemesh O, Ross JC, Deen WM, Grant GW, Myers BD (1986) Nature of the glomerular capillary injury in human membranous glomerulopathy. J Clin Invest 77:868-877
4. Bohrer MP, Baylis C, Humes HD, Glassock RJ, Robertson CR, Brenner BM (1978) Permselectivity of the glomerular capillary wall: facilitated filtration of circulating polycations. J Clin Invest 61:72-78
5. Bohrer MP, Baylis C, Humes HD, Glassock RJ, Robertson CR, Brenner BM (1977) Mechanisms of the puromycin-induced defects in the transglomerular passage of water and macromolecules. J Clin Invest 60:152-161
6. Olson JL, Rennke HG, Venkatachalam MJ (1981) Alterations in the charge and size selectivity barrier of the glomerular filter in aminonucleoside nephrosis in rats. Lab Invest 4:271-279
7. Deen WM, Satvat B (1981) Determinants of the glomerular filtration of proteins. Am J Physiol 241 (Renal Fluid Electrolyte Physiol 10):F162-F170

8. Parving H-H, Noer I, Deckert T, Ervin PE, Nielsen SL, Lygsoe J, Mogensen CE (1976) The effect of metabolic regulation on microvascular permeability to small and large molecules in short-term juvenile diabetes. Diabetologia 12:161-166

9. Vittinghus E, Mogensen CE (1982) Graded exercise and protein excretion in diabetic man and the effect of insulin treatment. Kidney Int 21:725-729

10. Viberti G, Mackintosh D, Keen H (1983) Determinants of the penetration of proteins through the glomerular barrier in insulin-dependent diabetes mellitus. Diabetes 32(Suppl 2):92-95

11. Deckert T, Feldt-Rasmussen B, Djurup R, Deckert M (1988) Glomerular size and charge selectivity in insulin-dependent diabetes mellitus. Kidney Int 33:100-106

12. Loon N, Nelson R, Myers BD (1989) Glomerular barrier abnormality in new onset NIDDM in Pima Indians. Proceedings of the 22nd Annual Meeting of the American Society of Nephrology Washington, USA p 325A

13. Nakamura Y, Myers BD (1988) Charge selectivity of proteinuria in diabetic glomerulopathy. Diabetes 37:1202-1211

14. Friedman S, Jones HW III, Golbetz HV, Lee JA, Little HL, Myers BD (1983) Mechanisms of proteinuria in diabetic nephropathy II. Diabetes 32(Suppl 2):40-46

15. Tomlanovich S, Deen WM, Jones III HW, Schwartz HC, Myers BD (1987) Functional nature of glomerular injury in progressive diabetic glomerulopathy. Diabetes 36:556-565

16. Deen WM, Bridges CR, Brenner BM, Myers BD (1985) Heteroporous model of glomerular size selectivity: application to normal and nephrotic humans. Am J Physiol 249 (Renal Fluid Electrolyte Physiol 18):F374-F389

17. Meyer TW, Rennke HG (1988) Increased single-nephron protein excretion after renal ablation in nephrotic rats. Am J Physiol 255:F1243-F1248

18. Mauer SM, Steffes MW, Ellis EN, Sutherland DER, Brown DM, Goetz FC (1984) Structural-functional relationships in diabetic nephrology. J Clin Invest 74:1143-1155

19. Chavers BM, Bilous RW, Ellis EN, Steffes MW, Mauer SM (1989) Glomerular lesions and urinary albumin excretion in type I diabetes without overt proteinuria. N Engl J Med 320:966-970

20. Kanwar YS (1984) Biology of disease: Biophysiology of glomerular filtration and proteinuria. Lab Invest 51:7-21

21. Østerby R, Anderson AR, Gundersen HJ, Jorgensen HE, Mogensen CE, Parving HH (1984) Quantitative studies of glomerular ultrastructure in type I diabetics with incipient nephropathy. Diabetic Nephrol 3:95-100

22. Ellis EN, Steffes MW, Chavers B, Mauer SM (1987) Observations of glomerular epithelial cell structure in patients with type I diabetes mellitus. Kidney Int 32:736-741

23. Parving H-H, Andersen AR, Smidt UM, Hommel E, Mathiesen ER, Svendsen PA (1987) Effect of antihypertensive treatment on kidney function in diabetic nephropathy. Br Med J [Clin Res] 294:1443-1447

24. Parving H-H, Hommel E, Smidt UM (1988) Protection of kidney function and decrease in albuminuria by captopril in insulin dependent diabetics with nephropathy. Br Med J [Clin Res] 297:1086-1091

25. Zatz R, Dunn BR, Meyer TW, Anderson S, Rennke HG, Brenner BM (1986) Prevention of diabetic glomerulopathy by pharmacological amelioration of glomerular capillary hypertension. J Clin Invest 77:1925-1930

26. Morelli E, Loon N, Meyer TW, Peters W, Myers BD (to be published) Effects of converting enzyme inhibition on barrier function in diabetic glomerulopathy. Diabetes

27. Viberti GC, Pickup JC, Jarrett RJ, Keen H (1979) Effect of control of blood glucose on urinary albumin excretion and β_2-microglobulin in insulin-dependent diabetes. N Engl J Med 300:638-41

28. KROC Collaborative Study Group (1984) Blood glucose control and the evolution of

diabetic retinopathy and albuminuria: A preliminary multicenter trial. N Engl J Med 311:365–372

29. Feldt-Rasmussen B, Mathiesen ER, Hegedus L, Deckert T (1986) Kidney function during 12 months of strict metabolic control in insulin-dependent diabetic patients with incipient nephropathy. N Engl J Med 314:665–670

30. Viberti GC, Bilous RW, Mackintosh D, Bending JJ, Keen H (1983) Long-term correction of hyperglycemia and progression of renal failure in insulin dependent diabetes. Br Med J [Clin Res] 286:598–602

31. Anderson S (1990) Low protein diets and diabetic nephropathy. Semin Nephrol 10:287–293

32. Mogensen CE (1984) Microalbuminuria predicts clinical proteinuria and early mortality in maturity-onset diabetes. N Engl J Med 310:356–360

33. Ballard DJ, Humphrey LL, Melton III LJ, Frohnert PP, Chu C-P, O'Fallon WM, Palumbo PJ (1988) Epidemiology of persistent proteinuria in type II diabetes mellitus. Population-based study in Rochester, Minnesota. Diabetes 37:405–412

34. Kunzelman CL, Knowler WC, Pettitt DJ, Bennett PH (1989) Incidence of proteinuria in type 2 diabetes mellitus in the Pima Indians. Kidney Int 35:681–687

35. Fabre J, Balant LP, Dayer PG, Fox HM, Vernet AT (1982) The kidney in maturity onset diabetes mellitus. Kidney Int 21:730–738

36. Uusitupa M, Siitonen O, Penttila I, Aro A, Pyorala K (1987) Proteinuria in newly diagnosed type II diabetic patients. Diabetes Care 10:191–194

Management of Advanced Nephrotic Disease in Diabetics: Short-term and Long-term Effects of Angiotensin Converting Enzyme (ACE)-Inhibitors and a New Trial Using Camostat Mesilate

Yoshio Taguma, Mitsunobu Matsubara, Osamu Hotta, and Kosei Kurosawa[1]

SUMMARY. Two studies of the management of nephrotic diabetics were performed. Captopril (37.5 mg/day, $n=16$), decreased urinary protein excretion from 9.6 ± 1.6 to 4.9 ± 1.0 g/day, $P < 0.05$ (M $\pm$ SEM) and significantly decreased total cholesterol. No significant adverse effect was observed. Camostat mesilate (600 mg/day, $n=15$) decreased urinary protein from 4.8 ± 0.6 to 2.9 ± 0.4 ($P < 0.01$). Elevated plasma fibrinogen level and noticeably enhanced urinary fibrin degradation product (FDP) excretion were also attenuated by this medication. No serious adverse effect was noted. These types of medication, particularly when combined, seemed promising for the treatment of nephrotic diabetics. The long-term effect of ACE-I was retrospectively analyzed in 56 azotemic diabetics, of whom almost all had noninsulin-dependent diabetes mellitus (NIDDM). The patients were divided into two groups (group A: treated with ACE-I, $n=27$; group B: without ACE-I, $n=29$). The inverse creatinine deteriorated by 0.023 per month in group B and by 0.012 in group A. Although the mean blood pressure was kept at a similar level, HBA1c differed significantly. In an additional study, ACE-I slowed the progression rate in 10 patients with nephrosclerosis. Taking these observations into consideration, it is suggested that ACE-I might slow the progression rate of advanced diabetic nephropathy.

Introduction

The management of diabetic patients with advanced nephropathy is not easy, because such patients tend to have the nephrotic syndrome and to have severe damage in many organs. This nephrotic syndrome is believed to accelerate the progression of nephropathy and to further accelerate damage in other organs. Consequently, it would be of great value to try and alleviate the massive proteinuria which is char-

---

[1]Department of Nephrology, Sendai Shakaihoken Hospital, 3-16-1 Tsutsumimachi Aobaku, Sendai, 981 Japan

acteristic of this condition. In this regard, we studied the effect of two kinds of drugs; captopril and camostate mesilate. We will discuss the advantages of these drugs in the treatment of advanced diabetic nephropathy.

Our greatest concern is whether or not long-term ACE-inhibition slows the progression rate of nephropathy. In order to investigate whether an ACE-inhibitor has such an effect, we retrospectively analyzed the clinical course of our patients with advanced diabetic nephropathy and hypertensive nephrosclerosis.

Methods

The Effects of Captopril on the Nephrotic Syndrome in Advanced Diabetic Nephropathy

This study was performed while patients were hospitalized. Sixteen NIDDM patients (8 men and 8 women, mean age of 49 years), were the subjects. All patients had azotemia and proliferative retinopathy. During the control period of more than two weeks, their hypertension was controlled by conventional antihypertensive drugs and their clinical variables were confirmed to be relatively constant. Thereafter, captopril, at 37.5 mg a day, was administered and the patients were observed for 8 weeks.

The Effects of Camostat Mesilate

This study was performed while patients were hospitalized. Fifteen patients (13 men and 2 women, mean age of 57 years) were the subjects. All patients had NIDDM and proliferative retinopathy; fourteen of them had azotemia. During the control period an ACE-inhibitor had been used to control their hypertension and massive proteinuria, and the clinical variables were confirmed to be almost constant. Thereafter, camostat mesilate, at 600 mg a day, was administered and the patients were observed for a minimum of 4 weeks.

The Long-term Effects of ACE-Inhibition

The clinical courses of 56 azotemic diabetics and 10 patients with hypertensive nephrosclerosis were analyzed. The azotemic diabetics were divided into two groups, according to whether or not ACE-inhibitors had been used. Twenty-seven patients (16 men and 11 women, mean age of 49), had been treated with an ACE-inhibitor for more than twelve months. In the remaining 29 patients (19 men and 10 women, mean age of 51), hypertension had been controlled using only conventional antihypertensive drugs. Patients who developed any acute complications were excluded from this study. Of the 56 patients, only two had insulin-dependent diabetes mellitus (IDDM).

The clinical courses of ten patients with hypertensive nephrosclerosis, who fell into the following category, were analyzed: azotemia was present at the initial point of observation, during the following twelve months no ACE-inhibitor was used, and thereafter we started administration of this drug. We examined the slopes of inverse creatinine in each period.

Table 1. The effects of captopril (37.5 mg a day) in 16 azotemic diabetics

		Before	After	
Urinary protein	(g/day)	9.6 ± 1.6	4.9 ± 1.0*	
Serum total protein	(g/dl)	5.8 ± 0.2	6.1 ± 0.2	ns
Serum total cholesterol	(mg/dl)	228 ± 13	177 ± 8**	
Serum creatinine	(mg/dl)	4.4 ± 0.5	4.6 ± 0.5	ns
Serum potassium	(mEq/L)	4.5 ± 0.1	4.7 ± 0.1	ns
Mean blood pressure	(mmHg)	108 ± 3	100 ± 4	ns
HBA1c	(%)	6.3 ± 0.4	5.9 ± 0.4	ns

Values are expressed as M ± SEM. $**P < 0.01$, $*P < 0.05$: ns, not significant

Results

The Effects of Captopril

Table 1 shows the result of this study. Urinary protein excretion of 9.6 grams a day decreased to about half by the end of the study. The increase in total protein concentration did not reach statistical significance, but the total cholesterol level decreased significantly. On the whole, neither serum creatinine nor serum potassium showed any significant increments. However, in one case acute worsening of azotemia was observed; this patient was excluded from the study. Mean blood pressure and level of HBA1c did not change significantly.

The Effects of Camostat Mesilate

Table 2 shows the result of this study. Urinary protein decreased significantly and serum albumin concentration increased. Serum creatinine was unchanged. Plasma fibrinogen concentration was abnormally high during the control period and fell to a normal level after this drug was administered. A large amount of urinary total-FDP, which is not excreted in the urine of healthy people, was observed during the control period, and decreased significantly after this drug was administered. In addition, no worsening in retinal hemorrhage was observed in any patient.

Table 2. The effects of camostat mesilate (600 mg a day) in 15 patients with advanced diabetic nephropathy

		Before	After	
Urinary protein	(g/day)	4.8 ± 0.6	2.9 ± 0.4**	
S-Albumin	(g/dl)	2.7 ± 0.2	2.9 ± 0.2**	
S-creatinine	(mg/dl)	3.8 ± 0.7	3.8 ± 0.1	ns
Plasma fibrinogen	(mg/dl)[a]	420 ± 42	307 ± 28**	
Urinary total-FDP	(μg/day)	26100 ± 9700	18100 ± 7100*	

[a]Normal range for plasma fibrinogen is 160–400 mg/dl.
Values are expressed as M±SEM. $*P < 0.05$, $**P < 0.01$; ns, not significant

Table 3. Profiles of our 56 patients with advanced diabetic nephropathy

I] Type of diabetes
IDDM 2   NIDDM 54
II] Historical data for 54 NIDDM patients
Proteinuria present at the onset/detection of diabetes
12 (22%)
Preceding hypertension
Present 26 (48%)
Absent 28 (52%)

Long-term Effects of ACE-inhibition

The profile of the 56 diabetic patients who were the subjects of this study are shown in Table 3. It seemed noteworthy that most of the patients were those with NIDDM, and that in about half of them, hypertension preceded diabetes. The patients' clinical courses were analyzed and they were divided into two groups according to whether or not an ACE-inhibitor had been used. Figure 1 shows the time course of inverse creatinine, mean blood pressure, and levels of HBA1c in these two groups. A regression line for the slope of inverse creatinine in each patient was drawn, and the calculated mean of this line was expressed for each group. The dots represent the mean values of each period of time for each group. The levels in mean blood pressure were kept at a similar range in the two groups, though the levels in HBA1c differed almost constantly throughout the observed period. Therefore, even though there was a significant difference in the deteriorating rate in renal function between these two groups, we should not draw a definite conclusion.

Figure 2 shows the time course of progression of 10 patients with hypertensive nephrosclerosis. During the first twelve months, when patients had been treated with conventional antihypertensive drugs, a further declining tendency in renal function was observed. The mean blood pressure tended to rise, and then, depending on the result, ACE-inhibitor was administered to each patient. During the following twelve months, the declining tendency seemed to disappear. The differences in the slopes of inverse creatinine during, before, and after ACE-inhibition, were statistically significant.

Discussion

Since we reported in 1985 that captopril had an effect on reducing massive proteinuria in advanced diabetic nephropathy patients some controversy was evoked [1]. But now it seems to be indisputable that ACE-inhibitors have a definite effect in reducing urinary protein excretion in various renal disorders [2,3]. This effect is thought to be brought about through attenuation of glomerular hyperfiltration. Glomerular hyperfiltration is suspected to be one of the factors responsible for the initiation and the progression of diabetic nephropathy [4]. Our result would be regarded as supporting evidence for this hypothesis.

In any type of renal disease, particularly in diabetes, the development of the nephrotic syndrome is considered to be an accelerating factor in the progression of

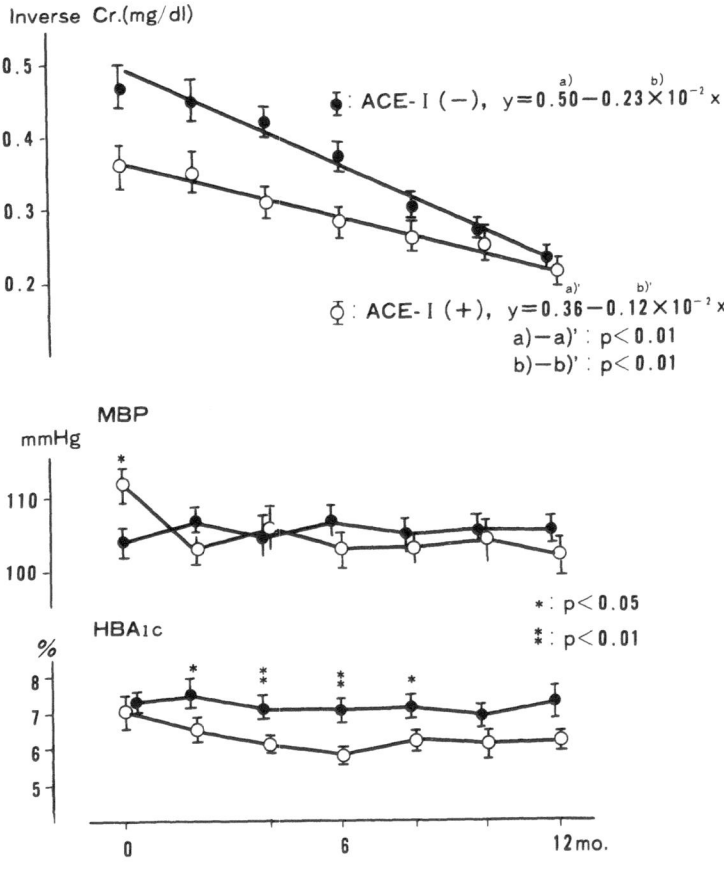

Fig. 1. Clinical course of azotemic diabetics treated with ACE-I ($n=27$) and without ACE-I ($n=29$). The *lines* drawn for the slope of inverse creatinine represent the calculated regression line for each group. The *dots* represent the mean values (M $\pm$ SEM) of each group in each time-period

nephropathy and in the damage in other organs [5]. Many factors other than hyper-filtration might also be responsible for the massive proteinuria which occurs in advanced diabetics [6], therefore, various therapeutic interventions would be necessary to alleviate this condition. At this juncture, we performed a new trial using camostat mesilate. Camostat mesilate is a derivative of gabexate mesilate, which is now used world-wide for the treatment of acute pancreatitis and disseminated intra-vascular coagulation. We recently found that use of this drug was advantageous in the treatment of heavy proteinuria in various nephropathies, including diabetic nephropathy [7,8]. The results of this study could be regarded as beneficial, in that massive proteinuria was reduced and also in that hypercoagulability was amelio-rated. The long-term effects and the precise in vivo action of this drug remain to be elucidated. In any case, by using an ACE-inhibitor and camostat mesilate, we could

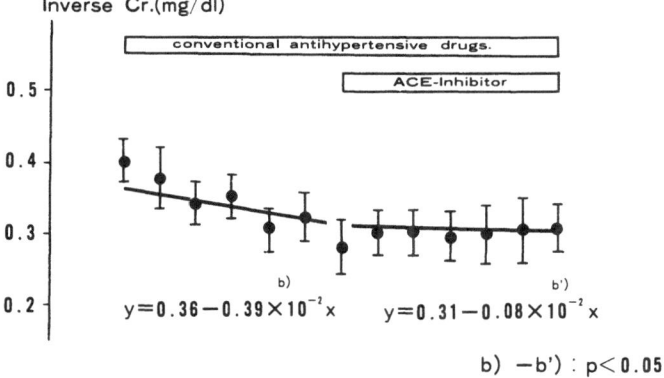

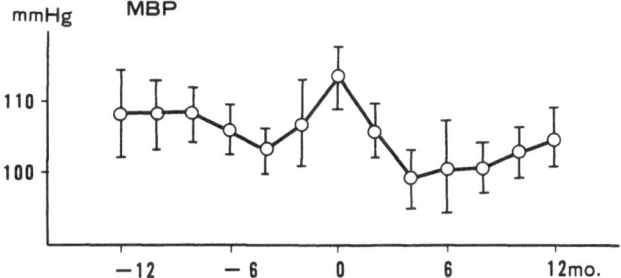

Fig. 2. Time course of progression before and after ACE-inhibition in 10 azotemic patients with hypertensive nephrosclerosis. The *lines* drawn for the slope of inverse creatinine represent the calculated regression line for each period. The *dots* represent the mean values of each time-period

alleviate the nephrotic syndrome in most patients with advanced diabetic nephropathy. Therefore, we may suppose that this combination therapy would be promising in improving the prognosis of these patients.

The pathogenesis of nephropathy in NIDDM is not clearly understood when compared to that in IDDM. The high prevalence rates, noted in our patients, of proteinuria and of hypertension preceding the detection of diabetes, seem to be one of the characteristics of NIDDM. This characteristic would be considered to be related to the concept of "insulin resistance" [8]. Another simpler explanation for this phenomenon is that, to some extent, arterionephrosclerosis precedes the development of diabetic glomerulosclerosis in some NIDDM patients. Figure 3 represents a schema of our line of thought in this direction. If we presume such a condition, we could expect to see similar effects of ACE-inhibitors in patients with hypertensive nephrosclerosis and in those with NIDDM. As was indicated by this study and by other researchers [9], an ACE-inhibitor slowed the progression rate in patients with hypertensive nephrosclerosis. Concerning advanced diabetic nephropathy, a similar beneficial effect, albeit not a definite one, was suggested by this study. Many factors might

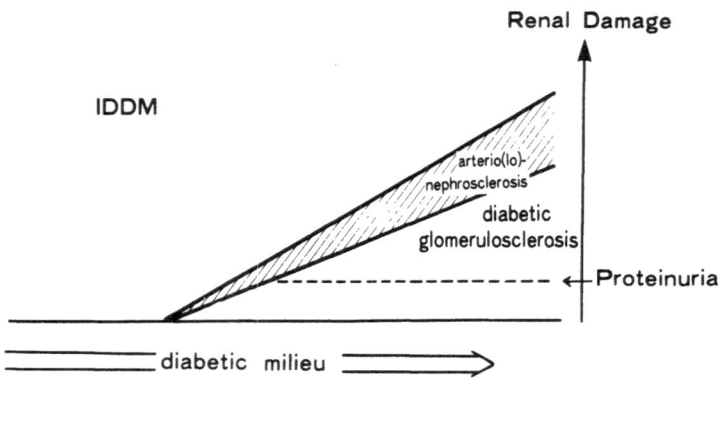

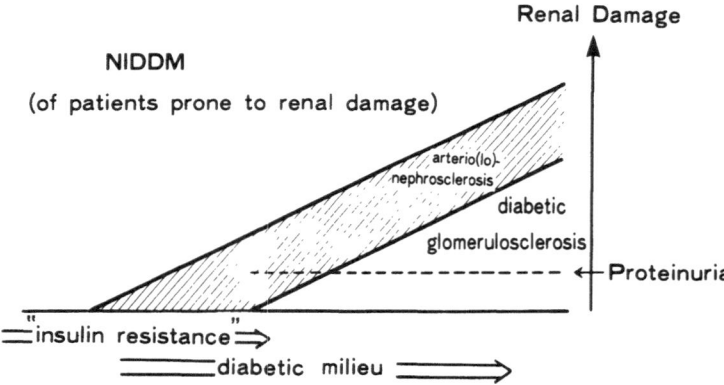

Fig. 3. A proposed schema of the pathophysiological alteration which takes place during the development of nephropathy in patients with IDDM and in NIDDM patients who are prone to renal damage

be responsible for the progression of diabetic glomerulosclerosis; ACE-inhibition alone would not be enough to stop the progression. We have to wait for future research before we can further improve the prognosis of advanced diabetic nephropathy.

Acknowledgment. We thank Ms Emiko Sakai for technical assistance.

References

1. Taguma Y, Kitamoto Y, Futaki G, Ueda H, Monma H, Ishizaki M, Takahashi H, Sekino H, Sasaki Y (1985) Effect of captopril on heavy proteinuria in azotemic diabetics. N Engl J Med 313:1617–1620
2. Hommel E, Parving HE, Mathiesen E, Edsberg B, Nielsen MD, Giese J (1986) Effect of captopril on kidney function in insulin-dependent diabetic patients with nephropathy. Br Med J [Clin Res] 293:467–470

3. Heeg JE, DeJong PE, Hem GK, Zeeum D (1987) Reduction of proteinuria by angiotensin converting enzyme inhibition. Kidney Int 32:78–83
4. Hostetter TH, Rennke HG, Brenner BM (1982) The case for intrarenal hypertension in the initiation and progression of diabetic and other glomerulopathies. Am J Med 72:375–380
5. Bernard DB (1982) Metabolic abnormalities in nephrotic syndrome: pathophysiology and complications. In: Brenner BM, Stein JH (eds) The nephrotic syndrome. Churchill Livingstone, New York, pp 85–120
6. Hostetter TH (1986) Pathogenosis of diabetic nephropathy. In: Mitch WE, Brenner BM, Stein JH (eds) The progressive nature of renal disease. Churchill Livingstone, New York, pp 149–166 (Contemporary issues in nephrology vol 14)
7. Matsubara M, Taguma Y, Kurosawa K, Hotta O, Suzuki K, Futaki G (1989) Effect of camostat mesilate on heavy proteinuria in various nephropathies. Clin Nephrol 32:119–123
8. Matsubara M, Taguma Y, Kurosawa K, Hotta O, Suzuki K, Ishizaki M (to be published) Effect of camostat mesilate for the treatment of advanced diabetic nephropathy. J Lab Clin Med
9. Reaven GM (1988) Role of insulin resistance in human disease. Diabetes 37:1595–1607
10. Jenkins AC, Dreslinski GR, Tardos SS, Groel JT, Fand R, Herczeg SA (1985) Captopril in hypertension: Seven years later. J Cardiovasc Pharmacol 7:S96–101

Transport of Organic Molecules

Chair: Karl J. Ullrich (FRG)
Takeshi Hoshi (Japan)

Transport of Organic Molecules

K.J. ULLRICH[1]

Introduction

If we consider the transport processes in the proximal renal tubule, this symposium deals with the majority of transport agencies which are present there (Fig. 1): The transporter for glucose, luminally Na^+-dependent, contraluminally not so: the transporters for amino acids and for sulfate, again luminally Na^+-dependent, contraluminally not; Na^+-dependent transport processes for dicarboxylate at both cell sides; and then the two secretory systems a] for organic anions, contraluminally in exchange for α-ketoglutarate and luminally partially electrogenic, partially working as exchanger and b] for organic cations contraluminally driven by an electrogenic exchange and luminally driven by an H^+-organic cation antiport.

Since I personally have been working for eight years now with the stop flow peritubular capillary perfusion method to characterize contraluminal anion and cation transport systems, you expect at least a short message from me: As Fig. 2 shows, the *para*-aminohipporate (PAH) transporter likes substrates with a negative charge and a hydrophobic core. The negative charge may be one ionic negative charge or a partial negative charge. However, there can be a second ionic or partial negative charge. In each case a hydrophobic core is needed. When two ionic negative charges, or one ionic negative charge and a partial negative charge are 5-9 Å apart on a molecule, then the molecule is a substrate for the dicarboxylate transporter and if the negative charges are 3-7 Å apart then it is a substrate for the contraluminal sulfate/oxalate transporter. If the substrates for the dicarboxylate and sulfate transporter have, in addition, a hydrophobic core then they are also substrates for the PAH transporter. Thus, many substrates interact with two or with all three contraluminal anion transporters. The contraluminal organic cation transporter requires a positive ionic charge

---

[1]Max-Planck-Institut für Biophysik, 6000 Frankfurt 70, Federal Republic of Germany

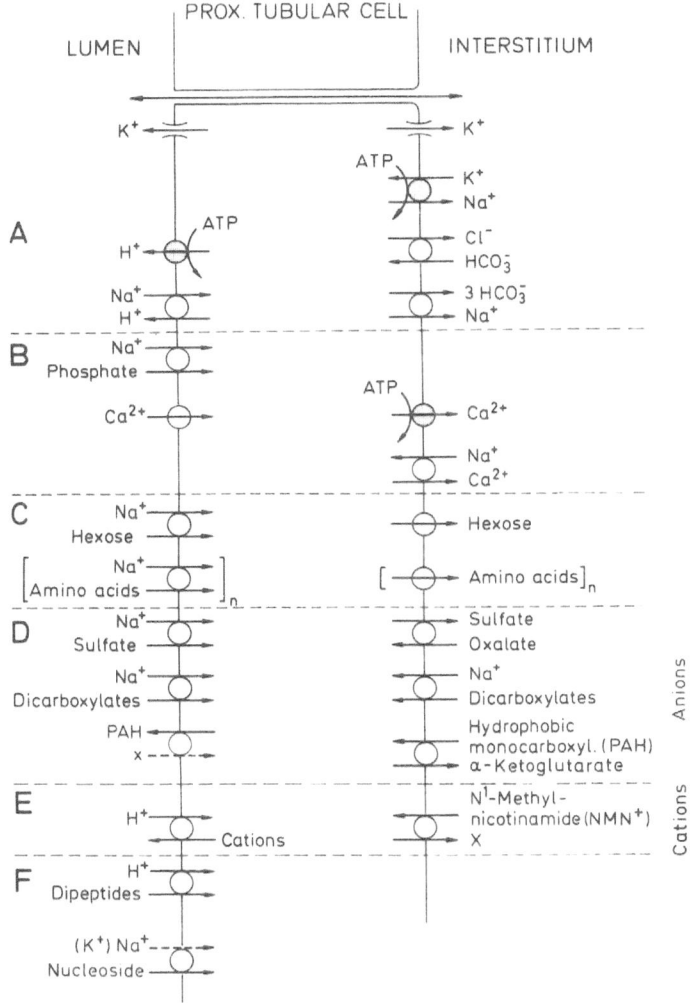

PROX. TUBULAR CELL

LUMEN   INTERSTITIUM

Fig. 1. Sidedness of the transport processes in the proximal renal tubule

and a hydrophobic core. If a substrate has two positive charges its interaction with the transporter is reduced.

Table 1 shows specific inhibitors of contraluminal anion and cation transport: The PAH transport, which has a K_m of 0.08 mmol/l, can be specifically inhibited by benzoylbutyrate, apalcillin, cyano-hydroxycinnamate and nitroazidophenyl-alanine with a K_i of 0.01–0.02 mmol/l. *Sulfate transport*, which has a rather high K_m of 1.4 mmol/l, can be specifically inhibited by thiosulfate, although the K_i, at 0.33 mmol/l, is also relatively high. *For dicarboxylate*, a specific substrate does not seem to exist. Thus, succinate and the best inhibitor, tetrafluorosuccinate, also interact

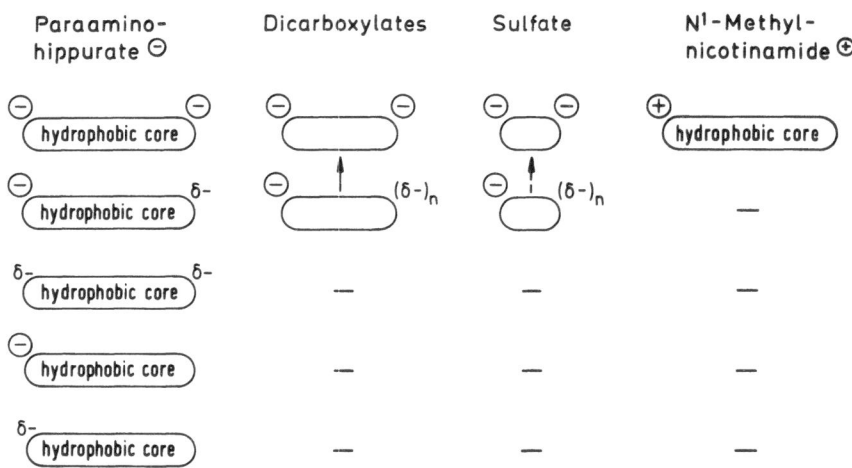

Fig. 2. Schematic specificity pattern of the PAH, dicarboxylate, and sulfate contraluminal organic anion transport systems, and the organic cation N^1-methylnicotinamide transport system, in the proximal renal tubule

with the PAH transporter, although with a much higher K_i value, i.e., much lower affinity. Contraluminal transport for *N^1-methylnicotinamide* (K_m 0.54 mmol/l) can be inhibited by a number of tetraalkylammonium compounds and methylnicotinamide analogues with a K_i around 0.1 mmol/l. Only one compound interacts much better than N^1-methylnicotinamide: a heptafluorobutyroxy-analogue of N^1-methylpyridinium.

Table 1. Specific inhibitors for contraluminal *anion and cation transport* in the proximal renal tubule (K_i and K_m in mmol/l)

	PAH $K_{i,PAH}$	Succinate $K_{i,Succ}$	Sulfate $K_{i,SO4^{2-}}$
PAH	0.08 (K_m)	1.9	NS
Benzoylbutyrate	0.02	NS	NS
Apalcillin	0.02	NS	NS
2-Cyano-3-hydroxy-cinnamate	<0.01	NS	4.45
2-Nitro-4-azido-phenylalanine	<0.01	NS	NS
Sulfate	NS	NS	1.4 (K_m)
Thiosulfate	NS	NS	0.33
Succinate	1.3	0.09 (K_m)	NS
Tetrafluor-succinate	1.4	0.05	NS

	N^1-methylnicotinamide $K_{i,NMN}$
N^1-Methylnicotinamide	0.54 (K_m)
Tetraethylammonium Cl⁻	0.07
Tetrapropylammonium Cl⁻	0.08
Tetrabutylammonium Cl⁻	0.09
N'-Trifluoroethyl-N^1-methylnicotinamide	0.14
N^1-Trifluorobenzyl-nicotinamide	0.12
N^1-Methyl-2-methyl-4-heptafluoro-butyroxy-pyridinium	0.02

Table 2. Non-specific and relatively specific inhibitors of contraluminal *anion transport* in the proximal renal tubule (K_i and K_m in mmol/l)

	$K_{m,PAH}$ 0.08 $K_{i,PAH}$	$K_{m,Succ}$ 0.09 $K_{i,Succ}$	$K_{m,SO_4^{2-}}$ 1.4 $K_{i,SO_4^{2-}}$
Probenecid	0.03	NS	7.9
Tienilic acid	0.01	NS	2.7
Indomethacin	0.05	NS	1.4
Diisothiocyanato-dihydrostilbene- disulfonate (H_2DIDS)	0.02	1.8	0.4
Eosinthiocyanate	0.04	0.75	0.19
8-Anilinonaphthalene-1 sulfonate (8-ANS)	0.04	0.5	0.09
Bromphenol-blue	0.13	2.5	0.11
Orange G	0.15	NS	0.02

You might have missed your favorite inhibitors for organic anion transport: probenecid, indomethacin, DIDS, and 8-ANS. As is evident from Table 2 they unfortunately interact not only with the PAH transporter with rather high affinity (low app. K_i values), but also with the sulfate transporter, and some interact with the dicarbosylate transporter. Fortunately the affinity of probenecid for the sulfate transporter is low, so that probenecid could be considered as a rather specific inhibitor for PAH transport. More care must be taken with indomethacin, DIDS, and the other compounds listed because their affinity for PAH and sulfate transport might be equal. At the bottom is Orange-G which has a 7 times higher affinity for sulfate than for PAH transport. Thus, at 0.01 mmol/l, Orange-G can be considered as a specific inhibitor for contraluminal sulfate transport.

Strategies for Evaluating the Molecular Structure of Membrane Transport Systems

ERNEST M. WRIGHT[1]

SUMMARY. The strategies that have been successfully employed to identify and characterize the brush border Na$^+$/glucose cotransporter are summarized. These include the use of photoaffinity and covalent reagents, expression cloning, polyclonal antibodies to defined domains of the predicted sequence, and cDNA probes. The successful application of these strategies to renal membrane proteins will significantly advance the study of transporters for organic molecules.

Introduction

Over the past 30 years much effort has been directed at describing the non-electrolyte transport across epithelial cells. The transport systems involved have been carefully delineated and characterized kinetically. Particular progress has been achieved in understanding the underlying role of Na$^+$ pumps in the active transport of organic molecules across epithelia. The renal Na$^+$/K-pump (Na/K-ATPase) has been isolated, purified, reconstituted, cloned, and sequenced. The availability of antibodies and cDNA probes for the α and β subunits has revolutionized research on Na/K pumps. The importance of the pump for the transport of organic molecules is that it provides the energy ($\Delta \bar{\mu}_{Na}$) for secondary active transport of many solutes.

In the case of organic substances, much less progress has been realized, and this is due to (1) the low amounts of transport proteins in epithelial membranes (typically less than 0.1% of the membrane protein) and the attendant difficulty in isolating and purifying rare hydrophobic membrane proteins; (2) the general absence of high affinity inhibitors and specific covalent probes. So, despite the fact that a dozen or so epithelial transporters have been described over the past 30 years, only a few have been identified, and only one has been cloned, sequenced, and expressed.

In this report I will describe the strategies that have been employed in the identification, characterization, and cloning of the intestinal brush border Na$^+$/glucose

[1]Department of Physiology, UCLA School of Medicine, Los Angeles, CA 90024-1751, USA

cotransporter. This is the archetypical eukaryote Na^+ cotransporter, and it has an advantage in that a high affinity competitive inhibitor, phlorizin, is available.

The first clues to the identity of the Na^+/glucose cotransporter came from a study by Semenza's group, using a H^3-azidophlorizin as a photoaffinity probe [1]. Despite a very high background incorporation of the label into brush border proteins, protection experiments with D-glucose and cold phlorizin revealed specific labeling of a 70–75 kDa polypeptide. This was subsequently confirmed by Semenza's group, using a monoclonal body [2], and by our group, using covalent group-specific reagents.

Our strategy with group-specific reagents was simply to screen reagents for their effect on Na^+/glucose cotransport in brush border vesicles, and then to attempt to protect against inhibiting reagents with Na^+ and D-glucose [3,4]. We first found that the lysine reagent phenylisothiocyanate (PITC) was a potent inhibitor and that the transporter was protected by the presence of Na^+ *and* D-glucose (or phlorizin). Neither Na^+ nor D-glucose alone protected, and the requirement for Na^+ and D-glucose was specific. The next step was to label the protein; the approach was, first, to react the membranes with PITC in the presence of Na^+ and D-glucose (to derivatize all exposed lysine residues), then to wash the membranes free of PITC, Na^+, and D-glucose, and finally, to label the membranes with a fluorescent PITC derivative (FITC). The brush borders were then subjected to SDS-PAGE analysis and the gel was sliced and assayed for FITC. We found a single band of protein, 70–75 kDa, labeled with FITC, and this labeling was blocked when the FITC labeling was conducted in the presence of Na^+ and D-glucose. Similar experiments carried out with tyrosine group-specific reagents, e.g., N-acetyl-imidazole, also labeled the 70–75 kDa band, and this was specifically blocked with physiological levels of Na^+. We concluded that lysines were near the D-glucose binding site and that tyrosine residues were near the Na^+ binding site on the polypeptide.

Using this differential labeling approach with fluorescent or non-fluorescent group-specific reagents, the Na^+/proline and Na^+/phosphate intestinal brush border cotransporters were identified as 100 kDa and 140 kDa polypeptides, respectively [5,6]. In principle, this approach can be employed to identify other intestinal and renal transport proteins. Given success in labeling membrane transporters, it should then be possible to isolate and purify the polypeptide to homogeneity. The intestinal Na^+/glucose cotransporter has been partially purified by chromatofocusing (pI ~ 5.3) [7]. More recently, it has apparently been purified to homogeneity in an active form, although no conventional purity criteria (e.g., amino acid composition, N-terminal microsequencing) have been presented [8].

Two successful studies have been reported in which Na^+-cotransporters were identified using functional assays. The brain Na/Cl/GABA-cotransporter was purified, using reconstitution of transport activity in liposomes as an assay [9], and this provided a reagent for the conventional molecular cloning of the GABA transporter cDNA [10]. An alternative approach, involving expression cloning, was employed by our group to identify the intestinal Na^+/glucose cotransporter [11]. The starting point was the observation that the rabbit intestinal Na^+/glucose cotransporter could be expressed in a functional form in *Xenopus* oocyte plasma membrane after the injection of intestinal mRNA. The mRNA was enriched by electrophoresis (in a 2.3 kb fraction), a cDNA library was made in an expression plasmid (Bluescript), and the clones were screened by injected RNA synthesized from the clones, using the T_3 and

T$_7$ promoters. A single 2.3 kb clone was isolated that coded for the classical Na$^+$/glucose cotransporter. The advantage of expression cloning is that a functional clone is isolated, which may be expressed (using a suitable vector) in cultured cells (oocytes, COS-7 cells, fibroblasts, etc.) [12].

The clone was sequenced and found to code for a 662 amino acid polypeptide with a predicted molecular weight of 73 kDa. The sequence showed no homology to any other eukaryote protein, but had high homology to the *E. coli* Na$^+$/protein cotransporters [13]. Again, in principle, this expression cloning strategy may be used to clone other transport proteins. So far, we have expressed renal transporters for lysine, alanine, phenylalanine, and succinate in oocytes, and found that all are coded by 2–3 kb RNA fractions [14]. The next step is to construct a cDNA library from this mRNA fraction and to screen the library.

Once a transporter has been cloned and sequenced, it is then possible to generate antibodies to the protein. Short peptides (10–20 residues), corresponding to specific domains on the predicted secondary structure of the cloned protein, can be synthesized and these are used to raise polyclonal antibodies. We have, so far, obtained two useful antibodies to the intestinal Na$^+$/glucose cotransporter (B.A. Hirayama, unpublished results). Using Western analysis, these antibodies have been found to recognize the cotransporter both in intestinal brush borders, from alligator to man, and in renal brush borders (pig, rabbit, human). These results have been confirmed using Northern analysis [15]. We have also used cDNA probes to isolate clones for the human intestinal [13] and rabbit renal [15] Na$^+$/glucose cotransporters.

In the case of the brush border Na$^+$/glucose cotransporter, we are now poised to map the human gene, examine the genetic defect in glucose-galactose malabsorption, and to probe the structure/function relations of the transport protein. We anticipate that similar biochemical and molecular approaches will be used to great advantage to unravel the secrets of organic solute transport by the kidney.

References

1. Hosang M, Vasella A, Semenza G (1981) Specific photoaffinity inactivation of the D-glucose transporter in small intestinal brush border membrane using new phlorizin analogues. Biochemistry 20:5844–5854
2. Schmidt UM, Eddy B, Frazer CM, Venter CJ, Semenza G (1983) Isolation of (a subunit of) the Na$^+$/D-glucose cotransporter(s) of rabbit intestinal brush border membranes using monoclonal antibodies. FEBS Lett 161:279–283
3. Peerce BE, Wright EM (1984) Sodium-induced conformational changes in the glucose transporter of intestinal brush borders. J Biol Chem 259:14105–14112
4. Peerce BE, Wright EM (1985) Evidence for tyrosyl residues at the Na$^+$ site on the intestinal Na$^+$/glucose cotransporter. J Biol Chem 260:6026–6031
5. Wright EM, Peerce BE (1984) Identification and conformational changes of the intestinal proline carrier. J Biol Chem 259:14993–14996
6. Peerce BE (1989) Identification of the intestinal Na$^+$/phosphate cotransporter. Am J Physiol 256:6645–6652
7. Peerce BE, Wright EM (1986) Distance between substrate sites on the glucose/glucose cotransporter by fluorescence energy transfer. Proc Natl Acad Sci USA 83:8092–8096
8. Peerce BE, Clarke RD (1990) Isolation and reconstitution of the intestinal Na$^+$/glucose cotransporter. J Biol Chem 265:1731–1736

9. Radian R, Bendahan A, Kanner BI (1986) Purification and identification of the functional sodium- and chloride-coupled γ-aminobutyric acid transport glycoprotein from rat brain. J Biol Chem 261:15437–15441
10. Guastella J, Nelson N, Nelson H, Czyzyk L, Keynan S, Miedel MC, Davidson N, Lester HA, Kanner BI (1990) Cloning and expression of a rat brain GABA transporter. Science 249:1303–1306
11. Hediger MA, Coady MJ, Ikeda TS, Wright EM (1987) Expression cloning and cDNA sequencing of the Na$^+$/glucose cotransporter. Nature 330:379–381
12. Birnir B, Lee H-S, Hediger MA, Wright EM (1990) Expression and characterization of the intestinal Na$^+$/glucose cotransporter in COS-7 cells. Biochim Biophys Acta 1048:100–104
13. Hediger MA, Turk E, Wright EM (1989) Homology of the human intestinal Na$^+$/glucose and *Escherichia coli* Na$^+$/proline cotransporters. Proc Natl Acad Sci USA 86:5748–5752
14. Coady MJ, Pajor AM, Toloza EM, Wright EM (1990) Expression of mammalian renal transporters in *Xenopus laevis* oocytes. Arch Biochem Biophys 283:130–134
15. Coady MJ, Pajor AM, Wright EM (1990) Sequence homologies amongst intestinal and renal Na$^+$/glucose cotransporters. Am J Physiol (Cell Physiol) 259:C605–C610

p-Aminohippurate Uptake Across the Basolateral Membrane of Rat Proximal Tubule Cells: Specificity and Mode of Energetization

GERHARD BURCKHARDT, CHRISTIANE SCHMITT, and KARL JULIUS ULLRICH[1]

SUMMARY. Uptake of [³H]PAH (*p*-aminohippurate) across the basolateral membrane of rat proximal tubule cells was studied in intact kidneys and membrane vesicles to determine biologically and pharmacologically important substrates of the PAH transporter and its energization by ion gradients. Effective inhibition of in situ [³H]PAH uptake by *trans*-2-decanoate, α-ketoglutarate, prostaglandin E_2, 11-dehydrocorticosterone, and dibutyryl cyclic GMP suggests an involvement of the PAH transporter in cellular entry and exit of metabolic products, selected hormones and second messengers. The high affinity for N-acetyl-, N-benzoyl-, N-acetylcysteine-, sulfate- and glucuronide-conjugates supports the role of the PAH transporter in renal excretion of metabolites. Among the drugs, apalcillin proved an inhibitor of high affinity (app. $K_{i,PAH}$ 0.02 mM) and selectivity for the PAH transporter. The nephrotoxic agents, ochratoxin A, orellanin, and β-amanitin, also inhibited in situ [³H]PAH uptake indicating that their cellular uptake proceeds *via* the PAH transporter. In vesicles, glutarate and an out > in Na^+ gradient, but not a Na^+ gradient alone, drove uphill [³H]PAH accumulation. Stimulation of [³H]PAH uptake was half-maximal at 10.8 μM glutarate and 2.3 mM Na^+ with 3 Na^+ ions being involved. These results reflect the kinetic properties of the $(Na^+)_3$-dicarboxylate cotransporter and prove its role in uphill PAH transport. Glutarate/PAH exchange is electroneutral, suggesting either exchange of one glutarate for two PAH molecules, or the involvement of hitherto undefined ions in the exchange process. In conclusion, PAH uptake across the basolateral membrane occurs through exchange with α-ketoglutarate, which is itself intracellularly accumulated by the Na^+-coupled dicarboxylate transporter.

Introduction

The kidney has the capability to excrete a large number of endogenous and exogenous organic anions. Many of these compounds undergo filtration in the glomeruli and net

[1]Max-Planck-Institut für Biophysik, Kennedyallee 70, D-6000 Frankfurt 70, Federal Republic of Germany

secretion in the proximal tubules [1–3]. Secretion involves uptake of organic anions across the contraluminal (basolateral) membrane into the cell and exit from the cell into the tubulus lumen via the luminal (brush-border) membrane. Transport across the cell membranes in turn involves interaction of the anions with specialized transport systems. Using homologous series of substrates three organic anion transport systems with overlapping specificities have been found in the basolateral membrane of rat proximal tubule cells [4,5]: *First*, an anion exchanger accommodating sulfate, oxalate, HCO_3^-, and organic anions which bear two negative charges, or one negative and a partial negative charge, at less than 7 Å distance; *second*, a Na^+-coupled dicarboxylate transporter interacting with Krebs cycle intermediates as well as with organic anions carrying two negative charges, or one ionic and one partial negative charge, at 5–9 Å distance; *third*, the "*p*-aminohippurate (PAH) transporter" which accepts substrates with one or two partial, or one or two ionic negative charges at 6–10 Å distance and having a hydrophobic domain of at least 4 Å length.

Uptake of PAH across the basolateral membrane occurs "uphill" and requires energy. As reviewed recently [6] PAH uptake into renal cortical cells was impaired by anaerobic conditions, uncouplers of oxidative phosphorylation, lowering of temperature, addition of cyanide, as well as by removal of Na^+ or K^+, or addition of ouabain. Taken together these data suggested that intact metabolism is needed to create transmembrane gradients of Na^+ which drive uphill PAH transport presumably via a Na^+/PAH symporter. Pritchard [6,7] and Shimada et al. [8] suggested another mechanism for uphill transport of PAH. As indicated above, the basolateral membrane possesses a Na^+-coupled transport system for dicarboxylates. Since the PAH transporter shows affinity for some dicarboxylates too, both systems could cooperate through exchanging common substrates. Indeed, glutarate can be accumulated in basolateral membrane vesicles in the presence of an out > in gradient of Na^+, and can be subsequently exchanged for external labeled PAH. Thereby, the Na^+ gradient drives PAH uptake indirectly, i.e. via accumulation of glutarate, rather than by acting directly on the PAH transporter.

In this contribution we tested endogenous and pharmacologically important compounds as possible substrates of the PAH transporter, including those Krebs cycle intermediates that could serve for driving uphill PAH transport at the basolateral membrane. We also performed experiments with basolateral membrane vesicles to offer additional evidence for the involvement of the Na^+-coupled dicarboxylate transporter during PAH accumulation.

Methods

Experiments on the Intact Kidney

The details of measuring contraluminal influx of radioactively labeled substrates from the interstitium into the cells, and the mode of evaluating the transport parameters have been described elsewhere [9]. In essence, immediately after clamping the renal artery and vein, a blood capillary was punctured with an oil-filled sampling pipette. At 100–140 μm distance another blood vessel was impaled by a filling pipette containing tritiated PAH or methyl-succinate, and [^{14}C]inulin as a reference substance for estimation of the extracellular space. Besides 0.1 mM

[³H]PAH, the solution in the filling pipette contained (in mM): 150 Na⁺, 4 K⁺, 154 gluconate, at pH 7.4. When dicarboxylate uptake was tested the filling pipette contained (in mM): 0.15 [³H]-methyl-succinate, 136 Na⁺, 4 K⁺, 1.5 Ca²⁺, 1 Mg²⁺, 120 Cl⁻, and 25 HCO₃⁻, gassed with 95% O₂/5% CO₂. The test solutions were rapidly injected into the capillary and withdrawn after 2 s through the sampling pipette. The recovered radioactivity was determined by liquid scintillation counting. To screen for inhibitors of transport 1–10 mM of test anions were applied together with the labeled substrates. Using previously determined K_m values for PAH (0.08 mM [10]) an apparent K_i was determined from the degree of inhibition of contraluminal uptake, assuming competitive inhibition.

Experiments on basolateral membrane vesicles. Vesicles were prepared from the cortex of rat kidneys by the Percoll density gradient technique described by Scalera et al. [11]. They were preloaded with 150 mM KCl, 20 mM Hepes buffered with Tris to pH 7.4, adjusted to a protein concentration of 10 mg/ml, and stored in liquid nitrogen. For the experiment, 5 µl of vesicle suspension was added to 95 µl prewarmed (37°C) incubation medium containing (in mM) 0.05 [³H]PAH, 150 NaCl, KCl, or tetramethylammonium chloride, respectively, and 20 Hepes/Tris, pH 7.4. Further additions are indicated in the legends. Uptake was stopped by addition of 1 ml ice-cold solution containing 150 mM NaCl, 20 mM Hepes/Tris, at pH 7.4, and separation of vesicles from the medium by rapid filtration. The radioactivity remaining with the vesicles on the filters was determined by liquid scintillation counting. The figures show means ± SD from 4–5 determinations.

Results and Discussion

At low concentrations, PAH is handled by a single transport system in the basolateral membrane, the PAH transporter (apparent K_m, 0.08 mM [10]). The interaction with the (Na⁺)₃-dicarboxylate cotransporter is weak (inhibition of succinate uptake with an apparent K_i of 1.9 mM [12]) and that with the sulfate transporter not detectable [5]. Although a selective test anion, PAH is not the natural substrate of the PAH transport system. Searching for putative endogenous substrates we screened previously tested compounds for those having the highest affinities towards the PAH transporter. These compounds are listed in Table 1. Fatty acids such as, e.g., *trans*-2-decanoate, or dicarboxylates of intermediate chain length, e.g., α-ketoglutarate, interact strongly with the PAH transporter. Their affinity for the PAH transporter is nearly three times that of PAH. Comparably high affinities are displayed by hormones (prostaglandin E₂ and 11-dehydro-corticosterone) as well as by a derivatized second messenger, dbcGMP. The naturally occurring second messengers, cAMP and cGMP, also interact with the PAH transporter although with lower affinities (apparent K_i, 2.6 and 0.34 mM, respectively [13]). Another metabolite strongly inhibiting PAH transport is 3,7-diketo-cholate, an oxidized form of the unconjugated bile salt cholate. These results suggest that the PAH transporter may be involved in the exit and entry of fatty acids, some Krebs cycle intermediates, and, notably, the exit and entry of some hormones and second messengers. Whether the PAH transporter is thus involved in paracrine functions in the kidney and, possibly, in other cells remains an interesting question to be solved in the future.

Table 1. Biologically and pharmacologically important compounds which interact with the PAH transport system in the basolateral membrane

Compounds	$K_{i,PAH}$ (mM)
A. Metabolites and hormones	
Trans-2-decanoate	0.03
α-Ketoglutarate	0.03
Prostaglandin E_2	0.08
Dibutyryl-cyclic GMP	0.04
11-Dehydro-corticosterone	0.02
3,7-Diketo-cholate	0.17
B. Conjugates	
L-tryptophyl-L-tryptophan	0.21
N-α-acetyl-L-glutamate	0.17
N-α-benzoyl-D-glutamate	0.04
Pentachlorobutadienyl-L-cysteine	0.07
Pentachlorobutadienyl-N-acetyl-L-cysteine	0.07
Taurolithocholate-sulfate	0.17
Lithocholate-glucuronide	0.15
C. Drugs	
Probenecid	0.03
3,4-Dichlorophenoxy-acetate	0.03
Apalcillin	0.02
Cephodizime	0.22
Glycine-salicylate (salycuric acid)	0.03
Mercaptoethanedisulfide	0.25

The compounds listed have been tested as inhibitors of [3H]PAH uptake in the intact kidney. (From [13,14,16,31,32])

Table 1, B, lists conjugates with high affinities for the PAH transporter. These consist of a dipeptide, N-acetylated and N-benzoylated L-glutamate, cysteine- and N-acetyl-cysteine-conjugates of pentachlorobutadiene, and the sulfate- and glucuronide-conjugates of litho- and taurolithocholate. It should be emphasized that the unconjugated compounds, L-tryptophan, L-glutamate, pentachlorobutadiene, lithocholate and taurolithocholate interact weakly or not at all with the PAH transporter [14,15] either because they are too hydrophilic (amino acids) or too hydrophobic. Therefore, conjugation plays an important role in rendering compounds acceptable for the PAH transporter and, thus, for their disposal by renal excretion. Among the drugs listed in Table 1, C, the antibiotic apalcillin may prove suitable to specifically inhibit the PAH transporter, since it displays a high affinity for this system and does not interact with the sulfate and dicarboxylate carriers [16].

Table 2 lists compounds which are known to damage proximal tubule cells. The metabolite of *Aspergillus* and *Penicillium* fungi, ochratoxin A, occurs as contaminant in grain and is involved in the development of Balkan nephritis [17]. Other nephrotoxic agents are the mushroom toxins, orellanin [18], and amanitin [19]. These toxins as well as the carcinogen, aflatoxin B_1, inhibit PAH uptake with apparent K_i values ranging between 0.02 and 2.3 mM, suggesting that these compounds enter proximal tubule cells and are accumulated to toxic levels by the PAH transporter. The primary location of lesions in proximal tubules is in accordance with this assumption.

Table 2. Interaction of nephrotoxic agents with the PAH transporter

Compounds	$K_{i,PAH}$ (mM)
Ochratoxin A	0.02
Aflatoxin B_1	0.41
Orellanin	0.13
α-Amanitin	2.3
β-Amanitin	0.7

Data for amanitins are from [14]; the other results are from unpublished observations

Since α-ketoglutarate inhibits [³H]PAH uptake from the blood into the cell (cf Table 1) the ability of other Krebs cycle intermediates to interact with the PAH transporter was tested; the result is shown in Fig. 1, top. Only α-ketoglutarate strongly inhibits the PAH transporter. In contrast, all dicarboxylates proved to be efficient inhibitors of the Na⁺-coupled dicarboxylate transporter, whereas the tricarboxylates, citrate and isocitrate, inhibit less (Fig. 1, bottom). Thus, of all the intermediates, α-ketoglutarate has a high affinity for both PAH and dicarboxylate transporter, and should therefore be suited to energize PAH uptake across the basolateral membrane. This was tested in the experiment for which results are shown in Fig. 2. Basolateral membrane vesicles were loaded with KCl and suspended at zero time in a buffer containing NaCl and [³H]PAH without or with 10 μM glutarate. In the absence of glutarate, [³H]PAH was not accumulated above the equilibrium value, indicating that the Na⁺ gradient alone cannot drive uphill PAH uptake. In the presence of glutarate (or α-ketoglutarate [20]), however, PAH uptake was markedly stimulated and transiently exceeded the equilibrium value. This result, which is in agreement with our and Pritchard's earlier observations [7,8,20], indicates Na⁺-coupled uptake of glutarate (or α-ketoglutarate) into the vesicles and subsequent exchange of intravesicular glutarate for extravesicular [³H]PAH.

In order to substantiate the cooperation of Na⁺-coupled dicarboxylate transporter and PAH/dicarboxylate exchanger, the effect of Li⁺, which inhibits the dicarboxylate transporter was tested [12,21]. Li⁺ had no effect on PAH/[³H]PAH exchange but inhibited [³H]PAH uptake driven by external glutarate and Na⁺ [7,8]. This result indicates that glutarate is taken up by the Li⁺-sensitive dicarboxylate transporter and subsequently exchanges for PAH via the Li⁺-insensitive PAH transporter. A further argument for the involvement of the Na⁺-coupled dicarboxylate transporter during PAH accumulation in basolateral membrane vesicles is provided by the results of the experiment shown in Fig. 3. Here, the dependence of [³H]PAH uptake was tested as a function of glutarate and Na⁺ concentration in the medium. At a fixed Na⁺ concentration (150 mM) increasing glutarate concentrations caused an increasing stimulation of PAH uptake. Corrected for [³H]PAH uptake observed in the absence of glutarate, this stimulation follows Michaelis-Menten kinetics, exhibiting an apparent K_m of 5.1 μM. In three experiments of this type, a mean K_m of 10.8 μM (SE 2.9) was found. This K_m value reflects the high affinity for its substrates of the dicarboxylate transporter in basolateral membrane vesicles [21,22]. At a fixed glutarate concentration (10 μM, Fig. 3, right panel), increasing Na⁺ concentrations stimulate [³H]PAH uptake. As opposed to glutarate, stimulation by Na⁺ does not follow simple

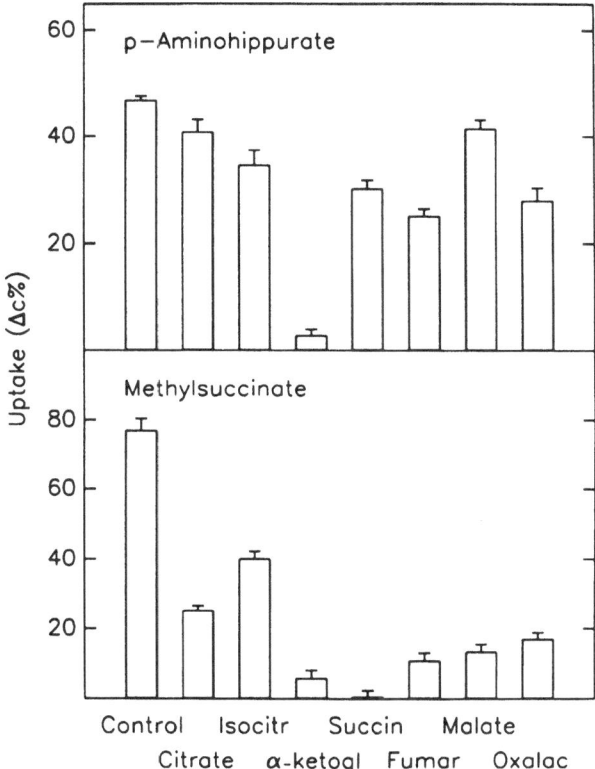

Fig. 1. Interaction of Krebs cycle intermediates with the renal contraluminal transporters for PAH and dicarboxylates. [³H]PAH and [³H]methyl-succinate uptake across the basolateral membrane was measured in the intact kidney. The indicated Krebs cycle intermediates were added at 10 mM concentration to the test solutions containing 0.1 mM [³H]PAH (*top panel*) or 0.15 mM [³H]methyl-succinate (*bottom panel*). Controls received the labeled substrates without added intermediates. The ordinate shows the decrease in [³H]PAH and [³H]methyl-succinate concentrations in the capillaries within 2 s incubation time. (Data from [12,31])

Michaelis-Menten kinetics. The data can, rather, be fitted to an equation taking the interaction of 3 Na⁺ ions with the carrier into account [23]. A half-maximal effect of Na⁺ is observed at 2.3 mM. The interaction of more than one sodium ion is typical for the dicarboxylate transporter; kinetic experiments and its electrogenicity [21,22] suggest that three sodium ions are cotransported with one doubly negatively charged dicarboxylate (surplus of one positive charge during cotransport). Taken together, the data shown in Fig. 3 reflect the properties of the (Na⁺)₃-dicarboxylate cotransporter and thus prove its involvement in Na⁺ and (α-keto)glutarate-stimulated [³H]PAH uptake into basolateral membrane vesicles.

Next, we investigated whether the exchange of glutarate (two negative charges) for PAH (one negative charge) was electrogenic or electroneutral. As a control, we tested the influence of changes in membrane potential on PAH/[³H]PAH exchange. Vesicles

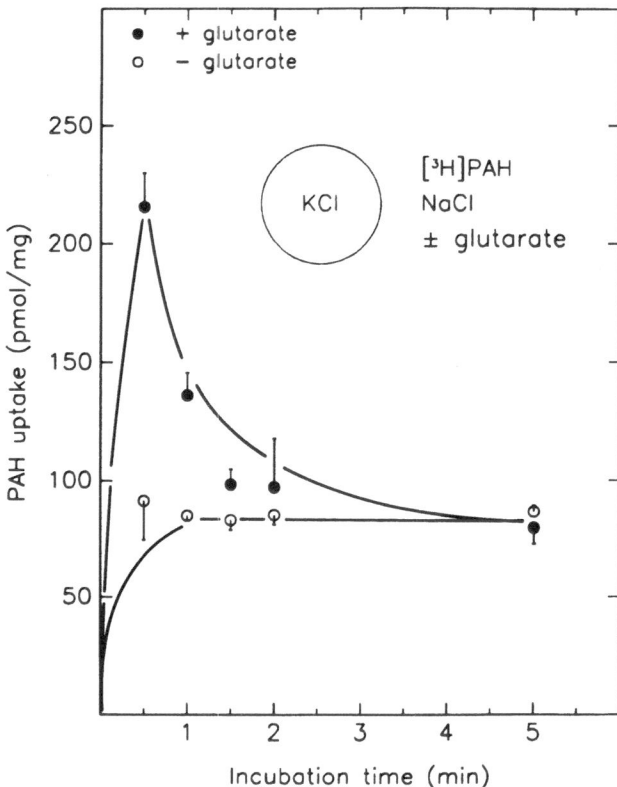

Fig. 2. Effect of glutarate and a Na⁺ gradient on PAH uptake into rat renal basolateral membrane vesicles. The vesicles were loaded with KCl and suspended in buffers containing NaCl, 0.05 mM [³H]PAH, and no (*open circles*) or 0.01 mM glutarate (*closed circles*). Uptake was terminated after the time periods indicated at the abscissa

were preloaded with KCl and either 1 mM PAH (for PAH/[³H]PAH exchange) or 1 mM glutarate (for glutarate/[³H]PAH exchange). At zero time the vesicles were diluted into media containing labeled PAH, the K⁺ ionophor valinomycin, and either KCl or tetramethylammonium chloride (TMA Cl). In this setting, the imposition of an in > out K⁺ gradient creates an inside negative K⁺ diffusion potential. This potential does not influence PAH/[³H]PAH exchange, as shown in Fig. 4, left panel (compare open bars with hatched bars). Surprisingly, the exchange of intravesicular glutarate for extravesicular [³H]PAH was also not influenced by the K⁺ diffusion potential, indicating an electroneutral exchange process (Fig. 4, right panel).

Electroneutral exchange can occur if one glutarate plus a proton is exchanged with PAH. In this case the hydrogen ion would compensate one negative charge of glutarate. Such an exchange should be favored by lowering pH, i.e., by increasing hydrogen ion concentration. Such a decrease in pH, however, rather decreased the rate of glutarate/PAH exchange (data not shown). Thus, we must assume that either

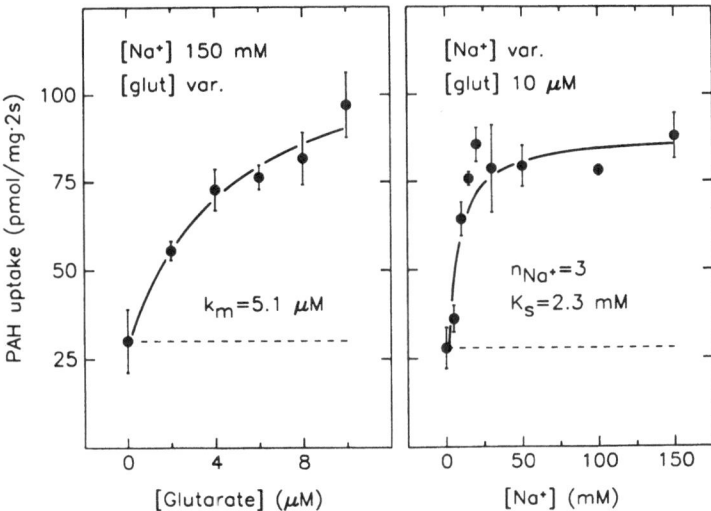

Fig. 3. Kinetics of cis-stimulation by glutarate and Na$^+$ of PAH uptake into basolateral membrane vesicles. *Left panel:* Vesicles loaded with KCl were added to media containing 150 mM NaCl, 0.05 mM [^{3}H]PAH, and 0–10 μM Na$_2$ glutarate. The curve fitted to the experimental results was calculated using a Michaelis-Menten equation with the parameters, K$_m$, 5.1 μM and V$_{max}$, 91.3 pmol/mg 2s. The dashed line shows [^{3}H]PAH uptake in the absence of glutarate. *Right panel:* Vesicles were suspended in buffers containing 0–150 mM NaCl, 150–0 mM tetramethylammonium Cl, 0.05 mM [^{3}H]PAH, and 0.01 mM glutarate. The curve was fitted to the data points considering the interaction of 3 Na$^+$ ions and using the kinetic parameters K$_s$ 2.3 mM and V$_{max}$ 60.1 pmol/mg 2s. The dashed line indicates [^{3}H]PAH uptake in the absence of Na$^+$

2 PAH molecules are exchanged for one glutarate, or that a hitherto unknown intravesicular (intracellular) cation or extravesicular (extracellular) anion is also involved in the exchange process.

Conclusions and Outlook

Experimental evidence indicates that uphill PAH uptake across the basolateral membrane of proximal tubule cells requires the cooperation of three transport systems. The (Na$^+$ + K$^+$)-ATPase maintains an out > in Na$^+$ gradient across the basolateral membrane and an in > out K$^+$ gradient, which in turn is responsible for the inside negative electrical potential difference across the basolateral membrane. The electrogenic (Na$^+$)$_3$-dicarboxylate cotransporter utilizes the electrochemical gradient for Na$^+$ ions for uptake and intracellular accumulation of α-ketoglutarate. In a final step, α-ketoglutarate exchanges for extracellular PAH (or other suitable organic anions). Thus, uphill PAH transport is indirectly energized by the Na$^+$ gradient (tertiary active transport). From our studies α-ketoglutarate seems to be the

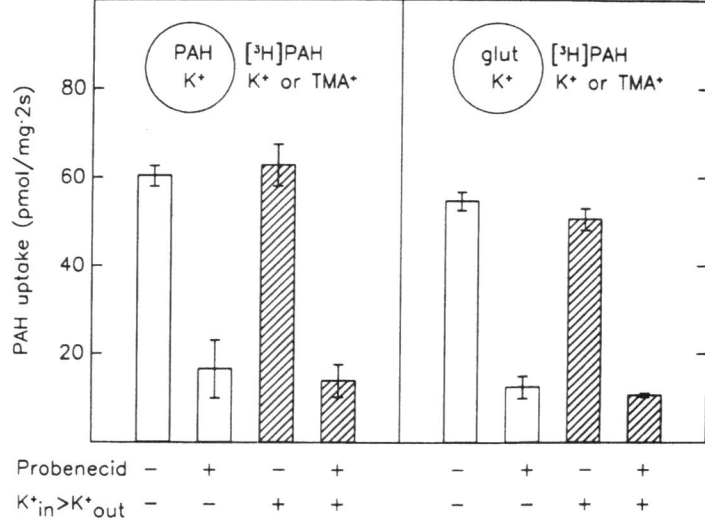

Fig. 4. Lack of effect of membrane potential on PAH/[³H]PAH (*left*) and glutarate/[³H]PAH exchange (*right*). Basolateral membrane vesicles were loaded with 150 mM KCl, either 1 mM PAH or glutarate, and suspended in 150 mM KCl or 150 mM tetramethylammonium (*TMA⁺*) chloride ($K^+_{in} > K^+_{out}$) containing 5 μM valinomycin, 0.05 mM [³H]PAH, and 0 or 1 mM probenecid. Uptake of [³H]PAH was stopped after 2 s incubation time

only naturally occurring dicarboxylate which can be utilized in the coupled action of dicarboxylate and PAH transporters.

Data presented in this contribution suggest a physiologic role of the PAH transporter in translocation of long chain fatty acids, some steroid hormones and second messengers. The pharmacologically important role of this transport system relies on its ability to accept anionic xenobiotics and drugs and/or their metabolic products. The PAH transporter also plays an important pathophysiological role in cellular uptake and in the intracellular accumulation of toxic compounds which subsequently damage proximal tubule cells.

One of the questions remaining is the definition of PAH exit from the cell across the luminal membrane. Rabbit and pig proximal tubule cells possess in their brush-border membrane a conductive transport system for PAH [24,25]. Thereby, the inside electrical potential difference across this membrane can be utilized to drive PAH (and urate) out of the cell into the lumen. In brush-border membrane vesicles from rat and dog, however, a transport system has been found which can exchange PAH for succinate [26]. Since the rat renal brush-border membrane contains also a Na⁺-coupled dicarboxylate transporter [27,28], PAH uptake would be favored rather than secretion, similar to the situation in the basolateral membrane. Net secretion may yet occur, due to different kinetic properties (affinities, maximal velocities) of the PAH transporters in the two membranes [29], or due to different substrate specificities, e.g., PAH/Cl⁻ and PAH/lactate exchange, in the brush-border [7,26,30], but not in the basolateral membrane. A detailed knowledge of organic anion uptake across the basolateral membrane and exit across the brush-border membrane may help in understanding and in preventing, the intracellular accumulation of nephrotoxic compounds.

Acknowledgments. The authors thank B. Moewes and G. Rumrich for their excellent technical assistance.

References

1. Despopoulos A (1965) A definition of substrate specificity in renal transport of organic anions. J Theor Biol 8:163–192
2. Møller JV, Sheikh MI (1983) Renal organic anion transport system: Pharmacological, physiological, and biochemical aspects. Pharmacol Rev 34:315–358
3. Weiner IM (1985) Organic acids and bases and uric acid. In: Seldin DW, Giebisch G (eds) The Kidney: Physiology and Pathophysiology. Raven, New York, pp 1703–1724
4. Fritzsch G, Rumrich G, Ullrich KJ (1989) Anion transport through the contraluminal cell membrane of renal proximal tubule. The influence of hydrophobicity and molecular charge distribution on the inhibitory activity of organic anions. Biochim Biophys Acta 978: 249–256
5. Ullrich KJ, Rumrich G (1988) Contraluminal transport systems in the proximal renal tubule involved in secretion of organic anions. Am J Physiol 254:F453–F462
6. Pritchard JB (1987) Luminal and peritubular steps in renal transport of *p*-aminohippurate. Biochim Biophys Acta 906:295–308
7. Pritchard JB (1988) Coupled transport of *p*-aminohippurate by rat kidney basolateral membrane vesicles. Am J Physiol 255:F597–F604
8. Shimada H, Moewes B, Burckhardt G (1987) Indirect coupling to Na⁺ of *p*-aminohippuric acid uptake into rat renal basolateral membrane vesicles. Am J Physiol 253:F795–F801
9. Fritzsch G, Haase W, Rumrich G, Fasold H, Ullrich KJ (1984) A stopped flow capillary perfusion method to evaluate contraluminal transport parameters of methylsuccinate from interstitium into renal proximal tubular cells. Pflügers Arch 400:250–256
10. Ullrich KJ, Rumrich G, Fritzsch G, Klöss S (1987) Contraluminal para-aminohippurate transport in the proximal tubule of the rat kidney. I. Kinetics, influence of cations, anions, and capillary preperfusion. Pflügers Arch 409:229–235
11. Scalera V, Huang Y-K, Hildmann B, Murer H (1981) A simple isolation method for basal-lateral membranes from rat kidney cortex. Membr Biochem 4:49–61
12. Ullrich KJ, Fasold H, Rumrich G, Klöss S (1984) Secretion and contraluminal uptake of dicarboxylic acids in the proximal convolution of rat kidney. Pflügers Arch 400:241–249
13. Ullrich KJ, Rumrich G, Papavassiliou F, Klöss S, Fritzsch G (to be published) Contraluminal para-aminohippurate transport in the proximal tubule of the rat kidney. VII. Specificity: Cyclic nucleotides, eicosanoids. Pflügers Arch
14. Ullrich KJ, Rumrich G, Wieland Th, Dekant W (1989) Contraluminal para-aminohippurate transport in the proximal tubule of the rat kidney. VI. Specificity: Amino acids, their N-methyl-, N-acetyl and N-benzoylderivatives; glutathione- and cysteine conjugates, di- and oligopeptides. Pflügers Arch 415:342–350
15. Ullrich KJ, Rumrich G, Mark G, Dekant W (1990) Transformation and transport: How does metabolic transformation change the affinity for the renal contraluminal anion and cation transporters? In: International Symposium on "Renal Disposition and Nephrotoxicity of Xenobiotics." Toxicol Lett 53:19–27

16. Ullrich KJ, Rumrich G, Klöss S (1989) Contraluminal organic anion and cation transport in the proximal renal tubule: V. Interaction with sulfamoyl- and phenoxy diuretics, and with β-lactam antibiotics. Kidney Int 36:78–88

17. Cooper P (1979) The kidney and ochratoxin A. Food Cosmet Toxicol 17:406–408

18. Prast H, Pfaller W (1988) Toxic properties of the mushroom *Cortinarius orellanus (Fries)*. II. Impairment of renal function in rats. Arch Toxicol 62:89–96

19. Fiume L, Marinozzi V, Nardi F (1969) The effect of amanitin poisoning on mouse kidney. Br J Exp Pathol 50:270–276

20. Burckhardt G, Ullrich KJ (1989) Organic anion transport across the contraluminal membrane – dependence on sodium. Kidney Int 36:370–377

21. Burckhardt G (1984) Sodium-dependent dicarboxylate transport in rat renal basolateral membrane vesicles. Pflügers Arch 401:254–261

22. Wright SH, Wunz TM (1987) Succinate and citrate transport in renal basolateral and brush-border membranes. Am J Physiol 253:F432–F439

23. Wright SH, Kippen I, Wright EM (1982) Stoichiometry of Na^+-succinate cotransport in renal brush-border Membranes. J Biol Chem 257:1773–1778

24. Martinez F, Manganel M, Montrose-Rafizadeh C, Werner D, Roch-Ramel F (1990) Transport of urate and *p*-aminohippurate in rabbit renal brush-border membranes. Am J Physiol 258:F1145–F1153

25. Werner D, Martinez F, Roch-Ramel F (1990) Urate and *p*-aminohippurate transport in the brush border membrane of the pig kidney. J Pharmacol Exp Ther 252:792–799

26. Guggino SE, Martin GJ, Aronson PS (1983) Specificity and modes of the anion exchanger in dog renal microvillus membranes. Am J Physiol 244:F612–F621

27. Kahn AM, Branham S, Weinman EJ (1984) Mechanism of L-malate transport in rat renal basolateral membrane vesicles. Am J Physiol 246:F779–F784

28. Sheridan E, Rumrich G, Ullrich KJ (1983) Reabsorption of dicarboxylic acids from the proximal convolution of rat kidney. Pflügers Arch 399:18–28

29. Kinsella JL, Holohan PD, Pessah NI, Ross CR (1979) Transport of organic ions in renal cortical luminal and antiluminal membrane vesicles. J Pharmacol Exp Ther 209:443–450

30. Kahn AM, Aronson PS (1983) Urate transport via anion exchange in dog renal microvillus membrane vesicles. Am J Physiol 244:F56–F63

31. Ullrich KJ, Rumrich G, Fritzsch G, Klöss S (1987) Contraluminal para-aminohippurate transport in the proximal tubule of the rat kidney. II. Specificity: Aliphatic dicarboxylic acids. Pflügers Arch 408:38–45

32. Ullrich KJ, Rumrich G, Klöss S (1987) Contraluminal para-aminohippurate transport in the proximal tubule of the rat kidney. III. Specificity: monocarboxylic acids. Pflügers Arch 409:547–554

Organic Cation Transport in the Renal Brush-Border and Basolateral Membranes

Ken-ichi Inui[1], Mikihisa Takano, and Ryohei Hori[2]

SUMMARY. To characterize the specific membrane events underlying the secretion of organic cations in the proximal tubules, the transport of tetraethylammonium (TEA), a prototype cation, has been studied, using brush-border and basolateral membrane vesicles isolated from rat renal cortex. TEA is transported across basolateral membranes via a carrier-mediated system, and this system is stimulated by an inside-negative membrane potential. The transport of TEA across brush-border membranes is driven by an H^+ gradient via an electroneutral H^+/organic cation antiport system. Aminocephalosporins such as cephalexin (an amphoteric molecule) share a common carrier transport system with TEA in brush-border membranes. The H^+/organic cation antiport system is very sensitive to pH (optimum pH 7.0), in contrast to organic anion and D-glucose transport systems. Sulfhydryl groups and histidine residues are essential for the H^+/organic cation antiport system in renal brush-border membranes.

Introduction

The function of the proximal tubule is to reabsorb solutes such as glucose and amino acids from the glomerular filtrate, and to secrete organic ions. Active secretion of organic ions in the proximal tubules is viewed as a means of eliminating many drugs and their metabolites from the body. The sequence of movement of organic ions is transport across basolateral membranes, accumulation in the cell, followed by efflux from the cell across brush-border membranes into the tubular fluid. Although the molecules secreted by the organic cation secretory mechanism have a variety of chemical structures, all contain a nitrogen atom carrying a positive charge at the

[1]Department of Hospital Pharmacy, School of Medicine, Tokyo Medical and Dental University, Bunkyo-ku, Tokyo, 113 Japan
[2]Department of Pharmacy, Kyoto University Hospital, Faculty of Medicine, Kyoto University, Sakyo-ku, Kyoto, 606 Japan

physiological pH. Numerous techniques have been used for studying the renal excretion of cations, including in vivo renal clearance and in vitro cortical slices. These techniques have generated a great deal of information about the overall sequence of events. However, it has been difficult to characterize the specific membrane events underlying the transepithelial transport of organic cations. In addition, transport studies with organic cations in intact tissues are limited because these compounds often lead to circulatory disturbances.

In recent years, a methodology has been developed for isolating the brush-border and basolateral membrane vesicles from renal cortex; the membrane vesicles have been used for the analysis of tubular transport of nutrients and organic ions in well-controlled conditions [1]. To obtain precise information about the mechanisms of tubular secretion of organic ions, we have studied the transport characteristics of p-aminohippurate (anion), tetraethylammonium (cation), and aminocephalosporin antibiotics (zwitterion) in brush-border and basolateral membranes. This article deals with the characteristics of organic cation transport systems in renal brush-border and basolateral membranes.

Organic Cation Transport Systems in Brush-Border and Basolateral Membranes

Brush-border and basolateral membrane vesicles were isolated from rat renal cortex by the methods of calcium precipitation and Percoll density gradient centrifugation, respectively [2].

To characterize organic cation transport systems, the uptake of tetraethylammonium, a prototype cation, was studied using brush-border and basolateral membrane vesicles [3]. In the concentration dependence of [^{3}H]tetraethylammonium uptake, the relationship between concentration and uptake rate was nonlinear in both membranes, providing evidence for saturability. After correction for the nonsaturable component, the kinetic values of K_m and V_{max} were 0.8 mM and 7.4 nmol/mg protein per min for brush-border membranes, and 2.5 mM and 5.6 nmol/mg protein per min for basolateral membranes, respectively. Vesicles preloaded with a high concentration of unlabeled tetraethylammonium showed enhancement of [^{3}H]tetraethylammonium accumulation by countertransport in brush-border and basolateral membranes. The countertransport effect, or trans-stimulation, is a criterion for carrier-mediated transport. These data suggest the contribution of a carrier-mediated transport system for tetraethylammonium in brush-border and basolateral membranes.

To obtain further information concerning the driving force of the transport, we studied the effect of various ionic conditions on the uptake of tetraethylammonium. Although ionic conditions had no effect on tetraethylammonium uptake in basolateral membranes, the presence of an outward sodium gradient stimulated the tetraethylammonium uptake by brush-border membrane vesicles; sodium chloride was inside the vesicles and potassium chloride was outside. Furthermore, by monitoring the changes in fluorescence of Acridine orange, we confirmed the intravesicular acidification of brush-border membrane vesicles with sodium inside and potassium outside. Therefore, the H$^+$ gradient was tested as to whether it could drive the active transport of tetraethylammonium.

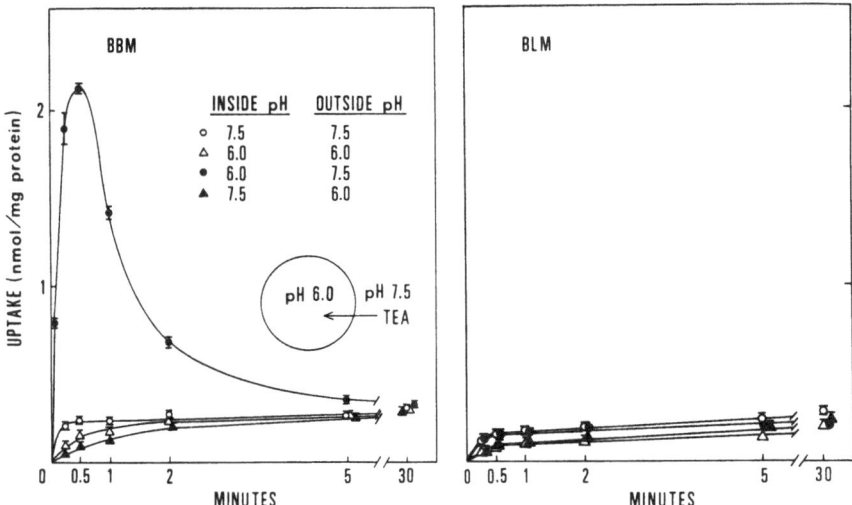

Fig. 1. Effect of H⁺ gradient on tetraethylammonium (*TEA*) uptake by brush-border (*BBM*) and basolateral membrane (*BLM*) vesicles. (From [3] with permission)

Figure 1 shows the effect of H⁺ gradient on tetraethylammonium uptake by brush-border and basolateral membrane vesicles [3]. In brush-border membranes, the presence of an outward H⁺ gradient (inside pH 6.0, outside pH 7.5) induced a transient uphill transport of tetraethylammonium (overshoot phenomenon), while an inward H⁺ gradient resulted in the lowest uptake. The final levels of uptake were all identical, indicating that the pH gradient did not affect vesicle size. In contrast, the H⁺ gradient was ineffective in the transport of tetraethylammonium in basolateral membranes. These data strongly suggest that tetraethylammonium transport across brush-border membranes is driven actively by an outward H⁺ gradient: that is, an H⁺/organic cation antiport system.

It is important to clarify the role of membrane potential as a driving force in tetraethylammonium uptake by brush-border and basolateral membrane vesicles. To produce an inside-negative membrane potential, the potassium ionophore valinomycin was employed in the presence of an outward potassium gradient. Tetraethylammonium uptake by brush-border membrane vesicles was unaffected by valinomycin. In contrast, a valinomycin-induced inside-negative membrane potential significantly stimulated the initial rate of tetraethylammonium uptake by basolateral membrane vesicles.

These data suggest that tetraethylammonium is transported across basolateral membranes via a carrier-mediated system, which is stimulated by an inside-negative membrane potential. Tetraethylammonium transport across brush-border membranes is driven by an H⁺ gradient via an electroneutral H⁺/organic cation antiport system. These characteristics of an organic cation transport system are very different from those of an organic anion transport system [4–6].

Furthermore, the transport of other widely used drugs was examined in relation to the organic cation transport system. Cimetidine, a potent histamine H₂-receptor antagonist, is a weak organic base and its major route of elimination is in the urine. Cimetidine inhibited tetraethylammonium uptake by brush-border and basolateral membrane vesicles. In agreement with the tetraethylammonium transport mechanisms found in brush-border membranes, the presence of an outward H^+ gradient induced a marked stimulation of cimetidine uptake against its concentration gradient, and this concentrative uptake was inhibited by tetraethylammonium. These results suggest that cimetidine shares a common carrier system with tetraethylammonium in brush-border and basolateral membranes [7].

Aminocephalosporin antibiotics such as cephalexin are amphoteric molecules, having both amino and carboxyl groups, and, at physiological pH, are ionized mostly as zwitterions and anions. It has been thought that most cephalosporin antibiotics are actively secreted into the proximal tubules via an organic anion transport system. However, during the course of our studies of cephalosporin transport, we found that aminocephalosporins can be transported via H^+/organic cation antiport systems in renal brush-border membranes [8]. Cephalexin uptake by brush-border membrane vesicles was markedly stimulated in the presence of an outward H^+ gradient, and was inhibited in the presence of tetraethylammonium.

In addition, it was noted that apical membranes isolated from the LLC-PK_1 pig kidney epithelial cell line retained tetraethylammonium transport characteristics similar to those observed in renal brush-border membranes [9].

pH Sensitivity of the H^+/Organic Cation Antiport System in Renal Brush-Border Membranes

The time course of tetraethylammonium uptake was examined in the presence of various H^+ gradients, with a fixed extravesicular pH of 7.2 [10]. In spite of the increase of an outward H^+ gradient, the initial uptake rate of tetraethylammonium decreased at pH 5.7 and 5.2, compared with that at pH 6.2. These results suggest that pH, as well as an H^+ gradient, is an important factor in regulating the activity of the H^+/organic cation antiport system. To verify this possibility, we studied the pH profile of tetraethylammonium uptake by brush-border membrane vesicles in the absence of an H^+ gradient. As shown in Fig. 2, the uptake of tetraethylammonium for 30 s was maximum at pH 7.0, and at an acidic pH or an alkaline pH the uptake decreased [10]. However, the uptake for 30 min did not change in the indicated pH regions. Therefore, the inactivation was not considered to be due to the decrease in intravesicular space, but to the decrease in the activity of the H^+/organic cation antiport system.

We also examined the pH dependence of tetraethylammonium uptake by basolateral membrane vesicles compared with that in brush-border membranes. The uptake of tetraethylammonium for 30 s and 30 min did not change in the neutral pH regions, but decreased similarly in the acidic pH regions. Thus, the pH dependence of tetraethylammonium uptake in basolateral membranes was very different from that in brush-border membranes.

The uptake of tetraethylammonium, p-aminohippurate, and D-glucose in the absence of an H^+ gradient was compared at pH 6.0, 7.0, and 8.0. The transport of p-aminohippurate and D-glucose had no optimum pH in the range of 6.0–8.0. These results suggest that the H^+/organic cation antiport system, exclusively, is sensitive to pH, and is activated at pH 7.0.

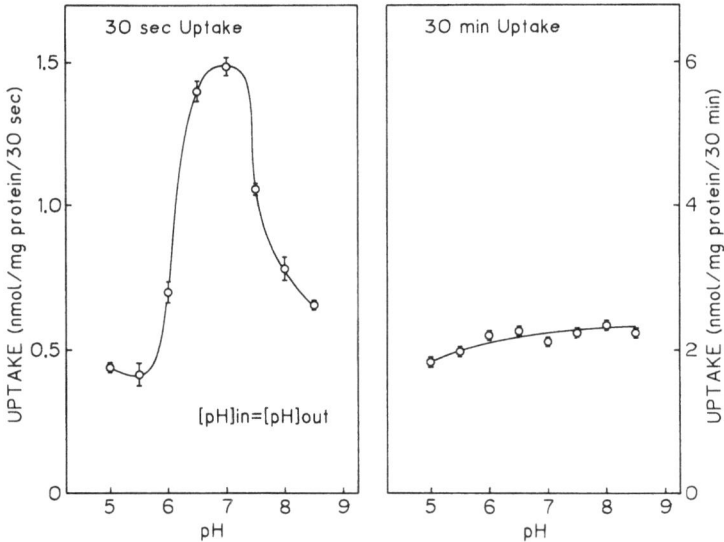

Fig. 2. pH Dependence of tetraethylammonium uptake by brush-border membrane vesicles (without H⁺ gradient). (From [10] with permission)

For the kinetic parameters at an acidic pH, the K_m value increased significantly without any change in V_{max} value, compared with the values at pH 7.0. In contrast, at an alkaline pH, the V_{max} value decreased significantly without any change in K_m value. From these data, the activity of the H⁺/organic cation antiport system was considered to be inhibited at an acidic pH due to the increase in K_m value, and was considered to be inhibited at an alkaline pH due to the decrease in V_{max} value.

Effect of Chemical Modifiers on the H⁺/Organic Cation Antiport System

We examined the uptake of tetraethylammonium, in the absence of H⁺ gradient, by brush-border membrane vesicles pretreated with p-chloromercuribenzene sulfonate (PCMBS), a sulfhydryl reagent, at various concentrations [11]. The initial rate of tetraethylammonium uptake decreased in a dose-dependent manner in the vesicles pretreated with PCMBS ($IC_{50} = 38$ μM). The inhibitory effect of PCMBS pretreatment was protected by preincubation with unlabeled tetraethylammonium.

The reversibility of the effect of PCMBS by subsequent treatment with thiols was examined. The inhibition of tetraethylammonium uptake was reversed almost to the control level by subsequent treatment of the vesicles with 10 mM dithiothreitol, glutathione, or cysteine. These results suggested that sulfhydryl reagent inhibits the transport of tetraethylammonium by specific interaction with the active sites of the carrier, and that sulfhydryl groups are essential as binding sites for substrate in the organic cation transport system in renal brush-border membranes. In the kidney,

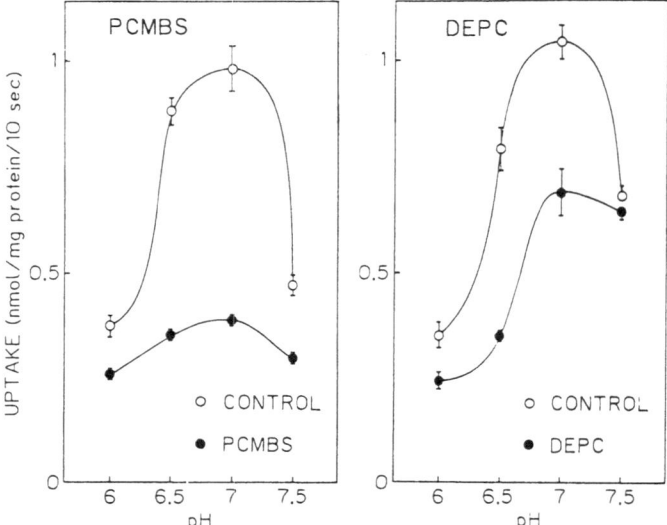

Fig. 3a,b. Tetraethylammonium uptake at various pH values by brush-border membrane vesicles pretreated with **a** p-chloromercuribenzene sulphonate (PCMBS) and with **b** diethyl pyrocarbonate (DEPC) (without H^+ gradient). (From [12] with permission)

glutathione is synthesized intracellularly and is translocated through the cell membranes. Therefore, endogenous thiols, such as glutathione and cysteine, may protect the functional sulfhydryl groups of the organic cation transport system against oxidative stress in vivo.

Furthermore, we studied the effect of diethyl pyrocarbonate (DEPC), a histidine modifying reagent, on the H^+/organic cation antiport system in brush-border membranes [12]. The overshoot uptake of tetraethylammonium was markedly inhibited by pretreatment of the vesicles with DEPC. We also examined tetraethylammonium uptake for 10 s and 30 min in the absence of an H^+ gradient using vesicles pretreated with DEPC. With DEPC pretreatment at concentrations of 0.01–1 mM, tetraethylammonium uptake for 30 min did not change but it decreased at higher concentrations. The uptake of tetraethylammonium for 10 s decreased in a concentration-dependent manner in vesicles pretreated with DEPC. The uptake decreased to 75% at 0.5 mM DEPC. These results indicate that DEPC directly inactivates the H^+/organic cation antiport system. The uptake of p-aminohippurate for 10 s and 30 min decreased when treated with DEPC only at the higher concentrations of 5 and 10 mM. Judging from the uptake for 30 min, the intravesicular space seemed to decrease when treated with 5 mM DEPC.

It has been reported that DEPC reacts not only with histidine residues, but also with sulfhydryl groups in some conditions, and that hydroxylamine can reverse the DEPC modification of histidine residues but not the DEPC modification of sulfhydryl groups. The inhibitory effect of DEPC pretreatment on tetraethylammonium uptake for 10 s was reversed significantly by subsequent treatment of the vesicles with 0.5 M hydroxylamine. However, there was no restoration of tetraethylammonium

Table 1. Characteristics of organic cation transport systems in renal brush-border and basolateral membranes

	Brush-border membrane	Basolateral membrane
Transport system	H$^+$/organic cation antiport	Carrier-mediated
Driving force	H$^+$ gradient	Membrane potential
Electrogenicity	Neutral	Electrogenic
Optimum pH	7.0	6.5 - 8.5
Functional moiety	Sulfhydryl groups	?
	Histidine residues	
	Carboxyl groups	
Substrate	Tetraethylammonium	Tetraethylammonium
	N^1-methylnicotinamde	N^1-Methylnicotinamide
	Cimetidine	Cimetidine
	Aminocephalosporins etc.	others

uptake on subsequent treatment with dithiothreitol, which could reverse the inhibition induced by PCMBS pretreatment. These results suggest that under the present experimental conditions DEPC reacted specifically with histidine residues, but not with sulfhydryl groups.

Figure 3 shows tetraethylammonium uptake, at various pH values, by brush-border membrane vesicles pretreated with DEPC and PCMBS [12]. Tetraethylammonium uptake for 10 s at pH 6.0–7.0, but not at pH 7.5, was inhibited by pretreatment with 1 mM DEPC (Fig. 3b), although the uptake for 30 min was not affected at various pH values by pretreatment with DEPC. In contrast, the uptake of tetraethylammonium for 10 s in the pH range used was inhibited by pretreatment with PCMBS (Fig. 3a). In the DEPC-pretreated vesicles, the V_{max} value of tetraethylammonium uptake at pH 7.0 decreased significantly without a change in the K_m value. Unlabeled tetraethylammonium had no protective effect on the inhibition of tetraethylammonium uptake by DEPC pretreatment. The data suggest that histidine residues in the carrier do not interact with the substrate, but may play a role in the regulation of H$^+$ transfer in this transport system.

Conclusion

Based on the data above, the characteristics of organic cation transport systems are summarized in Table 1. Tetraethylammonium is transported from blood to cell across basolateral membranes via a carrier-mediated system; this process is stimulated by the intracellular negative membrane potential. Tetraethylammonium transport from cell to urine across brush-border membranes is driven by an H$^+$ gradient via an electroneutral H$^+$/organic cation antiport system. The H$^+$ gradient can be created by a Na$^+$/H$^+$ antiport system and an ATP-driven H$^+$-pump in brush-border membranes. The H$^+$/organic cation antiport system in brush-border membranes is very sensitive to pH, in contrast to other transport systems in brush-border membranes and the organic cation transport system in basolateral membranes. Thus, pH is an important factor in regulating the activity of the H$^+$/organic cation antiport. Sulfhydryl groups and histidine residues are essential for the organic cation transport system in renal brush-border membranes. These studies provide new insight into our understanding of the regulatory mechanisms of organic cation transport in renal brush-border and basolateral membranes.

References

1. Murer H, Gmaj P (1986) Transport studies in plasma membrane vesicles isolated from renal cortex. Kidney Int 30:171–186
2. Inui K, Okano T, Takano M, Kitazawa S, Hori R (1981) A simple method for the isolation of basolateral plasma membrane vesicles from rat kidney cortex: Enzyme activities and some properties of glucose transport. Biochim Biophys Acta 647:150–154
3. Takano M, Inui K, Okano T, Saito H, Hori R (1984) Carrier-mediated transport systems of tetraethylammonium in rat renal brush-border and basolateral membrane vesicles. Biochim Biophys Acta 773:113–124
4. Hori R, Takano M, Okano T, Kitazawa S, Inui K (1982) Mechanisms of p-aminohippurate transport by brush-border and basolateral membrane vesicles isolated from rat kidney cortex. Biochim Biophys Acta 692:97–100
5. Inui K, Takano M, Okano T, Hori R (1986) Role of chloride on carrier-mediated transport of p-aminohippurate in rat renal basolateral membrane vesicles. Biochim Biophys Acta 855:425–428
6. Hori R, Takano M, Okano T, Inui K (1985) Transport of p-aminohippurate, tetraethylammonium and D-glucose in renal brush border membranes from rats with acute renal failure. J Pharmacol Exp Ther 233:776–781
7. Takano M, Inui K, Okano T, Hori R (1985) Cimetidine transport in rat renal brush border and basolateral membrane vesicles. Life Sci 37:1579–1585
8. Inui K, Takano M, Okano T, Hori R (1985) H^+ Gradient dependent transport of amino-cephalosporins in rat renal brush border membrane vesicles: Role of H^+/organic cation antiport system. J Pharmacol Exp Ther 233:181–185
9. Inui K, Saito H, Hori R (1985) H^+ Gradient-dependent active transport of tetraethylammonium cation in apical-membrane vesicles isolated from kidney epithelial cell line LLC-PK_1. Biochem J 227:199–203
10. Maegawa H, Kato M, Inui K, Hori R (1988) pH Sensitivity of H^+/organic cation antiport system in rat renal brush-border membranes. J Biol Chem 263:11150–11154
11. Hori R, Maegawa H, Okano T, Takano M, Inui K (1987) Effect of sulfhydryl reagents on tetraethylammonium transport in rat renal brush border membranes. J Pharmacol Exp Ther 241:1010–1016
12. Hori R, Maegawa H, Kato M, Katsura T, Inui K (1989) Inhibitory effect of diethyl pyrocarbonate on the H^+/organic cation antiport system in rat renal brush-border membranes. J Biol Chem 264:12232–12237

Urate Transport in Mammalian Nephron

FRANÇOISE ROCH-RAMEL and DOMINIQUE WERNER[1]

SUMMARY. The differences in renal handling of urate by mammals are discussed, focusing on the main role played by the proximal tubule, which is responsible for urate secretion, as well as for most urate reabsorption. The membrane mechanisms involved in urate transport are different in urate reabsorbing and urate secreting species. Brush-border membranes of rats and dogs (urate reabsorbers) possess a urate/anion exchanger which accepts various organic anions as well as chloride, bicarbonate, and hydroxyl ions. Pigs and rabbits (urate secreters) do not possess this anion exchanger, but have a potential-dependent facilitated mechanism which favors urate efflux from cell to lumen. The basolateral membranes of rats (urate reabsorbers) have urate/chloride exchangers, whereas those of pigs (urate secreters) have urate/2-oxoglutarate exchangers, which, coupled to the activity of the sodium dicarboxylate cotransport, allows urate to concentrate into the cells.

Introduction

In man and closely related primates, uric acid is the end product of purine metabolism, whereas in other mammals, it is further broken down to allantoin by uricase, an enzyme which is missing in man. Due to lack of uricase activity, the plasma concentration of uric acid in man is higher than in other mammals [1]. In all mammals, urate, being little bound to plasma proteins, is freely filtered; it then undergoes transtubular bidirectional transport. Depending on the relative importance of the secretory and reabsorptive fluxes, urinary excretion exceeds filtered load (net secretion) or is smaller than filtered load (net reabsorption) [1]. Thus, large species differences have been observed, fractional excretion of urate (Curate/GFR) varying from about 10% in man to 100%–300% in pigs [1] (for a more complete report, see [2]).

---

[1]Institut de Pharmacologie de l'Université de Lausanne, CH-1005 Lausanne, Switzerland

Even within one species, important variations have been reported. For example, a few patients with hypouricemia were observed to excrete urate by net secretion [3]. Also, the case of the Dalmatian coach hound which, in contrast to mongrel dogs, excretes urate by net secretion, is well known [4]. Hereafter, we shall call mammalian species which excrete urate by net secretion, at normal or slightly elevated concentrations of urate in the plasma "urate secreters", and mammals which excrete less urate than is filtered, "urate reabsorbers."

Tubular Handling of Urate

The net transport of urate along the nephron was investigated in vivo, in tubular micropuncture experiments.

"Urate Reabsorbers"

In anesthetized non-diuretic rats, at endogenous plasma concentration of urate (35–60 μM), the fractional excretion of urate is about 30%. By using a sensitive and specific method for urate determination (high-performance liquid chromatography (HPLC) and amperometric detection), the fractional delivery of urate to the late proximal convoluted tubules was shown to be about 35%–50%, while that to the early distal tubules was close to 35% [5,6]. Most of the reabsorption appears thus to occur before the convoluted distal tubule. The same is true for deep nephrons, since fractional delivery of urate to Henle's loop of deep nephrons (micropuncture at the tip of the papilla) is about 35% [6]. The lower parts of the nephron are little permeable to urate (for review see [2]). For ethical reasons, tubular micropuncture experiments can obviously not be done in man. However, such experiments were performed on the Cebus monkey, a mammal which, as does man, excretes only a small fraction of the filtered load (about 3–4% in nondiuretic state) [7]. As in rats, urate reabsorption occurs mainly before early distal convolutions (Fig. 1). In mongrel dogs, also, proximal tubule is the main site of urate reabsorption [4].

"Urate Secreters"

In the pig, the fractional delivery of urate to proximal convoluted tubules largely exceeds the filtered load (Fig. 2), demonstrating net secretion along the convoluted proximal tubule [8]. In the Dalmatian coach hound, net secretion occurs mainly along the pars recta [4].

Characterization of Unidirectional Fluxes of Urate

The proximal tubule being the main site of urate transport, attempts have been made to characterize the secretory and reabsorptive fluxes by using in situ or in vitro tubular microperfusion techniques (for review, see [9]). In situ experiments were performed only in rats, a species in which the kidney can be immobilized well enough

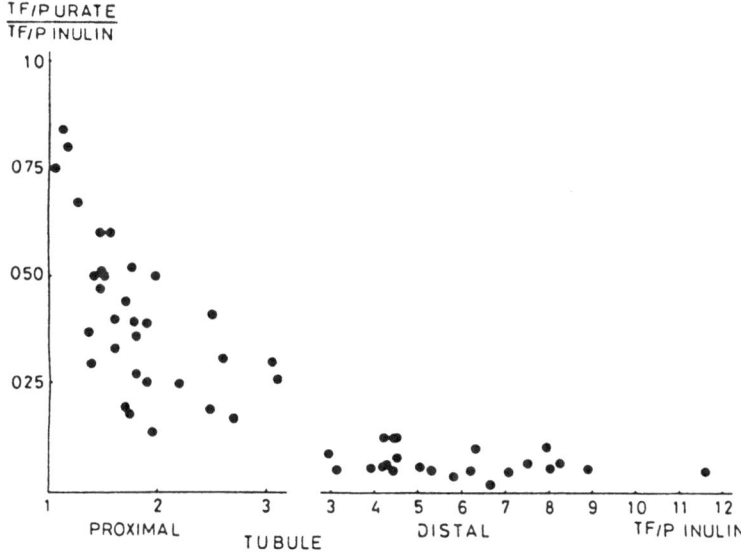

Fig. 1. Fractional deliveries of urate to proximal and distal tubules of Cebus monkeys. The fractional deliveries of urate ($TF/P_{urate}/TF/P_{inulin}$) to the sites of micropuncture are displayed as a function of TF/P_{inulin}. Mean endogenous urate concentration in the plasma was: 190 ± 30 μM. Fractional excretion of urate in the pelvic urine was: 3.3% $\pm$ 0.3% and that of water was: 1.4% $\pm$ 0.1%. At the end of the proximal convoluted tubule, about 75% of urate has already been reabsorbed as demonstrated by the low fractional delivery ($TF/P_{urate}/TF/P_{inulin} = 0.25$) to this site. At early distal convolutions, 90% of urate has been reabsorbed ($TF/P_{urate}/TF/P_{inulin} = 0.1$). TF/P_{urate}, ratio of urate concentrations in tubular fluid (*TF*) and in plasma (*P*); TF/P_{inulin}, ratio of inulin concentrations in TF and P. (From [7] with permission)

to allow microperfusion of tubular segments and of peritubular capillaries. In vitro perfusion experiments were performed on proximal tubules of rabbits and mice.

"Urate Reabsorbers" (Rats and Mice)

Reabsorption

In rats, it was clearly demonstrated that the reabsorption of urate is not directly coupled to that of sodium [10]. Urate reabsorption (see [9] for ref.) is saturable, but at rather high concentrations (about 0.5mM). It is inhibited by many organic anions, such as probenecid, pyrazinoate, furosemide, *para*-aminohippuric acid (PAH), as well as by SITS and DIDS when added to the tubular lumen (cis-inhibition) [9]. When added to the basolateral side by perfusion into peritubular capillaries, PAH stimulates urate reabsorption (trans-stimulation) [9], demonstrating that urate can be exchanged with PAH across the tubular epithelium. The characteristics of this exchange mechanism have been investigated independently in brush-border and basolateral membranes (see below).

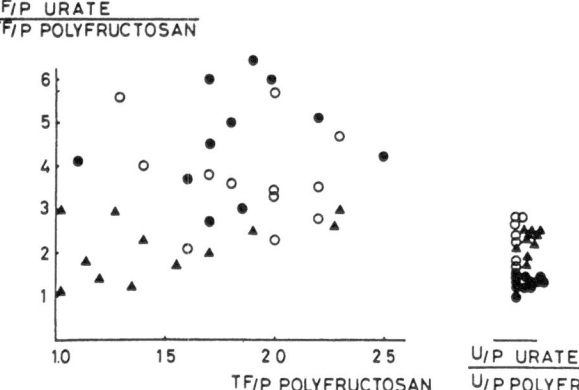

Fig. 2. Fractional excretion and fractional deliveries of urate to proximal tubules of pigs. The fractional deliveries of urate (TF/P$_{urate}$/TF/P$_{polyfructosan}$) to the sites of micropuncture in proximal tubules are displayed as a function of TF/P$_{polyfructosan}$ (polyfructosan is an analogue of inuline). Fractional excretion in pelvic urine is given by the U/P$_{urate}$/U/P$_{polyfructosan}$ ratio. Data are from 2 pigs, at endogenous concentration of urate in the plasma (3 μM, ●), 2 pigs at 21 μM (o), and 2 pigs at 95 μM (▲). At all plasma levels, fractional deliveries exceeded the filtration load (TF/P$_{urate}$/TF/P$_{polyfructosan}$ > 1), demonstrating net secretion. (Data from [8] with permission)

Reabsorption was measured in vitro in mice proximal tubule [11]. As in rats, probenecid inhibits urate reabsorption when added to the lumen. It also inhibits reabsorption when added to the basolateral site (bathing medium) as it penetrates into the tubular lumen by secretion.

Secretion

In rats, in vivo tubular microperfusion demonstrated that the urate secretory flux is saturable. As for reabsorption, saturation is observed at rather high concentrations of urate (1 mM) (for ref., see [9]). When added to the peritubular site, probenecid and PAH inhibit secretion (cis-inhibition) [9]. When added to the lumen, PAH stimulates urate secretion (trans-stimulation). SITS, which inhibits anion exchangers, decreased the urate secretory flux when applied in the lumen or at the peritubular site [9].

"Urate Secreters" (Rabbits)

Reabsorption

In the rabbit, urate reabsorption was measured in the S$_2$ segments of proximal tubules, using in vitro microperfusion techniques. The reabsorptive flux was found to be of low magnitude, temperature independent [12], and not sensitive to probenecid [13]. Such data would suggest that reabsorption occurs by simple diffusion. However, as urate is not liposoluble, reabsorption by transcellular simple diffusion seems unlikely, although a facilitated transport has not been demonstrated.

Secretion

The secretory flux of urate was measured in all three proximal segments (S_1, S_2, S_3) of the rabbit. This flux can occur against an electrochemical gradient, is saturable, inhibitable by probenecid, and is larger in S_2 than in S_1 and S_3 segments [13]. PAH inhibits the cellular accumulation of urate in non-perfused proximal tubule, showing that these 2 organic anions compete for the same transporter at the basolateral membrane, i.e., for the first step of urate secretion. The intracellular concentration of urate can exceed that in the incubation medium, showing active transport at the basolateral membrane [14]. Similar data were obtained in non-perfused proximal tubules of pigs [15].

Transport of Urate in Membrane Vesicles

Brush-Border Membranes

"Urate Reabsorbers"

In contrast to other endogenous compounds such as aminoacids, lactate, and glucose, no sodium urate cotransport has been demonstrated in brush border membranes of urate reabsorbers [16,17]. This lack of direct sodium-urate cotransport is in agreement with in vivo findings, as reported above.

Blomstedt and Aronson [18] first demonstrated the presence of a mediated transport for urate in brush border membrane vesicles prepared from dog renal cortex, which allowed urate/OH^- exchange (or urate/H^+-cotransport). Thus, the imposition of an outwardly directed hydroxyl ion gradient (pH in = 7.5, pH out = 6) stimulates urate uptake into vesicles (Fig. 3). Further studies demonstrated that this transport mechanism is a urate-anion exchanger having affinity for a wide variety of anions, including chloride, lactate, succinate, etc. [19,20]. Another mechanism was also demonstrated, which is dependent on the activity of a membrane associated uricase [21].

"Urate Secreters"

Urate transport into brush-border membrane vesicles was investigated in rabbits and pigs, two urate secreters. In these "urate secreters" no urate-anion exchanger was demonstrated. However, another transport mechanism was observed. It was demonstrated in the pig [22] that urate uptake into (BBMV) vesicles was stimulated and exceeded chemical equilibrium when an electropositive intravesicular space was created by applying an inwardly directed potassium gradient in the presence of the potassium ionophore, valinomycin (Fig. 4). The same was observed in rabbits, although the stimulation was much smaller and no overshoot in concentration was observed [23]. PAH appears to share this transport mechanism with urate. It should be mentioned that in dogs and rats, the stimulation of urate uptake by the creation of an electropositive intravesicular space, per se, has not been specifically studied. It might be that part of the stimulation of urate uptake observed in the presence of a pH gradient might be due to an effect of potential [16,17].

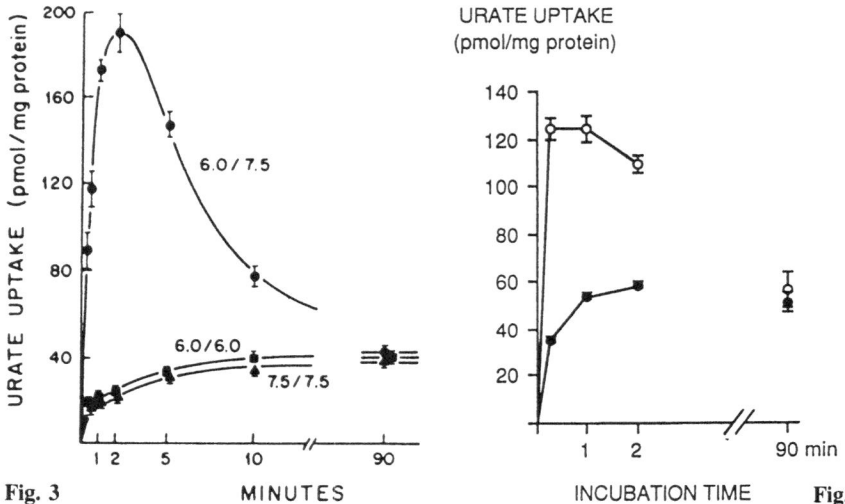

Fig. 3　　　　　　　　MINUTES　　　　　　INCUBATION TIME　　　Fig. 4

Fig. 3. Effect of an outwardly directed hydroxyl ion gradient on urate uptake by dog brush-border membrane vesicles (BBMV). ▲, 7.5/7.5: Membrane vesicles were preincubated for 120 min at 20°C in 170 mM mannitol, 42 mM Tris, 67 mM Hepes, 36 mM K^+, and 18 mM sulfate at pH 7.5, and then uptake of 22 µM urate was assayed in the presence of 155 mM mannitol, 8 mM Tris, 13 mM Hepes, 104 mM K^+, 4 mM sulfate, and 52 mM phosphate at pH 7.5; ●, 6.0/7.5: Membranes were similarly preincubated at pH 7.5, but urate uptake was assayed in the presence of 200 mM mannitol, 8 mM Tris, 13 mM Hepes, 60 mM K^+, 4 mM sulfate, and 52 mM phosphate at pH 6.0; ■, 6.0/6.0: Membranes were preincubated in 200 mM mannitol, 42 mM Tris, 67 mM Hepes, and 18 mM sulfate at pH 6.0, and then urate uptake was assayed in the presence of 180 mM mannitol, 8 mM Tris, 13 mM Hepes, 60 mM K^+, 4 mM sulfate, and 52 mM phosphate at pH 6.0. Each point represents the mean ± SE for three determinations. (Data are reproduced from the *Journal of Clinical Investigation* by copyright permission of the American Society for Clinical Investigation [18])

Fig. 4. Effect of an electropositive intravesicular space on urate uptake by pig brush-border membrane vesicles (BBMV). BBMV (prepared as described in [22]) were suspended in 300 mM mannitol and 20 mM HEPES-Tris at pH 7.4, with 6.0–8.0 µg of valinomycin per mg of protein (electropositive intravesicular space: o) or with an equivalent volume of ethanol (control: ●), and then uptake of 46 µM [14C] urate was assayed in the presence of 99 mM mannitol, 120 mM K^+ gluconate, and 20 mM HEPES-Tris at pH 7.4. Data represent the mean ± S.E. of three experiments

Basolateral Membranes

Urate transport into basolateral membrane vesicles has been studied in only two species: the rat (urate reabsorber) and the pig (urate secreter).

"Urate Reabsorbers"

In rat basolateral membrane, urate transport was shown to be mediated by a mechanism sensitive to probenecid and DIDS [24]. In addition, an outwardly directed chloride gradient resulted in an enhancement of urate uptake. This stimulation, which was not secondary to the creation of a chloride diffusion potential, is compatible with a chloride/urate exchange mechanism. This transport system, unlike the luminal exchanger, has no affinity for PAH. No sodium cotransport of urate was observed, urate uptake being not stimulated by applying an inwardly directed sodium gradient [24]. As in rat brush border membrane, a transport mechanism dependent on membrane associated uricase has also been reported in basolateral membrane [21].

"Urate Secreters"

Recently, in pig basolateral membrane vesicles obtained from renal outer cortex, we also found no *direct* coupling between sodium and urate. Thus, the replacement of 150 mM potassium from extravesicular medium by 150 mM sodium did not stimulate urate uptake. However, we observed that the presence of sodium in the extravesicular medium could influence urate uptake by an *indirect* effect. This effect is similar to that reported for PAH transport in rat basolateral membranes [25], i.e., the uptake occurs by the coupling of a sodium/dicarboxylate cotransport with a dicarboxylate/urate exchange [26]. The cis-addition of 150 μM 2-oxoglutarate to the extravesicular medium, in the presence of an inwardly directed sodium gradient, stimulated urate transport, compared to the control condition in the absence of 2-oxoglutarate [26]. Although of low magnitude, a concentrative urate uptake was observed. This stimulation was not the consequence of an ion diffusion potential, as a voltage clamp was applied. Thus, in the pig, the basolateral step of urate secretion might be, at least in part, mediated by the coupling of a sodium/2-oxoglutarate cotransport with a 2-oxoglutarate/urate exchange.

General Conclusions

Reabsorption and secretion in urate reabsorbers and secreters are summarized in Fig. 5.

Replaced in the intact proximal tubule, the physiological conditions are such that the urate/anion exchanger demonstrated in brush-border membranes of "urate reabsorbers" favors urate reabsorption, as evidenced by the low fractional delivery of urate to the late proximal tubule (see above). Urate entry into the cell might occur in exchange with bicarbonate or OH^-, as well as with cell metabolites such as succinate, pyruvate, or lactate, etc. The cellular efflux of urate might be facilitated at the basolateral membrane by an exchange with chloride (exchange with other anions has been little investigated).

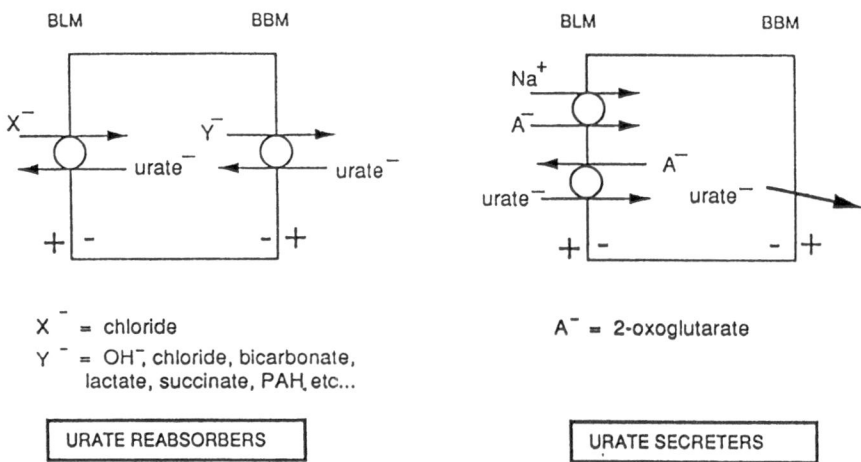

Fig. 5. Schematic representation of membrane mechanisms involved in urate transport BLM, basolateral membrane; BBM, brush-border membrane

The anion exchangers of each membrane can also allow the transport of urate in the secretory direction, depending on the anion present in the cell or in the lumen [20]. Anionic drugs, such as diuretics and uricosurics, might have affinity for the urate exchanger, and thus might favor reabsorption or secretion, depending on their concentrations in the lumen or in the blood capillaries.

In "urate secreters," the absence of the brush-border anion exchanger might explain the low rate of urate reabsorption. The mechanisms driven by electrical potential, demonstrated in pig and rabbit brush-border membranes, favor the efflux of urate into the lumen, which is positive compared to the cell. The physiological conditions are such that reabsorption is negligible. The anion exchanger present at the basolateral membrane, coupled to the activity of the Na$^+$/dicarboxylate cotransport, allows urate to concentrate into the cells.

References

1. Roch-Ramel F (1979) Renal excretion of uric acid in mammals. Clin Nephrol 12:1–6
2. Weiner IM (1979) Urate transport in the nephron. Am J Physiol 237:F85–F92
3. Sperling O (1989) Hereditary renal hypouricemia. In: Scriver CR, Beaudet AL, Sly WS, Valle D (eds) The metabolic basis of inherited disease, vol 1, 6th ed. McGraw-Hill, New York, pp 2605–2617
4. Roch-Ramel F, Wong NLM, Dirks JH (1976) Renal excretion of urate in mongrel and Dalmatian dogs: a micropuncture study. Am J Physiol 231:326–331
5. Roch-Ramel F, Granges F, Roth L, Widmer J, Weiner IM (1979/80) Renal handling of urate by nondiuretic and diuretic rats. HPLC-amperometric determination of urate concentrations. Renal Physiol 2:122–129
6. Frommer JP, Sheth AU, Senekjian HO, Babino H, Weinman EJ (1982) Free-flow micropuncture study of renal urate transport in the Munich-Wistar rat. Min Electrol Metab 7:324–330

7. Roch-Ramel F, Diezi-Chométy F, Roth L, Weiner IM (1980) A micropuncture study of urate excretion by Cebus monkeys employing high performance liquid chromatography with amperometric detection of urate. Pflugers Arch 383:203–207

8. Roch-Ramel F, White F, Vowles L, Simmonds HA, Cameron JS (1980) Micropuncture study of tubular transport of urate and PAH in the pig kidney. Am J Physiol 239:F107–F112

9. Kahn AM, Weinman EJ (1985) Urate transport in the proximal tubule: in vivo and vesicle studies. Am J Physiol 249:F789–F798

10. Kahn AM (1989) Indirect coupling between sodium and urate transport in the proximal tubule. Kidney Int 36:378–384

11. Lang F, Gstrein E, Geibel J, Rehwald W, Völkl H, Oberleithner H (1983) 605-redox microelectrodes for the continuous recording of organic substances in renal tubular fluid. Bioelectrochem. Bioenerg. 11:365–372

12. Senekjian HO, Knight TF, Weinman EJ (1981) Urate transport by the isolated perfused S_2 segment of the rabbit. Am J Physiol 240:F530–F535

13. Shimomura A, Chonko A, Tanner R, Edwards R, Grantham J (1981) Nature of urate transport in isolated rabbit proximal tubules. Am J Physiol 241:F565–F578

14. Schäli C, Roch-Ramel F (1980) Accumulation of [^{14}C]urate and [^{3}H]PAH in isolated proximal tubular segments of the rabbit kidney. Am J Physiol 239:F222–F227

15. Schäli C, Roch-Ramel F (1981) Uptake of [^{3}H]PAH and [^{14}C]urate into isolated proximal tubular segments of the pig kidney. Am J Physiol 241:F591–F596

16. Kahn AM, Aronson PS (1983) Urate transport via anion exchange in dog renal microvillus membrane vesicles. Am J Physiol 244:F56–F63

17. Kahn AM, Branham S, Weinman EJ (1983) Mechanism of urate and p-aminohippurate transport in rat renal microvillus membrane vesicles. Am J Physiol 245:F151–F158

18. Blomstedt JW, Aronson PS (1980) pH gradient-stimulated transport of urate and p-aminohippurate in dog renal microvillus membrane vesicles. J Clin Invest 65:931–934

19. Guggino SE, Martin GJ, Aronson PS (1983) Specificity and modes of the anion exchanger in dog renal microvillus membranes. Am J Physiol 244:F612–F621

20. Guggino SE, Aronson PS (1985) Paradoxical effects of pyrazinoate and nicotinate on urate transport in dog renal microvillus membranes. J Clin Invest 76:543–547

21. Abramson RG, King VF, Reif MC, Leal-Pinto E, Baruch SB (1982) Urate uptake in membrane vesicles of rat renal cortex: effect of copper. Am J Physiol 242:F158–F170

22. Werner D, Martinez F, Roch-Ramel F (1990) Urate and p-aminohippurate transport in the brush border membrane of the pig kidney. J Pharmacol Exp Ther 252:792–799

23. Martinez F, Manganel M, Montrose-Rafizadeh C, Werner D, Roch-Ramel F (1990) Transport of urate and p-aminohippurate in rabbit renal brush-border membranes. Am J Physiol 258:F1145–F1153

24. Kahn AM, Shelat H, Weinman EJ (1985) Urate and p-aminohippurate transport in rat renal basolateral vesicles. Am J Physiol 249:F654–F661

25. Shimada H, Moewes B, Burckhardt G (1987) Indirect coupling to Na^+ of p-aminohippuric acid uptake into rat renal basolateral membrane vesicles. Am J Physiol 253:F795–F801

26. Werner D, Roch-Ramel F (1990) Urate transport across the basolateral membrane of the pig renal proximal tubule (abstract). Experientia 46:A54

Pump, Leak and Metabolism: Postproximal Handling of Amino Acids in the Kidney

S. Silbernagl, M. Gekle, K. Völker[1], E. Braun, and W.H. Dantzler[2]

Summary. (1) During portal venous perfusion of the isolated non-filtering kidney of the toad (*Xenopus laevis*) with solutions containing 65 µM L-citrulline (L-Cit), urinary excretion of L-Cit was 2.25 nmol/2h. In the absence of NaCl or in the presence of 20 mM L-phenylalanine (L-Phe) in the perfusate, this value dropped to about 10% of the control value. The same was true for D-Cit excretion if L-Cit in the perfusate was replaced by D-Cit. Thus, secretory AA fluxes in the tubule seem to be carrier-mediated to at least 90%. (2) Rat kidney short loops of Henle were microperfused continuously in vivo et in situ with solutions containing ^{3}H-inulin and ^{14}C-amino acids. Fractional ^{14}C-reabsorption (FR) in the loop of Henle was high (glycine (Gly) 0.95; L-alanine (L-Ala) 0.97) at low concentrations (0.21 and 0.15 mM, respectively) but dropped to 0.24 (Gly) if 50 mM L-phenylalanine (L-Phe) or L-proline (L-Pro) was present. At 5 mM (L-arginine (L-Arg), L-glutamine (L-Glu) and at 50 mM (Gly, L-Phe, L-Pro), FR was 0.43, 0.74, 0.59, 0.50, and 0.18, respectively. At 0.6 mM, FR of L- and D-Ala was 0.97 and 0.84, respectively, but was 0.27 (L-Ala) and 0.74 (D-Ala) at 50 mM. The latter value dropped to 0.43 ($P < 0.005$) in the presence of D-AA oxidase inhibitors. FR of ^{14}C-mannitol was 0.05 ± 0.07 SEM. In conclusion, resorptive fluxes in short loops of Henle are mediated by high-capacity carriers. For D-alanine, D-AA oxidase is a metabolic sink accelerating D-Ala resorption to a value higher than that for L-Ala. (3) Tissue serine concentrations in antidiuretic rat kidney are 2- to 30-fold (cortex to papilla) higher than in systemic plasma and 7- to 125-fold higher than in urine. The total intracellular AA concentration in the anti-diuretic papilla is > 100 mM contributing substantially to the intracellular osmolyte concentration.

[1]Department of Physiology, University of Würzburg, D-8700 Würzburg, Federal Republic of Germany
[2]Department of Physiology, University of Arizona, Tucson, AZ 85724, USA

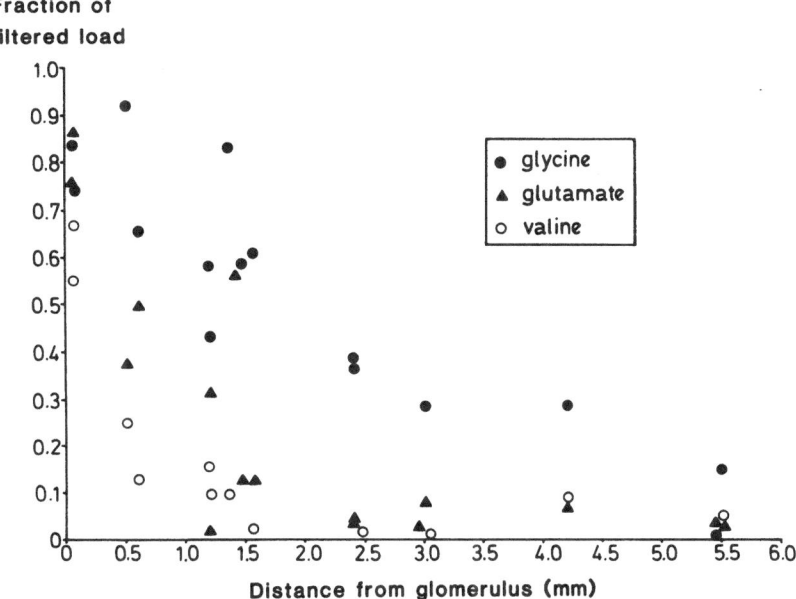

Fig. 1. Fractions of filtered loads of three amino acids found in samples collected by free-flow micropuncture along superficial proximal convoluted tubules of rat kidney. The mean endogenous plasma concentrations of glycine, glutamate, and valine during these experiments were 282, 117, and 278 μM, respectively. On the abscissa 5.5 mm represents the mean distance of the last accessible loop of the proximal convoluted tubule in 250 g rats

Introduction

It is well established that amino acids filtered at the glomerulus are reabsorbed rapidly along the proximal tubule (for review see [1]). With some exceptions, less than 1% of their filtered load is excreted in the final urine. Micropuncture data, obtained under endogenous free flow conditions, show that there are distinct values for the proximal reabsorption of different amino acids (see Fig. 1): Glycine is slowly reabsorbed, whereas more than 90% of the filtered load of glutamine [2], glutamate⁻, valine (Fig. 1), and many other amino acids has already disappeared after about one fifth of the total length of the proximal tubule of these rats. The dots at the bottom of Fig. 1, however, show that the fractional delivery does not decrease further in this quasi-exponential manner. Depending on the amino acid, there is still some 2%–5% left even at a distance of 6 mm from the glomerulus. This phenomenon has been explained by the establishment of a pump-leak concentration in the later parts of the proximal tubule. "Pump" usually means secondary-active Na⁺-Cotransport (dibasic amino acids may be an exception [3,4]), but what does "leak" mean? Is it a paracellular leak (see [5] and [1] for discussion) or do the amino acids use the brush-border carriers in the "wrong" direction if the transmembranal gradients toward the lumen are steep enough? This latter possibility is not unlikely, because many brush-border

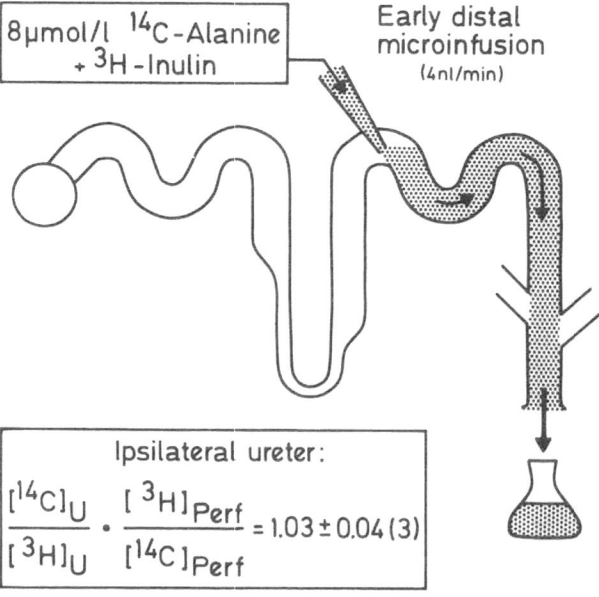

Fig. 2. Relative urinary recovery of ^{14}C-L-alanine microinjected into early superficial loops of distal convoluted tubules of rat kidney. The value does not differ significantly from that in Fig. 1, indicating that L-alanine does not leave the lumen in sections distal to the puncture site. Similar results have been obtained by Bergeron and Morel [8] for several other L-amino acids and by ourselves for D-alanine (S. Silbernagl et al. unpublished results)

membrane vesicle studies (see review in [1]) demonstrate that these carriers can be transstimulated. The first part of this study was designed to answer this question by investigating amino acid (citrulline) secretion in the non-filtering toad kidney.

What happens in the loop of Henle and in the distal nephron? As can be seen from Fig. 1, the fractional delivery of amino acids to the last accessible loop of the proximal convolution amounts to several percent, e.g., about 3% for alanine [6,7]; these values differ significantly from the fractional excretion of the respective amino acid (alanine 0.06–0.13% [6,7]). This may be explained by a high-affinity reabsorption and a relatively low leak of amino acids in the straight part of the proximal tubule, as shown with isolated perfused tubules (review, [5]). However, nearly the same amount (3%–4%) of filtered alanine was found in the superficial nephrons of the early distal tubule (short loops) [6,7]. Are amino acids reabsorbed in the distal nephron? The answer is "no" for superficial nephrons [7,8] (see Fig. 2), and "yes" for juxtamedullary nephrons [9,10]. In the second part of this study, we tested whether the zero net flux in the short loops of Henle was the result of opposed unidirectional fluxes of about the same size. As the answer to this question was "yes," we also characterized the unidirectional reabsorptive flux of several amino acids, including the D-isomer of alanine. In preliminary experiments we also measured the amino acid concentrations in six zones of the kidney situated between the cortex and the papilla to look for gradients that might favor one or the other of the unidirectional fluxes.

Methods

Isolated Perfused Non-Filtering Toad Kidney

Blood enters the toad kidney not only through the aorta but also through the portal vein [11]. We decapitated the toad (*Xenopus laevis*, male, 50–60 g BW), destroyed the spinal cord, opened the abdomen, and ligated all vessels to and from the kidney, except for the portal veins and the caval vein. We perfused the kidney only through the portal vein at a rate half as high as normal (2 ml/h into each portal vein). Under these conditions, venous volume recovery was 90%–100% and the inulin added to the perfusate did not reach the urine. Therefore, this preparation could be regarded as a non-filtering kidney, i.e., the perfusate reaches only the peritubular side of the tubule cells. Besides studying peritubular uptake and the metabolism of citrulline [12], we measured the urinary excretion of citrulline (column chromatography, see below) during perfusion of the kidneys with Ringer's solution containing inulin as well as citrulline and aspartate at the physiological concentrations of 65 and 35 μmol/l, respectively. p-Aminohippurate (2 mmol/l) was added to the perfusate in order to increase urinary flow.

Microperfusion of Short Loops of Henle

Male Wistar rats (200–250 g BW) were anesthetized with Inactin (120 mg/kg BW i.p.) and the left kidney was prepared and immobilized for micropuncture [13]. The perfusate, containing the ^{14}C-labelled amino acid and ^{3}H-inulin, was microperfused continuously in vivo et in situ [14] into the last accessible loop of the proximal convoluted tubule at a rate of 20 nl/min and was collected from the first accessible loop of the early distal convolution of the same nephron. Radioactivity was measured by liquid scintillation counting.

Measurement of Amino Acid Concentrations in Renal Tissue

In this preliminary experiment, a male antidiuretic Wistar rat (320 g BW) was anesthetized and the urinary bladder was punctured to obtain urine. The kidney was clamped, the hilus was cut, and, within about 5 s after clamping, the kidney was immersed in liquid nitrogen. Blood was obtained by subsequent heart puncture. Within several days, the kidney was warmed up to about -5 °C and 6 pieces (10–40 mg each) were cut out (as shown in Fig. 3) in a cooled room. The frozen pieces were weighed (in preweighed vials) and were deep-frozen at -70 °C. For amino acid determination, the cells of the tissue were destroyed by adding a buffer containing 1% Triton 100. After deproteinization with trichloracetic acid (100ml/l), amino acids were measured by ultramicro column chromatography (Kontron, Chromacon 500).

Results

Secretory Fluxes of Citrulline in the Toad Kidney

During perfusion of the toad kidney with a solution containing 65 μM L-citrulline, urinary excretion of this amino acid was about 2.5 nmol/2h (see Fig. 4). Replace-

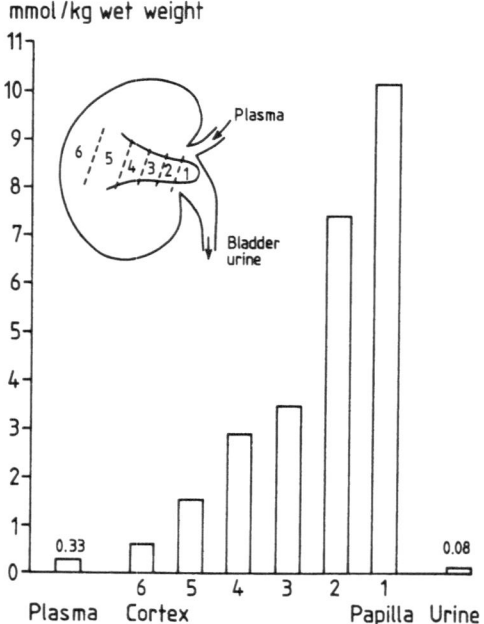

Fig. 3. Distribution of serine in kidney, systemic plasma, and bladder urine in one antidiuretic male rat of 326 g BW. Urine osmolality was 1400 mosm/l. A similar concentration gradient from cortex to papilla was found for all other amino acids. This results in a total amino acid concentration in the papilla (layer 1) of more than 100 mmol/kg wet weight

ment of NaCl with mannitol in the perfusate resulted in a dramatic drop of citrulline excretion to about 10% of the control value. Similarly, little excretion was found if 65 μM D-Citrulline was used or if 20 mM L-phenyl-alanine was added to the L-citrulline solution (see Fig. 4). These results clearly indicate that citrulline enters the urinary space nearly exclusively on a route which is stereospecific, inhibitable by another neutral amino acid, and Na(Cl)-dependent.

Unidirectional Amino Acid Fluxes in Short Loops of Henle in the Rat

As shown in Table 1, the radiolabels of glycine and L-alanine are nearly completely reabsorbed in the short loops of Henle if the initial concentration is small (0.21 and 0.15 mM, respectively), i.e., at about physiological concentrations. Fractional recovery is only 0.051 or 0.029, respectively, of the amount perfused. These non-reabsorbed fractions rise to 0.41 and 0.73, respectively, at the extremely high initial concentration of 50 mM; this indicates a significant but not full saturation of the reabsorptive process. Similar values are obtained with L-arginine, L-glutamate, L-phenylalanine and L-proline at high concentrations. As in the proximal convoluted tubule [1], L-proline and L-phenylalanine are potent inhibitors of glycine reabsorption (Table 1). At an initial concentration of 0.6 mM, D-alanine is reabsorbed more slowly than its L-isomer. This was to be expected. What is surprising, however, is

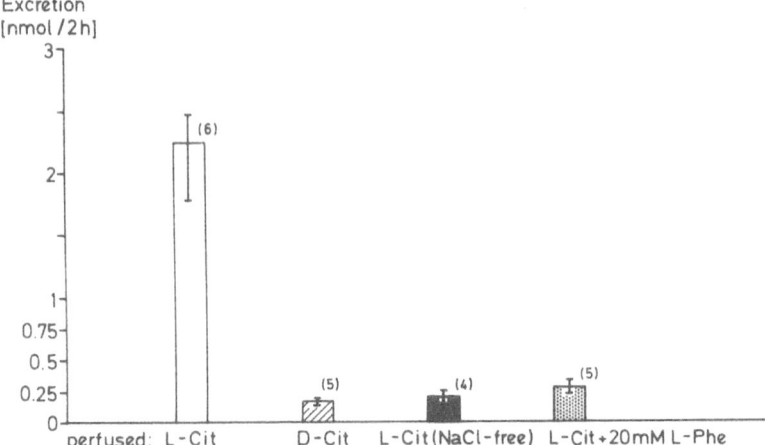

Fig. 4. Urinary excretion of L- and D-citrulline (*Cit*) during 2-hour portal-venous perfusion of isolated non-filtering kidneys of the toad (*Xenopus laevis*). The perfusion fluid contained L- or D-citrulline, respectively, in a concentration of 65 μM, i.e., the endogenous citrulline concentration that we found in the plasma of these toads. p-aminohippurate was added to the perfusate in order to increase urinary volume flow. Inulin was also added to the perfusion fluid. Under this condition, the absence of inulin in the urine proved the absence of glomerular filtration. The perfusion rate was 2 ml/h per portal vein. Phe, phenylalanine

that 84% of the D-alanine is reabsorbed. As 50 mM D-alanine inhibits the reabsorption of the radiolabel of 0.15 mM L-alanine (Table 1), this can be explained by assuming that the D-form is accepted by the carrier involved but possesses a lower affinity for it. It is even more surprising that, at high initial concentrations (50 mM), D-alanine is reabsorbed to a much greater extent (74%) than the L-form (27%) (see Table 1). This rapid reabsorption of D-alanine is partly blocked ($P < 0.005$) if benzoate and indole carboxylic acid are added to the perfusate (5 mM each). Both compounds are well-known inhibitors of D-amino acid oxidase [15], suggesting that this enzyme is involved in the quick removal of D-alanine from the tubule lumen.

Tissue Concentrations of Free Amino Acids in the Kidney

As described in the methods and as shown for serine in Fig. 3, overall amino acid concentrations (mmol/kg wet weight) are higher in the cortex than in the plasma. In the renal medulla the overall tissue concentration is even higher and increases further toward the papilla where the serine concentration amounts to more than 10 mmol/kg. In contrast, the urine (1400 mosm/kg H_2O), although excreted in the very neighborhood of the papillary tissue, contains only 0.08 mM serine. As all other amino acids measured in this experiment (data not shown) also show a high amino acid concentration gradient toward the papilla (papillary values in mmol/kg wet weight: taurine 4.7, aspartate⁻ 8.8, threonine 7.5, glutamate⁻ 14.0, etc.) they add up to a total

Table 1. Continuous microperfusion of the short loops of Henle of rat kidneys in vivo et in situ at a rate of 20 nl/min. ^{14}C-labeled amino acids, listed in the first row, and tritiated inulin were added to the perfusion fluid. Fractional delivery (*FD*) of the ^{14}C-label as compared to the ^{3}H-activity was determined in the collected samples. Fractional reabsorption, $(1 - FD)$

[14]C-compounds (mM)	added (mM)	FD ± SEM (*n*)
L-arginine (5)	–	0.57 ± 0.05 (10)
L-glutamate (5)	–	0.26 ± 0.04 (14)
Glycine (0.21)	–	0.051 ± 0.006 (6)
Glycine (50)	–	0.41 ± 0.04 (9)
Glycine (0.21)	L-Phe (50)	0.76 ± 0.05 (9)
Glycine (0.21)	L-Pro (50)	0.76 ± 0.05 (9)
L-phenylalanine (50)	–	0.50 ± 0.10 (7)
L-proline (50)	–	0.82 ± 0.09 (5)
L-alanine (0.15)	–	0.029 ± 0.008 (6)
L-alanine (0.15)	D-Ala (50)	0.14 ± 0.03 (7)
L-alanine (0.6)	–	0.029 ± 0.009 (6)
D-alanine (0.6)	–	0.16 ± 0.03 (17)
L-alanine (50)	–	0.73[a] ± 0.03 (8)
D-alanine (50)	–	0.26* ± 0.04 (15)
D-alanine (50)	[b]	0.57 ± 0.08 (8)
Mannitol (0.68)	–	0.95 ± 0.07 (10)**

[a]More than 95% of this ^{14}C-activity was intact L-alanine
*Significantly different from the foregoing value ($P < 0.005$)
[b]The D-amino acid oxidase inhibitors benzoate and indole carboxylic acid (5 mM each) were added to the perfusate
**Not significantly different from one

amino acid tissue concentration in the papilla of about 100 mmol/kg wet weight. Within the cells, these concentrations should be even higher (see Discussion).

Discussion

Our microperfusion experiments show (Table 1) that the short loops of Henle have a very high capacity to reabsorb amino acids which may have escaped reabsorption in earlier parts of the proximal tubule or which may stem from intraluminal peptide degradation (review, [1]). The fact that net reabsorption in the short loops is zero [6,7] shows, however, that amino acids leak into the lumen to a great extent. The fact that citrulline virtually completely enters the lumen of the non-filtering tubule of the toad on a route which is stereospecific and Na(Cl)-dependent and can be inhibited by another neutral amino acid (Fig. 4) suggests that this entry is a transcellular pathway involving the well-known peritubular and luminal amino acid carriers in the "wrong" direction. Thus, a nonspecific leak does not play a significant role here, if no great differences can be assumed between the toad and rat kidney in this regard. This view is confirmed by the fact that the radiolabel of mannitol, which has a molecular size comparable to that of the amino acids, is not reabsorbed from the lumen of rat short loops of Henle to a significant extent (see Table 1).

If secretory fluxes of amino acids are mediated nearly exclusively by the membrane carriers of the tubule cells in humans also, the tubule defects in inherited specific hyperaminoacidurias have to be reconsidered. In some of these diseases ("classic" cystinuria, "acidic" hyperaminoaciduria), net secretion of cystine and "acidic" amino acids (glutamate⁻ and aspartate⁻), respectively, has been observed (review, [1]). Consequently, this would mean that amino acid binding and transport by the carriers involved are intact, as they are still able to transport in the "wrong" direction. What might be defective in the kidneys of these patients is the ability of the carrier to be energized by the sodium gradient which normally drives the secondary-active amino acid transport in the opposite direction. A defect at the Na^+-binding site of the carriers involved is one possible explanation. This hypothesis, however, needs to be tested in further studies.

Returning to the discrepancy between zero net flux and high unidirectional fluxes of amino acids in the short loops of Henle, it seems feasible that the unexpectedly high early distal amino acid recovery might be even higher if there were no potent reabsorptive pump mechanisms in the loops of Henle. Thus, the main business of these pump mechanisms may not be to reabsorb amino acids overflowing from the proximal convolution, but it may be, instead, to counteract the leak driven by the extremely high medullary amino acid concentrations found in this study (see Fig. 3). These tissue concentrations are most probably underestimated because the volume of the cortex, the outer stripe, and the inner medulla contains about 25% tubule lumina and collecting ducts [16], where the amino acid concentrations are relatively low and, therefore, do not contribute significantly to the overall amino acid concentration. Although luminal amino acid concentrations in the inner medullary sections of the long loops of Henle (as well as in inner medullary vasa recta) are higher than in the systemic plasma [10], they are still much lower than the values we found in the whole tissue: e.g., 0.6 −2 mM for serine (entire tissue 7–10 mM) or 0.1–0.3 mM for aspartate (whole tissue 6–8 mM). In view of the fact that the total concentration of amino acids found in the papillary tissue in this study (about 100 mM) is an underestimation of the intracellular concentration, amino acids seem to contribute quite significantly to the high osmolality in medullary cells during antidiuresis. (This 100 mM compares, e.g., with 65–110 mM glycerophosphorylcholine, 35–74 mM betaine and 60 mM sorbitol.)

Confirming earlier in vitro data obtained with luminal membrane vesicles of rabbit proximal tubules [17], our microperfusion data with L- and D-alanine show (see Table 1) that the D- and L-isomers of alanine seem to share one carrier in the wall of the loop of Henle, because (a) the D-alanine reabsorption rate is not very much different from that of the L-isomer and (b) the high concentrations of D-alanine inhibit reabsorption of the L-form to some extent. The result showing that, at high concentrations, the radiolabel of L-alanine is reabsorbed significantly more slowly than that of the D-form, could be explained by re-secretion of a (still radiolabelled) metabolite of L-alanine into the lumen. We therefore identified the compound to which the ^{14}C-label was bound in the collected samples of this series by combining column chromatography and scintillation counting. It turned out that more than 95% of the radio-label represented L-alanine. This result shows that D-alanine is indeed reabsorbed faster than the L-form. The significant retardation of the reabsorption of D-alanine by D-amino acid oxidase inhibitors shows that D-alanine has access to this intracellular enzyme, which has been localized mainly in the straight part of the proximal tubule [18]. This phenomenon suggests that this enzyme provides a metabolic sink for D-alanine and also, perhaps, for other substrates of this enzyme. Besides other D-amino acids, glycine also belongs to this group.

Acknowledgments. We thank Ms. Olga Brokl for her great encouragement and support during the time S.S. spent his sabbatical in the lab at the University of Arizona. We also thank Ms. Margit Schulze for drawing the figures and Ms. Angelika Reuβ for secretarial help. Supported in part by NATO Collaborative Research Grant 0104/88 and by National Institute of Health Grant DK 16294.

References

1. Silbernagl S (1988) The renal handling of amino acids and oligopeptides. Physiol Rev 68:911–1007
2. Silbernagl S (1980) Tubular reabsorption of L-glutamine studied by free flow micropuncture and microperfusion of rat kidney. Int J Biochem 12:9–16
3. Schwegler JS, Heuner A, Silbernagl S (1989) Electrogenic transport of neutral and dibasic amino acids in a cultured opossum cell line (OK). Pflugers Arch 414:543–550
4. Schwegler JS, Schömig E, Heuner A, Silbernagl S (1990) Development of high-capacity, low-affinity L-arginine transport in a proximal tubular cell line during differentiation. In: Lubec G, Rosenthal GA (eds) Amino acids. Chemistry, biology and medicine. ESCOM, Leiden, pp 1017–1028
5. Schafer JA, Barfuss DW (1980) Membrane mechanisms for transepithelial amino acid absorption and secretion. Am J Physiol 238:F335–F346
6. Eisenbach GM, Weise M, Stolte H (1975) Amino acid reabsorption in the rat nephron. Free flow micropuncture study. Pflugers Arch 357:63–76
7. Günther R, Silbernagl S, Deetjen P (1979) Maleic acid induced aminoaciduria studied by free flow micropuncture and continuous microperfusion. Pflugers Arch 382:109–114
8. Bergeron M, Morel F (1969) Amino acid transport in rat renal tubules. Am J Physiol 216:1139–1149
9. Dantzler WH, Silbernagl S (1988) Amino acid transport by juxtamedullary nephrons: distal reabsorption and recycling. Am J Physiol 255:F397–F407
10. Dantzler WH, Silbernagl S (1990) Amino acid transport: microperfusion and micropuncture of Henle's loop and vasa recta. Am J Physiol 258:F504–513
11. Hayman JM Jr (1928) Notes on the arrangement of blood vessels of the frog's kidney together with some measurements of blood pressure in the renal portal and renal veins. Am J Physiol 86:331–339
12. Gekle M, Grimme M, Silbernagl S (1989) Peritubular transport, tubular metabolism, and transcellular secretion of L-citrulline in the isolated perfused kidney of the frog (*Xenopus laevis*). Kidney Int 36:311
13. Lang F, Greger R, Lechene C, Knox FG (1978) Micropuncture techniques. In: Martinez-Maldonado M (ed) Methods in pharmacology, renal pharmacology. Plenum, New York, pp 75–103
14. Sonnenberg H, Deetjen P (1964) Methode zur Durchströmung einzelner Nephronabschnitte. Pflugers Arch 278:669–674
15. Bartlett GR (1948) The inhibition of D-amino acid oxidase by benzoic acid and various monosubstituted benzoic acid derivatives. J Am Chem Soc 70:1010–1011
16. Pfaller W (1982) Structure function correlation in rat kidney. Quantitative correlation of structure and function in the normal and injured rat kidney. In: Pfaller W (ed) Advances in anatomy, embryology and cell biology, vol. 70. Springer, Berlin
17. Jessen H, Vorum H, Jørgensen KE, Sheikh MI (1988) Characteristics of D-alanine transport by luminal membrane vesicles from pars convoluta and pars recta of rabbit proximal tubule. Biochim Biophys Acta 942:262–270
18. Chan AWK, Perry SG, Burch HB, Fagioli S, Alvey TR, Lowry OH (1979) Distribution of two aminotransferases and D-amino acid oxidase within the nephron of young and adult rats. J Histochem Cytochem 27:751–755

Optical Techniques for Studying Kidney Cell Function

Chair: Walter F. Boron (USA)
Kenneth R. Spring (USA)

Optical Approaches for Studying Intracellular pH in Epithelial Cells

WALTER F. BORON[1]

Introduction

Ten years ago, the only practical approach for continuously monitoring intracellular pH (pH$_i$) in epithelial cells was to employ pH-sensitive microelectrodes with a recessed glass sensor [1]. Although these electrodes are extremely accurate and stable, they require skill to fabricate and use. Moreover, although they can be used with modestly small cells (e.g., amphibian proximal-tubule cells), the electrode response time increases with the sharpness of the electrode tip. In the ensuing years, the introduction of improved "proton cocktails" [2] for liquid-membrane electrodes has greatly simplified the preparation of pH-sensitive microelectrodes and, to a lesser extent, has increased the sharpness of their tips. Nevertheless, although it is relatively easy to use these pH-sensitive microelectrodes with amphibian renal tubules, it remains rather difficult to extend the technology to mammalian tubules. It is for this reason that we have devoted considerable effort during the past decade to developing three optical techniques for monitoring pH$_i$ in isolated renal tubules and even in single cells. The first technique exploits photodiode array technology for measuring the absorbance spectrum of an intracellular pH-sensitive dye. It has been applied to isolated renal tubules from amphibians [3] and mammals [4], as well as to single cells [5]. The second technique is the use of an epifluorescence microscope to monitor the fluorescence of a pH-sensitive dye. Once again, this approach has been applied both to single cells [6] and to isolated mammalian tubules [7]. Finally, the approach on which we have devoted our most recent efforts is an extension of the earlier fluorescence technique in which the detector is an image-intensifier/TV-camera rather than a photomultiplier tube. Digital image processing makes it possible to monitor pH$_i$ transients in multiple individual cells, or even in portions of a single cell.

[1]Department of Cellular and Molecular Physiology, Yale University School of Medicine, New Haven, CT 06510, USA

Before beginning a description of these techniques, I should make two points. First, the use of optical techniques for monitoring pH, requires good dyes. In our absorbance measurements, we employ dimethylcarboxyfluorescein (Me_2CF). The dye is introduced into the cell by exposing the latter to a diacetate-ester derivative of Me_2CF. This ester is hydrolyzed intracellularly by native esterases, forming Me_2CF, which is relatively trapped inside the cell. Such ester derivatives of various fluorescein compounds were used to assess cell viability before it was recognized that these compounds could also be employed for measuring pH, [8]. Probably the best of these fluorescein derivatives is 2,7-biscarboxyethyl-5(6)-carboxyfluorescein (BCECF); both it and its acetoxymethylester derivative were developed by Roger Tsien and his colleagues [9], who have pioneered several other dyes as well. The second point worth noting is that abandoning the microelectrode approach for optics has not come without a price: a loss of a continuous record of membrane voltage. The latter, which is a byproduct of every pH-sensitive microelectrode measurement, has proven extremely useful in characterizing electrogenic processes [10]. Thus, it would be desirable to supplement pH-sensitive dye measurements with either microelectrode or dye measurements of membrane voltage.

Absorbance Measurements

Theoretical Considerations

When a molecule absorbs a photon of energy hv, where h is Planck's constant and v is the frequency, the molecule is raised to an excited state. The excited molecule can return to the ground state in any of three ways. First, through random collisions (*quenching*), it can transfer all or part of its excess energy to other molecules, which can in turn undergo a variety of reactions. Second, it can emit one or more photons. If the single emitted photon has the same wavelength as the exciting photo, the process is termed *resonance radiation*. If the emitted photon has less energy (i.e., a higher wavelength) than the exciting photon, the process is termed *fluorescence*. The remainder of the energy can be dissipated either by emitting another photon, or by transferring energy by random collisions. The third possible fate of an excited molecule is to fragment. Regardless of the mechanism by which the molecule returns to its ground state, the molecule must absorb light. The amount of absorbed light is termed the *absorbance*, which is defined as

$$A = -\log \frac{I}{I_o},$$

where A is the absorbance, I_o is the intensity of the beam of light as it enters the sample, I is the intensity as the light leaves the sample. According to Beer's law, the absorbance is proportional to the thickness of the sample (l) and the concentration of the molecule (c):

$$A = \varepsilon l c,$$

where ε is the *molar extinction coefficient*.

In general, ε is a function of wavelength (λ). For pH-sensitive dyes, such as Me_2CF, ε is also a function of pH. Thus, the shape of the absorbance spectrum is

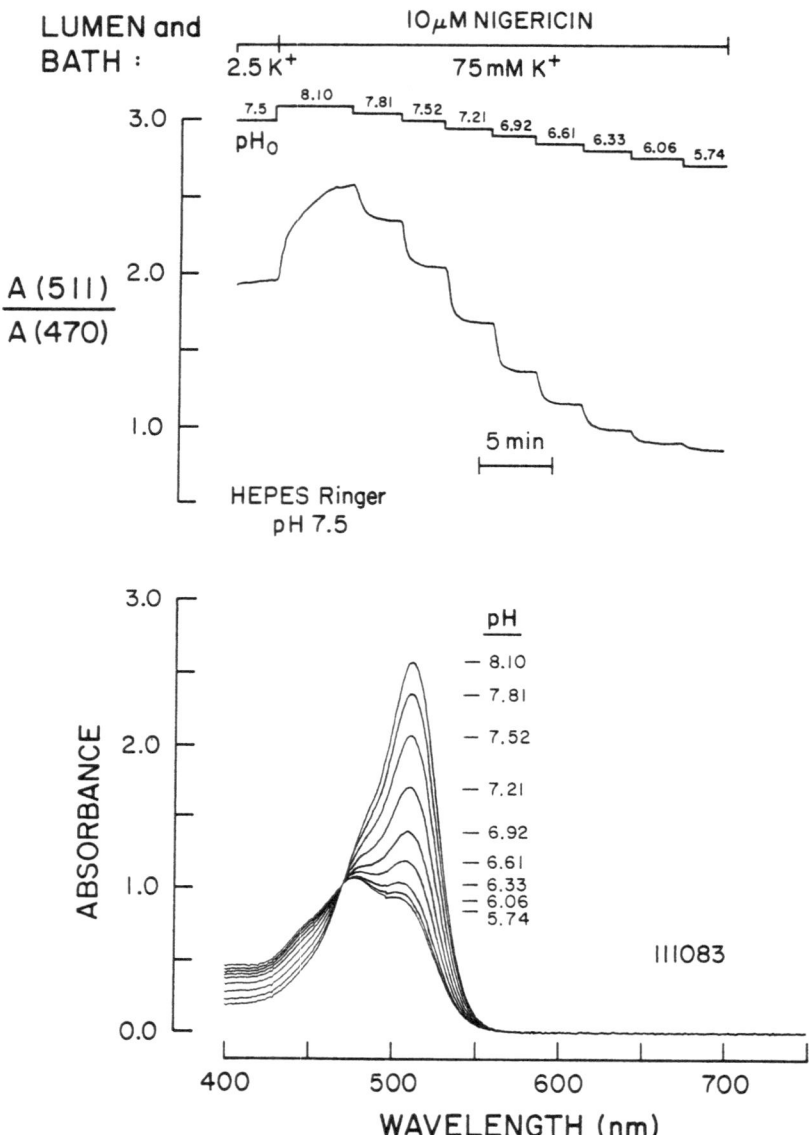

Fig. 1. pH dependence of the absorbance spectrum of in vitro dimethylcarboxyfluorescein. The data are normalized to unity at 470 nm, the isosbestic wavelength. The *inset* shows the ratio of absorbance at 505 nm (the peak) to that at 470 nm as a function of pH. (From [3] by permission of The Rockefeller University Press)

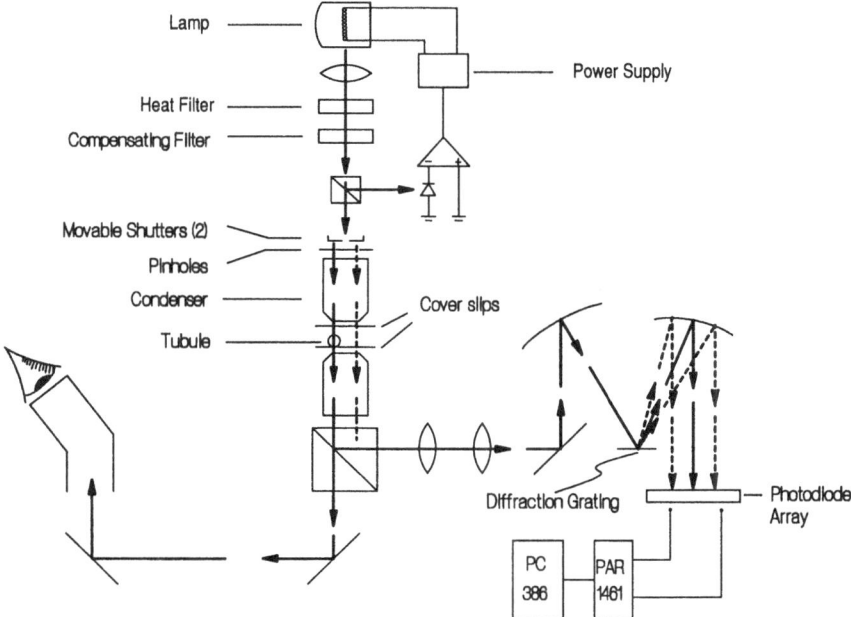

Fig. 2. Schematic diagram of the apparatus used in measuring the optical absorbance of pH sensitive dyes. In brief, white light is passed either next to (providing I_o) or through (providing I) an isolated tubule or a single cell. The intensity spectrum of this light is obtained by creating a spectrum with a diffraction grating, and focusing the spectrum on an array of 1024 photodiodes. The photon signal on each diode is read into the computer with 14-bit resolution (1 part in 16384). The absorbance spectrum is computed from the intensity spectra of the incident and transmitted light. (Redrawn from [3])

pH sensitive, as indicated in Fig. 1. Under the conditions employed in the experiment summarized in Fig. 1, the in-vitro absorbance of Me_2CF is most pH sensitive at a wavelength of 505 nm (the peak), and is not pH sensitive at all at 470 nm. Although it might be tempting to compute pH from the absorbance at the peak wavelength, this is not possible. A is not a unique function of pH; A is also dependent on c and l. If intracellular dye concentration changes during an experiment (it almost always drifts downward due to dye leakage and/or bleaching), or if the optical path length through the cell changes, A would change even if pH_i were to remain constant. A solution to this problem is to divide A_{505} by A_{470}, which has the effect of canceling out the contributions of l and c. A_{505} is chosen because this is the most pH sensitive wavelength. A_{470} is chosen for convenience because this value can be used to independently compute dye concentration, assuming that the path length and intracellular ε are known. However, it should be emphasized that in principle any pair of wavelengths could be used for computing the ratio. Some wavelength pairs are more sensitive to pH changes than others, but all provide an index of the pH-sensitive spectral shape change.

Measuring the Absorbance of an Intracellular pH Sensitive Dye

Fig. 2 is a schematic representation of the apparatus used in our laboratory to measure the absorbance of intracellular dyes. Me_2CF can be loaded into the cells as described above. The ionophore nigericin can be used in high-K^+ solutions to approximately clamp pH_i to pH_o, the limitations of which have been described previously [3]. When intracellular absorbance spectra are obtained, it is immediately obvious that intracellular Me_2CF behaves differently from the dye in the cuvette. As summarized in Fig. 3a, when both intra- and extracellular spectra are normalized to unity at 470 nm, the intracellular spectrum is shorter and broader. In addition, the peak absorbance of the intracellular spectrum is red shifted (i.e., shifted to higher wavelengths) by ~6 nm. When the A_{peak}/A_{470} ratios are compared as a function of pH (Fig. 3b), we see that the pK is shifted to more alkaline values by ~0.4 pH units. Some discrepancy between the spectral properties of intra- vs. extracellular dye can be accounted for by the higher concentrations of Me_2CF inside the cell. However, the majority is probably due to interactions of the dye with intracellular constituents. The combination of the red-shifted spectrum and the alkali-shifted calibration curve could lead to errors of as much as 0.5 pH units if extracellular calibration/spectral data were used to compute pH_i. Fig. 3 emphasizes the importance of obtaining intracellular calibration and spectral information.

Single-Cell Fluorescence Measurements

In our laboratory, we have found pH_i values derived from absorbance spectra of mammalian renal tubules to have outstanding signal to noise ratio. This is achievable because the cells are loaded with mM concentrations of the dye, and have a rather large total optical path length (through two cell layers). Although we have had some success in applying the absorbance approach to single LLC-PK1 cells in culture [5], the experiments are more difficult owing to the much smaller path length. Therefore, our group has explored methods for using the fluorescence excitation spectrum of fluoroscein dyes to compute pH_i, as previously employed by J. A. Thomas et al. [8]. The approach is to alternately excite the dye with light at a wavelength (e.g., 490 nM) at which the emitted fluorescent light (e.g., at 530 nm) is very pH sensitive, and at a wavelength at which the emitted light is less pH sensitive or even has the reverse pH sensitivity (e.g., 440 nm). The ratio I_{490}/I_{440} is thus very pH sensitive, but is relatively insensitive to parameters such as dye concentration.

Our apparatus, summarized in Fig. 4, is based on an inverted microscope with epi-illumination. A single cell or a small portion of a renal tubule typically is illuminated with a 10-µm diameter beam of 490-nm or 440-nm light. Light of the two wavelengths is generated by using a system of dichroic mirrors, band-pass filters and computer-controlled shutters. This is not the only approach for generating two wavelengths of light. Several laboratories select wavelengths by moving into the light path filters mounted on a linear or rotary actuator. In an ingenious approach introduced by Kurtz [11], light beams of the two desired wavelengths are chopped at different frequencies and then combined by a dichroic mirror, so that the preparation is simultaneously excited by light of the two different wavelengths. The emission-intensity data from the independent excitation wavelengths are extracted by using a

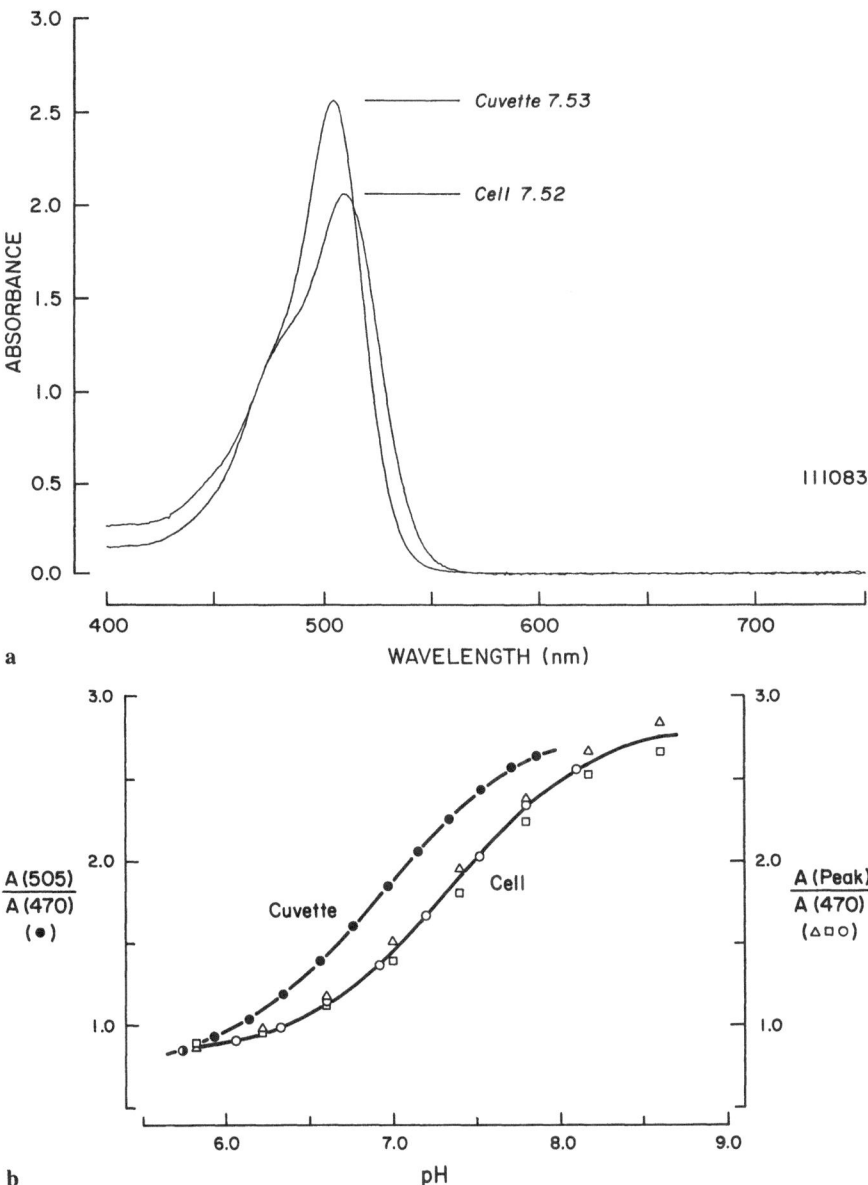

Fig. 3. Comparison of spectral properties of intra- and extracellular Me$_2$CF. **a** Comparison of absorbance spectra at a pH value of ~7.5. The curve labeled "cuvette" was obtained at a [Me$_2$CF] of 10 μM, that labeled "cell," at a [Me$_2$CF] in the mM range. **b** pH calibrations obtained from spectra similar to those shown in **a**. (From [3] by permission of The Rockefeller University Press)

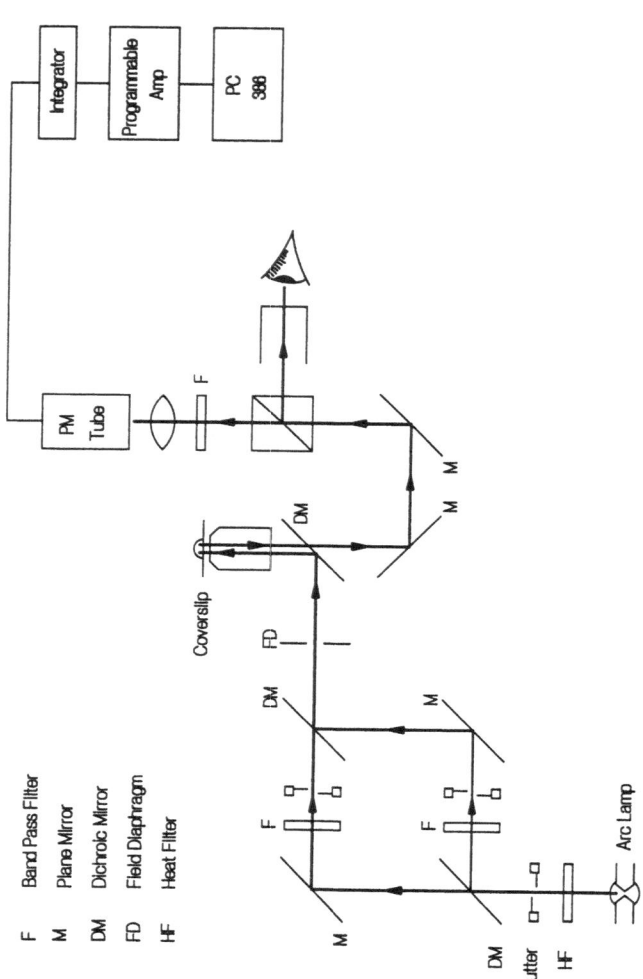

F Band Pass Filter
M Plane Mirror
DM Dichroic Mirror
FD Field Diaphragm
HF Heat Filter

Fig. 4. Schematic diagram of the apparatus used in measuring the fluorescence excitation ratio of an intracellular dye. In brief, light from an arc lamp is split by a 470-nm short-pass dichroic mirror into one path that is filtered at 440 nm and another that is filtered at 490 nm. A series of computer-controlled shutters determines whether 440-nm light, 490-nm light or no light at all illuminates the cell(s) as a 10-μm beam on the microscope stage. The emitted light is filtered at 530 nm and sensed by a photomultiplier tube. (Redrawn from [6])

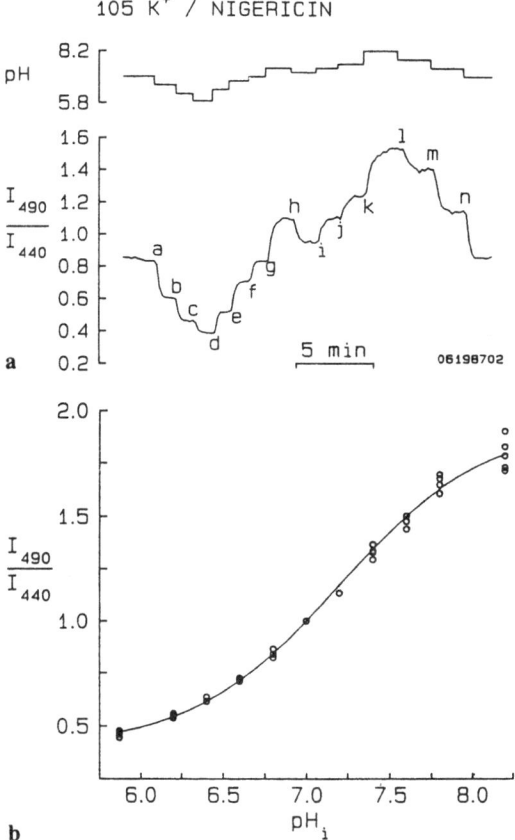

Fig. 5. Intracellular pH calibration of the fluorescence excitation ratio of BCECF. **a** Time course of I_{490}/I_{440} for a single renal mesangial cell exposed to high-K^+ solutions containing 10 μM nigericin, and titrated to various pH values, as indicated. **b** Summary of the pH dependence of I_{490}/I_{440} data from 6 experiments. The curve drawn through the points is the result of a non-linear least-squares curve fit, and has an apparent pK of 7.19. (From [6] by permission of The American Physiological Society)

lock-in amplifier. In our preliminary experiments, we found that two major problems were stray light and bleaching/photodynamic damage. We minimized bleaching/ photodynamic damage by keeping the cells in the dark for most of the time; a cell is typically illuminated with 440-nm light for 200 ms, 490-nm light for another 200 ms, and then is in the dark until another cycle begins. The fluorescence signal is optimized by programming the amplifier to adjust its gain to the magnitude of the expected signal at each of the two wavelengths. During the experiment, the operator monitors I_{440}, which is a good approximation of intracellular dye concentration, as well as the ratio I_{490}/I_{440}, which is an estimate of pH,.

As is the case with absorbance experiments, it is essential to calibrate the dye inside the cell(s). A typical intracellular calibration experiment is shown in Fig. 5a

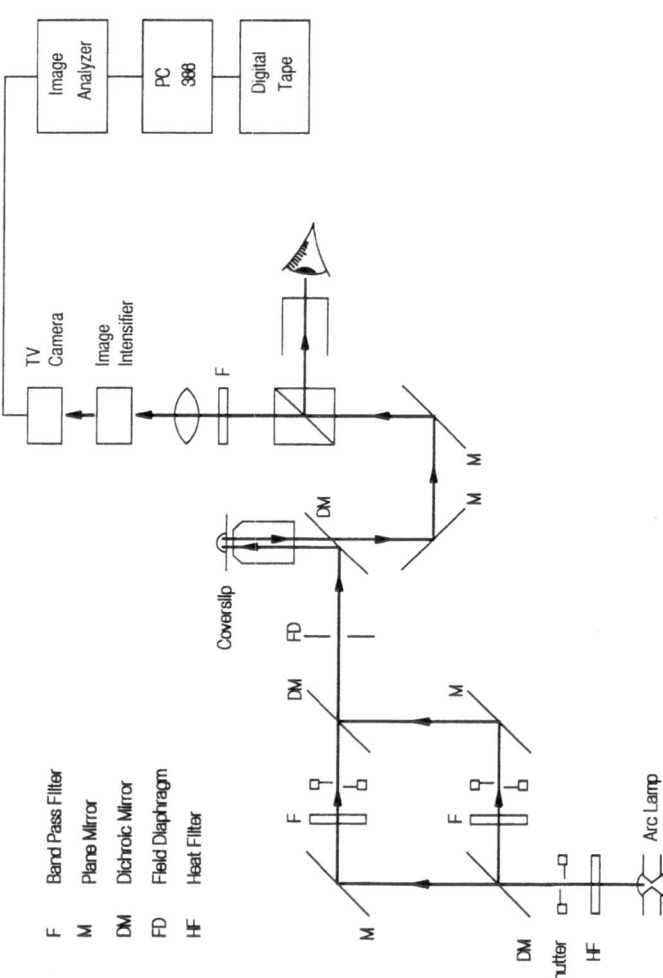

Fig. 6. Schematic diagram of the digital imaging system used in measuring the fluorescence excitation ratio of an intracellular dye. The apparatus is similar to that summarized in *Fig. 4*, except that the photomultiplier tube is replaced by an image intensifier and a television camera

for a single renal mesangial cell. The data from several cells is summarized in Fig. **5b**. We have used this fluorescence technique with single cultured cells of several different types [6,12], as well as with isolated rabbit proximal tubules [7].

Fluorescence Imaging

The approach outlined in the previous section provides the pH_i of a single cell or the average pH_i of a small group of cells. In a heterogeneous cell population, it would be advantageous to monitor, simultaneously, the pH_i of multiple cells. In addition, it might also be desirable to measure apparent pH_i values in different regions of a single cell. This can be achieved by imaging fluorescence signals, an approach used by others before us [13-18]. The approach used in our laboratory is similar to that used in single-cell fluorescence experiments, except that the photodetector is an image intensifier/television camera instead of a photomultiplier tube. In addition, we use a digital image processor to digitally analyze our fluorescence images. The apparatus is summarized in Fig. 6.

In preliminary experiments we found that, as expected, a major problem in imaging experiments was a shortage of photons at the pixel (picture element) level (Eisen and W. Boron, unpublished work). Because the limiting signal-to-noise ratio is proportional to the square root of the number of photons, the signal-to-noise ratio for a single pixel is extremely high [19]. However, we have found that if we group the pixels corresponding to a large part of a cell, the signal-to-noise ratio can approach that of the single-cell fluorescence technique, with a usable pH_i precision of ~ 0.02. We have employed digital analysis of fluorescence images to monitor pH_i transients with single osteoclasts (very large multinucleate cells), up to six simultaneous mesangial cells (moderately large cells, when in culture), and over 30 simultaneous MDCK cells (Eisen and W. Boron, unpublished work).

Acknowledgments. This work was supported by a grant from the NIH (DK30344). I acknowledge the dedicated efforts of Dr. J. Richard Chaillet and Mr. Andrey Yeatts, who developed the absorbance apparatus; Dr. Gregory Boyarsky, Dr. John P. Geibel, Mr. Andrey Yeatts and Mr. Vic Pantani, who developed the fluorescence apparatus; and Dr. Thomas D. Eisen and Mr. Duncan Wong, who developed the imaging system.

References

1. Thomas RC (1974) Intracellular pH of snail neurones measured with a new pH-sensitive glass microelectrode. J Physiol 238:159-180
2. Ammann D, Lanter F, Schulthess P, Shijo Y, Simon W (1981) Neutral carrier based hydrogen ion selective microelectrode for extra- and intracellular studies. Anal Chem 53:2267-2269
3. Chaillet JR, Boron WF (1985) Intracellular calibration of a pH-sensitive dye in isolated perfused salamander proximal tubules. J Gen Physiol 86:765-794
4. Nakhoul NL, Lopes AG, Chaillet JR, Boron WF (1988) Intracellular pH regulation in the S3 segment of the rabbit proximal tubule in HCO_3^--free solutions. J Gen Physiol 92:369-393

5. Chaillet JR, Amsler K, Boron WF (1986) Optical measurement of intracellular pH in single LLC-PK1 cells: demonstration of $Cl^-HCO_3^-$ exchange. Proc Natl Acad Sci USA 83:522–526

6. Boyarsky G, Ganz MB, Sterzel B, Boron WF (1988) pH regulation in single glomerular mesangial cells. I. Acid extrusion in absence and presence of HCO_3. Am J Physiol 255:C844–C856

7. Geibel JP, Giebisch G, Boron WF (1989) Basolateral sodium-coupled acid-base transport mechanisms of the rabbit proximal tubule. Am J Physiol 257:F790–F797

8. Thomas JA, Buchsbaum RN, Zimniak A, Racker E (1979) Intracellular pH measurements in Ehrlich ascites tumor cells utilizing spectroscopic probes generated in situ. Biochemistry 81:2210–2218

9. Rink TJ, Tsien RY, Pozzan T (1982) Cytoplasmic pH and free Mg^{+2} in lymphocytes. J Cell Biol 95:189–196

10. Boron WF, Boulpaep EL (1983) Intracellular pH regulation in the renal proximal tubule of the salamander: basolateral HCO_3^- transport. J Gen Physiol 81:53–94

11. Kurtz I (1987) Apical Na^+/H^+ antiporter and glycolysis-dependent H^+-ATPase regulate intracellular pH in the rabbit S3 proximal tubule. J Clin Invest 80:928–935

12. Boyarsky G, Ranson BR, Schlue W-R, Davis M (1989) Anomalous stimulation of pH regulation by ethylisopropyl amiloride in cultured mammalian astrocytes. Society for Neuroscience Abstracts 15:15

13. Ambler SK, Poenie M, Tsien RY, Taylor P (1988) Agonist-stimulated oscillations and cycling of intracellular free calcium in individual cultured muscle cells. J Biol Chem 263:1952–1959

14. Spring KR (1985) The study of epithelial function by quantitative light microscopy. Pflugers Arch 405:S23–S27

15. Kruskal BA, Shak S, Maxfield FR (1986) Spreading of human neutrophils is immediately preceded by a large increase in cytoplasmic free calcium. PNAS 83:2919–2923

16. Paradiso AM, Machen TE (1987) Digital image processing of intracellular pH in gastric oxyntic and chief cells. Nature 325:447–450

17. Negulescu PA, Harootunian A, Minta A, Tsien RY, Machen TE (1988) Intracellular sodium regulation in rabbit gastric glands determined using a fluorescent sodium indicator. J Gen Physiol 92:26a

18. Jacob R, Merritt JE, Hallam TJ, Rink TJ (1988) Repetitive spikes in cytoplasmic calcium evoked by histamine in human endothelial cells. Nature 335:40–45

19. Spring KR (To be published) Quantitative imaging at low light levels: differential interference contrast and fluorescence microscopy without significant light loss. Digitized Video Microscopy

Cell pH Regulation in Collecting Tubules

MICHIO KUWAHARA, SEI SASAKI, and FUMIAKI MARUMO[1]

SUMMARY. We measured the single cell pH of principal cells (PC) and intercalated cells (IC) in the outer stripe of the outer medullary collecting duct (OMCDo) of the rabbit using fluorescence ratio imaging.

1. It was suggested that single cell fluorescence measurement is influenced by fluorescence from neighboring, out-of-focus cells.
2. To minimize the effect of out-of-focus cells:
   a) in PC, a cell that is minimally surrounded by IC should be carefully selected.
   b) in IC, luminal dye loading is useful.
3. Using these techniques, HCO_3^--independent mechanisms of pHi regulation were examined. Our results suggest that:
   a) in PC, basolateral Na^+/H^+ exchange, and
   b) in IC, the luminal N-ethylmaleimide (NEM)- and N-N'-dicyclohexylcarbodiomide (DCCD)-inhibitable H^+ pump, and basolateral Na^+/H^+ exchange, contribute to cell pH regulation in rabbit OMCDo.

Introduction

A renal tubule is cylindrical in shape and contains hundreds of cells per mm of its length. It has been demonstrated that fluorescence measurement in a single cell in a three-dimensional tissue is influenced by fluorescence derived from surrounding out-of-focus cells [1]. Thus, to measure intracellular pH (pHi) of a single tubule cell accurately, special care should be taken to eliminate (or minimize) this "out-of-focus" effect.

The outer stripe of the outer medullary collecting duct (OMCDo) is one of the important sites of renal acidification [2,3]. In this segment HCO_3^- is absorbed con-

---

[1]Second Department of Internal Medicine, Tokyo Medical and Dental University, Tokyo, 113 Japan

sistently [3]. OMCDo consists of principal cells (PC) and intercalated cells (IC) [4–6]. Because there are morphological and functional differences between these two cell types [4–7], different mechanisms might be involved in pHi regulation. However, pHi regulation of individual cells in this segment has not been studied so far.

We measured single cell pHi of PC and IC in rabbit OMCDo, using fluorescence ratio imaging microscopy. In the first half of this paper, we describe detailed methods for pHi measurement in the tubule cell. In the latter half, we describe the HCO_3^--independent mechanisms of pHi regulation which were examined using these techniques.

Methods

Kidneys from Japanese white rabbits (2.0–2.5kg) were cut in coronal slices. Segments of OMCDo (300–600 um in length) were dissected and transferred to a thermo-regulated bath of 150ul volume. This bath was set on the stage of an inverted epifluorescence microscope (Olympus IMT-2, Japan) which was placed on a vibration-proof plate (Visolator, Meiritsu, Japan). After tubules were mounted between perfusion and holding pipettes, the lumen was perfused as described previously [8]. The perfusion rate was maintained at > 10nl/min. In some protocols, an isolated OMCDo was split with fine forceps along the long axis and a cell monolayer was made. The monolayer was also mounted between holding pipettes. The bath solution was pre-heated at 37°C and was exchanged at 10ml/min by gravity. The control perfusion and bath solutions were identical and contained (in mM) 134 NaCl, 5 KCl, 1.0 NaH_2PO_4, 1.2 $MgSO_4$, 1.0 $CaCl_2$, 5.5 glucose, 6.0 L-alanine, and 20 HEPES.

After tubules were perfused 20–30 min for equilibration, the acetoxymethyl derivative of 2'-7'-bis (carboxyethyl)-5(6)-carboxyfluorescein (BCECF-AM) was loaded to tubules from the lumen or the bath. For the luminal loading, tubules were perfused with 20–30 μM BCECF-AM for 15–20 min. For the basolateral loading, bath flow was stopped and tubules were bathed with 7–10 μM BCECF-AM for 15–20 min.

Tubule cells were viewed with a 40 × objective (Olympus DPlan Apo, Japan, NA=0.85) and a silicon-intensified target camera (Hamamatsu Photonics C2400-08H, Japan), and were displayed on a TV monitor with 483 × 512 pixels (SONY Trinitron PVM-1371Q, Japan). The final magnification on the TV monitor was 1400 ×. The area of each cell contained 800–2000 pixels at this magnification. One tubule image was recorded in 1/30 s and was stored in an image processor (ARGUS 100, Hamamatsu Photonics, Japan).

Fluorescence was excited using a 75-W xenon lamp. Excitation light was attenuated by neutral density filters. For pHi measurement with BCECF, 490 ± 10 nm and 440 ± 10 nm interference filters, a 520 nm dichroic mirror, a > 520 nm cut-on filter, and a 535 ± 6 nm bandpass filter were used. Background images were recorded before taking fluorescent images. Tubules were excited alternately at 490 and 440 nm by moving the interference filters placed on a computer-assisted slider. Each image was an average of 4 sequential 1/30 s images; a pair of images (490 and 440 nm excitation) were taken in 1s. After the background signal was subtracted, the 490 nm image was divided by the 440 nm image. For pHi measurement, a rectangular measuring area (15 × 15 pixels) was set on the center of each tubule cell. pHi was determined in 1–5 cells from one tubule.

The in vivo BCECF calibration curve was obtained by the nigericin high K^+ method [9]. The calibration solution contained (in mM) 105 KCl, 30 phosphate, 1.2 $MgSO_4$, 20 HEPES, 40 NMDG, 5.5 glucose, 6 alanine, 1.0 $CaCl_2$, and 10 μM nigericin. The solution pH was adjusted to 7 different pHs (pH 5.8 − 8.2) by KOH or HCl. The fluorescence ratios in PC were 0.68 ± 0.02 (means ± SE of 12 cells from 5 tubules) at pH 5.8; 0.86 ± 0.03 at pH 6.2; 1.04 ± 0.04 at pH 6.6; 1.35 ± 0.04 at pH 7.0; 1.73 ± 0.03 at pH 7.4; 2.03 ± 0.03 at pH 7.8; and 2.36 ± 0.04 at pH 8.2. The ratios in IC were higher than PC by 0.01 − 0.06 at any pH, although differences in values were not significant in these two cell types. Because the fluorescence ratio-pH relationship was approximately linear between pH 5.8 and 6.6 and between pH 6.6 and 7.8 in both PC and IC, linear conversion formulas (the ratio of 490/440 nm = a + b × pHi) were made separately for these two pH ranges. These calibrations were used to convert the ratios to pHi.

Because this study was focused on HCO_3^--independent mechanisms of pHi regulation, all experiments were performed in the absence of extracellular CO_2/HCO_3^-. pHi regulation processes were examined by analyzing the time course of pHi recovery from intracellular acid load, using the NH_4Cl pre-pulse technique [10]. Five to ten min after BCECF-AM removal, 20mM NH_4Cl was added to the bath (replaced by 20mM NaCl in the control solution) for 3min, and then NH_4Cl was rapidly removed. The time course of pHi was monitored at a 5 or 10 s interval. In response to NH_4Cl withdrawal, pHi decreased for 10–20s; this was followed by a gradual pHi recovery. pHi recovery rate ($dpHi/dt$, pHU/s × 10^3) was calculated from data points during 20s of the initial recovery phase. Similar experiments were carried out in the absence of Na^+ (replaced by $NMDG^+$). Acid loading was done by substituting 20mM $NMDG^+$ for NH_4^+. Data for pHi of 1–5 cells were obtained from one tubule.

The results are expressed as means ± SE. Student's t-test and an analysis of variance were used, when appropriate, to determine statistical significance. Values of $P < 0.05$ were considered significant.

Results and Discussion

Measurement of Single Cell pHi

Because the OMCDo is cylindrical, a single cell fluorescence measurement would be affected by neighboring cells [1]. Before starting experiments with tubule cells, we tested this issue in our experimental system. A glass capillary of 5μm diameter (similar in size to a single cell in rabbit OMCDo) was filled with 200μM BCECF. The fluorescence intensity of this capillary sample was measured at various focus levels. When the focus was adjusted just at the level of the capillary, the fluorescence was detected virtually right on the sample (Fig. 1). This result indicates that the influence from neighboring cells could be negligible if fluorescence was measured in a flat sheet. Some protocols were performed with a cell monolayer made by splitting an isolated OMCDo (Fig. 2c). Fluorescence was also measured at 10μm, 20μm and 30μm above the capillary level (Fig. 1). Fluorescence was detected not only right above the sample but also around the sample. These results suggested

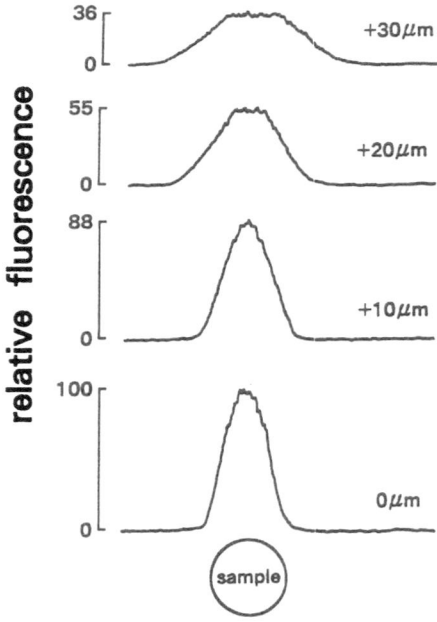

Fig. 1. Out-of-focus effect on fluorescence measurement. A glass capillary (5μm in diameter) was filled with 200μM BCECF and fluorescence was detected at various focus levels.

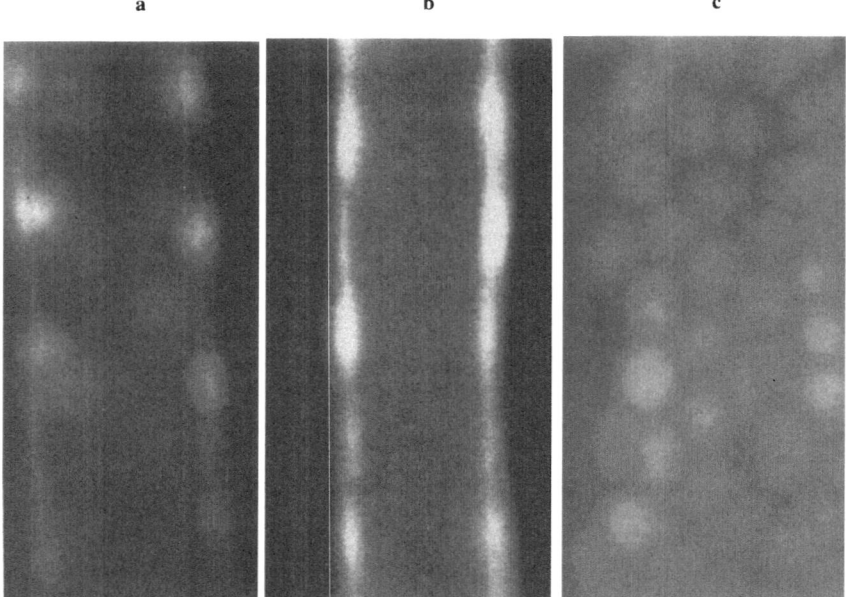

Fig. 2a-c. Fluorescent images of OMCDo perfused in vitro (400x). BCECF was loaded from the lumen (**a**) or the bath (**b**). **c** A fluorescent image of a cell monolayer that was made by splitting an isolated OMCDo. × 400

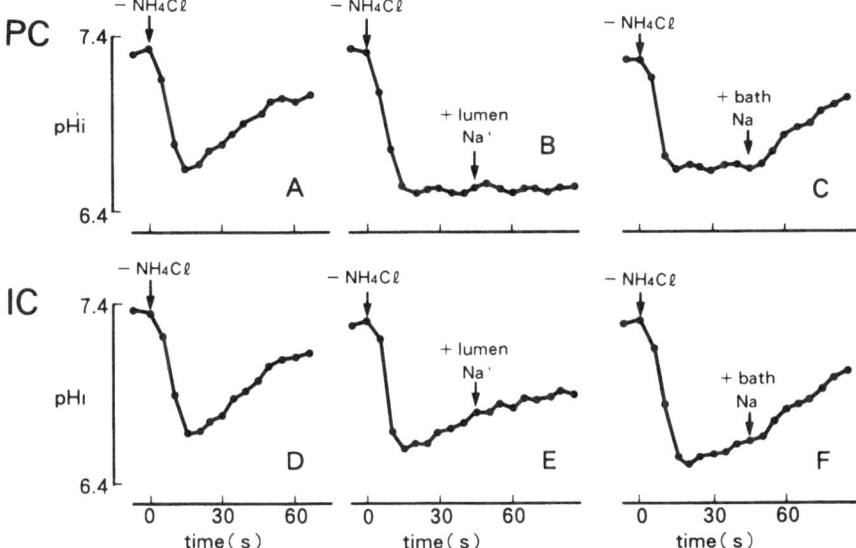

Fig. 3a-f. Time courses of pHi recovery from intracellular acid load in PC (**a-c**) and in IC (**d-f**) in the absence of extracellular HCO_3^-. NH_4Cl was removed from the bath at time zero. See text for details. PC, principal cells; IC, intercalated cells

that single cell fluorescence measurement in the intact tubule would be influenced by out-of-focus cells.

Cell identification was basically dependent on morphological criteria originally described in cortical collecting tubule (CCT) cells by Strange and Spring [11]. In most cases cells were identified without differential interference contrast optics. When BCECF was loaded from the lumen, only IC were intensely stained (Fig. 2a), a finding consistent with a recent report by Weiner and Hamm [12]. Because the fluorescence of PC was very weak, the interference from surrounding PC would be small. Thus, luminal loading was used in the pHi measurement of IC. In contrast, all cells were brightly stained with basolateral loading of BCECF (Fig. 2b). IC were slightly (< 50%) brighter than PC. To avoid the influence of IC fluorescence in the pHi measurement of PC, we carefully chose PC that were minimally surrounded by IC (the ratio of the number of PC and IC is about 4:1 in OMCDo (see [4]). As will be shown later, pHi data obtained in intact tubule and monolayer preparations were in general quite similar for both PC and IC.

pHi Recovery from Intracellular Acid Load

To examine HCO_3^--independent mechanisms of pHi regulation, time courses of pHi upon acid load were observed in the absence of extracellular HCO_3^- (Fig. 3). Figs. 3a and 3d show experiments with monolayer cells. After NH_4Cl was removed from the bath at time zero, the pHi of PC (Fig. 3a) and IC (Fig. 3d) decreased promptly and recovered gradually thereafter. In PC dpHi/dt was 12.3 ± 0.9 (10 cells) and in IC it

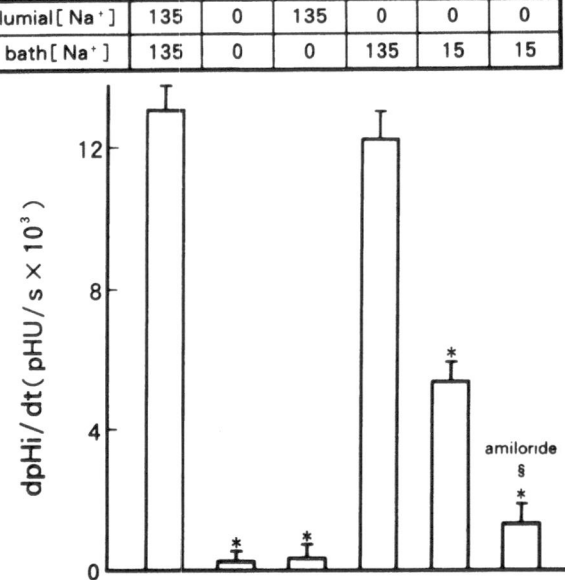

| lumial[Na⁺] | 135 | 0 | 135 | 0 | 0 | 0 |
| bath[Na⁺] | 135 | 0 | 0 | 135 | 15 | 15 |

Fig. 4. pHi recovery rates ($dpHi/dt$) of PC at various [Na⁺] (in mM). Each *bar* represents means ± SE of 10–21 cells from 4–11 tubules. amiloride; 1mM amiloride was added to the bath at the NH₄Cl removal. *P < 0.001 compared with the control, §P < 0.01 compared with the absence of amiloride

was 11.5 ± 1.0 (10 cells). Similar values of dpHi/dt were obtained in the intact tubule study (13.8 ± 0.7 in 15 PC; 12.7 ± 0.9 in 12 IC). The advantage of the experiment with the cell monolayer is that single cell fluorescent measurement would be free from the effect of ambient cells shown above. However, the localization (luminal or basolateral) of pHi regulation processes was not detected in this preparation because the solutions of both luminal and basolateral sides were altered simultaneously at bath fluid change. Thus most of the following experiments were performed in the intact tubule preparation.

Na⁺ dependence was examined under nominally Na⁺-free conditions. At NH₄Cl loading, Na⁺ was eliminated from the lumen and the bath. pHi recovery was absent in PC (Figs. 3b and 3c). The addition of 135mM luminal Na⁺ had no effect on the acidified pHi (Fig. 3b). pHi started to increase in response to 135mM bath Na⁺ (Fig. 3c). A significant pHi recovery was observed in IC in the absence of Na⁺ (Figs. 3e and 3f). Luminal Na⁺ did not change dpHi/dt (Fig. 3e), whereas bath Na⁺ further increased dpHi/dt (Fig. 3f). These results in PC and IC are summarized in Figs. 4 and 5, respectively.

Similar bath Na⁺ effect was seen in the monolayer cells. In response to basolateral addition of Na⁺, dpHi/dt increased from 0.6 ± 0.5 to 11.9 ± 1.5 in 15 PC, and from 9.1 ± 0.8 to 12.3 ± 0.9 in 11 IC.

To further examine the basolateral Na⁺-dependent pHi recovery process, the effect of amiloride, a Na⁺/H⁺ exchanger inhibitor [13–16] was tested in PC. pHi recovery

lumial [Na $\cdot$]	135	0	135	0	0	0	0	0
bath [Na $\cdot$]	135	0	0	135	15	15	0	0

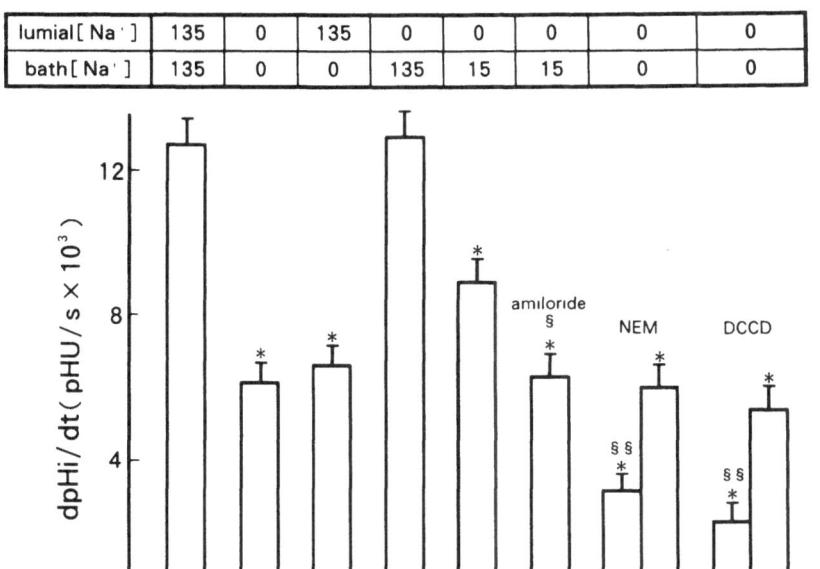

Fig. 5. pHi recovery rates (dpHi/dt) of IC at various [Na$^+$] (in mM). Each *bar* represents means ± SE of 8–24 cells from 4–12 tubules. Amiloride, 1mM amiloride was added to the bath at the NH$_4$Cl removal; NEM, DCCD 0.5mM NEM or DCCD was added to the lumen (*L*) or the bath (*B*) 10min before the experiment. *P < 0.01 compared with the control, §P < 0.05 compared with the absence of amiloride, §§P < 0.01 compared with the absence of H$^+$-ATPase inhibitor

induced by 15mM bath Na$^+$ was lower in the presence of 1mM basolateral amiloride (dpHi/dt = 1.4 ± 0.5) than in its absence (5.4 ± 0.5, P<0.01) (Fig. 4). A similar amiloride effect was seen on the bath Na$^+$-dependent pHi recovery in IC (Fig. 5). These results suggest the presence of a basolateral Na$^+$/H$^+$ exchanger in both PC and IC.

In the renal collecting duct, Chaillet et al. [13] first demonstrated the basolateral Na$^+$/H$^+$ antiporter in CCT. This antiporter has also been found in cultured inner medullary collecting duct (IMCD) cells [14,15] and in the inner stripe of OMCD (OMCDi) cells [16]. The physiological role of the peritubular Na$^+$/H$^+$ antiport in relation to transepithelial transport of H$^+$/HCO$_3^-$ and other solutes is not clear at present. In contrast to findings in the basolateral membrane, evidence of the presence of luminal Na$^+$/H$^+$ was not detected, a finding consistent with previous studies in the collecting duct [13,17].

The pHi of IC consistently recovered from cellular acidification in the absence of Na$^+$ (Figs. 3 and 5). ATP-dependent H$^+$ secretion has been shown in collecting duct cells [2,14,18–20]. To determine whether H$^+$-ATPase is associated with the Na$^+$-independent pHi recovery, a known H$^+$-ATPase inhibitor, N-ethylmaleimide (NEM) [21–23] was added at 0.5 mM to the lumen or the bath 10 min before the experiment. The results are summarized in Fig. 5. In the presence of bath NEM dpHi/dt (6.1 ± 0.5, 10 cells) was not significantly different from dpHi/dt in its absence (6.4 ± 0.3, 24 cells). In contrast, dpHi/dt was significantly lower in the presence of luminal NEM (3.3 ± 0.6, 11 cells). Similar results were obtained with another H^+-ATPase inhibitor, N,N'-dicyclohexylcarbodiomide (DCCD) [21,24] at 0.5 mM (Fig. 5). These results suggest that a luminal H^+-ATPase is involved in Na^+-independent pHi recovery in IC. Our finding supports the view that most of the IC in rabbit OMCDo are type A [8,25]. Our finding is also compatible with the recent work done by Brown et al. [26], in which the luminal membrane of IC in OMCDo was heavily labeled with antibodies to bovine kidney H^+ pump.

Luminal 0.5 mM NEM or DCCD did not totally inhibit the Na^+-independent pHi recovery of IC (Fig. 5). This result shows the possibility of the presence of another pHi recovery process besides that of H^+-ATPase. In fact, Wingo [27] has recently shown functional evidence for the presence of omeprazole-sensitive, NEM-insensitive H^+-K^+-ATPase in the rabbit OMCDi. We did not test this possibility in the present study.

Acknowledgments. The authors thank Dr. Tomita for encouragement of this work. The authors are grateful to Miss Mayumi Mirokuji for her excellent secretarial assistance.

This work was supported by a Grant-in-Aid from the Ministry of Education, Science, and Culture, Japan.

References

1. Agard DA, Hiraoka Y, Shaw P, Sedat JW (1989) Fluorescence microscopy in three dimensions. In: Taylor DL, Wang Y-L (eds) Methods in Cell Biology, vol 30. Fluorescence microscopy of living cells in culture, part B. Academic Press, pp 379–398
2. Schwartz GJ, Al-Awqati Q (1985) Carbon dioxide causes exocytosis of vesicles containing H^+ pumps in isolated perfused proximal and collecting tubules. J Clin Invest 75:1638–1644
3. McKinney TD, Davidson KK (1987) Bicarbonate transport in collecting tubules from outer stripe of outer medulla of rabbit kidneys. Am J Physiol 253 (Renal Fluid Electrolyte Physiol 22):F816–F822
4. LeFurgey A, Tisher CC (1979) Morphology of rabbit collecting duct. Am J Anat 155:111–124
5. Kaissling B, Kriz W (1979) Structural analysis of the rabbit kidney. Adv Anat Embryol Cell Biol 56:1–123
6. Ridderstrale Y, Kashgarian M, Koeppen B, Giebisch G, Stetson D, Ardito T, Stanton B (1988) Morphological heterogeneity of the rabbit collecting duct. Kidney Int 34:655–670
7. Koeppen BM (1986) Conductive properties of the rabbit outer medullary collecting duct: outer stripe. Am J Physiol 250 (Renal Fluid Electrolyte Physiol 19):F70–F76
8. Kuwahara M, Sasaki S, Marumo F (to be published) Intracellular pH regulation in rabbit outer medullary collecting duct cells: mechanisms and localization of HCO_3^--independent processes. Am J Physiol
9. Thomas JA, Buchsbaum RN, Zimniak A, Racker E (1979) Intracellular pH measurements in Ehrlich ascites tumor cells utilizing spectroscopic probes generated in situ. Biochemistry 18:2210–2218
10. Roos A, Boron WF (1981) Intracellular pH. Physiol Rev 61:296–434
11. Strange K, Spring KR (1987) Cell membrane water permeability of rabbit cortical collecting duct. J Membr Biol 96:27–43

12. Weiner ID, Hamm LL (1989) Use of fluorescent dye BCECF to measure intracellular pH in cortical collecting tubule. Am J Physiol 256 (Renal Fluid Electrolyte Physiol 25):F957–F964
13. Chaillet JR, Lopes AG, Boron WF (1985) Basolateral Na-H exchange in the rabbit cortical collecting tubule. J Gen Physiol 86:795–812
14. Kleinman JG, Blumenthal SS, Weissner JH, Reetz KL, Lewand DL, Mandel NS, Mandel GS, Garanics JC, Cragoe EJ Jr (1987) Regulation of pH in rat papillary tubule cells in primary culture. J Clin Invest 80:1660–1669
15. Wall SM, Muallem S, Kraut JA (1987) Detection of a sodium-hydrogen antiporter in cultured rat renal papillary collecting duct cell. Am J Physiol 253 (Renal Fluid Electrolyte Physiol 22):F889–F895
16. Breyer MD, Jacobson HR (1989) Regulation of rabbit medullary collecting duct pH by basolateral Na^+/H^+ and Cl^-/base exchange. J Clin Invest 84:996–1004
17. McKinney TD, Burg MB (1978) Bicarbonate absorption by rabbit cortical collecting tubules in vitro. Am J Physiol 234 (Renal Fluid Electrolyte Physiol 3):F141–F145
18. Graber ML, Bengele HH, Schwartz JH, Alexander EA (1981) pH and PCO_2 profiles of the rat inner medullary collecting duct. Am J Physiol 241 (Renal Fluid Electrolyte Physiol 10):F659–F668
19. Prigent A, Bichara M, Paillard M (1985) Hydrogen transport in papillary collecting duct in rabbit kidney. Am J Physiol 248 (Cell Physiol 17):C241–C246
20. Zeidel ML, Silva P, Seifter JL (1986) Intracellular pH regulation and proton transport by rabbit renal medullary collecting duct cells: role of plasma membrane proton adenosine triphosphatase. J Clin Invest 77:113–120
21. Gluck S, Al-Awqati Q (1984) An electrogenic proton-translocating adenosine triphosphatase from bovine kidney medulla. J Clin Invest 73:1704–1710
22. Kaunitz JD, Gunther RD, Sachs G (1984) Characterization of an electrogenic ATP and chloride-dependent proton translocating pump from rat renal medulla. J Biol Chem 260:11567–11573
23. Ait-Mohamed AK, Marsy S, Barlet C, Khadouri C, Doucet A (1986) Characterization of N-ethylmaleimide-sensitive proton pump in the rat kidney: localization along the nephron. J Biol Chem 261:12526–12533
24. Stone DK, Xie X-S, Wu LT, Racker E (1984) Proton translocating ATPases of clathrin-coated vesicles, renal medulla, and Ehrlich ascites tumor cells. In: Forte JG, Warnock DG, Rector FC Jr (eds) Hydrogen transport in epithelia. John Wiley and Sons, New York, pp 219–230
25. Schwartz GJ, Satlin LM, Bergmann JE (1988) Fluorescent characterization of collecting duct cells: a second H^+-secreting type. Am J Physiol 255 (Renal Fluid Electrolyte Physiol 24):F1003–F1014
26. Brown D, Hirsch S, Gluck S (1988) Localization of a proton-pumping ATPase in rat kidney. J Clin Invest 82:2114–2126
27. Wingo CS (1989) Active proton secretion and potassium absorption in the rabbit outer medullary collecting duct: functional evidence for proton-potassium-activated adenosine triphosphatase. J Clin Invest 84:361–365

Ultramicro-Analysis of Tubular Fluid by Continuous-Flow Methodology

MARK A. KNEPPER[1]

SUMMARY. The measurement of net transepithelial fluxes in isolated perfused tubule experiments requires highly sensitive analytical methods, capable of precise determination of solute concentrations in 1–30 nanoliter samples of collected fluid. The continuous-flow approach to ultramicro-analysis of small aqueous samples, developed by Vurek in the early 1980s, has provided the sensitivity, precision, and speed necessary to dramatically enhance the efficiency of transepithelial flux measurements in isolated perfused tubules. The instruments used, a continuous-flow colorimeter and a continuous-flow fluorometer, are extremely versatile, allowing measurement of any of the major osmotically-active components of either plasma or urine in nanoliter volume samples. Specifically, these two instruments have been used to measure chloride, bicarbonate, sodium, potassium, ammonium, urea, creatinine, glucose, raffinose, lactate, calcium, magnesium, phosphate, and acetaminophen concentrations in 1–30 nanoliter samples with a coefficient of variation in the range 2%–4%. This paper reviews the design and application of these continuous-flow instruments.

Introduction

In vitro perfusion of renal tubules, a technique developed by Burg and his colleagues in the late 1960s [1], remains one of the mainstays of renal physiological research. This technique has allowed detailed investigation of the transport properties of renal tubule segments not accessible to micropuncture and other in vivo approaches. Furthermore, the ability to maintain well-controlled conditions in isolated perfused tubule experiments, free of the complexity of the normal in vivo environment, has led to substantial progress in the understanding of transport processes and their control, even in renal tubule segments that can be studied in vivo.

---

[1]Laboratory of Kidney and Electrolyte Metabolism, National Heart, Lung and Blood Institute, National Institutes of Health, Bethesda, MD 20892, USA

1438

Table 1. Ultramicroanalytical methods using the continuous-flow colorimeter

Solute	Chemistry	Detection limit (pmol)	Coefficient of variation[a]	Reference
Chloride	Ferric thiocyanate	5	2%–3%	[8]
Sodium	Macrocylic ionophore	57	3%–5%	[5]
Potassium	Macrocylic ionophore	8	3%–5%	[5]
Creatinine	Alkaline picrate	2	2%–3%	[9]
Calcium	Methylthymol blue	1	3%–4%	[2]
Magnesium	Calmagite	0.2	2%–3%	[3]
Phosphate	Ammonium molybdate	1	3%–4%	[3]
Acetominophen	Sodium nitrate	2	4%–5%	[10]

[a]Standard deviation divided by mean for 4–5 repeat determinations using as standards the usual range of sample sizes from isolated perfused tubule collections

Measurement of transepithelial fluxes in isolated perfused tubules generally requires the collection and analysis of the fluid exiting the tubule lumen. Depending on the flow rates required to measure the appropriate fluxes, the volumes of the collected samples typically range from 2–100 nl. Success in such studies has required the availability of precise methods for the analysis of these small tubule fluid samples. In the early years of isolated perfused tubule studies, most flux measurements were achieved using radio-isotopic tracers. This approach yields unidirectional solute fluxes, i.e., bath-to-lumen or lumen-to-bath fluxes. Estimates of net fluxes from radio-isotopic flux measurements have usually been achieved by subtracting one unidirectional flux from the other. The precision of such net flux measurements is therefore somewhat limited. Consequently, renal physiologists began very early to search for sensitive ultramicroanalytical methods capable of measuring solute concentrations in nanoliter volume fluid samples, thus permitting direct determination of net solute fluxes. In the early 1980s, Vurek introduced a new "continuous-flow" approach for the ultramicroanalysis of tubule fluid samples [2–4]. This approach has dramatically broadened the utility of the isolated perfused tubule technique. Vurek's continuous-flow approach has been further developed to allow the determination, in nanoliter-range samples, of concentrations of virtually all of the osmotically-important solutes normally present in urine or plasma [5] (Tables 1 and 2).

The continuous-flow method is diagrammed in Fig. 1. It consists of four elements. A *reagent reservoir* contains the appropriate reagent to allow conversion of the target

Table 2. Ultramicroanalytical methods using the continuous-flow fluorometer

Solute	Enzyme(s)	Detection limit (pmol)	Coefficient of variation[a]	Reference
Ammonium	Glutamic dehydrogenase	0.50	3%–5%	[7]
Urea	Urease/glutamic dehydrogenase	0.25	3%–5%	[11]
Bicarbonate	PEP carboxylase/malic dehydrogenase	0.50	3%–5%	[12]
Glucose	Hexokinase/glucose-6-phosphate dehydrogenase	0.25	3%–5%	–
Lactate	Lactic dehydrogenase	0.25	4%–6%	[13]
Raffinose	Galactosidase/galactose dehydrogenase	0.75	4%–5%	[14]

[a]Standard deviation divided by mean for 4–5 repeat determinations using as standards the usual range of sample sizes from isolated perfused tubule collections

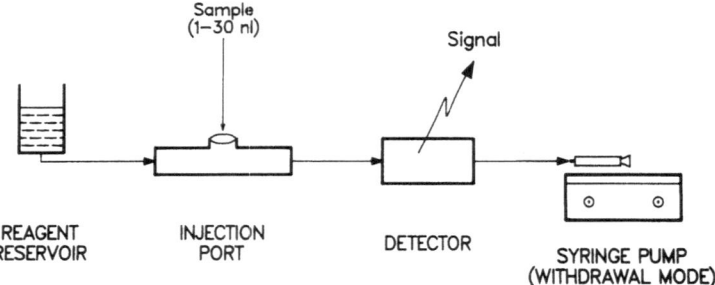

Fig. 1. *General scheme for continuous-flow instruments.* Typically, one to thirty nanoliter samples are injected into the flowing reagent stream. The appropriate chemical reaction occurs while the injected sample flows toward the detector to form a colored or fluorescent product. The detector is either a miniature colorimeter (Fig. 2) or a miniature fluorometer (Fig. 3). (From [4] with permission)

substance into a colored or fluorescent product. A precision *syringe pump* fitted with a Teflon-tipped gas tight syringe draws the reagent through the *injection port* and the *detector element* at a constant rate. Typically a 1–30 nanoliter volume sample is injected into the flowing reagent stream via the injection port. The appropriate color-producing or fluorescence-producing chemical reaction takes place as the sample bolus flows toward the detector. The detector element is essentially a scaled-down colorimeter or fluorometer, capable of accurately measuring either the absorbance or the fluorescence of the reaction product. It contains a sensitive photo-detector, either a silicon photodiode [6] or a photomultiplier tube [7], which converts an optical signal to an electronic signal (see below). Generally, the output is available within 2–5 minutes of sample injection, allowing measurements to be made as the samples are collected from the perfused tubules.

In the following sections, we discuss first the design and application of the continuous-flow *colorimeter.* Then, we describe the design and application of the continuous-flow *fluorometer.*

Continuous-Flow Colorimeter

Figure 2 is a diagram of the detector element for the continuous-flow colorimeter [5]. The cuvet is a U-tube fashioned from a small-bore glass capillary which is connected to the injection port at one end and the syringe pump at the other. An incandescent lamp containing a built-in lens is oriented so as to send a beam of broad-spectrum light along the shaft of the cuvet. Thus, when the colored reaction product flows into the cuvet, light is absorbed, resulting in a measurable reduction in the amount of light exiting the cuvet. The emerging light is filtered by an appropriate band-pass interference filter that passes only the wavelengths corresponding to the absorption maximum of the reaction product. The optical signal is measured using a sensitive silicon photodiode. A simple electronic circuit utilizing a low cost operational amplifier is used to convert the change in resistance of the photodiode to an amplified voltage

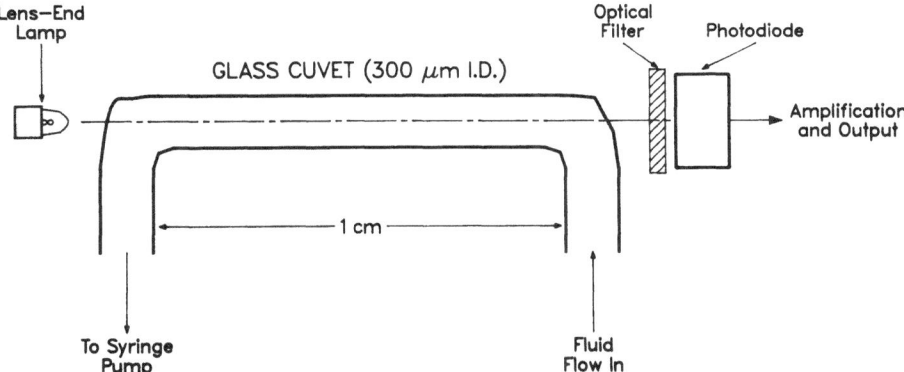

Fig. 2. *Detector system for ultramicro-colorimeter.* The colored reaction product flows through the light path, decreasing the amount of light impinging on the silicon photodiode. (From [4] with permission)

signal [6]. The output can then be read out on a linear chart recorder or can be fed to an analog-to-digital converted to allow a computer to carry out digital filtering and peak integration [5].

As described in Table 1, the continuous-flow colorimeter has been used successfully for the ultramicro-analysis of several solutes including chloride, sodium, potassium, creatinine, calcium, magnesium, phosphate, and acetaminophen. These methods have allowed the detection of as little as 5–10 pmol of some solutes, while at the same time affording a high degree of precision. When working in the optimal range of sample sizes (generally about 5–10 fold above the detection limit), the coefficient of variation (standard deviation/mean × 100%) for repeat injections of standards is generally in the range 2%–3%. Reaction times vary among the assay methods, ranging from a virtually instantaneous reaction for the magnesium method to about 10 minutes for the sodium method. Most of the reactions are complete within 3–4 minutes, allowing samples to be injected into the apparatus as they are collected from the perfused tubule. It is relatively easy to switch from the analysis of one solute to the analysis of another within 5–10 minutes by changing the reagent in the reagent reservoir and replacing the optical filter with the appropriate one to match the absorbance spectrum of the reaction product.

Continuous-Flow Fluorometer

Figure 3 is a diagram of the detector element for the continuous-flow fluorometer. As with the colorimeter, the fluorometer cuvet is a small-bore U-tube connected at one end to the injection port and at the other end to the withdrawal pump. Ultraviolet excitation light from a Hg-Xe lamp is delivered to the cuvet via a fused-silica optical fiber inserted into the side of the cuvet. The fluorescent reaction product is excited as it passes through the cuvet, resulting in an emission signal proportional to the amount of fluorescent material. The emitted light is filtered by an appropriate long-

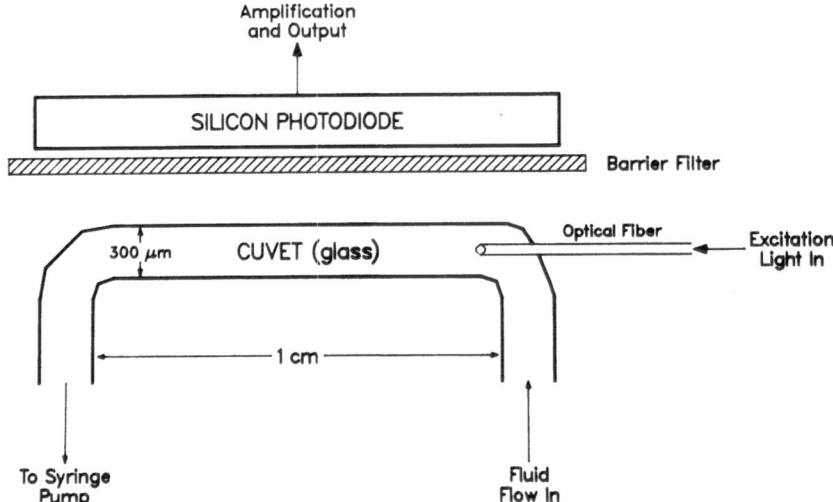

Fig. 3. *Detector system for ultramicro-fluorometer.* The fluorescent reaction product (generally NADH) flows past the tip of a fused-silica optical fiber carrying ultraviolet excitation light from a Mercury-Xenon lamp. The emitted light passes through a barrier filter to impinge on a silicon photodiode

pass optical filter and impinges on a silicon photodiode. Amplification of the photodiode output and processing of the amplified signal is accomplished in a manner nearly identical to the approach used for the continuous-flow colorimeter.

As described in Table 2, the continuous-flow fluorometer has been used successfully for the ultramicroanalysis of several solutes including ammonium, urea, bicarbonate, glucose, lactate, and raffinose. All of these methods depend on the use of various dehydrogenase enzymes, which catalyze oxidation-reduction reactions coupled to the simultaneous reduction of NAD or oxidation of NADH. Since NADH is fluorescent and NAD is not, the enzyme-catalyzed chemical reactions result in either an increase or a decrease in the fluorescent signal, which is proportional to the amount of the substrate injected into the reagent stream. Thus, a variety of substances can be assayed with a single instrument that measures the concentration of NADH, simply by changing the enzymes that are placed in the reagent stream. Because fluorescence measurements are intrinsically more sensitive that absorbance measurements, the methods shown in Table 2 have detection limits considerably lower than those shown in Table 1 (generally less than 1 pmol). When working in the optimal range of sample sizes (generally about 5–50 fold above the detection limit), the coefficient of variation (standard deviation/mean $\times 100\%$) for repeat injections of standards is generally in the range 3%–4%. The reaction time depends on the amount of enzyme added to the reagent stream. Generally, it is possible to add enough enzyme to enable the appropriate chemical reaction to go to completion within 2 minutes of injection, permitting samples to be run every 2–3 minutes. Consequently, as for the colorimetric methods, it is generally feasible to analyze tubule fluid samples during the course of a perfused tubule experiment. Because the specificity of the fluorescent assay depends only on the enzymes that are placed in the reagent reservoir, the same instrument can be used for the measurement of any of the solutes shown on Table 2.

Discussion

The continuous-flow methods discussed in this paper afford the investigator an unprecedented degree of precision in the analysis of 1–30 nanoliter volume tubule fluid samples. A coefficient of variation in the range 2%–4% is typical when the instruments are set up to measure quantities of solutes in the optimal range (generally 5–10 times greater than the detection limit). This high degree of reproducibility is the consequence of the mechanical simplicity of the instruments; the only moving mechanical component is the stepping-motor syringe pump which, when used with a clean gas-tight syringe, can produce extremely steady flow rates through the instruments. The method is quite insensitive to the injection technique, allowing even inexperienced operators to attain a high degree of reproducibility.

The continuous-flow techniques are very rapid. The collected fluid samples can generally be injected directly into the instrument immediately after collection and the output is available within 2–5 minutes of injection. Consequently, the investigator obtains immediate feedback which allows him to adjust the rate of tubule perfusion or other conditions to optimize the accuracy of flux measurements. With other assay methods (radio-isotope measurement and older chemical analytical techniques) it was generally necessary to accumulate samples during experiments and to complete the measurements either later in the day or overnight. Because of the speed and simplicity of the measurements, the efficiency of the isolated perfused tubule technique has improved, i.e., we are generally able to obtain a greater yield of successful experiments.

The continuous-flow methods are also very inexpensive to run. Most of the reagents needed for the assays are available commercially as relatively inexpensive analytical kits. Because of the small volume of reagent needed (2–4 ml per day), one kit often lasts several weeks or months. The instruments are now commercially available for under $6000 (Sewell Machine Shop, Birmingham, Ala.). Several tubule perfusion laboratories in the United States and Japan are presently using either the commercial version of the continuous-flow instruments or custom-built instruments made locally.

The continuous-flow instruments described in this paper have been divided into two classes (colorimetric and fluorometric) depending on the type of detector utilized. Other types of continuous-flow instruments can be devised based on other methods of detection. For example, Garvin [15] has recently introduced a continuous-flow method for measuring potassium using a potassium-selective electrode as the detection element.

References

1. Burg MB, Grantham JJ, Abramow M, Orloff J (1983) Preparation and study of fragments of single rabbit nephrons. Am J Physiol 210:1293–1298

 2. Vurek GG (1981) Calcium measurement: picomole quantitiation by continuous-flow colorimetry. Anal Biochem 114:288–293
 3. Vurek GG (1981) Flow-through nanocolorimeter for measurement of picomole amounts of magnesium and phosphate. Anal Letters 14:261–269
 4. Vurek GG (1982) Nanoliter-volume flow-through fluorometer. Anal Chem 54:840–842
 5. Terada Y, Knepper MA (1989) Continuous-flow quantitation of Na⁺ and K⁺ in nanoliter samples using chromogenic macrocyclic ionophores. Am J Physiol 257:F893–F898
 6. Vurek GG, Knepper MA (1982) A colorimeter for measurement of picomole quantities of urea. Kidney Int 21:656–658
 7. Good DW, Vuek GG (1983) Picomole quantitation of ammonia by flow-through fluorometry. Anal Biochem 130:199–202
 8. Star RA, Burg MB, Knepper MA (1985) Bicarbonate secretion and chloride absorption by rabbit cortical collecting ducts. J Clin Invest 76:1123–1130
 9. Knepper MA, Good DW, Burg MB (1985) Ammonia and bicarbonate transport by rat cortical collecting ducts perfused in vitro. Am J Physiol 249:F870–F877
10. Chou C-L, Sands JM, Nonoguchi H, Knepper MA (1990) Concentration dependence of urea and thiourea transport in rat inner medullary collecting duct. Am J Physiol 258:F486–F494
11. Sands JM, Knepper MA (1987) Urea permeability of mammalian inner medullary collecting duct system and papillary surface epithelium. J Clin Invest 79:138–147
12. Star RA (1990) Quantitation of total carbon dioxide in nanoliter samples by flow-through fluorometry. Am J Physiol 258:F429–F432
13. Bagnasco S, Good D, Balaban R, Burg M (1985) Lactate production in isolated segments of the rat nephron. Am J Physiol 248:F522–F526
14. Garvin JL, Burg MB, Knepper MA (1985) Ammonium replaces potassium in supporting sodium transport by the Na⁺-K⁺-ATPase of renal proximal straight tubules. Am J Physiol 249:F785–F788
15. Garvin JL (1989) Picomole quantitation of potassium using a continuous-flow apparatus. Kidney Int 36:726–729

Optical Methods for Quantifying Cell Volume Changes in Isolated Nephron Segments

KEVIN STRANGE[1]

SUMMARY. Animal cell volume is determined by extracellular and intracellular solute content. Measurements of cell volume changes induced by osmotic, ionic, electrophysiological and/or pharmacological manipulations can therefore provide important and often unique insights into membrane solute and water transport properties. In addition, volume measurements allow the elucidation of cell volume regulatory mechanism. The purpose of this brief review article is to describe the requirements for measuring volume changes in isolated nephron segments and to illustrate the types of questions that can be addressed using this powerful approach.

Introduction

Water is in thermodynamic equilibrium across animal cell membranes and cell volume is therefore determined by extracellular and intracellular solute content. This fundamental characteristic can be exploited as an experimental tool. Measurements of cell volume changes induced by osmotic, ionic, electrophysiological, and/or pharmacological manipulations provide important and often unique insights into membrane solute and water transport properties. The purpose of this article is to describe briefly the requirements for measuring volume changes in isolated nephron segments and to illustrate the types of questions that can be addressed using this powerful approach. For a more extensive discussion of the use of optical techniques to study epithelial function, the reader is referred to a recent excellent review by Foskett [1].

MacRobbie and Ussing [2] were the first to employ cell volume measurements to study epithelial function. These investigators monitored experimentally-induced changes in the thickness of isolated frog skin by light microscopy and demonstrated that the mucosal and serosal membranes were permeable to NaCl and KCl, respec-

[1]The Children's Hospital, Division of Nephrology, Harvard Medical School, Boston, MA 02115, USA

tively, and that the mucosal membrane was the site of antidiuretic hormone (ADH) action. The capacity of epithelial cells to regulate their volume following osmotic perturbations was also revealed in these early studies. In the late 1970s and early 1980s, Spring and co-workers established the technical and conceptual foundations necessary for rapid and continuous volume measurements in living epithelial cells using high resolution differential interference contrast (DIC) microscopy, video recording methods, and computer image processing techniques [3].

The development of the isolated perfused tubule preparation by Burg and co-workers [4] revolutionized renal physiology and provided the first step toward utilizing volume measurements to study nephron cell function. In a very general sense, observations of cell volume are an inherent component of all perfusion studies. Because of the small size of nephron segments, tubule perfusion is necessarily done under microscopic examination. As such, cell volume changes during experimental manipulations have frequently been reported, beginning with the earliest in vitro studies. For example, Burg et al. [5] noted that addition of glucose and alanine to the luminal perfusate caused marked cell swelling in the proximal convoluted tubule. These studies provided direct evidence for the existence of apical organic solute transport pathways in this nephron segment.

The earliest measurements of nephron cell volume were carried out using conventional brightfield microscopy and photography or measuring devices such as reticules and image-splitting eyepieces. A major advance was made when DIC microscopy was applied to in vitro perfusion methods. Horster and Gundlach [6] were the first to utilize this approach, noting that it generated images with high resolution and contrast, provided optical sectioning capabilities, and allowed for rapid recording of morphology changes. Shortly thereafter, video enhancement and recording methods were combined with both DIC and conventional brightfield microscopy to quantify rapid, experimentally-induced changes in nephron cell volume [7–8].

Video Methods for Measuring Cell Volume

There are many methods for measuring cell volume in both fixed and living tissues. For the purposes of this review, however, I will restrict my discussion of methodology to video techniques combined with light microscopy. Video methods allow the continuous monitoring of rapid cell volume changes and low cost video recording and analysis equipment is now readily available and commonplace in many research laboratories. The advantages afforded by combining video technology with the light microscope are numerous and include image contrast enhancement, ease and speed of data storage and playback, and the ability and ease of digitizing images for processing and analysis.

Two main approaches for quantifying renal tubule cell volume changes by video methods have been taken. In nephron segments composed of a single cell type, tubule length and inner and outer diameter are measured. The tubule geometry is approximated as a cylinder and total epithelial volume is calculated (e.g., [9–10]). This method has three potential sources of error. First, it is assumed that changes in interspace volume do not occur or do not contribute significantly to total epithelial volume. In most nephron segments this assumption is valid, but it should be assessed for each experimental situation. As discussed by Strange and Spring [11], failure to correct for interspace distension has caused significant overestimates of cell swelling during ADH-induced water flow in the cortical collecting tubule (CCT). Second, changes in tubule length accompanying volume perturbations need to be monitored and corrected for, or volume perturbations should be minimized so that length changes do not occur. With respect to the latter approach, a number of investigators have reported that small volume changes have no effect on tubule length [9]. Third, Kirk et al. [9] have noted that significant curvature of the apical surface will invalidate the assumption of a cylindrical tubule geometry. This error has been assessed in the proximal straight tubule [9] and medullary thick ascending limb [10] and found to be less than 1% of the measured cell volume.

Tubule length and diameter can be measured manually from recorded video images using precision calipers [12]. Individual video fields have been analyzed by this method, providing for a maximum image acquisition rate of 60 images/s. Welling et al. [12] have claimed that this method can detect tubule diameter changes of 0.05 µm. Tubule diameters have also been measured by digitizing video images and tracing tubule inner and outer borders using a computer-generated cursor and image analysis software [9–10]. This approach is capable of detecting volume changes of approximately 2% [13].

A fully automated procedure for monitoring cell volume has been described by Whittembury and co-workers [7,14]. In this approach, perfused or nonperfused tubules are imaged so that the video scan lines are oriented perpendicular to the longitudinal tubule axis. For on-line volume determinations, high contrast tubule images are generated by vital staining of the cells or by addition of dye (FDC green) to the perfusate, followed by suitable filtering of the transmitted light. Each video scan line is converted to a binary signal by one or two analog comparators with appropriate threshold settings. Measurement of the duration of binary pulses passing through the cellular or luminal compartment is a measurement of the cell and lumen diameter, respectively. This method can analyze 50–60 images/s and can detect a 1% change in tubule diameter.

For heterogeneous nephron segments such as the CCT, it is necessary to quantify volume changes at the single cell level. Cells can be imaged either en face or in the lateral tubule wall [8]. In both cases it is essential to use DIC microscopy to generate high contrast images and to be able to visualize lateral, apical, and basal cell borders.

Imaging in the en face mode allows the determination of cell volume directly by optical sectioning methods [8]. In this approach, high numerical aperture objective and condenser lenses are used to obtain high resolution in the vertical axis (i.e., shallow depth-of-field). The microscope is step focused through the cell, either manually or under computer control by a stepping motor. At the bottom of the cell and at predetermined levels of focal displacement, video images are recorded. The cross-sectional area of each optical "slice" of the cell is then determined at a later time by tracing the cellular outline on a video monitor with a planimeter [15] or with a computer-generated cursor and image analysis software [16]. Cell volume is calculated from the area measurements and the known distance between each image [16].

Optical sectioning has been used to monitor cell volume in the rabbit CCT [16]. In this nephron segment, minimum volume changes of only 5%–7% can be detected with this method and approximately 2–4 seconds are required to complete an optical sectioning scan of a single cell [8,16]. Because of the high cellular surface area-to-

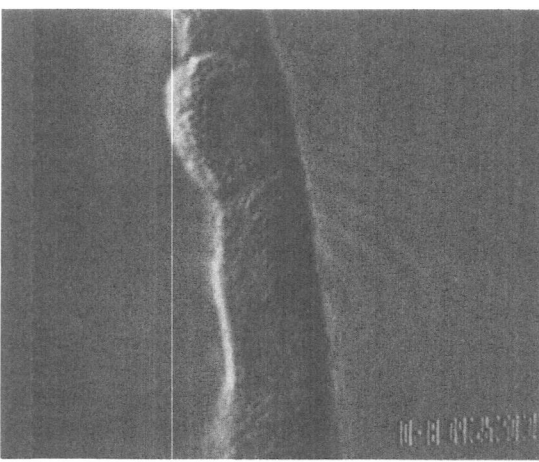

Fig. 1. Video-enhanced DIC image of a principal (*bottom cell*) and an intercalated cell in the lateral wall of the rabbit CCT. Apical surface is to the *left*

volume ratio of most mammalian nephrons, experimentally-induced volume changes can often be complete in less than 1 second (e.g., [16]; Fig. 2). Thus, optical sectioning does not have sufficient speed and resolution to detect initial rates of cell volume change under many experimental conditions. The preferred approach for monitoring the volume of single nephron cells is to image random cellular cross sections in the lateral tubule wall (see Fig. 1). Lateral wall images can be recorded at video framing rates (i.e., 30 images/s). Images are digitized at a later time and cellular outlines are traced on a television monitor with a computer-generated cursor and image analysis software. Relative volume changes are quantified by monitoring changes in cross-sectional area (see [8] for a detailed discussion). Minimum volume changes of 2%–3% can be detected by this approach [16].

Optical and Video Equipment Requirements

The minimum requirements for video quantification of cell volume include a microscope, a video camera, and a measuring system. For tubule perfusion studies, an inverted microscope with a focusable nosepiece is essential. We have used the Nikon Diaphot (Nikon Inc., Garden City, New Jersey) extensively for our studies of the CCT. Optical component micromanipulators are used to mount tubule perfusion V-tracks (White Instrument Co., Suitland, Md.) directly to the microscope stage (see [8,16]), which is equipped with a low-mounted coaxial control arm. This arrangement allows the entire tubule to be scanned simply by translating the stage in the x and y directions.

For many types of volume measurements, the microscope must be equipped with DIC optics. The merits of various DIC systems have been described in detail previously [17]. Our studies of the CCT have utilized calcite polarizer and analyzer prisms (Zeta International Corp., Mt. Prospect, Ill.), a quartz ¼ wave plate (Esco Products Inc., Oak Ridge, N.Y.), and matched Wollaston prisms (Carl Zeiss Inc., New York, N.Y.; see [8] for details). Tubules are imaged using a Zeiss Neofluar 63X (1.25 N.A) lens as the objective and a Leitz 32X (0.4 N.A.) lens as the condenser.

A wide variety of high resolution, research-grade video cameras are readily available from a number of different manufacturers. Inoue has discussed in detail the numerous considerations that go into the choice of a camera for a given microscopy application [17]. For measurements of cell volume, tube-type cameras are generally preferred because of their higher resolution compared to most solid-state imagers. Our studies of the CCT have utilized a Dage camera (Model NC-65S; Dage-MTI Inc., Michigan City, Ind.) equipped with a Newvicon tube. This camera has low geometric distortion, a horizontal resolution of approximately 800 lines, adequate sensitivity for brightfield illumination, electronic magnification capability (Insta-View option), and automatic gain and black level control. It is advantageous to use cameras that allow manual control over gain and black levels for certain types of volume measurements such as the real-time area-tracker described by Whittembury and co-workers [7,14].

The quality of incoming video images can be significantly improved by edge enhancement using a differentiating circuit (e.g., Model IV-530; FOR-A Corp., West Newton, Mass.) or digital image processing. This is particularly useful when DIC microscopy is employed. Some camera systems can be purchased with built-in analog edge enhancement features (e.g., Dage-MTI).

Additional hardware needed for quantifying cell volume changes is dependent on the type of measuring system utilized. The real-time area-tracker method [7] requires construction of an analog image processing circuit. Lindemann has described this circuitry in detail and has published the necessary circuit diagrams [14]. All other methods require the recording of video images for later analysis. Currently, we use an optical disc recorder (Model TQ-2028F; Panasonic Industrial Co., Secaucus, N.J.), which is capable of recording video images in real-time with a horizontal resolution of 450 lines. Video tape recorders can also be employed, but they should be research or broadcast quality instruments with high resolution and they should allow for frame-by-frame analysis of images. In the stop frame mode, the images must be free of excessive jitter, particularly if computer digitization and analysis is to be used.

Image acquisition and analysis systems have undergone tremendous development during the last 10 years. Complex image processing algorithms can now easily be carried out on a personal computer (PC). My laboratory has extensively utilized IBM-AT and compatible machines. A wide variety of high quality data acquisition and image digitizing hardware and software is available for these instruments. We quantify cell volume changes off-line at a data analysis station separate from the experimental setups. Recorded video images are digitized using an image processing computer board with $512 \times 512 \times 8$-bit resolution (Model FG-100-AT; Imaging Technology Inc., Woburn, Mass.). Cell borders are traced on a high resolution video monitor (Model 8831; Aydin Controls, Fort Washington, Pa.) using a 12×12 inch graphics tablet (SummaSketch; Summagraphics Corp., Fairfield, Conn.).

An important consideration in the development of a cell volume measuring system is the type of image analysis software that will be employed. Custom programming can be done by the user, or commercial software can be purchased. Numerous PC-based software packages are available that provide an extensive array of menu-driven image processing routines. For volume measurements, where the user is digitizing and tracing a large number of sequential video images, menu-driven software can be tedious to use. The software package purchased should include the capability to develop custom programs via macro routines or by providing the source code to image processing algorithms. If macros are used, the program should allow easy retrieval and storage of data in ASCII format.

General Experimental Requirements

It is necessary to rigorously fulfill several experimental requirements when cell volume changes are used to characterize epithelial membrane water and solute transport. First, the preparation must have good mechanical stability to prevent shifts in focal position during volume measurements. Second, unstirred layers must be minimized and/or corrected for in data analysis. Third, bath and perfusate composition changes need to be made at rates significantly faster than the time constant of the solute and/or water flow under study. Fourth, the image acquisition and recording system utilized must have sufficient spatial and temporal resolution so that initial rates of volume change can be quantified.

For our studies of the CCT, we designed and constructed a rapid laminar flow bath chamber [8]. This chamber provides excellent mechanical stability and allows for peritubular solution changes with half-times of 50–60 ms. Peritubular unstirred layer thickness, measured by observing the flow pattern of latex beads and liposomes, is less than the thickness of the basal lamina. A recent modification of this chamber design allows simultaneous electrophysiological and optical measurements [19].

Apical unstirred layers in isolated nephron segments are negligible due to the small luminal diameter and the laminar flow characteristics of the perfusate. Rapid changes in perfusate composition can be carried out using double barrelled pipets, a retractable pipet assembly, or a conventional exchange pipet arrangement (reviewed in [8]).

Cell Membrane Water Permeability

One of the earliest applications of cell volume measurements in the isolated nephron was the determination of apical and basolateral membrane water permeability. Membrane water flow is characterized by making "step" changes in extracellular osmolality and then monitoring the initial rate of cell swelling or shrinkage (Fig. 2). Water permeability (L_p) is calculated according to the equation,

$$J_v = L_p \, \sigma \, \Delta \, \pi$$

where J_v is the rate of cell volume change (i.e., rate of transmembrane water flow), σ is the solute reflection coefficient and $\Delta\pi$ is the experimentally-induced osmotic pressure difference.

Determination of apical or basolateral L_p in the nephron is complicated by water flow across the opposing membrane [16]. Water flow needs to be blocked at the

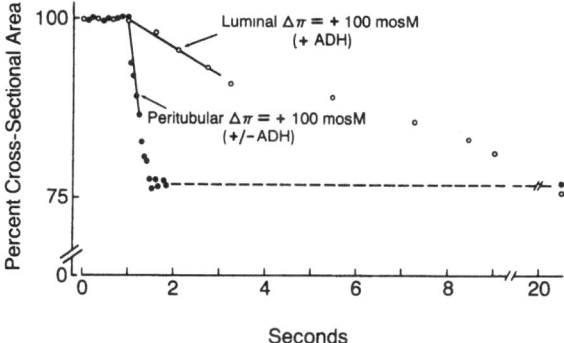

Fig. 2. Volume changes in rabbit CCT principal cells induced by raising luminal or peritubular osmolality from 290 mOsm to 390 mOsm. Luminal osmolality was changed shortly after replacing the peritubular bath with silicone oil [16]. Rates of volume change reflect the total water permeability of each membrane. ADH, antidiuretic hormone

opposing membrane if it has an L_p similar to or greater than the membrane under study. This is usually done by replacing the bath or perfusate with oil [7,16].

Measurement of membrane water permeability is crucial for understanding the routes and mechanisms of transepithelial water flow. Video measurements of membrane L_p (e.g., [12,20]) and solute reflection coefficients [21] have been carried out in the proximal tubule. These studies have demonstrated that both the apical and basolateral membranes of this nephron segment have extremely high water permeabilities and that high rates of transcellular water reabsorption can be driven by osmotic gradients of less than 1–2 mOsm. Recent investigations also indicate that the paracellular pathway may play a significant role in proximal tubule water reabsorption [20]. Guggino et al. [15] measured membrane L_p values in the *Amphiuma* distal tubule and demonstrated that the apical membrane is a major barrier to water flow. This is a result of both an intrinsically low apical bilayer L_p and a greatly reduced apical membrane surface area. Strange and Spring [16] measured water permeability in the rabbit CCT and demonstrated directly that the apical membrane was the site of ADH action and was rate limiting for water reabsorption. In addition, these investigators demonstrated that apical and basolateral membranes had similar *intrinsic* water permeabilities in the presence of ADH. The basolateral membrane, however, had a much higher *total* L_p (see Fig. 2) due to a greatly amplified surface area. This asymmetry has important physiological consequences; it prevents excessive cell swelling and intracellular dilution during ADH-stimulated water reabsorption [11].

Transepithelial Solute Transport Pathways

Optical methods have been particularly powerful in defining solute transport pathways in perfused nephron segments. For example, Guggino et al. [15] demonstrated that ouabain-induced cell swelling in *Amphiuma* distal tubule could be blocked by

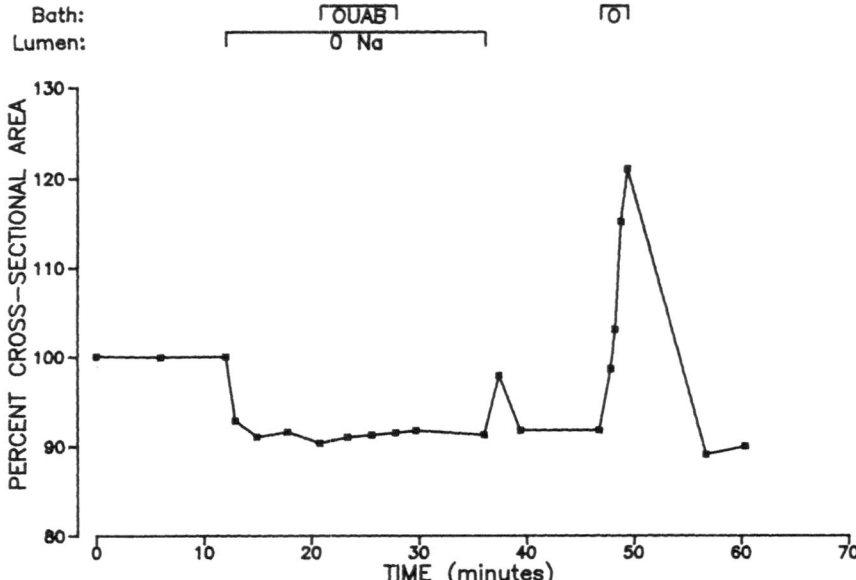

Fig. 3. Effects of luminal Na⁺ removal on ouabain (*Ouab*)-induced swelling in a rabbit CCT principal cell [25]

luminal furosemide, suggesting that apical $Na^+/K^+/2Cl^-$ cotransport was the major pathway for cellular NaCl entry. Sun et al. [22] have recently shown that ouabain-induced swelling in the mouse medullary thick ascending limb is blocked by luminal Na^+ removal or furosemide addition, but is unaffected by luminal K^+ deletion. When the tubules were treated with ADH, however, removal of luminal K^+ dramatically inhibited ouabain-swelling. These results indicate that in the unstimulated tubule the apical cotransporter functions in a NaCl uptake mode. ADH modifies the pathway to become K^+-dependent and function as a $Na^+/K^+/2Cl^-$ cotransporter. In mineralo-corticoid-treated CCT, ouabain causes rapid swelling in principal cells ([23]; Fig. 3). This swelling is inhibited by luminal Na^+ removal (Fig. 3) or by addition of low concentrations of amiloride, indicating that the major pathway for cellular Na^+ uptake is via apical amiloride-sensitive channels. Luminal Cl^- removal or addition of Cl^- transport inhibitors in the CCT causes significant principal cell shrinkage and also inhibits ouabain-swelling [23]. These results argue for the presence of an apical Cl^- transport pathway and suggest that this cell type plays a role in Cl^- reabsorption. Volume measurements in the rabbit proximal convoluted tubule have indicated the presence of apical Na^+/H^+ and Cl^-/formate exchangers that mediate transepithelial NaCl movement [24].

Basolateral solute transport pathways have also been elucidated by volume measurements. For example, Strange [19] recently demonstrated that peritubular K^+ elevation causes rapid swelling in CCT principal cells, which is completely blocked by bath Cl^- removal or addition of 5.0 mM Ba^{2+} (Fig. 4). These and previous results [23]

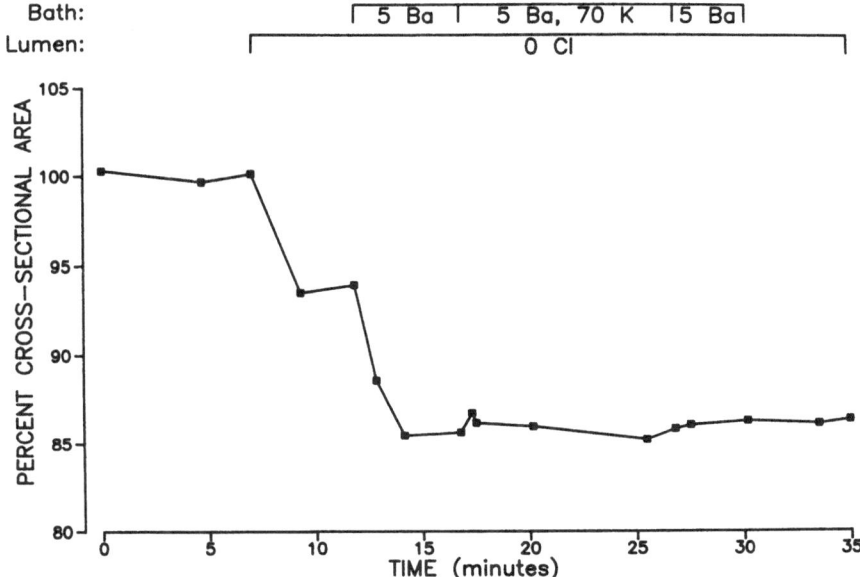

Fig. 4. Effects of 5.0 mM $BaCl_2$ on K^+-induced swelling in a principal cell of a CCT dissected from a desoxycorticosterone acetate (DOCA)-treated rabbit. Principal cells normally swell at a rate of 106%/min when peritubular K^+ concentration is raised from 5 mM to 70 mM [19]. As shown here, this swelling is completely blocked by peritubular $BaCl_2$. The cell shrinkage observed during Ba^{2+} addition most likely reflects inhibition of conductive, basolateral K^+ entry in the presence of continued basolateral and/or apical net solute efflux (discussed in [19])

indicate that the major pathways for basolateral K^+ movement are via the Na^+ pump and K^+ channels.

Studies of Cell Heterogeneity

Cell volume measurements are particularly valuable for defining the functional properties of specific cell types in heterogeneous epithelia. This approach was first used by O'Neil and Hayhurst [25] to study the rabbit CCT. These investigators observed that passage of current pulses across the epithelium had no effect on intercalated cell volume, but caused significant swelling in principal cells. Current-induced swelling could be blocked by luminal amiloride and Ba^{2+}, indicating the presence of apical Na^+ and K^+ channels in this cell type. Similar findings have been made using ouabain-induced cell swelling measurements [23]. Volume measurements by Strange and Spring [16] demonstrated that the apical membrane of both the CCT principal and intercalated cell has an extremely low L_p under resting conditions. Furthermore, their results demonstrated directly that ADH increases the water permeability of this membrane in principal and possibly in intercalated cells. In the *Amphiuma* distal tubule, Guggino [26] noted the presence of two populations of cells that exhibit distinctly different rates of swelling when bath K^+ was elevated. Electrophysiological measurements demonstrated that cells with the highest rate of swelling also had a high basolateral conductance to K^+ and Cl^-. The cells with the lower rate of swelling, however, were poorly conductive to these ions, suggesting the presence of an electroneutral basolateral KCl entry pathway. Measurements of the volume of macula densa cells in the cortical thick ascending limb have demonstrated the presence of an apical furosemide-sensitive NaCl cotransport process [27]. Finally, studies of hypertonic volume regulation in the CCT have revealed the presence of two physiologically distinct populations of intercalated cell [16]. One cell type shows almost complete volume recovery following shrinkage while the other has no hypertonic volume regulatory capabilities. The relationship between these physiological characteristics and the so-called type "A" and type "B" intercalated cell morphology and function is unknown.

Cell Volume Regulation

Renal tubule cells are normally faced with constant challenges to their volume and ionic composition. In medullary nephron segments, extracellular osmolality fluctuates with the diuretic state of the animal, leading to cell swelling or shrinkage. Variations in transcellular transport rates can also lead to cell volume changes. For some time, it has been clear that renal tubule cells respond to such volume perturbations by activating volume regulatory solute loss or accumulation pathways. The development and utilization of optical methods for quantifying cell volume have been essential in understanding the mechanisms by which this occurs. A lengthy discussion of volume regulation, however, is not warranted here. Interested readers should consult the recent review by Montrose-Rafizadeh and Guggino [28] and several articles published elsewhere in these proceedings (see List of Contributors).

Future Perspectives

Optical technology continues to evolve at a rapid pace. The development of higher resolution television monitors, recording devices, and digitization hardware may significantly improve the quality of nephron cell video images and be of value in cell volume studies. Utilization of so-called ultrathin optical sectioning techniques [18] may also enhance image quality. The combination of fluorescence and brightfield microscopy will allow simultaneous [29] or rapid, sequential [30] imaging of cell volume and fluorescent probes for membrane potential and intracellular ions. This, in turn, will provide a detailed understanding of the driving forces, ionic fluxes, and intracellular messengers involved in nephron salt and water transport and cell volume regulation.

References

1. Foskett JK (1990) Optical studies of ion and water transport in single cells. In: Foskett JK, Grinstein S (eds) Noninvasive techniques in cell biology. Wiley-Liss, New York, pp 237–272

2. MacRobbie EAC, Ussing HH (1961) Osmotic behaviour of the epithelial cells of frog skin. Acta Physiol Scand 53:348–365
3. Spring K (1985) The study of epithelial function by quantitative light microscopy. Pflugers Arch 405:S23–S27
4. Burg MB (1972) Perfusion of isolated renal tubules. Yale J Biol Med 45:321–326
5. Burg M, Patlak C, Green N, Villey D (1976) Organic solutes in fluid absorption by renal proximal convoluted tubules. Am J Physiol 231:627–637
6. Horster M, Gundlach H (1979) Application of differential interference contrast with inverted microscopes to the in vitro perfused nephron. J Micro 117:375–379
7. Whittembury G, Lindemann B, Carpi-Medina P, Gonzalez E, Linares H (1986) Continuous measurements of cell volume changes in single kidney tubules. Kidney Int 30:187–191
8. Strange K, Spring KR (1986) Methods for imaging renal tubule cells. Kidney Int 30: 192–200
9. Kirk KL, Schafer JA, DiBona DR (1987) Cell volume regulation in rabbit proximal tubule perfused in vitro. Am J Physiol 252:F922–F932
10. Hebert SC, Sun A (1988) Hypotonic cell volume regulation in mouse medullary thick ascending limb: effects of ADH. Am J Physiol 255:F962–F969
11. Strange K, Spring KR (1987) Absence of significant cellular dilution during ADH-stimulated water reabsorption. Science 235:1068–1070
12. Welling LW, Welling DJ, Ochs TJ (1983) Video measurements of basolateral membrane hydraulic conductivity in the proximal tubule. Am J Physiol 245:F123–F129
13. Kirk KL, Dibona DR, Schafer JA (1984) Morphologic response of the rabbit cortical collecting tubule to peritubular hypotonicity: quantitative examination with differential interference contrast microscopy. J Membr Biol 79:53–64
14. Lindemann B (1984) Real-time area-tracker records cellular volume changes from video images. Rev Sci Instrum 55:1788–1790
15. Guggino WB, Oberleithner H, Giebisch G (1985) Relationship between cell volume and ion transport in the early distal tubule of the *Amphiuma* kidney. J Gen Physiol 86:31–58
16. Strange K, Spring KR (1987) Cell membrane water permeability of rabbit cortical collecting duct. J Membr Biol 96:27–43
17. Spring KR (1985) The study of epithelial function by quantitative light microscopy. Pflugers Arch 405:S23–S27
18. Inoue S (1986) Video microscopy. Plenum, New York
19. Strange K Volume regulatory Cl⁻ loss following Na⁺ pump inhibition in CCT principal cells. Am J Physiol, in press
20. Carpi-Medina P, Whittembury G (1988) Comparison of transcellular and transepithelial water permeabilities (P_{os}) in the isolated proximal straight proximal tubule (PST) of the rabbit kidney. Pflugers Arch 412:66–74
21. Welling LW, Welling DJ, Ochs TJ (1987) Video measurement of basolateral NaCl reflection coefficient in proximal tubule. Am J Physiol 253:F290–F298
22. Sun A, Grossman EB, Lombardi M, Hebert SC (to be published) Vasopressin alters the mechanism of apical Cl⁻ entry from Na:Cl to Na:K:2Cl cotransport in mouse medullary thick ascending limb
23. Strange K (1989) Ouabain-induced cell swelling in rabbit cortical collecting tubule: NaCl transport by principal cells. J Membr Biol 107:249–261
24. Schild L, Aronson PS, Giebisch G (1990) Effects of apical membrane Cl⁻ formate exchange on cell volume in rabbit proximal tubule. Am J Physiol 258:F530–F536
25. O'Neil RG, Hayhurst RA (1985) Functional differentiation of cell types of cortical collecting duct. Am J Physiol 248:F449–F453
26. Guggino WB (1986) Functional differentiation in the early distal tubule of the *Amphiuma* kidney: evidence for two modes of Cl⁻ and K⁺ transport across the basolateral cell membrane. Am J Physiol 250:F430–F440

27. Gonzalez E, Salomonsson M, Muller-Suur C, Persson AEG (1988) Measurements of mac-
    ula densa cell volume changes in isolated and perfused rabbit cortical thick ascending limb.
    I. Isosmotic and anisosmotic cell volume changes. Acta Physiol Scand 133:149–157
28. Montrose-Rafizadeh C, Guggino WB (1990) Cell volume regulation in the nephron. Annu
    Rev Physiol 52:761–772
29. Foskett JK (1988) Simultaneous Nomarski and fluorescence imaging during video
    microscopy of living cells. Am J Physiol 255:C566–C571
30. Spring KR (to be published) Differential interference contrast and fluorescence
    microscopy without significant light loss. In: Herman B, Jacobsen K (eds) Optical
    microscopy in biology. Alan R. Liss, New York

Management of Childhood Nephrotic Syndrome

Chair: Alan M. Robson (USA)
Sunao Maki (Japan)

Steroids and Cytotoxic Drugs in the Treatment of Minimal Change Nephrotic Syndrome

JOHANNES BRODEHL[1]

SUMMARY. Treatment of minimal change nephrotic syndrome has 3 aims: to induce remission, to prevent relapses, and to avoid side-effects. Initial treatment with prednisone should be intensive, because it can be shown that the more intense the initial treatment, the lower the relapse rate thereafter. Therefore, it is recommended to extend the initial treatment to 6 weeks of continuous prednisone and 6 weeks alternate-day prednisone. Relapses do not respond better to intensified treatment and, therefore, should be treated in a standard way. Alkylating drugs are indicated in frequent relapser and steroid dependent cases who have developed steroid-toxicity. Drug of choice is cyclophosphamide, which should be given for 8 weeks in cases without steroid-dependency, and for 12 weeks in steroid-dependent cases.

Introduction

Minimal change nephrotic syndrome (MCNS) is the most frequent type of idiopathic nephrotic syndrome in childhood. It is briefly defined as a nephrotic syndrome of unknown etiology with a characteristic course, responsiveness to glucocorticoids, alkylating agents, and cyclosporine A, a high tendency to relapse, an absence of progressive renal deterioration, and a minimal morphological finding by light- and immunomicroscopy. There is much evidence that the disease is of pathoimmunological origin [1]. The association of MCNS with allergy and with genetic markers of immune responsiveness, as well as the excellent response of proteinuria to immunosuppressive agents has suggested a causal relationship between the immunological and the renal abnormality. However, the exact nature of this relationship is still uncertain.

[1]Medizinische Hochschule Hannover, Kinderklinik, Abteilung Pädiatrische Nephrologie, D-3000 Hannover 61, Federal Republic of Germany

Treatment

The treatment of MCNS has a threefold aim: (1) a remission should be induced as soon as possible, since the nephrotic state is associated with a high rate of dangerous and even fatal complications, such as infections, thromboembolism and vascular collapse. (2) Relapses of the nephrotic syndrome should be prevented as much as possible, since each relapse endangers the patient by new complications and side-effects of treatment. (3) The treatment should avoid side-effects as much as possible, since the disease can run a long relapsing course, which could potentiate the side-effects.

Glucocorticoids have been used for more than 40 years in the treatment of MCNS and are generally considered to be the drug of first choice. The steroid derivative most widely used is prednisone. Therefore, the following statements will be related to prednisone exclusively. There are no convincing data available which can claim that other derivatives of glucosteroids are more advantageous than prednisone or prednisolone in the treatment of MCNS.

Initial Treatment

The initial attack of MCNS is very sensitive to prednisone, as shown from the data of the International Study of Kidney Disease in Children (ISKDC) [2]. Ninety-three percent of cases with MCNS responded to an eight week course of prednisone, which means that almost 72% of all children with the nephrotic syndrome were steroid-responsive (Table 1). Of all other histological categories of the nephrotic syndrome, only focal global glomerulosclerosis (FGGS) exhibited a similar high response rate, while all other categories did not respond to prednisone, i.e., remained steroid-resistant.

The response to prednisone does not occur very promptly; it takes a delay time of one to two weeks before a urinary remission can be observed [3]. In the cooperative study of the Arbeitsgemeinschaft für Pädiatrische Nephrologie (APN) urinary remission was defined as the disappearance of significant proteinuria (< 4 mg/m2/h) for at least 3 consecutive days under prednisone treatment. After 8 days, 50% of cases had urinary remission; the great majority had urinary remission after 14 days. A

Table 1. Steroid response in children with the nephrotic syndrome (ISKDC 1981)

Histopathological category	Number patients = n	Responder		Percentage of Σ N
		n	(%)	
MCNS	363	338	(93.1)	71.8%
FGGS	8	6	(75.0)	1.3%
DMH	9	5	(55.6)	1.1%
FSGS	37	11	(29.7)	2.3%
PROLIF GN	12	3	(25.0)	0.6%
MPGN	29	2	(6.9)	0.4%
Miscellaneous	13	3	(23.0)	0.6%

ISKDC, International study of kidney disease in children; *MCNS*, minimal change nephrotic syndrome; *FGGS*, focal global glomerulosclerosis; *DMH*, diffuse mesangial hypercellularity; *FSGS*, focal segmental glomerulosclerosis; *PROLIF GN*, proliferative glomerulonephritis; *MPGN*, membrano proliferative glomerulonephritis

Table 2. Initial prednisone treatment in children with N.S. (studies of APN)

	Continuous 60 mg/m2/per day	Alternate–day 40 mg/m2/per 48 h days
Long	42	42
Standard	28	28
Short	14 ± 6	16 ± 8

complete remission was defined as the normalization of serum albumin ($\geq$ 35 g/l), it followed the urinary remission after two further weeks of treatment. Thus, a complete remission in children with MCNS, i.e., the first stated aim of treatment, could be achieved after 4 weeks of prednisone treatment.

The question is whether four weeks of prednisone in the initial treatment are enough to achieve the second aim of therapy, i.e., the prevention of subsequent relapses. In order to test the efficacy of the initial treatment the APN conducted comparative, randomized trials with 3 types of initial treatment: the short versus standard regimen [3], and the standard versus long treatment (Arbeitsgemeinschaft für Pädiatrische Nephrologie 1990, unpublished). The duration and dosage of prednisone treatment are shown on Table 2. In the short regimen 81% of patients experienced a relapse within the first 12 months after cessation of continuous prednisone; in the standard regimen 61% experienced such relapses, and in the long regimen only 36% experienced these relapses (Table 3). Not only the number of patients with relapses, but also the number of relapses which occurred in these patients, was highest after the short treatment. This is recognizable by the percentage of patients defined as infrequent relapsers (less than 2 relapses within 6 months) and frequent relapsers ($\geq$ 2 relapses within 6 months). More than twice as many of the patients became frequent relapsers after the short than after the long therapy (Table 3). Thus, the risk of becoming a frequent relapser is much higher after a short than after a long regimen of initial treatment.

In actuarial life table analysis for 24 months the difference between the three initial prednisone treatment groups becomes quite obvious (Fig. 1). The cumulative percentage of patients in sustained remission is highest after long treatment, and significantly lower after short treatment, while the standard treatment lies in between.

From the results it is obvious that the intensity of the initial treatment has a decisive influence on the subsequent rate of relapse. The more intense the initial prednisone treatment is, the lower the relapse rate thereafter, and the longer the subsequent remission will last.

Table 3. Percentage of patients with relapses within 12 months after cessation of continuous initial prednisone therapy

Regimen		Total patients	Infrequent relapsers	Frequent relapsers	Both
Long	(12w)	33	21%	15%	36%
Standard	(8w)	66	44%	17%	61%
Short	(4w)	32	47%	34%	81%

(from Arbeitsgemeinschaft für Pädiatrische Nephrologie 1990)

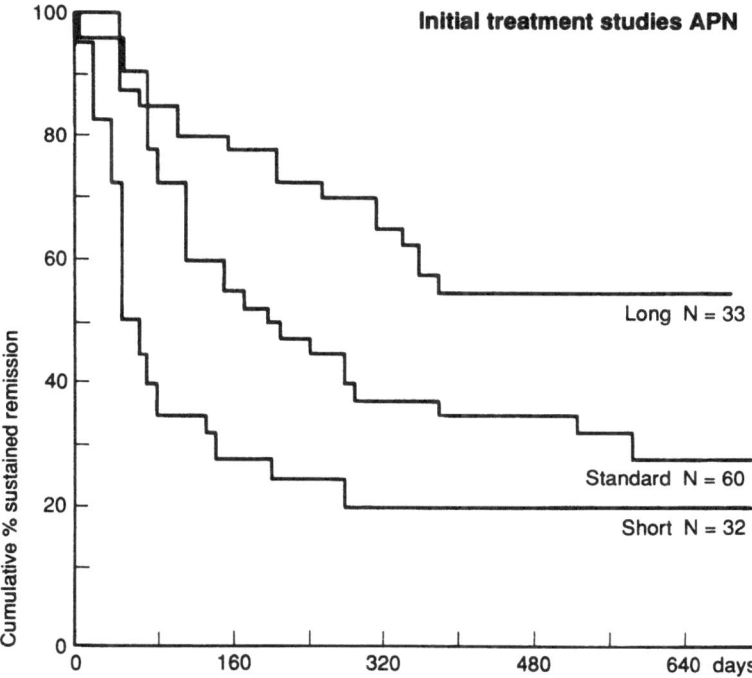

Fig. 1. Cumulative percentage of patients with sustained remission after 3 different prednisone regimens of initial treatment. Long, 12 weeks; standard, 8 weeks; and short, 4 weeks. (Preliminary data from Arbeitsgemeinschaft für Päediatrische Nephrologie)

It should be pointed out that this phenomenon can be only observed after the initial attack. If a relapse occurs, it usually is as steroid responsive as the initial attack. However, the length of the treatment and the dosage of prednisone no longer has any influence on the subsequent relapse rate [3,4]. This is shown in Table 4, which compares the mean duration of remissions after the initial attack and after the first and second relapse in those patients who relapsed [3]. There was a significantly longer remission after standard treatment of the initial attack than after short treatment. However, there were no differences after the relapse treatment, whether this was short or standard.

Table 4. Mean duration of remission after initial attack and relapses (APN 1988)

		Short prednisone therapy	Standard prednisone therapy	Significance*
Days after				
initial attack	(SD)	79 (74)	169 (143)	P = 0.004
first relapse	(SD)	58 (34)	84 (57)	ns
second relapse	(SD)	66 (36)	61 (46)	ns

*Mann-Whitney test; ns, not significant
APN Arbeitsgemeinschaft für Päediatrische Nephrologie

Table 5. Side effects of initial prednisone treatment (APN 1990)

	Standard (8 w)		Long (12w)	
	n = 33	(%)	n = 32	(%)
Steroid-Cushing	11	(33)	11	(34)
Steroid-Cushing with striae	2	(6)	6	(19)
Hypertrichosis	2	(6)	6	(19)
Psycho-emot. disturbances	2	(6)	3	(9)
Path.slit lamp	2/15	(13)	0/9	(0)
Other	3	(9)	1	(3)

Other, convulsions, pseudomotor cerebri, hypertension, thromboembolism, severe infection, osteochondritis etc

APN, Arbeitsgemeinschaft für Päediatrische Nephrologie

Thus, the second aim of MCNS treatment, i.e., the prevention of relapses, is approached best with an intensification of the initial treatment. However, before a definitive recommendation for the initial treatment can be issued, one has to evaluate the side-effects of the treatment according to the third aim of treatment, i.e., the avoidance of side-effects of drugs. It is self evident that the side-effects of steroids will increase, along with the dosage and length of treatment. Well known side-effects of steroids are cushingoid appearance, striae, hypertension, osteoporosis, cataracts, and, especially in children, growth retardation and psychosocial disturbances. The APN study, therefore, tried to evaluate the side-effects of long-prednisone treatment as compared with the standard treatment. The results are listed in Table 5. From these data it was concluded that the risk of a 12-week prednisone course is not essentially higher than that of an 8-week course. The members of APN, therefore, believed that the advantages of a prolonged initial prednisone treatment outweighed the risks, and therefore recommended the 12-week prednisone course for the initial treatment (Table 6). Since there was no benefit from a prolonged prednisone treatment of a relapse, the recommendation for relapse therapy remains the same as that proposed some years ago [5].

The majority of children with MCNS can be managed by this procedure. There are, however, a few who are, or become, steroid resistant, and others who turn out to be frequent relapsers or steroid-dependent.

Steroid-Resistant MCNS

Initial steroid resistance in MCNS is rare (see Table 1). Even if there is no remission after 8 weeks of prednisone treatment, there is still a good chance that prolonged

Table 6. Recommended treatment for initial attack and relapse of nephrotic syndrome in children (APN 1990)

Initial: Continuous **prednisone** 60 mg/m2 per day in 3 divided doses (not more than 80 mg/day) for
             6 weeks followed by
             alternate-day **prednidsone** 40 mg/m2 per 48h for 6 weeks

Relapse: Continuous **prednisone** 60 mg/m2 per day in 3 divided doses (not more than 80 mg/day) until
             urine protein free for 3 days followed by
             alternate-day **prednisone** 40 mg/m2 per 48h for 4 weeks

APN, Arbeitsgemeinschaft für Päediatrische Nephrologie

Table 7. Steroid resistance of children with MCNS. Percentage of total cases according to histological subcategories (ISKDC 1981)

Subcategory	Weeks after initial prednisone			
	8	26	52	104 (n)
Nil	4.7	1.4	0.9	0.9 (2)
FGO	7.8	3.3	2.2	2.2 (2)
MMT	6.3	6.3	0.0	0.0 (0)
FTC	14.3	10.7	3.6	0.0 (0)
MMH	14.8	14.8	7.4	7.4 (2)
DMH	45.5	18.2	9.1	9.1 (1)
Total	31/383	16/383	8/383	7/383
	=8.1%	=4.2%	=2.1%	=1.8%

ISKDC, International Study of Kidney Disease in Children
Abbreviations for subcategories of minimal change nephrotic syndrome (*MCNS*): Nil, nil - disease; FGO, focal global obsolescence; MMT, mild mesangial thickening; FTC, focal tubular changes; MMH, mild mesangial hypercellularity; DMH, diffuse mesangial hypercellularity

treatment with steroids or the addition of a cytotoxic agent can produce a final remission. As can be seen in Table 7, almost all subcategories of MCNS responded to treatment after 2 years, and only 7 cases out of 383 were left unresponsive to treatment [6]. It is, therefore, our policy in histologically proven cases of MCNS, after an 8–12 week course of prednisone, to continue immunosuppressive treatment, either with a combination of prednisone plus cyclophosphamide, or with a combination of prednisone plus cyclosporine A. To our knowledge, there are no controlled studies available which could indicate which type of treatment would be superior.

Frequent Relapsing and Steroid-Dependent MCNS

The rate at which children with MCNS will become frequent relapsers or steroid-dependent is partially determined by the initial treatment, as described above. There are no serological, laboratory, or morphological criteria which could be predictive of the future course of the disease. It is, therefore, necessary to conduct the treatment in a standardized way because this is the only way which helps to classify the patient according to the severity of the disease.

We speak of a frequent relapser without steroid dependency as a patient who responds initially to prednisone, but has two relapses within six months of his initial response, or 4 relapses within a one year period, without fulfilling the criteria of steroid-dependency [7]. The criterion for steroid-dependency is fulfilled when two consecutive relapses occur during the standard relapse therapy or within 14 days after cessation of steroid therapy—which then is called "fast relapse"– or when 2 out of 4 relapses in a period of 6 months are fast relapses.

Children with frequent relapses or steroid dependency are endangered by steroid toxicity, since steroids have to be administered for long periods and in high doses. Review of the literature reveals that in larger series of steroid treated children with glomerulopathies, more than 5% of patients died due to steroid complications, and not because of the renal disease [8]. Therefore, in the cases of frequent relapse and steroid-dependency an alternative immunosuppressive treatment is mandatory.

It has been known for many years that such alkylating substances as nitrogen mustard, cyclophosphamide, and chlorambucil are effective in MCNS. The majority of physicians prefer cyclophosphamide, since its longlasting toxicity within the immunosuppressive therapeutic range seems to be less than that of chlorambucil. Therefore, most experience has been accumulated with cyclophosphamide.

In our experience cyclophosphamide is indicated in children with frequent relapses or with steroid dependency who develop signs of steroid toxicity due to prolonged steroid application, and in children in whom a steroid contraindication exists, as in diabetes mellitus. The action of cyclophosphamide can be described thus [9]:

1) Cyclophosphamide induces remissions of MCNS in all patients who respond to steroids.
2) In addition, cyclophosphamide is also effective in some cases of steroid-resistant MCNS.
3) The time sequence until remission is achieved is somewhat slower than after steroids.
4) Remissions after cyclophosphamide are often long-lasting, even if cyclophosphamide is administered in steroid-induced remission.
5) The subsequent relapse rate is dependent on dosage and/or on length of cyclophosphamide treatment.

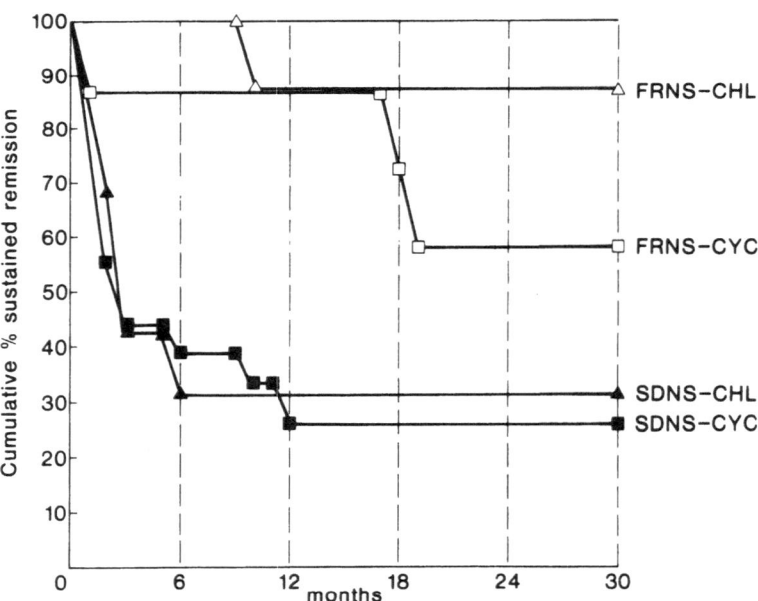

Fig. 2. Cumulative percentage of sustained remission in frequent relapser (*FRNS*) and steroid depender (*SDNS*) treated either with chlorambucil (*CHL*) or cyclophosphamide (*CYC*). (Data from [7])

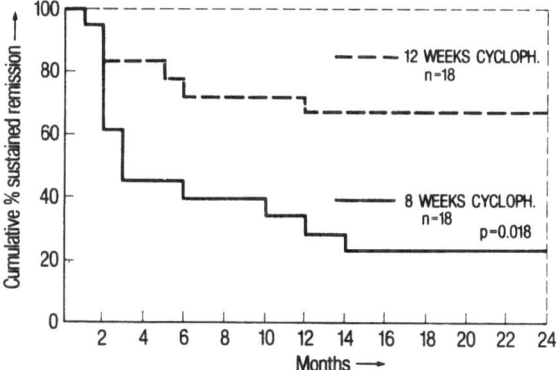

Fig. 3. Cumulative percentage of sustained remission in steroid-dependent minimal change nephrotic syndrome (*MCNS*): comparison of eight weeks with 12 weeks treatment with cyclophosphamide after 2 years. (From [10] with permission)

6) The efficacy of cyclophosphamide in repeated courses is uncertain (beware side-effects!).

The Arbeitsgemeinschaft für Pädiatrische Nephrologie has compared the efficacy of cyclophosphamide with that of chlorambucil in nephrotic children with and without steroid dependency [7]. It was shown that cyclophosphamide in a dosage of 2 mg/kg per day was as effective as chlorambucil in a dosage of 0.15 mg/kg per day. Both drugs were administered for 8 weeks after remission had been induced by prednisone therapy. Children with frequent relapses, but without steroid dependency, gained so much from the treatment that about 70% of them remained in prolonged remission thereafter. In contrast, steroid-dependent cases did not gain enough from the treatment, since only 30% remained in prolonged remission (Fig. 2).

Therefore, in a further study, the steroid-dependent children were treated with cyclophosphamide for 12 weeks instead of 8 weeks [10]. By this it was shown that the percentage of patients with long-lasting remissions was increased to 70% (Fig. 3). Remissions usually persisted for at least 5 years, as a follow-up study determined [11]; no serious side-effects were observed. The cumulative dosage of cyclophosphamide amounted to 168 mg/kg, which is below the known toxic threshold for gonadal toxicity in prepubertal boys [12].

Immunosuppressive Action

Both steroids and alkylating substances are immunosuppressive agents, for which, however, the exact pharmacomechanism in MCNS is not known. Steroids interfere with gene transcription through binding of the glucocorticoid receptors to regulating DNA sequences, thereby abrogating gene expression of important monokines [13]. They obviously suppress the secretion of IL1, IL6, and IL8 [14], mainly in monocytes. It is not known whether this mechanism is responsible for the antiproteinuric effects in MCNS.

Table 8. Comparison of prednisone and cyclophosphamide in the treatment of MCNS

	Prednisone	Cyclophosphamide
Delay time until antiproteinuric effect	7–14	14–21 days
Dose-response	yes	yes
Additive effect	yes	yes
Sustained effect after discontinuation	no	yes
Effective in repeated courses	yes	no

MCNS, minimal change nephrotic syndrome

Alkylating substances are antimitotic. By alkylating DNA they cause nuclear damage which is irreversible and results in cytotoxicity. The whole range of lymphocytes is susceptible to cyclophosphamide, the descending order of sensitivity being suppressor T cells, B cells, helper T cells, and cytotoxic T cells [15, 16]. Whether functional changes of lymphocytes are induced by cyclophosphamide is not yet known.

If one compares the in vivo effects of both immunosuppressive substances in children with MCNS, one recognizes similarities and dissimilarities. These are shown in Table 8. Cyclophosphamide needs a little more time than steroids to produce urinary remission. Both substances exhibit additive effects, and it is noteworthy that cyclophosphamide can exert its longlasting effect even in the prednisone-induced remission state. While prednisone has no longlasting effect, i.e., it does not protect against relapses after discontinuation, this is not the case with cyclophosphamide. In this respect cyclophosphamide is superior to prednisone. Finally, prednisone is effective in repeated courses, while cyclophosphamide is probably not. However, because of the gonadal toxicity, this has not been extensively tested.

Conclusion

From the findings of multicenter studies the recommendation for immunosuppressive treatment of children with MCNS today is as follows:

1) The initial attack needs an intensive steroid treatment: prednisone 60 mg/m2 per day for 6 weeks, followed by alternate-day 40 mg/m2 per 48 h for 6 weeks.
2) Relapses should receive a standardized treatment: prednisone 60 mg/m2 per day until urine is protein free for 3 days, followed by 40 mg/m2 per 48h for 4 weeks. This should be repeated in cases of infrequent relapse.
3) Frequent relapses and steroid dependency with steroid-toxicity should receive alkylating drug treatment: cyclophosphamide 2 mg/kg per day for 8 weeks in frequent relapsers; for 12 weeks in steroid-dependency.
4) Frequent relapsers, after cyclophosphamide, should receive treatment with cyclosporine A 100–150 mg/m2 per day for 6–12 months or more.

References

1. Schnaper HW (1989) The immune system in minimal change nephrotic syndrome. Pediatr Nephrol 3:101–110

2. International Study of Kidney Disease in Children (1981) The primary nephrotic syndrome in children. Identification of patients with minimal change nephrotic syndrome from initial response to prednisone. J Pediatr 98:561–564

3. Arbeitsgemeinschaft für Pädiatrische Nephrologie (1988) Short versus standard prednisone therapy for initial treatment of idiopathic nephrotic syndrome in children. Lancet I:380–383

4. Arbeitsgemeinschaft für Pädiatrische Nephrologie (1979) Alternate day versus intermittent prednisone in frequently relapsing nephrotic syndrome. Lancet I:401–403

5. Brodehl J, Krohn HP, Ehrich JHH (1982) The treatment of minimal change nephrotic syndrome (lipoidnephrosis): cooperative studies of the Arbeitsgemeinschaft für Pädiatrische Nephrologie (APN). Klin Pädiatr 194:162–165

6. International Study of Kidney Disease in Children (1981) Primary nephrotic syndrome in children: clinical significance of histopathologic variants of minimal change and of diffuse mesangial hypercellularity. Kidney Int 20:765–771

7. Arbeitsgemeinschaft für Pädiatrische Nephrologie (1982) Effect of cytotoxic drugs in frequently relapsing nephrotic syndrome with and without steroid dependence. N Engl J Med 306:451–454

8. Brodehl J (1986) Nephrotic syndrome in children: diagnosis and treatment. World Pediatrics and Child Care 1:9–18

9. Brodehl J (1989) Effective drugs for MCNS and their implications on the pathophysiology. VIII Congress of Int Pediatr Nephrology Association. Pediatr Nephrol 3:C74

10. Arbeitsgemeinschaft für Pädiatrische Nephrologie (1987) Cyclophosphamide treatment of steroid dependent nephrotic syndrome: comparison of eight weeks with 12 weeks course. Arch Dis Child 62:1102–1106

11. Krohn HP, Brodehl J (1986) Cytotoxic drug study I of the APN: 5 years follow-up. Helv Paediatr Acta 41:107

12. Etteldorf JN, West CD, Pitcock JA, Williams DL (1976) Gonadal function, testicular histology and meiosis following cyclophosphamide therapy in patients with nephrotic syndrome. J Pediatr 88:206–212

13. Beato M (1989) Gene regulation by steroid hormones. Cell 56:335–344

14. Zanker B, Walz G, Wieder KJ, Strom TB (1990) Evidence that glucocorticosteroids block expression of the human interleukin-6 gene by accessory cells. Transplantation 49:183–185

15. Balow JZ, Hurley DL, Fauci AS (1975) Cyclophosphamide expression of established cell-mediated immunity. J Clin Invest 56:65–70

16. Feehally J, Beattle TJ, Brenchley PEC, Coupes BM, Houston IB, Mallick NP, Postlethwaite RJ (1984) Modulation of cellular immune function by cyclophosphamide in children with minimal change. N Engl J Med 310:415–420

New Therapies for the Treatment of Idiopathic Nephrotic Syndrome

Patrick Niaudet, Michel Broyer, and Renée Habib[1]

SUMMARY. The treatment of children with idiopathic nephrotic syndrome who have multiple relapses or who are steroid-resistant is a difficult issue. Alkylating agents are often proposed but they have several side effects, including gonadal toxicity, which limit their use. Treatment with levamisole may be efficient in steroid-dependent patients, allowing prednisone to be tapered or stopped in approximately 50% of cases. Cyclosporine has proved to be effective in 85% of steroid-dependent patients, but most patients relapse when cyclosporine is tapered or withdrawn. Thus, in these patients, cyclosporine may be required for long periods of time. Conversely, cyclosporine alone is less effective in steroid-resistant patients, as only 28% of these patients respond to the treatment. Cyclosporine in association with prednisone may be a better alternative as, in our experience, 14 out of 31 patients went into remission with such treatment. It should be stressed that response to cyclosporine is better correlated with initial steroid responsiveness than with histological category. Eighteen out of 43 patients with serial renal biopsies developed significant tubulo interstitial lesions which could be attributable to cyclosporine nephrotoxicity. The risk of developing chronic nephrotoxicity appears to be higher in steroid-resistant patients. Cyclosporine nephrotoxicity is not related to the duration of treatment and may develop in patients with normal renal function.

Introduction

Idiopathic nephrotic syndrome (INS), the most common glomerular disease in children, is defined by the combination of nephrotic syndrome and minimal change glomerular disease with foot process fusion seen on electron microscopy. No immunoglobulin deposits are seen on immunofluorescence. However, in some cases,

[1]Service de Néphrologie Pédiatrique and INSERM U192, Hôpital Necker Enfants Malades, 75743 Paris, France

diffuse mesangial proliferation or focal and segmental glomerulosclerosis may be seen on light microscopy and sometimes immunofluorescence reveals mesangial IgM or, less frequently, IgA deposits. Although several authors consider that minimal change disease, focal and segmental glomerulosclerosis, diffuse mesangial proliferation, and IgM nephropathy are distinct entities as the response to treatment and the clinical course can be different, there is in fact a clinical overlap between the different anatomical entities and INS should rather be considered as a syndrome with different clinical and histologic variants [1].

The clinical experience shows that the response to steroid therapy carries greater prognostic weight than the histological features seen on initial biopsy. In the vast majority of childhood cases (90%), INS is steroid-responsive but 60% of these steroid responders relapse as soon as steroid therapy is withdrawn or when the dosage is decreased. This constitutes steroid-dependent INS, the severity of which lies less in the risk of developing end stage renal failure, which is a very rare outcome, than in the complications of treatment. When the level of steroid therapy required to maintain remission is too high, the side effects force one to resort to other drugs such as immunosuppressive agents that are themselves not without risk.

In 10% of cases, INS is steroid-resistant. The severity of this condition lies essentially in the risk of developing end stage renal failure, which occurs in about half of the cases.

Alkylating agents, which achieve long lasting remission, have been used for some 20 years in INS [2]. The majority of studies have concentrated on their use in steroid-dependent patients and in relapsing steroid-responders. Their efficacy has been clearly demonstrated in such cases. The duration of remission depends on the severity of the disease and the duration of treatment. The limitation on longer use of alkylating agents lies in their long-term toxic effects, in particular the risks of cancer and leukemia and, in boys, the gonadal toxicity. The efficacy of alkylating agents in steroid-resistant INS is more open to question.

In this paper we will discuss the other therapeutic approaches besides corticosteroids and alkylating agents, that have been proposed for patients with INS, namely levamisole and cyclosporine.

Levamisole

Levamisole is an anthelmintic which has immunostimulatory activity in different experimental systems. It was first used by Tanphaichitr et al. [3] in 7 children with steroid-responsive nephrotic syndrome; the treatment induced a remission within 6 months in all of them. Mehta et al. [4] treated 25 children with relapsing steroid-responsive nephrotic syndrome; 13 of them went into remission and 12 went into partial remission. Mongeau et al. [5] found that levamisole was able to reduce the mean dose of prednisone by 60% and the monthly relapse rate from 0.35 to 0.13. Our experience concerns 71 patients with steroid-dependent nephrotic syndrome who were treated with levamisole given twice weekly at a dose of 2.5 mg/kg while the dose of prednisone was gradually decreased. Prednisone could be stopped without relapse in 17 patients (24%) on levamisole. In 32 patients (45%), prednisone therapy could be reduced but not withdrawn. In the remaining 22 patients (31%) prednisone could not be tapered. The majority of the children in whom levamisole had been effective relapsed after the treatment was stopped.

Cyclosporine and Steroid-Dependent INS

Cyclosporine, an immunosuppressive drug introduced in organ transplantation more than a decade ago, was found to be effective in the treatment of patients with idiopathic nephrotic syndrome by Meyrier et al. [6] and by Hoyer et al. [7]. In children, Hoyer et al. [7] treated five steroid-dependent patients who all responded to cyclosporine with fewer relapses and with reduced prednisone requirements. Capodicasa et al. [8] treated six steroid-dependent patients; in 5 of them cyclosporine induced long lasting remissions. Tejani et al. [9] treated 13 steroid-dependent children for eight weeks. Eleven patients remained in remission for over nine months after discontinuation of therapy.

Our experience concerns 45 patients with steroid-responsive and steroid-dependent INS. Histological examination of renal biopsy specimens obtained before initiation of cyclosporine therapy showed minimal change disease in 40 cases, diffuse mesangial proliferation in 2 cases, and focal and segmental glomerulosclerosis in 3 cases. The 45 steroid-responders had had their last relapse while receiving alternate-day prednisone within 3 months preceding cyclosporine treatment. They received cyclosporine for periods of at least 3 months. Fifteen patients were receiving daily prednisone treatment and 27 were receiving alternate-day prednisone when cyclosporine therapy was started. Three patients were no longer receiving prednisone.

Thirty-six of the 45 patients either went into remission or did not relapse at all during the period of full-dose cyclosporine, despite the fact that prednisone treatment was withdrawn. Among the 36 patients, 3 were protein-free at last examination, but they were still receiving cyclosporine. Thirty-three patients relapsed: 23 relapsed while receiving cyclosporine at tapering doses varying between 0.7 and 6.6 mg/kg; 10 patients relapsed 7–120 days after withdrawal of cyclosporine therapy. Cyclosporine was ineffective in 2 patients, who relapsed as soon as alternate-day prednisone therapy was started. The remaining 7 patients relapsed at withdrawal of prednisone treatment, and the association of cyclosporine with low-dose prednisone allowed remission to be maintained.

Between 1985 and 1989, the French Society of Pediatric Nephrology performed an open randomized controlled study which compared the efficacy and the tolerance of cyclosporine with those of chlorambucil in children with steroid-dependent nephrotic syndrome and signs of steroid toxicity. Forty children, 9 girls and 31 boys, were entered in the study. Twenty children received cyclosporine at an initial dose of 6 mg/kgBW; the dose was adjusted to obtain trough plasma levels of between 50 and 150 ng/ml (radio-immunoassay (RIA), polyclonal antibodies). After 3 months, cyclosporine was tapered off within the next 3 months. Twenty children received chlorambucil 0.2 mg/kgBW during 6–8 weeks, with a cumulative dosage of 8 mg/kg, a dose which avoids gonadal toxicity. The two groups did not show significant differences concerning the proportion of girls and boys, the age at onset of the disease, the duration of disease, the number of relapses and the histology (minimal change disease (MCD), focal and segmental glomerulosclerosis (FSGS), diffuse mesangial proliferation (DMP)).

Among the 20 patients who received cyclosporine, 2 relapsed before prednisone withdrawal, 9 relapsed after prednisone withdrawal, at doses of cyclosporine ranging from 0.9 to 8.5 mg/kg (mean 4.15 mg/kg), 8 relapsed 1 week–7 months after cyclosporine withdrawal, and only one patient remained in remission 18 months after cyclosporine withdrawal.

Among the 20 patients who received chlorambucil, 4 patients relapsed before prednisone withdrawal, 10 relapsed within 34 months after prednisone withdrawal, and the remaining 6 patients were still in remission 21–42 months after chlorambucil treatment.

In summary, cyclosporine made it possible to stop prednisone in 18 out of 20 children, but subsequent relapses occurred in 17 of the children during the tapering phase or after withdrawal of cyclosporine. Conversely, chlorambucil allowed the withdrawal of prednisone in 16 out of 20 patients, but 10 of these patients experienced further relapses. At last follow-up, after 21–42 months, 30% of the patients who received chlorambucil and only 5% of the patients who received cyclosporine were still in remission.

Cyclosporine and Steroid-Resistant INS

Cyclosporine has been given to children with steroid-resistant idiopathic nephrotic syndrome in several uncontrolled studies. Capodicasa et al. reported that 2 of 4 patients treated with a combination of cyclosporine and prednisone went into remission [8]. Similarly, Brandis et al. [10] found a beneficial effect of cyclosporine given alone in 4 patients. Conversely, Waldo and Kohaut [11] reported partial remission among 6 treated children, while Brodehl et al. [12] found 2 partial remissions out of 7 cases and Tejani et al. [9] reported 3 remissions out of 7 cases.

We treated 14 steroid-resistant patients, including 11 early non-responders and 3 late non-responders. Only one patient, a late non-responder, went into complete remission on cyclosporine alone, while a partial and transient remission was observed in 4 patients. The remaining 9 patients failed to respond to cyclosporine. Cyclosporine in association with prednisone induced a remission in 2 out of 4 patients.

This observation led us to start an open trial with the French Society of Pediatric Nephrology on the effect of cyclosporine in association with prednisone [13]. Thirty one patients, 13 girls and 18 boys, aged 1 month–14.3 years at onset of the disease and in whom renal biopsy had shown MCD in 19 cases and FSGS in 12 cases, received cyclosporine (150–200 mg/m²) in combination with daily prednisone (30 mg/m²) for one month and with alternate day prednisone, 30 mg/m², for 5 months thereafter. Fourteen patients (45%) went into complete remission, nine of them during the first two months of the treatment. Three patients had a partial remission and 14 failed to respond to the treatment. Interestingly, the response to cyclosporine and prednisone was not correlated with the histopathological findings, since among the 14 patients who responded to the treatment, 9 had MCD and 5 FSGS, whereas among the 14 patients who failed to respond 9 had MCD and 5 had FSGS.

Nephrotoxicity of Cyclosporine

Among the side effects of cyclosporine, nephrotoxicity is the most worrying. Nephrotoxicity is generally evidenced by deterioration of renal function. In idiopathic nephrotic syndrome, renal insufficiency may occur during a relapse or as end stage renal failure develops in steroid-resistant patients. In patients treated with cyclosporine, it may be difficult to determine to what extent deterioration of renal function is due to drug-induced nephrotoxicity or to renal insufficiency due to the renal disease itself. Furthermore, the two events may be superimposed on one another.

We observed an impairment of renal function in 10 patients. Four out of the 45 steroid-dependent patients had a transient increase in serum creatinine levels. The increase occurred during a relapse in 3 patients with low cyclosporine trough levels. In the other patients, the increase in plasma creatinine levels completely reversed after withdrawal of cyclosporine therapy. Six out of the 14 steroid-resistant patients had an impairment of renal function. This impairment was transient, with complete recovery in 4 of the patients. In two patients, the impairment in renal function was only partially reversible and deteriorated further following withdrawal of cyclosporine therapy.

In order to better evaluate the eventual nephrotoxicity of cyclosporine in these patients with INS, we undertook a prospective study concerning 43 patients in whom at least two renal biopsies were performed, including one before initiation of cyclosporine. Thirty seven patients were steroid-dependent and six were steroid-resistant. Initial biopsy had shown minimal change disease (MCD) in 34 patients (32 steroid-dependent and 2 steroid-resistant), diffuse mesangial proliferation (DMP) in 2 steroid-dependent patients, and focal and segmental glomerulosclerosis (FSGS) in 7 patients (3 steroid-dependent and 4 steroid-resistant). Cyclosporine was efficient in 33 steroid-dependent patients and in 3 steroid-resistant patients (29 MCD, 2 DMP, and 5 FSGS). The second renal biopsy was performed after a 2–20 month cyclosporine treatment period. The lesions observed on these biopsies were classified as follows: Grade 0 included 16 patients, all steroid-dependent, who had no modification of renal parenchyma. Grade I was diagnosed in 11 patients, 10 steroid-dependent and 1 steroid-resistant, who showed scattered atrophic tubules; grade II was diagnosed in 11 patients, 10 steroid-dependent and one steroid-resistant, who showed several foci of atrophic tubules within stripes of interstitial fibrosis; and grade III was diagnosed in 5 patients (1 steroid-dependent and 4 steroid-resistant) in whom confluent areas of interstitial fibrosis with atrophic or collapsed tubules were observed. A third biopsy was obtained in 13 patients, after 11–37 months of cyclosporine therapy. Of the 5 patients with grade 0 on second biopsy, 3 remained grade 0 and 2 progressed to grade I. Of the 5 patients with grade I, 3 remained grade I and 2 progressed to grade II. Finally, the 3 patients with grade II progressed to grade III. Among the 43 patients, only 3 showed an impairment of renal function which, in two of them, was reversible. This study shows that cyclosporine nephrotoxicity is not related to the duration of treatment. The risk of developing chronic nephrotoxicity appears to be higher in steroid-resistant patients than in steroid-dependent ones. Histological signs of nephrotoxicity can develop in patients with normal renal function. Renal biopsy seems, therefore, the only way of detecting patients who develop cyclosporine nephrotoxicity.

References

1. Habib R, Churg J (1984) Minimal change disease, mesangial proliferation glomerulonephritis and focal sclerosis: individual entities or a spectrum. In: RR Robinson (ed) Nephrology. Springer, New York, pp 634–644

2. Niaudet P, Habib R, Gagnadoux MF, Tête MJ, Broyer M (1988) Treatment of severe child-hood nephrosis. In: Grunfeld JP, Bach JF, Crosnier J, Funk-Brentano JL, Maxwell MH (eds) Advances in nephrology. Year Book Medical, pp 151–172
3. Tanphaichitr P, Tanphaichitr D, Sureesatanan J (1980) Treatment of nephrotic syndrome with levamisole. J Pediatr 96:490–493
4. Mehta K, Ali U (1987) New approach to relapsing nephrotic syndrome. Pediatr Nephrol 1:C46
5. Mongeau JG, Robitaille PO, Roy F (1988) Clinical efficacy of levamisole in the treatment of primary nephrosis in children. Pediatr Nephrol 2:398–401
6. Meyrier A, Simon P, Perret G, Condamin-Meyrier MC (1986) Remission of idiopathic nephrotic syndrome after treatment with cyclosporine A. Br Med J [Clin Res] 292:789–793
7. Hoyer PF, Krull F, Brodehl J (1986) Cyclosporine in frequently relapsing minimal change nephrotic syndrome. Lancet II:385
8. Capodicasa G, De Santo NG, Nuzzi F, Giordano C (1986) Cyclosporine A in nephrotic syn-drome of childhood. A 14 month experience. Int J Pediatr Nephrol 7:69–72
9. Tejani A, Butt K, Trachtman H, Suthanthiran M, Rosenthal CJ, Khawar MR (1988) Cyclosporine A induced remission of relapsing nephrotic syndrome in children. Kidney Int 33:729–734
10. Brandis M, Burghard R, Leititis J, Zimmerhackl B, Hildebrandt F, Helmcher U (1988) Cyclosporine A for treatment of nephrotic syndrome. Transplant Proc 20 (Suppl 4):275–279
11. Waldo FB, Kohaut EC (1987) Therapy of focal segmental glomerulosclerosis with cyclosporine A. Pediatr Nephrol 1:180–182
12. Brodehl J, Hoyer PF (1989) Cyclosporin in idiopathic nephrotic syndrome of children. Am J Nephrol 9 (Suppl 1):61–64
13. Niaudet P, the French Society of Pediatric Nephrology. (to be published) Steroid resistant idiopathic nephrotic syndrome and cyclosporine. Nephron

Nephrotic Syndrome in Japan and Other Asian Countries—Epidemiology and Treatment

Kazuo Yoshioka and Sunao Maki[1]

Epidemiology

Nephrotic syndrome (NS) is a common form of childhood renal disease in Asian, as well as in Western, countries. According to the multicenter clinical study on the epidemiology of NS in Japan [1,2], approximately 9000 children with renal disease were seen as in- or out-patients over the two-year period between 1984 and 1985. Of these patients, 14% had NS. Steroids were first used to treat the patients with primary NS, and 90% of the patients responded well, but subsequent relapse during steroid therapy, or shortly after stopping the therapy, was noticed in 33% of the patients. Proteinuria persisted in 9%. Renal biopsy was done on a quarter of the patients who showed good response to steroids, including frequently relapsing patients, and on 80% of the children who showed poor response to, or resistance to, steroids. Under these circumstances, minor abnormalities and diffuse mesangial proliferation were often seen in patients who responded well to steroids. Patients who responded poorly to steroids or were resistant to steroid therapy were prone to show diffuse mesangial prolification, focal segmental sclerosis, and membranoproliferative glomerulonephritis. Approximately 10% of the patients in this group had minor lesions. The majority of primary NS patients in Korea (Dr. KW Ko, Seoul, 1990, personal communication) and in China (Dr. P. Wang, Beijing, 1990, personal communication) had minimal change disease and proliferative glomerulonephritis. Focal segmental sclerosis was diagnosed in a significant number of Korean patients.

Initial Corticosteroid Therapy

Most of the children with primary NS responded well to corticosteroids, but many of them experienced subsequent relapses. In order to prevent frequent relapse, and to

---

[1]Department of Pediatrics, Kinki University, Osaka-sayama, 589 Japan

find a more effective and safer treatment, Dr. Ueda and coworkers in Japan compared two initial steroid therapy regimens, a long-term tapering regimen and a short-term intermittent regimen [3]. The latter was originally proposed by ISKDC. Dr. Ueda and coworkers found that the numbers of patients who had a relapse within 6 months after terminating initial therapy and the numbers of patients with frequent relapses or steroid-dependence were significantly higher in the group treated with the short-term intermittent protocol. They concluded that the long-term tapering regimen was safe and preferable, and that this regimen had a favorable effect on the subsequent clinical course of this disease. Currently, in Japan, this long-term prednisolone therapy is commonly used to treat children with NS. This is also the case in Korea and in China. According to our own experience, 4% of primary NS patients did not show any response to the initial oral prednisolone, but they successfully responded to intravenous methylprednisolone "pulse" therapy.

Cyclophosphamide Therapy

Hitherto, children classified as frequently relapsing NS patients were treated with repeated courses of steroids. When steroid toxicity developed, cytotoxic drugs were used. Cyclophosphamide therapy, for 8 weeks, was generally chosen. Several studies, and our own experience, have shown that a period of 8 weeks is not sufficient to reduce the relapse. We examined the relationship between duration of remission and the age when cyclophosphamide therapy began. There was a significant correlation between relapse within 2 years and age when cyclophosphamide was given. In other words, cyclophosphamide therapy, at a dosage of 3 mg/kg per day for 8 weeks, was not effective, particularly in young children.

We prospectively compared three different durations of cyclophosphamide administration. Group A was of 8-weeks duration, Group B, 10 weeks, and Group C, 12 weeks (Table 1). The patients also received a small dosage of prednisolone during the therapy. There was no difference between the three groups in age at onset of NS, age at entry to study, relapse rate during 1 year before the treatment, and duration of follow-up. Renal histology was either minimal change or mesangial proliferation. These factors were not significantly different between the groups. Figure 1 shows the

Table 1. Frequently relapsing nephrotic syndrome. Cyclophosphamide treatment 3 mg/kg per day

	Group A (8 weeks)	Group B (10 weeks)	Group C (12 weeks)
Total dose (mg/kg)	168	210	252
No. of patients	20	16	8
Male/female	14/6	12/4	7/1
Age when nephrotic syndrome diagnosed (year)	6.7 ± 3.7	6.5 ± 3.7	6.3 ± 3.3
Age at entry to study (year)	9.5 ± 4.2	9.1 ± 3.9	9.1 ± 3.9
Renal history			
Minimal change	13	15	6
Mesangial proliferation	7	1	2
Duration of follow-up (month)	111 ± 48	95 ± 47	71 ± 47

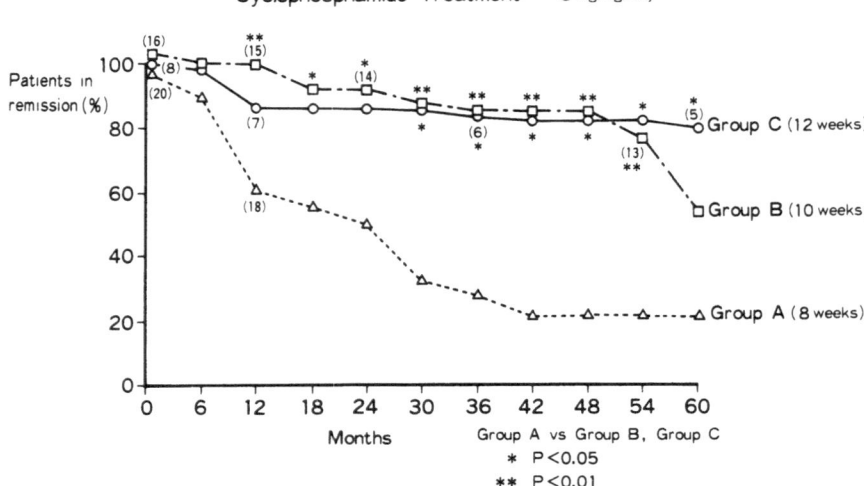

Fig. 1. Frequently relapsing nephrotic syndrome

rate of remission in the three groups. Significant difference between Group A and Group B was found at 12 months and subsequently. The difference between Group A and Group C was significant at 30 months and subsequently. There was no difference between Group B and Group C. No severe toxic effects of cyclophosphamide was observed during the treatment and the follow-up period. However, transient adverse effects, such as alopecia, leucocytopenia, gastrointestinal symptoms, mild elevation of transaminases, or hemorrhagic cystitis, developed in about 60% of the patients. The incidence of these complications was similar in the three groups. There was no correlation between the lowest leukocyte count and the remission period. Taken together, these observations suggest the efficacy and safety of the 10-week regimen. Toxicity to gonads should be monitored for long periods, even though such toxicity is difficult to assess.

Cyclosporin Therapy

Cyclosporin (CsA) therapy has recently been introduced into the treatment program for frequently relapsing NS patients. Several previous studies have shown the efficacy and minimal nephrotoxicity of CsA in nephrotic patients. In Japan, a clinical trial, comparing high and low doses of CsA in frequently relapsing NS patients, was recently carried out. When patients relapsed, CsA at 5 mg/kg per day (high dose) and 2.5 mg/kg per day (low dose) was begun. These dosages were administered for 6 months. Steroid therapy, similar to that given at the previous relapse, was given. Trough levels of CsA were monitored in whole blood and were adjusted to the optimal range of 100–500 ng/ml by polyclonal antibody radio-immunoassay (RIA) and 50–200 ng/ml by monoclonal antibody RIA.

Table 2. Cyclosporin therapy

Histology	Frequently relapsing NS		Steroid-resistant NS	
	High	Low	High	Low
Minimal change	12	8	7	4
Proliferative GN	1	1	6	2
Membranous nephropathy	0	0	0	3
Membranoproliferative GN	0	0	2	6
Focal segmental sclerosis	2	0	5	3
Biopsy, not done	9	10	1	0
Total	24	19	21	18

NS, nephrotic syndrome; GN, glomerulonephritis

Twenty four children received high doses of CsA, and 19 received low doses. Renal histology of the patients is shown in Table 2. Age, sex, duration of NS, relapse rate, and dosage of steroids used during the 6 months before CsA treatment were similar in the two groups. Relapse rate per patient decreased significantly after the therapy, when compared with the rates 6 months before and after starting CsA therapy (Fig. 2). A high dose of CsA significantly reduced the total dosage of steroids (Fig. 3), but a low dose of CsA did not significantly change the steroid dosage, because relapse occurred occasionally during low dose therapy.

In order to investigate whether CsA is effective on steroid-resistant NS, a multicenter study was also conducted. Again, high and low doses were used for 6 months. The histological classification of the patients is listed in Table 2. A high dose of CsA decreased proteinuria significantly 12 and 24 weeks after beginning the therapy (Fig. 4). In these patients, creatinine clearance did not change significantly.

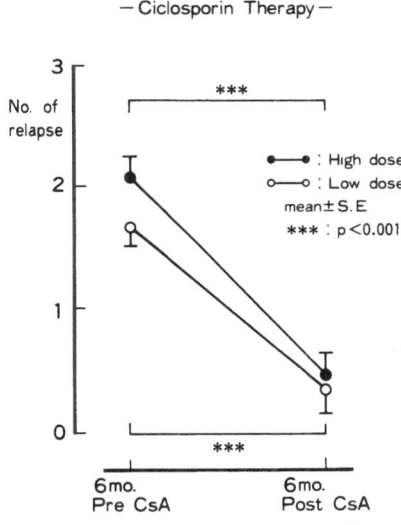

Fig. 2. Frequently relapsing nephrotic syndrome

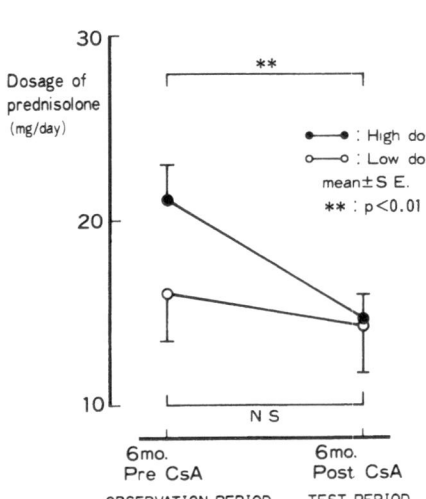

Fig. 3. Frequently relapsing nephrotic syndrome

Side effects of CsA, such as elevation of serum alkaline phosphatase, hypertension, hirsutism, and gastrointestinal symptoms, were observed frequently. Hypertension was controlled by decreasing the dose of CsA or by temporary administration of a Ca channel blocker. Renal function was temporariliy impaired in 3 (12%) patients with steroid-resistant NS. Most patients with frequently relapsing NS who were treated

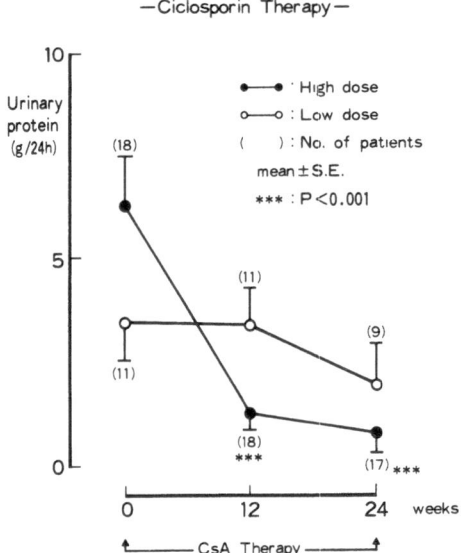

Fig. 4. Steroid-resistant nephrotic syndrome

with CsA relapsed shortly after the therapy had ended. Steroid-resistant patients obviously needed long-term CsA therapy.

In order to find out how long we can use CsA in nephrotic patients without causing nephrotoxicity, we are currently studying one-year CsA treatment. Our subjects are children with frequently relapsing NS, who have had severe steroid toxicity and have previously been treated with cyclophosphamide. In a total of 12 children, 5 mg/kg per day of CsA was administered with steroids. Trough levels of CsA were carefully monitored at least once a month. Significant decreases in the relapse rate and in the total dosage of steroids were observed. After CsA treatment, we biopsied four patients, and the results were compared with the biopsy findings which had been done prior to the therapy. In three out of four patients, no alterations suggesting CsA nephrotoxicity were found. In one patient with minimal glomerular changes, hypertrophy of the juxtaglomerular apparatus was observed in approximately half of the glomeruli. This patient was hypertensive at the beginning of CsA therapy, but he became normotensive thereafter. Renal function, urinary and serum Na concentration, and aldosterone and angiotensin II levels were normal at the time of biopsy. Plasma renin activity was slightly elevated. Taken together, these observations suggest that CsA therapy is effective and favorable for children, not only for those with frequently-relapsing NS, but also for those with steroid resistant NS. However, we need to conduct more research on this type of new therapy before we can use it for long periods with minimal CsA toxicity.

Acknowledgment. We appreciate the collaboration offered by Dr. K.W. Ko (Seoul National University, Children's Hospital, Korea) and Dr. P. Wang (First Hospital, Beijing Medical School, China) and permission to present CsA studies done by Dr. S. Tojo.

References

1. Kitagawa T, Sakai T (1985) Multicenter study on epidemiology of childhood renal diseases. In: Ishimaru T (ed) Annual report on study of prevention and treatment of childhood chronic renal diseases, pp 282–286
2. Kitagawa T, Sakai T (1986) Multicenter study on epidemiology of childhood renal diseases. In: Ishimaru T (ed) Annual report on study of prevention and treatment of childhood chronic renal diseases, pp 314–319
3. Ueda N, Chihara M, Kawaguchi S, Niinomi Y, Nonoda T, Matsumoto J, Ohnishi M, Yasaki T (1988) Intermittent versus long-term tapering prednisolone for initial therapy in children with idiopathic nephrotic syndrome. J Pediatr 112:122–126

Treatment of Childhood Steroid-Resistant Focal Segmental Glomerulosclerosis with Pulse Methylprednisolone and Alkylating Agents*

STANLEY A. MENDOZA[1], VIVIAN M. REZNIK[1], WILLIAM R. GRISWOLD[1], ALAN M. KRENSKY[2], PETER D. YORGIN[2], and BRUCE M. TUNE[2]

SUMMARY. In children, steroid-resistant nephrotic syndrome due to focal segmental glomerulosclerosis (FSGS) is frequently a progressive condition resulting in end-stage renal disease in spite of treatment. For the past several years, the Pediatric Nephrology services at the University of California, San Diego and Stanford University Schools of Medicine have treated these patients with a protocol involving infusions of high doses of methylprednisolone (MP), often in combination with oral alkylating agents. Twenty-three children have been treated in this manner with a follow-up of 55 ± 6 months. Thirteen of these children are in complete remission. Five have minimal to moderate proteinuria. Four children remain nephrotic. Each of these children has a normal glomerular filtration rate. One child developed chronic renal failure and subsequently died while on dialysis. These results appear better than those in previous series of children with FSGS. A controlled, multi-center trial of this protocol has been proposed.

Introduction

Focal segmental glomerulosclerosis (FSGS) is a cause of steroid-resistant nephrotic syndrome and chronic renal failure in childhood [1-7]. The incidence of renal failure is 20%–40% by 5 years after the onset of FSGS and increases further after 10 years. FSGS is the most common form of glomerular disease leading to chronic renal failure in children [8] and is seen in 10%–20% of children requiring dialysis or renal transplantation [9]. In recent years, the Pediatric Nephrology services at the Stanford and University of California, San Diego Schools of Medicine have treated these children

[1]Department of Pediatrics, University of California, San Diego, La Jolla, CA 92093, USA
[2]Department of Pediatrics, Stanford University School of Medicine, Stanford, CA, USA
*A manuscript describing this series of patients at a somewhat earlier time has been accepted for publication in *Pediatric Nephrology*

with a protocol involving intravenous infusions of high doses of MP, often in association with oral alkylating agents. Results of this treatment on the first seven patients have been described [10]. We now report the outcome of the first 23 patients treated with this protocol and followed for 55 ± 6 months.

Methods

Each of the patients included in this report presented with the nephrotic syndrome. The patients remained nephrotic after 4–8 weeks of treatment with oral prednisone at a dose of 2 mg/kg per day. Because of the steroid-resistance, a renal biopsy was done on each patient and was read as focal segmental glomerulosclerosis. The patients were 7.6 ± 0.95 years old at the time of entry into the protocol. Sixteen of the patients were male; seven were female. Eighteen of the children were steroid-resistant at the time of initial presentation (primary steroid-resistance); five initially responded to oral steroids, but were resistant later (secondary steroid-resistance).

Since this is a retrospective study, there were minor differences in the protocol from patient to patient. The protocol which was used most often is shown in Table 1. In some cases, the initial six MP infusions were given while the child was hospitalized. In most cases, all of the infusions were given by a nephrology nurse in an outpatient setting. If the patients either failed to respond to the initial 10 weeks of MP infusions or improved and later relapsed, they were restarted at the beginning of the MP protocol and given an 8–12 week course of therapy with an oral alkylating agent (cyclophosphamide 2 mg/kg per day or chlorambucil 0.2 mg/kg per day). Fifteen patients had at least one course of alkylating agent therapy. Seven patients received more than one course of treatment with alkylating agents. In general, multiple courses of alkylating agent therapy were given when a patient improved with the first course and subsequently relapsed.

The patients were seen frequently while they were receiving MP and/or alkylating agent therapy. In addition to routine clinical evaluation, serum creatinine concentrations and ratios of the concentrations of protein and creatinine in the urine were obtained. The glomerular filtration rate [GFR] was estimated using the height formula [11,12]. An estimated GFR greater than 80 ml/min per 1.73 m² was interpreted as normal. The magnitude of proteinuria was assessed by comparing the urinary concentrations of protein, in mg/dl, and creatinine, in mg/dl [13,14]. A urinary protein/creatinine ratio ≤ 0.20 was considered to be normal; a ratio of 0.21–0.5 was

Table 1. Usual FSGS protocol

Week	Methylprednisolone	Prednisone
1	30 mg/kg every other day X3	None
2	30 mg/kg every other day X3	None
3–10	30 mg/kg weekly	2 mg/kg qod (every other day)
11–18	30 mg/kg every other week	2 mg/kg qod
19–52	30 mg/kg monthly	2 mg/kg qod
53–78	30 mg/kg every other month	2 mg/kg qod

Methylprednisolone is then discontinued and oral prednisone tapered and discontinued

Table 2. Status of FSGS patients after 55 ± 6 months

In remission	13 (56.5%)
Minimal proteinuria	3 (13.1%)
Moderate proteinuria	2 (8.7%)
Nephrotic syndrome	4 (17.4%)
Renal failure	1 (4.4%)

called minimal proteinuria; a ratio of 0.51–2.0 was interpreted as moderate proteinuria; a ratio > 2.0 was seen in children with nephrotic levels of proteinuria. Data are presented as Mean ± SD.

Results

We have treated 23 patients with steroid-resistant nephrotic syndrome and biopsy-proven FSGS with MP infusions. The status of these patients at their most recent follow-up is summarized in Table 2. The mean follow-up is 55 ± 6 months. Twenty-two patients had a normal estimated GFR. One child progressed to end-stage renal failure (ESRD) and subsequently died. Thirteen patients were in complete remission (after 21–100 months). These patients were receiving no treatment when last seen. Three patients had minimally elevated urine protein excretion; 2 had moderately elevated urinary protein excretion without edema; and 4 children continued to have nephrotic levels of proteinuria. Three of these four nephrotic children had a urinary protein excretion at the time of their most recent follow-up which was more than 50% lower than that obtained before starting the MP protocol. The fourth child with persistent nephrotic levels of proteinuria had no change in his urinary protein excretion following MP therapy.

Side effects of the MP therapy have been acceptable to date, although no information is available regarding long-term side effects, such as sterility and oncogenesis. Five patients developed small cataracts which did not interfere with vision while receiving this treatment. In one child, the cataract improved after he went into remission and treatment was discontinued. In most children, growth during MP therapy was similar to the pretreatment growth rate. However, four children had significant growth retardation while receiving frequent MP infusions, alternate day oral prednisone, and several courses of treatment with oral alkylating agents. Eventually, each of these children went into remission. One of these patients subsequently had a period of "catch-up" growth. The other three remain growth-retarded. A number of children reported nausea during the MP infusions. This was particularly common when the interval between infusions was one month or longer. Four patients developed hypertension which required treatment during the MP protocol. The hypertension was easily controlled and resolved as the interval between MP infusions increased. Other complications of high dose steroid therapy such as striae, aseptic necrosis of the femoral head, diabetes, and pancreatitis were not observed.

No major adverse effects of alkylating agent therapy were observed in these patients. Three patients developed transient leukopenia during alkylating agent therapy, which led to an interruption of the treatment. In each case, the course of alkylating agent therapy was completed after the white blood count returned to normal.

Although fatal infections have been reported in patients treated with MP [15], we have not noted an increased incidence of serious infections in the FSGS patients treated with this protocol. Four of these patients had had an episode of bacterial peritonitis or sepsis before starting MP. Two patients had peritonitis while on this treatment. In addition, one patient had herpes zoster and another patient had cellulitis of the leg while receiving MP. Each patient recovered from his/her infection uneventfully.

Discussion

The prognosis of children with FSGS is poor [16]. It is estimated that 10%–20% of children who progress to dialysis or transplantation have FSGS [9]. In fact, FSGS is the most common form of glomerular disease leading to chronic renal failure in children [8]. In addition, there is a significant risk of recurrence of FSGS following renal transplantation [8,9,16].

In some series of children with FSGS, the prognosis of primary steroid-resistant patients and late steroid non-responders was equally poor [2,4]. Other authors have reported that FSGS patients with primary steroid-resistance progress to renal failure faster than late non-responders [5]. Eighteen of our 23 patients had primary steroid-resistance; 5 had secondary steroid-resistance. The numbers are too small to assess possible differences in outcome between primary and secondary steroid-resistant FSGS patients treated in this way.

The effect of alkylating agents in steroid-resistant FSGS is somewhat controversial. Several groups, including the International Study of Kidney Disease in Children, reported that cyclophosphamide does not improve the outcome in steroid-resistant children with FSGS [17,18]. In contrast, it has been reported that many children with FSGS and steroid-resistant nephrotic syndrome have a partial response to cyclophosphamide, which leads to an improved prognosis [19]. Recently, there has been interest in the use of cyclosporine A in the treatment of FSGS. Preliminary results with this agent have been disappointing, although somewhat variable [20–24].

We have reported previously that the initial response to the treatment of steroid-resistant nephrotic syndrome and FSGS with MP infusions appeared to be favorable [10]. Seven patients had been treated; disappearance of edema and improvement in serum and urine chemistries occurred within a short time after beginning MP therapy.

After a follow-up period of 55 ± 6 months, 56.5% of our 23 patients are in complete remission, 13.1% have minimal proteinuria, 8.7% have moderate proteinuria with no edema or hypoproteinemia, 17.4% remain nephrotic, and only one child [4.4%] developed ESRD. In Table 3, the outcome of our prednisone-resistant patients is compared with the outcome in other series of children with FSGS; series which include both prednisone-responsive and prednisone-resistant patients. Our patients had a strikingly lower incidence of ESRD and a markedly higher incidence of remission of their renal disease.

Side effects of the MP therapy have not been severe. We have not seen cardiac arrhythmias following MP infusions, but these have been reported by others [25,26]. We have seen a mild anaphylactoid reaction to MP [27] in a patient receiving the drug for a different reason, and we are aware of one child with FSGS who had an allergic reaction to intravenous MP (N.J. Siegel, personal communication).

Table 3. Outcome of FSGS in children in current and previous series

Series	No. patients	Follow-up (months)	ESRD or death	Remission
Habib [1]	64	61	31.2%	20.3%
Ito [28]	27	73	29.6%	N.S.
Arbus [4]	32	56	53.1%	N.S.
SPNSG [2]	75	57	21.0%	11.0%
Tejani [5]	24	114	62.5%	N.S.
Ellis [29]	32	62	37.5%	18.8%
Cameron [6]	12	N.S.	75.0%	0
Current series	23	55	4.4%	56.5%

N.S., Not stated in the manuscript; SPNSG, Southwest Pediatric Nephrology Study Group

In conclusion, this group of children with FSGS has done remarkably well following treatment with intravenous MP. The outcome of the patients in this study appears to be better than the outcome in each series of children with steroid-resistant nephrotic syndrome and FSGS of which we are aware. The authors are organizing a multi-center, randomized, controlled clinical trial of this protocol.

References

1. Habib R (1973) Focal glomerular sclerosis. Kidney Int 4:355–361
2. Southwest Pediatric Nephrology Study Group (1985) Focal segmental glomerulosclerosis in children with idiopathic nephrotic syndrome. A report of the Southwest Pediatric Nephrology Study Group. Kidney Int 27:442–449
3. Kohaut EC, Singer DB, Hill LL (1976) The significance of focal glomerular sclerosis in children who have nephrotic syndrome. Am J Clin Pathol 66:545–550
4. Arbus GS, Poucell S, Bacheyie GS, Bauman R (1982) Focal segmental glomerulosclerosis with idiopathic nephrotic syndrome: Three types of clinical response. J Pediatr 101: 40–45
5. Tejani A, Nicastri AD, Sen D, Chen CK, Phadke K, Adamson O, Butt KM (1983) Long-term evaluation of children with nephrotic syndrome and focal segmental glomerular sclerosis. Nephron 35:225–231
6. Cameron JS, Turner DR, Ogg CS, Chantler C, Williams DG (1978) The long-term prognosis of patients with focal segmental glomerulosclerosis. Clin Nephrol 10:213–218
7. Halevy J, Hayslett JP (1986) Clinical features and course of focal glomerulosclerosis. In: Mitch WE, Brenner BM, Stein JH (eds) The progressive nature of renal disease. Churchill Livingstone, New York, pp 189–201
8. Fine R (1987) Renal transplantation in children. Nephron 47:81–86
9. Broyer M, Gagnadoux MF, Guest G, Beurton D, Niaudet P, Habib R, Busson M (1987) Kidney transplantation in children: results of 383 grafts performed at Enfants Malades Hospital from 1973 to 1984. Adv Nephrol 16:307–333
10. Griswold WR, Tune BM, Reznik VM, Vazquez M, Prime DJ, Brock P, Mendoza SA (1987) Treatment of childhood prednisone-resistant nephrotic syndrome and focal segmental glomerulosclerosis with intravenous methylprednisolone and oral alkylating agents. Nephron 46:73–77
11. Schwartz GJ, Haycock GB, Edelmann CM Jr, Spitzer A (1976) A simple estimate of glomerular filtration rate in children derived from body length and plasma creatinine. Pediatrics 58:259–63

12. Schwartz GJ, Feld LG, Langford DJ (1984) A simple estimate of glomerular filtration rate in full-term infants during the first year of life. J Pediatr 104:849–854
13. Houser M (1984) Assessment of proteinuria using random urine samples. J Pediatr 104:845–849
14. Ginsberg JM, Chang BS, Matarese RA, Garella S (1983) Use of single voided urine samples to estimate quantitative proteinuria. New Engl J Med 309:1543–1546
15. Kozeny G, Quinn J, Bansal V, Vertuno L, Hano E (1987) Pneumocystis carinii pneumonia: a lethal complication of "pulse" methylprednisolone therapy. Int J Artif Organs 10(5):304–306
16. Sheldon CA, McLorie GA, Churchill BM (1987) Renal transplantation in children. Pediatr Clin North Am 34:1209–1232
17. International Study of Kidney Disease in Children (1982) Cyclophosphamide therapy in focal segmental glomerular sclerosis: A controlled clinical trial. Pediatr Res 16:320A
18. Mongeau J-G, Corneille L, Robitaille P, O'Regan S, Pelletier M (1981) Primary nephrosis in childhood associated with focal glomerular sclerosis: Is long-term prognosis that severe? Kidney Int 20:743–746
19. Geary DF, Farine M, Thorner P, Baumal R (1984) Response to cyclophosphamide in steroid-resistant focal segmental glomerulosclerosis: a reappraisal. Clin Nephrol 22:109–113
20. Trompeter RS (1987) Steroid resistant nephrotic syndrome: A review of the treatment of focal segmental glomerulosclerosis (FSGS) in children. In: Murakami K, Kitagawa T, Yabuta K, Sakai T (eds) Recent advances in pediatric nephrology. Elsevier Science, Amsterdam, pp 363–371
21. Tejani A, Butt K, Trachtman H, Suthanthiran M, Rosenthal CJ, Khawar MR (1988) Cyclosporine A induced remission of relapsing nephrotic syndrome in children. Kidney Int 33:729–734
22. Waldo FB, Kohaut EC (1987) Therapy of focal segmental glomerulosclerosis with cyclosporine A. Pediatr Nephrol 1:180–182
23. Niaudet P, Habib R, Tete M-J, Hinglais N, Broyer M (1987) Cyclosporin in the treatment of idiopathic nephrotic syndrome in children. Pediatr Nephrol 1:566–573
24. Brodehl J, Hoyer PF, Oemar BS, Helmchen U, Wonigeit K (1988) Cyclosporine treatment of nephrotic syndrome in children. Transplant Proc 20:269–274
25. Ueda N, Yoshikawa T, Chihara M, Kawaguchi S, Niinomi Y, Yasaki T (1988) Atrial fibrillation following methylprednisolone pulse therapy. Pediatr Nephrol 2:29–31
26. Bocanegra TS, Castaneda MO, Espinoza LR, Vasey FB, Germain BF (1981) Sudden death after methylprednisolone pulse therapy. Ann Intern Med 95:122
27. Preuss L (1985) Allergic reactions to systemic glucocorticoids: A review. Ann Allergy 55:772–775
28. Ito H, Yoshikawa N, Aozai F, Hazikano H, Sakaguchi H, Akamatsu R, Matsuo T, Matsuyama S (1984) Twenty-seven children with focal segmental glomerulosclerosis: Correlation between the segmental location of the glomerular lesions and prognosis. Clin Nephrol 22:9–14
29. Ellis D, Kapur S, Antonovych TT, Salcedo JR, Yunis EJ (1978) Focal glomerulosclerosis in children: Correlation of histology with prognosis. J Pediatr 93:762–768

Ca, Pi, PTH, and Vitamin D

Chair: Keith A. Hruska (USA)
Mordecai M. Popovtzer (Israel)

Towards Structural Identification of the Na$^+$/P$_i$-Cotransport System

HEINI MURER, ANDREAS WERNER, FRANÇOIS WUARIN,
STEPHAN J. RESHKIN, AND JÜRG BIBER[1]

SUMMARY. During the last several years different strategies have been developed for a structural identification of the renal proximal tubular Na$^+$/P$_i$-cotransport system. Such approaches can be related to the use of either "specific" (e.g., competitive) or "unspecific" inhibitors (e.g., amino-acid group-specific reagents) in combination with substrate protection and to labeling via specific cellular regulatory pathway (e.g., protein-phosphorylation or protein-turnover). As an additional strategy, expression cloning may be used for structural identification of Na$^+$/P$_i$-cotransport. Finally, the "functional" apparent molecular mass of the protein-complex(es) involved in Na$^+$/P$_i$-cotransport can be determined by radiation inactivation (target size) analysis.

Introduction

Renal proximal tubular phosphate reabsorption is under the control of a variety of hormonal and non-hormonal factors; the regulatory mechanisms seem, ultimately, to affect an apically located Na$^+$/P$_i$-cotransport system (for review see: [1–5]). Inhibition by parathyroid hormone (PTH) is the best studied example of hormonal control mechanisms; increases in Na$^+$/P$_i$-cotransport activity in response to low phosphate intake or to an increased phosphate demand may be examples of "non-hormonal" control mechanisms [1–5]. Over the years, rather specific regulatory cascades have been postulated to be involved, e.g., in PTH-dependent control (i.e., phosphorylation mechanisms) or in adaptive control (de novo synthesis or change in membrane fluidity) of Na$^+$/P$_i$-cotransport. Obviously, without structural identification of the Na$^+$/P$_i$-cotransport system, a detailed study of specific cellular mechanisms involved in the regulation of Na$^+$/P$_i$-cotransport is rather difficult and would provide only a working hypothesis which would remain to be proven.

---

[1]Department of Physiology, University of Zürich, Winterthurerstrasse 190, CH - 8057 Zürich, Switzerland

In this report we will briefly summarize present "knowledge" of the structural identity of the Na$^+$/P$_i$-cotransport system. Several very different approaches will be discussed, for which detailed descriptions of the methods will be not be included; the reader is referred to the original literature.

Experiments Involving Reconstitution and/or Measurements of Phosphate-Binding/Transport

Solubilization of brush border membrane proteins and protein separation followed by reconstitution into artificial lipid bilayers provided some evidence for a hydrophobic peptide ("phosphorin") which showed P$_i$-transport properties [6–9]; however, these activities were not Na$^+$-dependent processes [9], i.e., a participation in Na$^+$/P$_i$-cotransport was not documented. Similar phenomena were also reported for a protein of 155 kDa molecular weight, which under denaturing conditions shows a molecular weight of 70 kDa. P$_i$-binding to this protein was saturable (K$_D$ = 10 μM) as was Na$^+$-binding (K$_D$ = 7.5 mM); however, an effect of Na$^+$ on P$_i$-binding was not shown [10]. In all of the above-mentioned studies the basic function, i.e., N$^+$-gradient-dependent transport of P$_i$, was not documented; except for the observation, in a report by Kinne and Faust [11], of a small effect of a Na$^+$-gradient on P$_i$-uptake into liposomes which had been reconstituted from solubilized unfractionated brush border membrane protein and lipids isolated from renal cortex.

Experiments Using "Specific" or "Unspecific" Inhibitors

Phosphonoformic acid (PFA) is a competitive ("specific") inhibitor of Na$^+$/P$_i$-cotransport (e.g., [12]); this fact could offer the possibility of identifying the transporter in purification/separation experiments, as well as in affinity labeling/purification experiments [13,14]. However, until now this approach has not yet provided information on the molecular identity of the Na$^+$/P$_i$-cotransport system. We would like to add here some potential problems which could occur in the use of PFA as a ligand in experiments aiming to purify Na$^+$/P$_i$-cotransport: 1] the amount of "specific" Na$^+$-dependent, P$_i$-protectable PFA-binding is rather high and simple calculations assuming a molecular weight of 50–100 kDa (see below) for the Na$^+$/P$_i$-cotransport system would suggest that a rather high percentage of total brush border membrane protein is related to this transport activity; 2] recently it was shown that sulfate and phosphate interact with the same PFA-binding sites, documenting a lack of specificity of PFA-binding [15]. Furthermore, PFA also inhibits Na$^+$-dependent sulfate transport in brush border membrane vesicles [15].

As "unspecific" inhibitors, two amino acid group-specific reagents were used. Phenylglyoxal has been used to inhibit renal Na$^+$/P$_i$-cotransport, indicating the involvement of functionally important arginine groups; no attempts using phenylglyoxal for structural identification have been reported [16]. In our laboratory, we have found that N-acetylimidazole was able to inhibit P$_i$-transport via Na$^+$/P$_i$-cotransport in a P$_i$ protectable manner; subsequently it was possible to label membrane proteins by this procedure. It was concluded that proteins of 31, 53, 105, and/or 107 kDa may be important in mediating Na^+/P_i-cotransport across apical membranes of PTH-sensitive renal epithelial cells, i.e., OK cells [17], and rat renal proximal tubular cells (F. Wuarin, J. Biber, and H. Murer, unpublished work).

It should be mentioned that recent work on intestinal Na^+/P_i-cotransport using FITC-labeled phenylglyoxal or N-acetylimidazole provided evidence for an involvement of a 130 kDa protein in transmembrane transport of P_i in small intestine [18]. However, in view of the fundamental differences in kinetic behavior and regulatory control of intestinal vs renal Na^+/P_i-cotransport it cannot, a priori, be assumed that these transport pathways are structurally related [19].

Labeling Via Cellular Regulatory Pathways

In an attempt to identify the Na^+/P_i-cotransport system or proteins involved in its control, experiments on in situ labeling of apical membrane proteins either by PTH-dependent phosphorylation reactions, or on ^{35}S-L-methionine incorporation during phases of protein synthesis-dependent increases in Na^+/P_i-cotransport activity were also performed in OK cells. In the phosphorylation experiment a 105 kDa integral membrane protein turned out to be preferentially marked by high and low PTH concentrations as well as by pharmacological kinase A- and kinase C-activation ([120], SJ Reshkin, F Wuarin, and H Murer, manuscript in preparation). During protein synthesis-dependent increases in Na^+/P_i-cotransport (PTH removal and P_i-deprivation) preferential incorporation of radioactivity occurred in specific integral membrane proteins (J. Biber and H. Murer, manuscript in preparation). Further work on these proteins will determine at which level they are involved in Na^+/P_i-cotransport and/or its regulation.

Identification of Na^+/P_i-Cotransport via Expression Cloning

The only brush border membrane cotransport system which has been structurally identified up to now, the Na^+/D-glucose-cotransport system, was "obtained" by expression cloning using *Xenopus laevis* oocytes as an expression system [21]. In our laboratory we have applied a similar strategy for identification of the Na^+/P_i-cotransport system. A first success was the identification of a mRNA fraction from rabbit kidney cortex and OK cells which led, after injection into oocytes, to an increased Na^+/P_i-cotransport activity with kinetic properties similar to the transport pathway in the brush border membrane [22]. After cDNA-synthesis and insertion into a pBluescript-plasmid we could identify a single clone which, after in vitro mRNA transcription, produced a stimulation of Na^+/P_i-cotransport activity in mRNA-injected *Xenopus laevis* oocytes; the kinetics of expressed transport activity were different from the intrinsic activity of oocytes and similar to that in brush border membrane transport. The deduced amino acid sequence shows 489 amino acid residues and several putative transmembrane spanning regions (A. Werner, J. Biber and H. Murer, manuscript in preparation; M. Moore, N. Mantei, and G. Semenza, manuscript in preparation). On the basis of these results we conclude that we have cloned the renal proximal tubular brush border membrane Na^+/P_i-cotransporter.

Target-Size Analysis Na$^+$/P$_i$-Cotransport

Béliveau and his colleagues have determined the functional molecular weight (target size) of a protein complex apparently involved in Na$^+$/P$_i$-cotransport. Based on radiation inactivation analysis they concluded that a protein complex with an apparent molecular mass of 205 ± 36 kDa was involved in Na$^+$/P$_i$-cotransport [23]. For phosphate-protectable, Na$^+$-dependent PFA-binding the apparent molecular mass was 130 kDa [23]; as indicated above, it is not known at present whether PFA-binding and Na$^+$/P$_i$-cotransport activity are related properties [15].

Recently, a target size analysis of Na$^+$-dependent D-glucose transport has been reported for intestinal [24] and renal brush border membranes [25]; the apparent molecular mass was found to be 290 kDa for Na$^+$-dependent D-glucose transport in both membrane preparations. Taken together with the predicted molecular mass of 73 kDa from the cloning experiments, the suggestion was made that Na$^+$-dependent D-glucose transport operates as a homotetramer [21,24]. By analogy, the predicted molecular mass, around 50–60 kDa obtained for the Na$^+$/P$_i$-cotransport from our cloning experiment (A. Werner, J. Biber and H. Murer, manuscript in preparation; M. Moore, N. Mantei, and G. Semenza, manuscript in preparation), together with the target size of 205 ± 36 kDa [23,25] would suggest that N$^+$/P$_i$-cotransport also functions as a homotetramer.

Conclusions

In recent years renal proximal tubular Na$^+$/P$_i$-cotransport and its regulation based on analysis of function, i.e., transport activity, has been studied extensively. For a more precise analysis of Na$^+$/P$_i$-cotransport activity and its regulation a structural identification of the Na$^+$/P$_i$-cotransport system is mandatory. Different indirect and direct approaches, aiming for such identification, have been developed; none of these strategies have led to identification of the Na$^+$/P$_i$-cotransport system, although candidate-proteins for participation in Na$^+$/P$_i$-cotransport and/or its regulation could be identified. Recent progress in expression cloning has resulted in the identification of a 498 amino acid residue membrane protein which fulfills several criteria of being the renal proximal tubular Na$^+$/P$_i$-cotransport system. Thus, we hope that the availability of probes on the nucleic acid and protein level opens a new area in the study of renal Na$^+$/P$_i$-cotransport and its regulation.

Acknowledgments. The financial support of the Swiss National Science Foundation (Grant No. 3.851.088), the "Stiftung für wissenschaftliche Forschung an der Universität Zürich," the "Hartmann Müller Stiftung," the "Geigy-Jubiläumsstiftung" and the "Sandoz Stiftung" are gratefully acknowledged.

References

1. Biber J (1989) Cellular aspects of proximal tubular phosphate reabsorption. Kidney Int 36:360–369
2. Bonjour JP, Caverzasio J (1984) Phosphate transport in the kidney. Rev Physiol Biochem Pharmacol 100:161–214

3. Dennis VW (to be published) Phosphate homeostasis. In: Windhager EE, Giebisch G (eds) American Physiological Society, Bethesda (Handbook of Physiology)

4. Gmaj P, Murer H (1986) Cellular mechanisms of inorganic phosphate transport in kidney. Physiol Rev 66:36–70

5. Murer H, Biber J (to be published) Renal tubular phosphate transport: Cellular mechanisms. In: Seldin DW, Giebisch G (eds) The kidney. Raven, New York

6. Kessler RJ, Fanestil DD (1981) Identification of a phosphate-binding proteolipid in kidney brush border. In: Bronner F, Peterlik M (eds) Calcium and phosphate transport across biomembranes. Academic, New York, pp 123–126

7. Kessler RJ, Vaughn DA, Fensetil DD (1982) Phosphate-binding proteolipid from brush border. J Biol Chem 257:14311–14317

8. Kessler RJ, Vaughn DA (1984) Divalent metal is required for both phosphate transport and phosphate binding to phosphorin, a proteolipid isolated from brush-border membrane vesicles. J Biol Chem 259:9059–9063

9. Schaeli C, Vaughn DA, Fanestil DD (1986) Reconstitution of the partially purified renal phosphate (P_i) transporter. Biochem J 235:189–197

10. Debiec H, Lorenc R (1988) Identification of Na^+, P_i-binding protein in kidney and intestinal brush-border membranes. Biochem J 225:185–191

11. Kinne R, Faust RG (1977) Incorporation of D-glucose, L-alanine- and phosphate-transport systems from rat renal brush-border membranes into liposomes. Biochem J 168:311–314

12. Szczepanska-Konkel M, Yusufi ANK, Van Scoy M, Webster SK, Dousa TP (1986) Phosphonocarboxylic acids as specific inhibitors of Na^+-dependent transport of phosphate across renal brush border membrane. J Biol Chem 261:6375–6383

13. Lin JT, Dousa TP (to be published) Determination of Na^+-P_i symporters in solubilized renal brush border membranes (BBM) by ^{14}C-phosphonoformic acid (PFA) binding. Kidney Int 37:459

14. McKenna CE, Pham P, Hoppe A, Rassier ME, Dousa TP (to be published) Alpha-halophenyl (phosphonomethyl)-phosphinates as specific inhibitors of Na^+-P_i cotransport across renal BBM. Kidney Int 37:460

15. Tennenhouse HS, Lee J (to be published) Sulfate inhibits ^{14}C-phosphonoformic acid binding to renal brush-border membranes. Am J Physiol

16. Strevey J, Brunette MG, Béliveau R (1984) Effect of arginine modification on kidney brush border membrane transport activity. Biochem J 223:793–802

17. Wuarin F, Wu K, Murer H, Biber J (1989) The Na/P_i cotransporter of OK cells: Reaction and tentative identification with N-acethylimidazole. Biochim Biophys Acta 981:185–192

18. Peerce BE (1989) Identification of the intestinal Na-phosphate cotransporter. Am J Physiol 256:G645–G652

19. Danisi G, Murer H (to be published) Inorganic phosphate absorption in small intestine. In: M Field (ed) American Physiological Society, Bethesda (Handbook of Physiology)

20. Reshkin SJ, Wuarin F, Biber J, Murer H (1990) Parathyroid hormone induced alterations of apical membrane protein content and phosphorylation in opossum kidney cells. J Biol Chem 265:15261–15266

21. Hediger MA, Coady MJ, Ikeda TS, Wright EM (1987) Expression cloning and cDNA sequencing of the Na^+/glucose cotransporter. Nature 330:379–381

22. Werner A, Biber J, Forgo J, Palacin M, Murer H (1990) Expression of renal transport systems for inorganic phosphate and sulphate in *Xenopus laevis* oocytes. J Biol Chem 265:12331–12336

23. Béliveau R, Jette M, Demeule M, Potter M, Lee J, Tennenhouse HS (to be published) Different molecular size for Na^+-dependent phosphonoformic acid binding and phosphate transport in renal brush-border membrane vesicles. Biochim Biophys Acta

24. Stevens BR, Fernandez A, Hirayama B, Wright EM, Dempner ES (1990) Intestinal brush border membrane Na⁺/glucose cotransporter functions in situ as a homotetramer. Proc Natl Acad Sci USA 87:1456–1460
25. Béliveau R, Demeule M, Ibnoul-Khatib H, Bergeron M, Beauregard G, Potier M (1988) Radiation-inactivation studies on brush-border-membrane vesicles. General considerations, and application to the glucose and phosphate carriers. Biochem J 252:807–813

Insulin-Like Growth Factor I (IGF-I), Possible Mediator of the Stimulatory Effects of Growth Hormone on Renal Phosphate Transport and 1,25-Dihydroxyvitamin D3 Production

J. Caverzasio, C. Montessuit, and J.-P. Bonjour[1]

Introduction

Inorganic phosphate (Pi), which is a limiting factor in the stimulation of DNA synthesis by mitogenic agents [1], is an essential determinant of cellular growth and replication. In vivo, the level of extracellular Pi and thereby the amount of Pi available for cellular metabolism and growth, is mainly determined and regulated by the tubular reabsorption of Pi. This process is markedly influenced by the growth rate of the organism [2–4]. Thus, both the tubular reabsorption and the plasma concentration of Pi are maintained at a higher level in young growing, as compared to adult, individuals [2–4]. Likewise, tubular Pi reabsorption is lower in hypophysectomized than in intact counterparts [5]. Studies with brush border membrane vesicles isolated from rat renal cortex indicate that growth-related change in the tubular handling of Pi can be expressed at the level of the luminal membrane of the proximal tubule [6]. The mechanism responsible for this growth related enhancement in the tubular reabsorption of Pi is still not known. Growth hormone (GH) itself has been logically considered as a putative mediator. Indeed, a stimulation of the tubular capacity to reabsorb Pi, as assessed by determining the maximal rate of Pi reabsorption per unit volume of glomerular filtrate (maxTRPi/mlGFR or TmPi/GFR), can be observed both in human subjects and in experimental animals chronically treated with GH (7–9). Increased TmPi/GFR is also found in active acromegaly with excessive secretion of GH [2]. However, in animal experiments acute administration of GH failed for hours to stimulate the renal transport of Pi [10]. This lag time in the renal response suggested [11] that GH-induced stimulation of the tubular transport of Pi could, like other growth-related effects, be mediated by insulin-like growth factor I (IGF-I) [12,13]. Growth hormone can increase the circulating level of IGF-I, probably by enhancing its hepatic production [14]. Besides this classical endocrine pathway,

[1]Division of Clinical Pathophysiology, Department of Medicine, University Hospital of Geneva, CH-1211 Geneva 4, Switzerland

GH enhances the content of IGF-I in various tissues, suggesting the existence of autocrine and/or paracrine mechanisms [15]. Receptors specific for IGF-I have been identified in basolateral membranes of renal proximal tubules [16]. Therefore, change in the plasma level and/or in the renal production of IGF-I could mediate the effect of GH on the tubular transport of Pi. Interestingly, in many growth-related or GH-dependent physiological or pathophysiological conditions, changes in TmPi/GFR are associated with parallel alterations in the plasma level of 1,25-dihydroxyvitamin D3 (1,25(OH)2D3), a hormone implicated in the homeostasis of Pi [17–18]. As mentioned below, the mechanism responsible for this most intriguing parallelism could be IGF-I.

Stimulatory Effect of IGF-I in Vitro on Sodium-Dependent Pi Transport in Cultured Kidney Cells

In a first series of experiments [19] we speculated whether IGF-I could exert a direct effect on renal Pi transport. In order to examine this question we used kidney epithelial cell cultures, which have been shown to be an adequate system for in vitro study of the mechanisms regulating the renal transport of Pi [20–22]. The effect of recombinant IGF-I on Pi transport was studied in cultured opossum kidney (OK) epithelia. The results indicated that IGF-I (5.10^{-10} to 10^{-7} M) induced a dose-related stimulation of the Na-dependent Pi transport (NaPiT). A maximal response was observed at 10^{-7} M (IGF-I 1.64 ± 0.12; vehicle 0.90 ± 0.02 nmol/mg protein per 4 min, $P < 0.001$). Kinetic analysis of the stimulatory effect of IGF-I on NaPiT indicated an increase in Vmax and no change in Km. Insulin also stimulated NaPiT in OK epithelia, but only at concentrations about 2 orders of magnitude higher than IGF-I. The effect of IGF-I on NaPiT was detectable in less than 30 min, with a maximal response occurring after 4–5 h. The effect was selective for NaPiT, since the Na-dependent alanine transport was not affected by IGF-I. Inhibition of protein synthesis by either cycloheximide or cordycepin markedly attenuated the stimulatory effect of IGF-I on NaPiT. Cellular cAMP content was not modified by the growth factor. These results indicated that IGF-I selectively increases NaPiT through a mechanism that appears to involve de novo protein synthesis. These observations suggested that growth and growth hormone related stimulation of renal Pi transport could be mediated by IGF-I [19].

Stimulatory Effect of IGF-I in Vivo on Tubular Pi Transport and on Plasma 1,25(OH)2D3

In a second series of experiment [23], the influence of recombinant human IGF-I on renal Pi transport and on plasma 1,25(OH)2D3 was examined in hypophysectomized (HPX) rats. Infused by miniosmotic pump at a dose of 10 μg/h for 6 days, IGF-I significantly increased max TRPi/mlGRF: IGF-I 3.50 ± 0.16; vehicle 2.78 ± 0.14 μmol/mlGFR, $P < 0.005$. In brush border membrane vesicles isolated from renal cortex of HPX rats, the Na-dependent Pi transport was stimulated by IGF-I. Neither the Na-dependent glucose transport nor that of alanine was affected by the growth factor. Thus, as in OK epithelial culture [19], the in vivo effect of IGF-I on the Pi transport system localized in the luminal membrane of the proximal tubule cannot be ascribed to an unspecific alteration in the driving force generated by the transmembrane sodium gradient [23]. The stimulatory effect of IGF-I on maxTRPi/mlGFR was also expressed in thyroparathyroidectomized (TPTX) HPX rats (IGF-I 5.20 ± 0.29; vehicle 3.88 ± 0.37 µmol/mlGFR, $P < 0.025$). The increase in renal Pi transport was associated with a marked stimulation of plasma 1,25(OH)2D3 (IGF-I 409 ± 23; vehicle 208 ± 22 pmol/l, $P < 0.001$). As previously reported for GH, IGF-I also increased GFR and reduced urinary sodium excretion [23].

Thus, administration of IGF-I to HPX rats mimics the stimulatory effect of GH on maxTRPi/mlGFR and on plasma 1,25(OH)2D3. As described for GH [3], the IGF-I induced change in maxTRPi/mlGFR is mediated by a PTH independent mechanism and is expressed at the level of the luminal membrane of proximal tubules [24]. The fact that IGF-I simultaneously increases renal Pi transport and plasma 1,25(OH)2D3 levels raises the question of whether this peptide hormone might play a key role in Pi homeostasis in physiological and pathological conditions other than those associated with changes in growth and/or circulating GH. Parallel PTH-independent changes in renal Pi reabsorption and in plasma 1,25(OH)2D3 levels have been observed in many experimental and clinical conditions, particularly in relation to alterations in the Pi supply and demand of the organism [17,18,25]. From these results, obtained both in vitro [19] and in vivo [23], it is tempting to speculate that IGF-I, or an homologous protein, might be the common mediator influencing both the renal reabsorption of Pi and the production of 1,25(OH)2D3, which are two essential controlling elements of Pi homeostasis. The question arises as to whether the stimulatory effect of IGF-I on renal Pi transport could be directly mediated by the plasma level elevation of 1,25(OH)2D3. As mentioned in several reviews, a direct physiological role of 1,25(OH)2D3 on the renal transport of Pi has not been established, particularly in vitamin D-repleted animals [25–27]. According to the experimental conditions [25–29], 1,25(OH)2D3 has been shown variously to stimulate or to decrease the renal transport of Pi. Thus the possibility that 1,25(OH)2D3 could contribute to the stimulatory effect of IGF-I on tubular Pi reabsorption appears to be unlikely.

Conclusion

IGF-I stimulates the renal tubular transport of Pi and elevates the plasma level of 1,25(OH)2D3 in hypophysectomized rats. These findings and the results obtained in opossum cultured epithelia suggest that IGF-I mediates the renal effect of GH on tubular Pi transport. Thus, IGF-I might play an important role in the control of Pi economy, particularly in relation to growth.

Acknowledgments. Recent studies quoted in this report [19,23] were supported by the Swiss National Science Foundation (Grant No 3200-025.535) and by Ciba-Geigy, Basel, Switzerland.

References

1. Becker MA, Rozengurt E (1982) Inorganic phosphate is necessary for the stimulation of DNA synthesis in Swiss 3T3 cells by pure mitogenic agents. Exp Cell Res 139:431–436
2. Corvilain J, Abramow M (1972) Growth and renal control of plasma phosphate. J Clin Endocrinol Metab 34:452–459
3. Caverzasio J, Bonjour JP, Fleisch H (1982) Tubular handling of Pi in young growing and adult rats. Am J Physiol 242:F705–F710
4. Kiebzak, GM, Sacktor B (1986) Effect of age on renal conservation of phosphate in the rat. Am J Physiol 251:F399–F407
5. Caverzasio J, Faundez R, Fleisch H, Bonjour JP (1981) Tubular adaptation to Pi restriction in hypophysectomized rats. Pflugers Arch 392:17–21
6. Caverzasio J, Murer H, Fleisch H, Bonjour JP (1982) Phosphate transport in brush border membrane vesicles isolated from renal cortex in young growing and adult rats, comparison with whole kidney data. Pflugers Arch 394:217–221
7. Corvilain J, Abramow M (1962) Some effects of human growth hormone on renal hemodynamics and tubular Pi transport in man. J Clin Invest 41:1230–1235
8. Corvilain J, Abramow M (1964) Effect of growth hormone on tubular transport of Pi in normal and parathyroidectomized dogs. J Clin Invest 43:1608–1612
9. Hammerman MR, Karl IE, Hruska KA (1980) Regulation of canine renal vesicle Pi transport by growth hormone and parathyroid hormone. Biochim. Biophys. Acta 603:322–335
10. Westby GR, Goldfarb S, Goldberg M, Agus ZS (1977) Acute effects of bovine growth hormone on renal calcium and phosphate excretion. Metabolism 26:525–530
11. Ritz E, Kreusser W, Bommer J (1980) Effects of hormones other than parathyroid hormone on renal handling of phosphate. In: Massry SG, Fleisch H (eds) Renal handling of phosphate. Plenum, New York, pp 137–195
12. Froesch ER, Schmid C, Swander J, Zapf J (1985) Actions of insulin-like growth factors. Annu Rev Physiol 47:443–467
13. Underwood LE, D'Ercole AJ, Clemmons DR, Van Wyk J (1986) Paracrine functions of somatomedins. Clin Endocrinol Metab 15:59–77
14. Schalch DS, Heinrich UE, Draznin B, Johnson CJ, Miller LL (1979) Role of the liver in regulatory somatomedin activity: hormonal effects on the synthesis and release of insulin-like growth factor and its carrier protein by the isolated perfused rat liver. Endocrinology 104:1143–1151
15. D'Ercole AJ, Stiles AD, Underwood LE (1984) Tissue concentrations of somatomedin C: further evidence for multiple sites of synthesis and paracrine or autocrine mechanisms of action. Proc Natl Acad Sci USA 81:935–939
16. Hammerman MR, Gavin III JR (1986) Binding of IGF-I and IGF-I stimulated phosphorylation in canine renal basolateral membranes. Am J Physiol 251:E32–E41
17. Bonjour JP, Caverzasio J, Mühlbauer R, Trechsel U, Troehler U (1982) Are 1,25(OH)2D3 production and tubular phosphate transport regulated by one common mechanism which would be defective in X-linked hypophosphatemia rickets? In: Vitamin D, chemical, biochemical and clinical endocrinology of calcium metabolism. Walter de Gruyter, Berlin, pp 427–433
18. Lyles KW, Hasley DL, Friedman NE, Lobaugh B (1988) Correlations of serum concentrations of 1,25-dihydroxyvitamin D, phosphorus and parathyroid hormone in tumoral calcinosis. J Clin Endocrinol Metab 67:88–92
19. Caverzasio J, Bonjour JP (1989) Insulin-like growth factor I stimulates Na-dependent Pi transport in cultured kidney cells. Am J Physiol 257:F712–F717
20. Caverzasio J, Brown CDA, Biber J, Bonjour JP, Murer H (1985) Adaptation of phosphate transport in phosphate deprived LLC-PK1 cells. Am J Physiol 248:F122–F127

21. Caverzasio J, Rizzoli R, Bonjour JP (1986) Sodium-dependent phosphate transport inhibited by parathyroid hormone and cyclic AMP production in opossum kidney cell line. J Biol Chem 261:3233–3237
22. Malmström K, Murer H (1986) Parathyroid hormone inhibits phosphate transport in OK cells but not in LLC-PK1 and JTC-12P3 cells. Am J Physiol 251:C23–C31
23. Caverzasio J, Montessuit C, Bonjour JP (1990) Stimulatory effect of insulin-like growth factor-I on renal Pi transport and plasma 1,25-dihydroxyvitamin D3. Endocrinology 127:453–459
24. Hammerman MR, Karl IE, Hruska KA (1980) Regulation of canine renal vesicle Pi transport by growth hormone and parathyroid hormone. Biochim. Biophys. Acta 603:322–335
25. Bonjour JP, Caverzasio J (1984) Phosphate transport in the kidney. Rev Physiol Biochem Pharmacol 100:162–164
26. Knox FG, Haramati A (1984) Renal regulation of phosphate excretion. In: Seldin DW, Giebisch G (eds) Physiology and pathology of electrolyte metabolism. Raven, New York
27. Avioli LV (1980) Effects of vitamin D and its metabolites on renal handling of phosphate. In: Massry SG, Fleisch H (eds) Renal handling of phosphate. Plenum, New York, pp 197–207
28. Liang CI, Barnes J, Balakir R, Cheng L, Sacktor B (1982) In vitro stimulation of phosphate uptake in isolated chick renal cells by 1,25-dihydroxycholecalciferol. Proc Natl Acad Sci USA 79:3532–3536
29. Kurnik BRC, Hruska KA (1984) Effects of 1,25-dihydroxycholecalciferol on phosphate transport in vitamin D-deprived rats. Am J Physiol 247:F177–F182

Parathyroid Hormone Receptor Coupling to Phospholipase C is an Alternate Pathway of Signal Transduction in the Bone and Kidney

Keith Hruska, Robert Dunlay, Roberto Civitelli,
Akimitsu Miyauchi, Constanta Victoriea Dobre, and Ajay Gupta[1]

SUMMARY. The parathyroid hormone (PTH) receptor is coupled via guanine nucleo-tide-binding regulatory proteins (G proteins) to adenylate cyclase and phospholipase C (PLC). Activation of PLC with the subsequent hydrolysis of phosphatidylinositol 4,5-bisphosphate produces inositol 1,4,5-trisphosphate (IP_3) and diacylglycerol (DAG). Generation of IP_3 leads to the release of intracellular calcium stores, which produce an increase in the intracellular calcium concentration. DAG activates protein kinase C (PKC). Both IP_3 metabolites and PKC play roles in returning the intracellu-lar calcium concentration back to base line, by sequestering calcium within intracel-lular organelles and by stimulating the movement of calcium from the intracellular to the extracellular compartment. PKC appears to be important in the development of desensitization and down-regulation of the PTH receptor to PTH. Activation of PLC may be important in modulating the well-known effects of PTH on bone and kidney, and also less well-known actions, such as the role of PTH as an osteoblast and chondrocyte growth factor.

Introduction

Parathyroid hormone (PTH) is responsible for maintenance of calcium homeostasis and normocalcemia. Secretion of PTH is stimulated or suppressed by perturbations in the serum calcium level. The calciotropic effects of PTH are mediated primarily by the kidneys, where calcium resorption and phosphate excretion are increased, and by bone, where PTH-stimulated resorption releases calcium to the extracellular fluid.

Binding of PTH to its receptors on the plasma membranes of target cells leads to guanine nucleotide binding protein (G protein) regulated enhancement of enzyme activities which, in turn, generates second messengers that regulate cellular func-tions. Among the enzymes activated by PTH-receptor binding is adenylate cyclase.

[1]Department of Medicine (Nephrology), Jewish Hospital/Washington University, St. Louis, MO 63110, USA

1499

The result is an increase in the intracellular concentration of 3'5' cyclic adenosine monophosphate (cAMP), the classic second messenger for PTH. The final step in this sequence of events is phosphorylation of regulatory proteins by cAMP dependent protein kinases [1,2].

Recently, new mechanisms for generation of intracellular signals by the PTH-receptor have been identified. The best documentation of these is PTH activation of phospholipase C activity. In this report we will discuss our data regarding PTH mediated formation of second messengers by polyphosphoinositide hydrolysis; the possible role of G proteins in regulating this reaction; and the biologic effects of activating this system. Although PTH effects have been described in many organs, we will concentrate on its principal target tissues – bone and kidney.

Polyphosphoinositides and G Proteins

Phosphatidylinositol (PI) is formed in the plasma membrane from phosphatidic acid (PA) and inositol (Fig. 1). Stimulated by phosphatidylinositol kinase, PI then undergoes sequential phosphorylation to form phosphatidylinositol 4,5 bisphosphate (PIP$_2$). Initiation of signal transduction through the phospholipase C (PLC) system begins with agonist binding to its receptor, which, through a G protein (Gp), activates phospholipase C and leads to the hydrolysis of PIP$_2$. PIP$_2$ hydrolysis results in production of inositol 1,4,5 triphosphate (IP$_3$) and diacylglycerol (DAG). IP$_3$ acts through a specific receptor on the endoplasmic reticulum or calcisome, leading to opening of a Ca^{2+} channel and release of calcium stores – the phase I response. This produces an immediate and transient elevation of cytosolic Ca^{2+} ([Ca^{2+}]$_i$) which can be observed in the absence of extracellular Ca^{2+} [3,4]. Phosphorylation of the 4 and 5 positions of inositol is necessary for the interaction of IP$_3$ with the Ca^{2+} channel and the immediate production of a calcium transient [5]. The increase in [Ca^{2+}]$_i$ activates calmodulin-dependent protein kinases [6]. The [Ca^{2+}]$_i$ is rapidly lowered by calcium \ magnesium adenosine triphosphatases (Ca \ Mg \ ATPase), Ca^{2+} pumps which serve to transport Ca^{2+} uphill from the cytosol to the extracellular fluid and into the endoplasmic reticulum [7]. IP$_3$ disappears rapidly with a t^1/$_2$ of about four seconds; at least two relevant metabolism routes are available. First, IP$_3$ can undergo sequential dephosphorylation [8] to IP, and finally, to inositol, which may be recycled into PI. Alternatively [9], IP$_3$ can be phosphorylated to an intermediate compound, inositol 1,3,4,5 tetrakisphosphate (I 1,3,4,5 P$_4$), which then undergoes dephosphorylation to form inositol 1,3,4 trisphosphate (I 1,3,4 P$_3$). Both I 1,3,4,5 P$_4$ and I 1,3,4 P$_3$ may function as messengers in Ca^{2+} entry and Ca^{2+} release (see below). Note that in either degradation route the first dephosphorylation involves removal of a phosphate from either the 4 or 5 position. This precludes further stimulation of the endoplasmic reticulum receptor mediating the phase I response.

DAG remains within the plane of the plasma membrane, where it activates protein kinase C (PKC), which is translocated from the cytosol to the plasma membrane as a result of the increase in [Ca^{2+}]$_i$ during phase I [10]. In addition to DAG and calcium, PKC activity also requires the presence of phosphatidylserine. Characterization of the functions of PKC has been facilitated by the use of phorbol esters, which activate the enzyme in the presence of calcium. PKC phosphorylates various target proteins, including receptors, and also provides negative feedback to the polyphos-

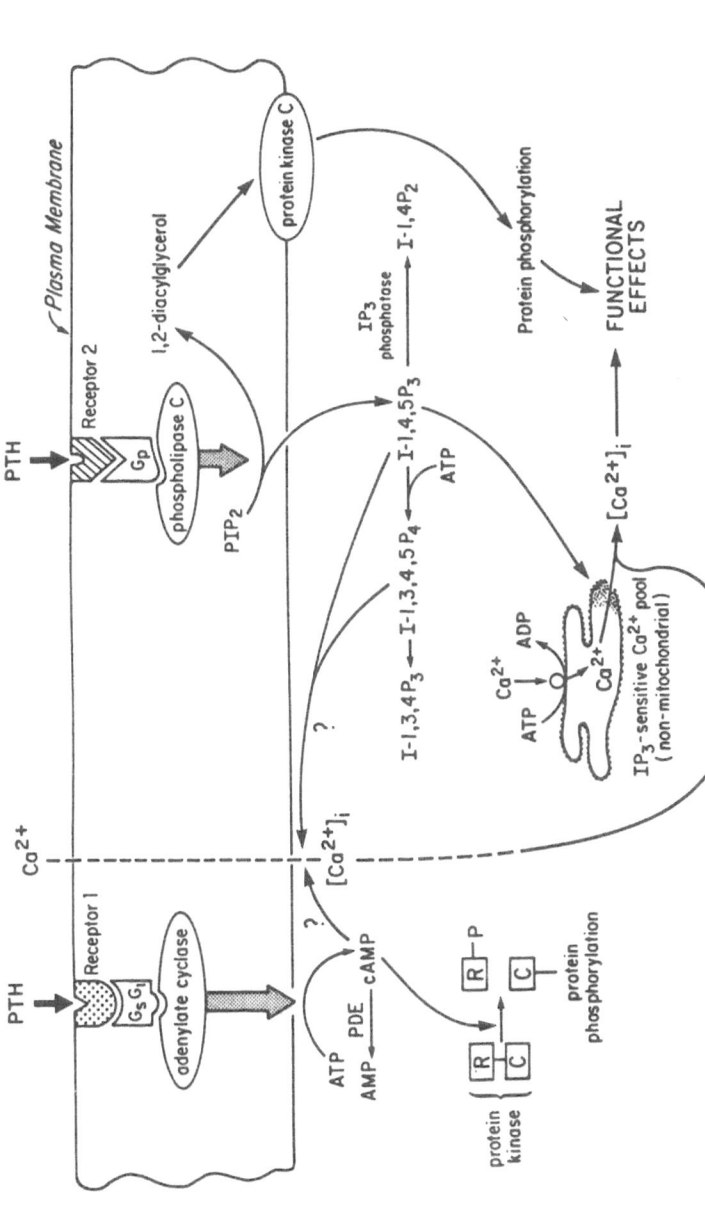

Fig. 1. Schematic concepts of parathyroid stimulated signal transduction in target cells based on a two receptor model (reproduced with permission from Dunlay and Hruska AJP 258:F223, 1990)

phoinositide cascade by phosphorylation of PLC, thus inhibiting the hydrolysis of PIP_2 [11]. Stimulation of PKC with phorbol esters increases the formation of PIP_2, as well as that of PA [12,13]. PKC also acts to decrease the elevated $[Ca^{2+}]_i$ found during the primary response by accelerating the exit of calcium across the plasma membrane [14].

During phase II, enhanced entry of calcium from the extracellular fluid replenishes intracellular calcium stores. I 1,3,4,5 P_4, as well as I 1,3,4 P_3, has been reported to facilitate this process [15]. A model proposed by Putney [16] requires no mediator; he suggests that depletion of calcium from the endoplasmic reticulum adjacent to the plasma membrane leads to calcium entry from the extracellular fluid without any change in the overall $[Ca^{2+}]_i$. Ongoing investigations should soon provide a better understanding of the phase II response.

G proteins are heterotrimers first described in association with receptors coupled to adenylate cyclase. They were initially characterized as either cholera (G stimulatory, Gs) or pertussis (G inhibitory, Gi) toxin sensitive [17]. The alpha subunit (M_r 39-52000) confers specificity for receptors and effectors. Upon receptor occupancy, the alpha subunit releases GDP, binds GTP, and dissociates from the beta and gamma subunits. The alpha subunit possesses intrinsic GTP hydrolytic activity, and interacts with its target effector protein until GTP is hydrolyzed to GDP; then, the heterotrimer reassembles. The G protein associated with PLC (Gp) is pertussis toxin sensitive in some, but not all, cells [6,18]. Gp appears to enhance PLC activity, but the exact mechanism by which this enhancement occurs is uncertain. The recent demonstration by Mattera et al. [19] that alpha subunits stimulatory for adenylate cyclase can also activate voltage regulated calcium channels has added greater complexity to the area of G protein regulation, as previously an alpha subunit had been thought to interact with only one effector protein. In recent years, several low molecular weight G proteins have been described, and their role requires further elucidation. We (Gupta and Hruska, submitted) have recently demonstrated several low molecular weight GTP-binding proteins in the microsomes of the proximal tubule. Their molecular weights range between 21 and 29 × 10^3 daltons. One is a botulinum toxin substrate, possibly rho and another is a ral. We are testing the hypothesis that PTH may stimulate binding of one of these low molecular weight G proteins to the PTH receptor, thus serving to amplify the number of potential signals emanating from a receptor class.

The Kidney

Parathyroid hormone increases turnover of phosphatidylinositol and the poly-phosphoinositides, PIP and PIP_2 [20,21]. The effect is also associated with increased turnover of diacylglycerol and phosphatidic acid, indicating that the Pi cycle has been activated. The stimulus begins with hydrolysis of PIP_2, which is detectable within seconds and maximal by 10 seconds [12]. The effect of PTH to reduce PIP_2 levels is overcome by phosphorylation of PI and PIP within 5 minutes. The product of PIP_2 hydrolysis, inositol 1,4,5 trisphosphate (IP_3) is detectably increased by 5–10 seconds of stimulation by parathyroid hormone (Fig. 2) [12]. IP_3 is rapidly phosphorylated to IP_4, which is then acted upon by a phosphatase to produce I 1,3,4 P_3. The production of I 1,3,4 P_3 accounts for the sustained elevation in IP_3 levels for several minutes after PTH stimulation. These actions of parathyroid hormone have

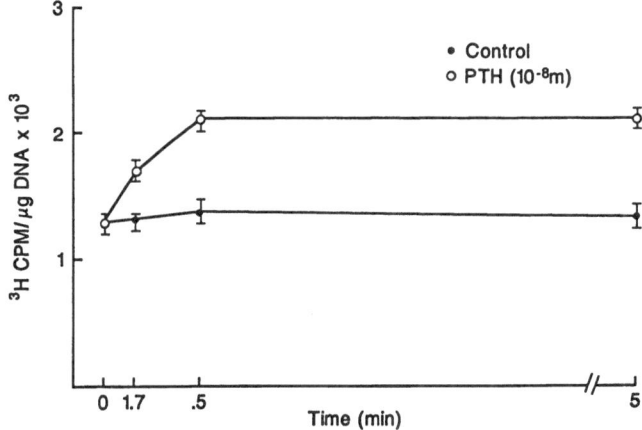

Fig. 2. Effect of parathyroid hormone on IP_3 production in opossum kidney (*OK*) cells. The initial effect represents an increase in I 1,4,5 P_3 which subsides within 1 min. The sustained elevation is due to I 1,3,4 P_3 which is produced by phosphatase activity on I 1,3,4,5 P_4 which is, in turn, a product of I 1,4,5 P_3 phosphorylation. I 1,3,4 P_3 has a longer half life than I 1,4,5 P_3, but its biologic role in the kidney is unclear. CPM, counts per minute

been observed in proximal kidney cells, in the primary cultures of the canine proximal tubule, and in basolateral membranes of the proximal tubular cells isolated from tubular segments in vitro. The dose response curve demonstrates a threshold at 10^{-10} M and a half-maximal effect at 10^{-9} M (Fig. 3).

The increase in IP_3 levels is associated with release of calcium from IP_3-sensitive intracellular stores and with the production of a rapid transient increase in $[Ca^{2+}]_i$. Parathyroid hormone also stimulates calcium entry across the plasma membrane, which contributes to the transient elevation in $[Ca^{2+}]_i$ following hormonal stimulation [22,3,4]. The mechanism of PTH-stimulated calcium entry is independent of the membrane potential and insensitive to Ca^{2+} channel antagonists. Data from isolated membrane vesicles suggest that the parathyroid hormone-stimulated Ca^{2+} entry is related to a receptor-operated Ca^{2+} channel, or is through a second-messenger-operated Ca^{2+} channel stimulated by IP_3 [23,24].

Activation of phospholipase C by parathyroid hormone in the basolateral membrane of the proximal tubule also results in the production of diacylglycerol. Measurement of DAG indicates a difference in the time course of stimulus, compared to IP_3 production. This may suggest that part of the DAG is derived from an effect of parathyroid hormone on phosphatidylcholine-specific phospholipase C, or possibly on phosphatidylethanolamine-specific phospholipase C. These studies will require further analysis. It is also possible that the observed increase in phosphatidic acid is derived from the stimulation of phospholipase D. This also requires further analysis.

The biologic effects of activation of the Ca^{2+} message system in the proximal tubule have been incompletely investigated. We have shown that parathyroid hormone produces dramatic shortening and rarefaction of proximal tubule and microvilli within one minute, with recovery after 5 minutes [25]. The effect of parathyroid hormone on brush border topography was associated with disappearance of micro-

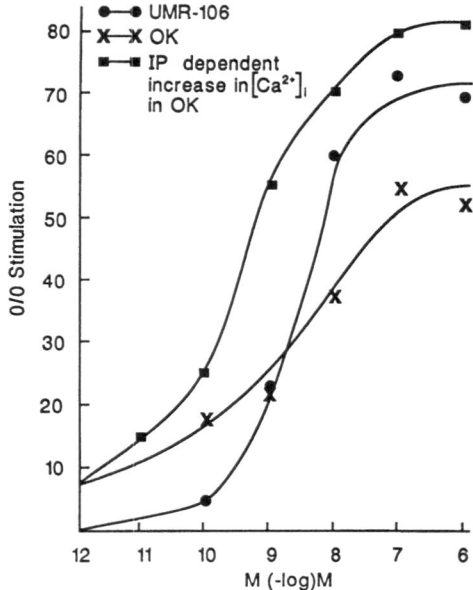

Fig. 3. Dose response of PTH stimulated IP$_3$ production in opossum kidney (*OK*) cells, UMR-106-01 cells, and IP$_3$ dependent stimulation of $[Ca^{2+}]_i$ in OK cells. $[Ca^{2+}]_i$ is a more sensitive measure of PTH stimulation of PLC activity than direct measurement of IP$_3$ production (reprinted with permission from Dunlay and Hruska AJP 258:F223, 1990)

villar core filaments, and it was abolished by a calmodulin inhibitor. Staining F-actin revealed that parathyroid hormone produced fragmentation of stress fibers.

Parathyroid hormone also stimulates proximal tubular gluconeogenesis; this effect is dependent upon $[Ca^{2+}]_i$ and can be stimulated by Ca^{2+} without participation of other second messengers, i.e., cAMP [26]. Stimulation of gluconeogenesis was observed with additions of parathyroid hormone, angiotensin-II and phenylephrine, all of which stimulated Ca^{2+} transients and whose gluconeogenic effect was inhibited by maptam, which prevented the production of the transient elevations in $[Ca^{2+}]_i$. Thus, elevations in $[Ca^{2+}]_i$ were a sufficient stimulus for glucose production and were also necessary for the effects of other second messengers.

The major effect of parathyroid hormone in the proximal tubule is inhibition of Na-dependent phosphate cotransport. The phosphaturic action of PTH is associated with an increase in intracellular cAMP and phosphorylation of proteins in the brush border membrane [2]. Recent studies [27] indicate that activation of protein kinase C may also participate in the inhibition of Na-dependent phosphate cotransport.

When two clones of opossum kidney cells were compared for their response to PTH [28] intriguing results were observed. Both clones (H and P) exhibited similar PTH binding and adenylate cyclase activation. However, the H clone was unresponsive to PTH when analyzed for stimulation of transient elevations in cytosolic calcium. On the other hand, PTH stimulated the P clone cells to produce IP$_3$ and elevate cytosolic calcium. The up-slope of these transient elevations in cytosolic calcium was

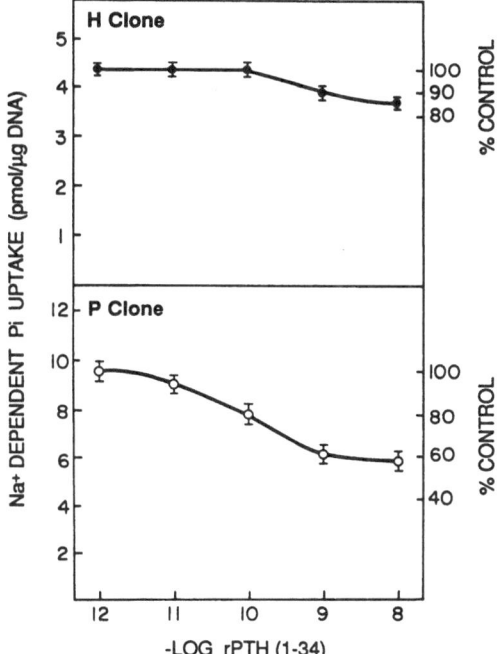

Fig. 4. Effect of PTH on Na⁺-Pi co-transport in OK clones (*OKP* and *OKH*). Experimental conditions: 1.5×10^4 cells/well of 12 well clusters, grown to confluency in DMEM with 7% fetal bovine serum; 72 h on serum-free DMEM; 4 hrs preincubation with rPTH-(1-34). ^{32}P uptake was performed in uptake buffer containing 0.1 mM Pi and 150 mM Na⁺. Means $\pm$ SE of five experiments in triplicate are presented (reprinted with permission from [28])

due in part to inositol trisphosphate-stimulated release of cytosolic calcium (Fig. 3). When sodium-dependent phosphate transport activity was analyzed in these two clones of opossum kidney cells, the H clone was nearly insensitive to the effects of PTH, while the P clone was extremely sensitive [28]. Half-maximal inhibition of phosphate transport was produced by 10^{-10} M PTH in P clone cells, similar to the half-maximal ability of PTH to stimulate increases in cytosolic calcium $(5 \times 10^{-10}$ M). This represents a greater concordance of the dose response curves for a biologic function and second messenger generation for the calcium message system than for stimulation of cAMP production. However, recent studies indicate that threshold levels of cAMP generation may represent sufficient levels to saturate protein kinase A. Nevertheless, in the opossum kidney cells, absence of PTH response to inhibition of phosphate transport was associated with absence of PTH-stimulated phospholipase C activity.

Thus, the mechanism of PTH-generated signal transduction in the renal tubule require further study. It is clear that multiple second messages are generated by the occupancy of the PTH receptor. The exact functional role of these messages should be elucidated in the future.

Bone

We have recently shown that parathyroid hormone increases $[Ca^{2+}]_i$ in a number of osteoblast-like cells, including the UMR-106 cell line, the ROS 17/2.8 cell line, and normal rat and human osteoblasts [29,30]. The effects have been confirmed in several laboratories [31,32]. We have shown that the Ca^{2+} transient stimulated by PTH is, in part, dependent upon Ca^{2+} release of IP_3-sensitive stores, and is, in part, due to both dihydropyridine-sensitive and -insensitive Ca^{2+} entry mechanisms. We have recently demonstrated the presence of L-type Ca^{2+} channels and non-specific stretch-activated cation channels in the plasma membrane of UMR-106 cells, which may be regulated by parathyroid hormone [33].

As expected from the nature of the transient elevation of $[Ca^{2+}]_i$ produced in osteoblast-like cells, we were able to demonstrate that parathyroid hormone elevated IP_3 production in the UMR-106 cells [29]. The effect was associated with increases in inositol 1,4,5 P_3, inositol 1,3,4 P_3, and inositol 1,3,4,5 teterakisphosphate. The effect was dose-dependent with the threshold dose being 10^{-10} M. It was pertussis toxin insensitive, similar to the opossum kidney cell where the PTH effect was also pertussis toxin insensitive [28,29].

In the plasma membrane of the UMR-106, we have characterized a phosphatidyl-inositol-specific phospholipase C activity which is stimulated by guanine nucleotides and is Ca^{2+} independent [34]. The characteristics of this PIP_2-specific phospholipase C suggest that it is the enzyme recoupled to the PTH receptor through G proteins. Recent investigations by Farndale et al. [35] and Babich [23] support these conclusions. Other studies have also indicated that PTH stimulates protein kinase C and its translocation to the plasma membrane [36].

The biologic effects of the parathyroid hormone-stimulated activation of the Ca^{2+}-protein kinase C message system in the regulation of bone remodeling are unclear. Parathyroid hormone induces both bone resorption and bone formation. The initial effect of parathyroid hormone on the osteoblast is to induce cell contraction, and this is likely to involve Ca^{2+} [22]. Parathyroid hormone also decreases osteoblast collagen production and may increase collagenase production. Parathyroid hormone stimulation of collagenase production can be demonstrated in UMR-106 cells, and in these cells, a participation of the Ca^{2+} message system in collagenase production has been demonstrated [37].

Conclusion

The available evidence indicates that the polyphosphoinositide pathway is stimulated in mediating the actions of PTH in both the kidneys and in bone. Many important issues remain, including: 1) characterization of the G protein modulating PLC activation in response to PTH binding to its receptor; 2) the possibility that different subclasses of PTH receptors coupled to different G proteins and effector proteins exist. Alternatively, if only one type of PTH receptor is found, activation of multiple G proteins or association with multiple effector proteins could explain the diverse messages produced by PTH.

Acknowledgments. This work was supported by NIH grants AR39561, AR32087, and DK09976 and a grant from the Shriner's Hospital (St. Louis Division).

References

1. Cochet C, Gill GN, Meisenhelder J, Cooper JA, Hunter T (1984) C-kinase phosphorylates the epidermal growth factor receptor and reduces its epidermal growth factor-stimulated tyrosine protein kinase activity. J Biol Chem 259:2553–2558

2. Hammerman MR, Hruska KA (1982) Cyclic AMP dependent protein phosphorylation in canine renal brush border membrane vesicles is associated with decreased phosphate transport. J Biol Chem 257:992–999

3. Hruska KA, Goligorsky M, Scoble J, Tsutsumi M, Westbrook S, Moskowitz D (1986) The effects of parathyroid hormone on cytosolic calcium in renal proximal tubular primary cultures. Am J Physiol 251:F188–F198

4. Prentki M, Wollheim CB, Lew PD (1984) Calcium homeostasis in permeabilized human neutrophils. J Biol Chem 259:13777–13782

5. Burgess GMK, Irvine RF, Berridge MJ, McKinney JS, Putney JW (1984) Actions of inositol phosphates on Ca pools in guinea-pig hepatocytes. Biochem J 224:741–746

6. Cohen P (1988) Protein phosphorylation and hormone action. Proc R Soc Lond [Biol] 234:115–144

7. Carafoli E (1987) Intracellular calcium homeostasis. Annu Rev Biochem 56:395–433

8. Connoly TM, Bross TE, Majerus PW (1985) Isolation of a phosphomonoesterase from human platelets that specifically hydrolyzes the 5-phosphate of inositol 1,4,5-triphosphate. J Biol Chem 260:7868–7874

9. Irvine RF, Letcher AJ, Heslop JP, Berridge MJ (1986) The inositol tris\tetrakisphosphate pathway-demonstration of Ins 1,4,5 3-kinase activity in animal tissues. Nature 320:631–634

10. Nishizuka Y (1984) The role of protein kinase C in cell surface signal transduction and tumour promotion. Nature 308:693–698

11. Berridge M (1987) Inositol triphosphate and diacylglycerol: Two interacting second messengers. Annu Rev Biochem 56:159–193

12. Hruska KA, Moskowitz D, Esbrit P, Civitelli R, Westbrook S, Huskey M (1987) Stimulation of inositol triphosphate and diacylglycerol production in renal tubular cells by parathyroid hormone. J Clin Invest 79:230–239

13. Taylor MV, Metcalfe JC, Hesketh TR, Smith GA, Moore JP (1984) Mitogens increase phosphorylation of phosphoinositides in thymocytes. Nature 312:462–465

14. Lagast H, Pozzan T, Waldvogel FA, Lew PD (1984) Phorbol myristate acetate stimulates ATP-dependent calcium transport by the plasma membrane of neutrophils. J Clin Invest 73:878–883

15. Irvine RF, Moor RM (1986) Micro-injection of inositol 1,3,4,5 tetrakisphosphate activates sea urchin eggs by a mechanism dependent on external calcium. Biochem J 240:917–920

16. Putney JW (1986) A model for receptor-regulated calcium entry. Cell Calcium 7:1–12

17. Stryer L (1986) G proteins: A family of signal transducers. Annu Rev Cell Biol 2:391–419

18. Fain JN, Wallace MA, Wojcikiewicz RJH (1988) Evidence for involvement of guanine nucleotide binding regulatory proteins in the activation of phospholipase by hormones. FASEB J 2:2569–2574

19. Mattera R, Graziano M, Yatani A, Zhou Z, Graf R, Codina J, Birnbaumer L, Gilman AG, Brown AM (1989) Splice variants of the alpha subunit of the G protein Gs activate both adenylyl cyclase and calcium channels. Science 243:804–807

20. Bidot-Lopez P, Farese R, Sabir M (1981) Parathyroid hormone and adenosine-3′,5′-monophosphate acutely increase phospholipids of the phosphatidate-polyphosphoinositide pathway in rabbit kidney cortex tubules *in vitro* by a cycloheximide-sensitive process. Endocrinology 108:2078–2081

21. Meltzer V, Weinreb S, Bellorin-Font E, Hruska KA (1982) Parathyroid hormone stimulation of renal phosphoinositide metabolism is a cyclic nucleotide independent effect. Biochim Biophys Acta 712:258–267

22. Goligorsky MS, Loftus D, Hruska KA (1986) Cytoplasmic Ca²⁺ in individual proximal tubular cells in culture: effects of parathyroid hormone. Am J Physiol 251:F938–F944
23. Scoble JE, Mills S, Hruska KA (1985) Calcium transport in canine renal basolateral membrane vesicles. J Clin Invest 75:1096–1105
24. Scoble JE, Civitelli R, Hruska KA (1988) Evidence for receptor operated Ca²⁺ chennels in basolateral membranes (BLM) of proximal tubular cells (PTC): Effects of inositol 1,4,5-trisphosphate (IP₃). Kidney Int 33:171A
25. Goligorsky MS, Menton DN, Hruska KA (1986) Parathyroid hormone-induced topography and cytoskeleton in cultured renal proximal tubular cells. J Membr Biol 92:151–162
26. Goligorsky MS, Osborne D, Howard T, Hruska KA, Karl IE (1987) Hormonal regulation of gluconeogenesis in cultured proximal tubular cells: role of cytosolic calcium. Am J Physiol 253:F802–F809
27. Cole JA, Forte LR, Eber S, Thorne PK, Poelling RE (1988) Regulation of sodium-dependent phosphate transport by parathyroid hormone in opossum kidney cells: Adenosine 3′,5′-monophosphate-dependent and -independent mechanisms. Endocrinology 122: 2981–2989
28. Miyauchi A, Dobre V, Rickmeyer M, Cole J, Forte L, Hruska KA (1990) Stimulation of transient elevations in cytosolic Ca²⁺ is related to inhibition of Pi transport in OK cells. Am J Physiol 259:F485–493
29. Civitelli R, Reid IR, Westbrook S, Avioli LV, Hruska KA (1988) PTH elevates inositol polyphosphates and diacylglycerol in a rat osteoblast-like cell line. Am J Physiol 255: E660–E667
30. Reid IR, Civitelli R, Halstead LR, Avioli LV, Hruska KA (1987) Parathyroid hormone acutely elevates intracellular calcium in osteoblastlike cells. Am J Physiol 252:E45–E51
31. Lowik CWGM, van Leeuwen JM, van der Meer JK, van Zeeland BAA, Scheven JPTM, Herrmann-Erlee MPM (1985) A two-receptor model for the action of parathyroid hormone on osteoblasts: a role for intracellular free calcium and cAMP. Cell Calcium 6:311–326
32. Yamaguchi DT, Hahn TJ, Iida-Klein A, Kleeman CR, Muallem S (1987) Parathyroid hormone-activated calcium channels in an osteoblast-like clonal osteosarcoma cell line. J Biol Chem 262:7711–7718
33. Duncan R, Misler S (1989) Voltage-activated and stretch-activated Ba²⁺ conducting channels in an osteoblast-like cell line (UMR 106). Elsevier Sci Pubs 251:17–21
34. Suzuki Y, Hruska KA, Reid I, Alvarez UM, Avioli LV (1989) Characterization of phospholipase C activity of the plasma membrane and cytosol of an osteoblast-like cell line. Am J Med Sci 296:135–144
35. Farndale RW, Sandy JR, Atkinson SJ, Pennington SR, Meghji S, Meikle MC (1988) Parathyroid hormone and prostaglandin E2 stimulate both inositol phosphates and cyclic AMP accumulation in mouse osteoblast cultures. Biochem J 252:263–268
36. Abdul-Badi A, Jueppner H, Westerberg D, Potts JT, Segre GV (1989) Parathyroid hormone causes translocation of protein kinase-C from cytosol to membranes in rat osteosarcoma cells. Endocrinology 124:1107–1113
37. Civitelli R, Hruska KA, Jeffrey JJ, Kahn JJ, Avioli LV, Partridge NC (1989) Second messenger signaling in the regulation of collagenase production by osteogenic sarcoma cells. Endocrinology 124:2928–2933
00. Cockroft S, Stutchfield J (1988) G-proteins, the inositol lipid signalling pathway, and secretion. Philos Trans R Soc Lond [Biol] 320:247–265
00. Babich M, King KL, Nissenson RA (1989) G protein-dependent activation of a phosphoinositide-specific phospholipase C in UMR-106 osteosarcoma cell membranes. J Bone Mineral Res 4:549–556

The Effects of Parathyroid Hormone (PTH) on Ca Transport

YUSUKE TSUKAMOTO[1]

SUMMARY. Parathyroid hormone (PTH) stimulates active Ca^{2+} reabsorption in the distal convoluted tubule of the rat and in the cortical connecting tubule, distal convoluted tubule, and granular portion of the cortical collecting tubule of the rabbit. The dominant mechanism of Ca^{2+} reabsorption in the proximal tubules is passive diffusion via the paracellular pathway and PTH does not stimulate this Ca^{2+} transport. The distal tubules are equipped with molecular mechanisms which favor active transcellular Ca^{2+} transport. $1,25(OH)_2D_3$ dependent calcium binding protein (CaBPr) facilitates Ca^{2+} diffusion in the cytosolic space and increases the supply of the Ca^{2+} pump. PTH regulates the Ca^{2+} pump directly by increasing the affinity for cytosolic Ca^{2+} and by facilitating Ca^{2+} extrusion from the cell. Lack of CaBPr makes the proximal tubule less capable of transcellular Ca^{2+} reabsorption.

Introduction

Parathyroid hormone (PTH) regulates various cellular functions other than Ca^{2+} transport in the kidney [1]. Firstly, PTH reduces the glomerular capillary ultrafiltration coefficient (Kf) and then decreases the glomerular filtration rate (GFR). PTH inhibits the Na/Pi antiporter at the brush-border membrane of proximal tubules and causes phosphaturia. PTH also inhibits the Na/H antiporter in this nephron to cause bicarbonaturia. PTH also alters water transport by acting as a partial agonist to ADH within the papillary collecting duct [2].

Other than participating in mineral transport, PTH also participates in the regulation of metabolism in the kidney. PTH stimulates 1δ-hydroxylation of $25(OH)D_3$ and increases the production of $1,25(OH)_2D_3$ in proximal tubular cells [3]. Gluconeo-

[1]Department of Medicine, Kitasato University School of Medicine, 1-15-1 Kitasato, Sagamihara, Kanagawa, 228 Japan

genesis is also stimulated by PTH in the proximal tubules and this stimulation is mediated by the Ca^{2+} messenger system [4].

These multifunctional aspects of PTH make the study of PTH regulation of renal calcium handling rather difficult. Furthermore, renal calcium transport mechanisms are not yet fully understood, either. A tremendous number of variable factors influence renal Ca^{2+} transport mechanisms. This is the reason why I would like to start this review with renal Ca^{2+} transport mechanisms. I believe this first part of the review makes the interpretation of PTH action on Ca^{2+} transport much easier and more comprehensive.

Calcium Transport Along the Nephron

In the case of interpretation of individual investigations, one should be aware of species difference. Rat and rabbit are frequently employed for this kind of study. In every species, the major part of Ca^{2+} reabsorption by the kidney takes place in the proximal tubules. In this segment, 60% of the filtered Ca^{2+} is reabsorbed. The paracellular permeability of Ca^{2+} in this segment is very high and is similar to the one for Na^+ [5]. Na^+ and water reabsorption through the paracellular pathway give enough energy as a solvent drug to carry a bulk of Ca^{2+} via the paracellular pathway. A Ca^{2+} concentration which is higher in the lumen than in the plasma at the end of rabbit S2 segment, and a positive lumen membrane potential favor the passive paracellular diffusion of Ca^{2+} in this segment. Ng et al. [6] concluded that virtually no portion of Ca^{2+} transport is operated by active transcellular reabsorption in rabbit proximal convoluted tubules. However, this conclusion does not completely agree with the results obtained from rats. Although paracellular passive diffusion accounts for a major portion of Ca^{2+} reabsorption in the rat proximal tubule, the active transcellular pathway accounts for about 25% of total reabsorption [7]. Bomsztyk [8] demonstrated that lumen HCO_3^- stimulates active transcellular Ca^{2+} reabsorption in the absence of net water movement, a process linked to tubule fluid acidification in rat proximal tubules.

In the rabbit straight proximal tubule, 10% of filtered Ca^{2+} is reabsorbed. Rouse et al. [9] showed that Ca^{2+} is actively transported against the electrochemical gradient in this segment. This Ca^{2+} reabsorption was inhibited by cooling and not by oubain, suggesting that the Na^+/Ca^{2+} exchange at the basolateral membrane did not operate this active transport. In contrasts, Sacks and Bourdeau concluded that diffusion is the primary mechanism in this section [10,11]; high transepithelial Ca^{2+} permeability in this segment is compatible with this result.

In the rabbit, Henle's loop, from the thin descending to the thin ascending limb, was found to be relatively impermeable to Ca^{2+} and no significant transport was found [9,12]. Then, beginning from the medullary thick ascending limb, the tubules become very permeable to Ca^{2+}. However, in the thick ascending limb of the rabbit Ca^{2+} transport is heterogenous. In the medullary segment, it is passive and paracellular, inhibited by furosemide [13]. In the cortical segment, however, Ca^{2+} transport appears to be a mixture of both active transcellular and passive paracellular types [13,14]. The passive component of Ca^{2+} transport in cortical thick ascending limb is driven by the lumen-positive transepithelial potential generated by active Cl^- transport [14].

In the distal convoluted tubules of the rat and in the cortical connecting tubule and the granular portion of the cortical collecting tubule of the rabbit, approximately 10% of the filtered Ca^{2+} is reabsorbed. These portions of the nephron, including the cortical thick ascending limb, are believed to be the main regulatory sites of renal Ca^{2+} reabsorption both in rabbit and in rat [15–19]. Ca^{2+} reabsorption in these segments has to be carried out against an electrochemical gradient; apparently the active transcellular pathway is dominant. In the rat, the distal tubule is morphologically heterogeneous. The early distal tubule consists mainly of distal convoluted tubule cells with a few intercalated cells; the late distal tubule consists of intercalated cells, connecting tubule cells, and principal cells [20]. Thiazide diuretics, which are known to be hypocalciuric, act preferentially on early distal tubules [21]. Thiazide inhibits Na^+ reabsorption and increases Ca^{2+} reabsorption in this segment, then dissociation of Ca^{2+} and Na^+ transport occurs. It is known that amiloride, another diuretic known to be an inhibitor of the Na^+/H^+ antiporter and the Na^+/Ca^{2+} exchanger, has an additive hypocalciuric effect on thiazide. However, this action of amiloride has been noted in late distal tubules [21]. This finding suggests that in the distal tubule the Ca^{2+} transport mechanism is heterogeneous; varying in type between the early and late portion or among different cell types. Actually, vitamin D-dependent calcium binding protein (CaBPr) and Ca pump have been located in the principal cells of rat kidney [22].

The last part of the nephron has not been studied extensively. In the light portion of the cortical collecting tubule of the rabbit, epithelial Ca^{2+} permeability is extremely low [19]. In the rat inner medullary collecting duct, Ca^{2+} transport is Na^+-independent and inhibited by verapamil, suggesting voltage-dependent passive diffusion [23].

Effect of PTH on Ca^{2+} Transport Along the Nephron

It is now clear that PTH stimulates active Ca^{2+} reabsorption in the distal nephron. It has been determined that PTH stimulates Ca^{2+} reabsorption in the cortical thick ascending limb [13,14,24] and cortical connecting tubules [24] of the rabbit, and in the distal convoluted tubules of the rat [18]. These are also the nephron segments in which active transport is the dominant mechanism of Ca^{2+} reabsorption. PTH-dependent adenylate cyclase activity is rich in these nephron segments [24] and the stimulation of Ca^{2+} transport is mediated via c-AMP in these segments. The hormonal regulation of Ca^{2+} transport is heterogenous along the thick ascending limb of the rabbit. Suki et al. demonstrated that calcitonin stimulates Ca^{2+} transport in the medullary part, whereas PTH stimulates Ca^{2+} transport in the cortical part of the thick ascending limb [13]. Besides PTH and calcitonin, glucagon has also been reported to stimulate both Ca^{2+} and Mg^{2+} reabsorption in the rat superficial distal convoluted tubule in which glucagon-dependent adenylate cyclase activity is rich [18].

PTH-dependent adenylate cyclase activity also locates in the proximal tubule in both rabbit and rat, although the activity is lower than that in the distal nephron [24]. It is still a matter of controversy whether PTH stimulates Ca^{2+} transport in the proximal tubule. In the 1970s, three studies reported different results of PTH action. Agus et al. [25] and Sutton et al. [26] reported that PTH inhibited both Ca^{2+} and Na^+ reabsorption proportionally in the proximal tubule of both normal and thyroparathyroidectomized (TPTX) dogs. In contrast, micropuncture technique revealed a 10%

increment of Ca^{2+} reabsorption with no augmentation of water movement induced by PTH infusion into the TPTX hamster [27]. In the rabbit, there is virtually no component of active Ca^{2+} transport in proximal convoluted tubule. However, an active transport might be operated to some extent in the rat proximal convoluted tubule. Although PTH could stimulate these active Ca^{2+} transports, it is very hard to determine whether this is true behind the large storm of passive Ca^{2+} flux associated with water and Na^+ reabsorption.

Cellular Mechanism of Renal Ca^{2+} Transport and the Role of PTH

When Ca^{2+} is reabsorbed from the ultrafiltrate to blood through the transcellular pathway, at least 3 modulators must exist. The first one is the barrier in the luminal plasma membrane which controls Ca^{2+} entry into the cell; the second one is the carrier or storage organelles which transfer and store Ca^{2+} in the cytosolic space; the third one is the barrier in the basolateral membrane which controls Ca^{2+} exit from the cell. When Ca^{2+} enters the cell through the luminal membrane, Ca^{2+} can be passively transported according to the favorable electrochemical gradient in both distal and proximal tubules. PTH has been shown to stimulate Ca^{2+} binding to the brush-border membrane, through the phosphorylation of phospholipids via a c-AMP-dependent pathway [28]. This phosphorylation is accompanied by the inhibition of Na^+/Pi cotransport in the proximal tubule [29]. In the distal nephron, the presence of a calcium channel on the luminal membrane has been investigated by using the fluorescent Ca^{2+} indicator, fura-2. In this study, Taniguchi et al. suggested that the voltage-independent calcium channel regulated passive Ca^{2+} entry in the rat cortical collecting tubules [30].

In contrast to its entry on the luminal side, Ca^{2+} must exit from the cell through the basolateral membrane against the electrochemical gradient. Ca^{2+} has to be pumped out by an active transport mechanism at this side of the plasma membrane. Two active transporters are identified in the basolateral membrane; the Na^+/Ca^{2+} exchanger and the ATP-dependent Ca^{2+} pump. Na^+/Ca^{2+} exchange is a secondary active transport, driven by the Na^+ gradient generated by $(Na^+ + K^+)$-ATPase. Recently, Ramachandran and Brunette [31] found that the Na^+/Ca^{2+} exchanger is located exclusively in the distal tubule of the rabbit. This exchanger transports Ca^{2+} very fast, in the order of seconds. This is an electrogenic and voltage-dependent process the same as the one found in excitable tissues [32]. Findings on the affinity that the Na^+/Ca^{2+} exchanger has for Ca^{2+} vary between studies. Jayakumar [33] and Scoble [34] reported 8 µM for rat and 10 µM for dog. This does not agree with the cytosolic Ca^{2+} concentration if this is the system for Ca^{2+} extrusion. In contrast, Van Heeswijk and Van Os reported 0.2 µM for the rat [35]. Although Van Os insisted that the difference in results could be attributed to the difference in Ca^{2+}-buffering systems employed, we also obtained a value similar to that of Jayakumar's study, using the EGTA buffer system which was also employed by van Heeswijk et al. In contrast to the different values found for Ca^{2+} affinity, all studies agree on the value for $[Na^+]_{0.5}$, which is around 15 mM [33]. This value is within the range of cytosolic Na^+ concentration. These studies strongly suggest that the Na^+/Ca^{2+} exchanger operates symmetrically in the kidney in the same way as it does in the heart sarcolemma. The Na^+/Ca^{2+} exchanger may be the system which operates Ca^{2+} entry most of the time.

Even if the Na^+/Ca^{2+} exchanger operates to extrude Ca^{2+} out of the cell, the capacity of this transporter is only 20% that of the ATP-dependent Ca^{2+} pump. This makes us believe that the ATP-dependent Ca^{2+} pump is the main system for the Ca^{2+} exit through the basolateral membrane. In the kidney, the ATP-dependent Ca^{2+} pump was first studied in the basolateral membrane vesicles of rat kidney cortex [36]. For a long time, it has been believed that this preparation of basolateral membrane vesicles originated from the proximal tubules. However, it has been found that the renal cortex contains not only PTH-dependent adenylate cyclase activity, but also ADH-dependent activity which locates only in the distal tubules [33]. Recently, we succeeded in obtaining the basolateral membrane vesicles separately, from proximal tubules and from distal tubules [37]. As a result, ATP-dependent Ca^{2+} pump activity in the tubules can be kinetically separated. The affinity of the Ca^{2+} pump is much higher in the distal tubules ($Ca^{2+} = 44.8$ nM) than in the proximal tubules ($Ca^{2+} = 80.4$ nM). Vmax is higher in the proximal tubules (9.18 nmol $^{45}Ca^{2+}$/min per mg) than in the distal tubules (3.26 nmol $^{45}Ca^{2+}$/min per mg). These Ca^{2+} pumps are apparently stimulated in a different fashion by PTH. Selective parathyroidectomy decreased the Vmax of the Ca^{2+} pump in the proximal tubules while it decreased the affinity of the Ca^{2+} pump in the distal tubules (unpublished data). The kinetic character of the Ca^{2+} pump is very suitable for active Ca^{2+} reabsorption in the distal tubules, because very high Ca^{2+} affinity forces the pump to operate continuously.

The molecular characteristics of the distal tubular cells strongly suggest that this segment is the main site of the regulation of Ca^{2+} transport by active transcellular Ca^{2+} reabsorption. The critical molecular difference between the proximal and distal tubules is that the latter possess $1,25(OH)_2D_3$-dependent CaBPr but the former do not [22]. Bronner [38] postulated that, in the presence of CaBPr, Ca^{2+} can diffuse in the cytosolic space without being trapped by calcium storage organelles at a speed 30 times faster than in the absence of this protein. For effective transcellular Ca^{2+} reabsorption, the Ca^{2+} extrusion pump at the basolateral membrane cannot work efficiently without a continuous supply of the substrate, Ca^{2+}. Kumar found that both the Ca^{2+} pump and CaBPr are located in the same cell, the principal cell of human distal tubules; this finding also supports the cooperative function of these two mechanisms [22]. Proximal tubule lacks this CaBPr, which makes transcellular Ca^{2+} movement least effective and indicates that it cannot be the dominant mechanism of Ca^{2+} reabsorption. Thus, the molecular findings strongly support the physiological findings.

From these results, I would like to propose a molecular mechanism for Ca^{2+} reabsorption and regulation by PTH. This is shown in Fig. 1. In the proximal tubules, most Ca^{2+} reabsorption takes place by a passive diffusion mechanism via the paracellular pathway. Neither PTH nor $1,25(OH)_2D_3$ directly regulates this passive diffusion. However, there is an influence of PTH on the Ca^{2+} flow indirectly, through water movement. In the rat, transcellular active transport also participates in a small proportion of Ca^{2+} reabsorption. There is a possibility that PTH might stimulate this active transport by increasing the Vmax of Ca^{2+} pump activity at the basolateral membrane. However, the capacity of this active transport is much less than the capacity of the active transport in the distal tubules, which possesses CaBPr. The distal tubules definitely have the main role in the regulation of Ca^{2+} reabsorption in the kidney. PTH stimulates 1δ-hydroxylation of $25(OH)D_3$ at the proximal tubules, and then the increased $1,25(OH)_2D_3$ level stimulates CaBPr production in the principal cell of the distal nephron. CaBPr facilitates Ca^{2+} diffusion inside the cell and increases the

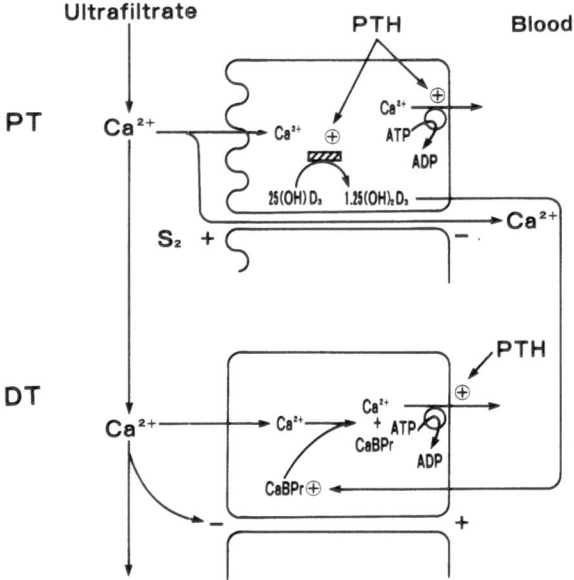

Fig. 1. Hypothesis for the molecular mechanisms of renal Ca²⁺ reabsorption and the effects of PTH

supply of Ca²⁺ to the Ca²⁺ pump. Then, the Ca²⁺ pump, whose affinity is stimulated by PTH, pumps an increased amount of Ca²⁺ out of the cell. Studies of molecular mechanisms support this hypothesis. However, we still lack direct investigation of the sequential movement of Ca²⁺ in native tubular cells, results of which could confirm this hypothesis.

References

1. Sutton RAL, Dirks JH (1986) Calcium and magnesium: Renal handlings and disorders of metabolism. In: Brenner BM, Rector FC Jr (eds) The kidney, 3rd edn. WB Saunders, Philadelphia, pp 551–618
2. Carney SL, Dirks JH (1988) Effect of parathyroid and antidiuretic hormone on water and calcium permeability in the rat collecting duct. Miner Electrolyte Metab 14:142–145
3. Kawashima H, Kurikawa K (1983) Unique hormonal regulation of vitamin D metabolism in the mammalian kidney. Miner Electrolyte Metab 9:227–235
4. Goligorsky MS, Osborne D, Howard T (1987) Hormonal regulation of gluconeogenesis in cultured proximal tubular cells: role of cytosolic calcium. Am J Physiol 253:F802–F809
5. Bomsztyk K, Wright FS (1982) Kidney Int 21:269–275
6. Ng RCK, Rouse D, Suki WN (1984) Calcium transport in the rabbit superficial proximal convoluted tubule. J Clin Invest 74:834–842
7. Ullrich KJ, Rumrich G, Kloss S (1976) Active Ca²⁺ reabsorption in the proximal tubule of the rat kidney. Dependence on sodium and buffer transport. Pflugers Arch 364:223–228

8. Bomsztyk K, Calaib MB (1988) Bicarbonate absorption stimulates active calcium absorption in the rat proximal tubule. J Clin Invest 81:1455–1461

9. Rouse D, Ng RCK, Suki WN (1979) Calcium transport in the pars recta and thin descending limb of Henle of the rabbit, perfused in vitro. J Clin Invest 65:37–42

10. Bourdeau JE (1986) Calcium transport across the pars recta of cortical segment 2 proximal tubules. Am J Physiol 251:F718–F724

11. Sacks P, Bourdeau JE (1989) Ca^{2+} absorption in the pars recta of cortical S2 rabbit proximal tubules: role of diffusion. Am J Physiol 257:F262–F267

12. Rocha AS, Magaldi JB, Kokko JP (1977) Calcium and phosphate transport in isolated segments of rabbit Henle's loop. J Clin Invest 59:975–983

13. Suki WN, Rouse D, Ng RCK, Kokko JP (1980) Calcium transport in the thick ascending limb of Henle. Heterogeneity of function in the medullary and cortical segments. J Clin Invest 66:1004–1009

14. Bourdeau JE, Burg MB (1980) Effect of PTH on calcium transport across the cortical thick ascending limb of Henle's loop. Am J Physiol 239:F121–F126

15. Suki WN, Rouse D (1981) Hormonal regulation of calcium transport in thick ascending limb renal tubules. Am J Physiol 241:F171–F174

16. Imai M (1981) Effects of parathyroid hormone and N_6,O_2-dibutyryl cyclic AMP on Ca^{2+} transport across the rabbit distal nephron segments perfused in vitro. Pflugers Arch 390:145–151

17. Shareghi GR, Stoner LC (1978) Calcium transport across segments of the rabbit distal nephron in vitro. Am J Physiol 235:F367–F375

18. Bailly C, Roinel N, Amiel C (1985) Stimulation by glucagon and PTH of Ca and Mg reabsorption in the superficial distal tubule of the rat kidney. Pflugers Arch 403:28–34

19. Bourdeau JE, Hellstrom-Stein RJ (1982) Voltage-dependent calcium movement across the cortical collecting duct. Am J Physiol 242:F285–F292

20. Kaissling B (1982) Structural aspects of adaptive changes in renal electrolyte excretion. Am J Physiol 243:F211–F226

21. Costanzo LS (1985) Localization of diuretic action in microperfused rat distal tubules: Ca and Na transport. Am J Physiol 248:F527–F535

22. Borkes JL, Caride A, Verma AK, Penniston JT, Kumar R (1989) Plasma membrane calcium pump and 28-kDa calcium binding protein in cells of rat kidney distal tubules. Am J Physiol 257:F842–F849

23. Magaldi AJ, van Baak AA, Rocha AS (1989) Calcium transport across rat inner medullary collecting duct perfused in vitro. Am J Physiol 257:F738–F745

24. Morrel F (1981) Sites of hormone action in the mammalian nephron. Am J Physiol 240:F159–F164

25. Agus ZS, Gardner LB, Beck LH, Goldberg M (1973) Effects of parathyroid hormone and renal tubular reabsorption of calcium, sodium, and phosphate. Am J Physiol 224:1143–1148

26. Sutton RAL, Wong NLM, Dirks JH (1976) Effects of parathyroid hormone on sodium and calcium transport in the dog nephron. Clin Sci Mol Med 51:345–351

27. Harris CA, Burnatowska MA, Seely JF, Sutton RAL, Quamme GA, Dirks JH (1979) Effects of parathyroid hormone on electrolyte transport in the hamster nephron. Am J Physiol 236:F342–F348

28. Hruska KA, Mills SC, Khalifa S, Hammerman MR (1983) Phosphorylation of renal brush border membrane vesicles. J Biol Chem 258:2501–2507

29. Hammerman MR, Hruska KA (1982) Cyclic AMP-dependent protein phosphorylation in canine renal brush-border membrane vesicles is associated with decreased phosphate transport. J Biol Chem 257:992–999

30. Taniguchi S, Marchetti J, Morel F (1989) Cytosolic free calcium in single microdissected rat cortical collecting tubules. Pflugers Arch 414:125–133

31. Ramachandran C, Brunette MG (1989) The renal Na⁺/Ca²⁺ exchange system is located exclusively in the distal tubule. Biochem J 257:259–264

32. Eisner DA, Lederer WJ (1985) Na-Ca exchange: stoichiometry and electrogenicity. Am J Physiol 248:C189–C202

33. Jayakumar A, Cheng L, Liang CT, Sacktor B (1984) Sodium gradient-dependent calcium uptake in renal basolateral membrane vesicles. Effect of parathyroid hormone. J Biol Chem 259:10827–10833

34. Scoble JE, Mills S, Hruska KA (1985) Calcium transport in canine renal basolateral membrane vesicles. J Clin Invest 75:1096–1105

35. Van Heeswijk MPE, Geertsen JAM, Van Os CH (1984) J Membr Biol 79:19–31

36. Gmaj P, Murer H, Kinne R (1979) Calcium ion transport across plasma membranes isolated from rat kidney cortex. Biochem J 178:549–557

37. Tsukamoto Y, Saka S, Saitoh M, Sugimura K (1990) Heterogeneity of calcium pump activity in proximal and distal tubules of rat kidney (abstract) Kidney Int 37:2471

38. Bronner F, Stein WD (1988) CaBPr facilitates intracellular Ca diffusion for Ca pumping in distal convoluted tubule. Am J Physiol 255:F558–F562

The Biology of Vitamin D-Dependent Calcium Binding Proteins

RAJIV KUMAR[1]

SUMMARY. Vitamin D-dependent calcium binding protein (CaBPs) are widely dispersed in many tissues that play an important role in calcium translocation. They are vitamin D-dependent in most tissues except for those in the central nervous system. The calcium binding proteins are co-localized with calcium pumps in many Ca^{2+} transporting tissues.

Introduction

Vitamin D_3, via its active metabolite $1,25(OH)_2D_3$, plays a crucial role in the active absorption of Ca in the intestine, the mobilization of bone and soft tissue Ca, the maintenance of normal serum Ca and phosphorus concentrations, and the normal mineralization of bone [1–5]. Although the hormone may not directly alter mineralization, many direct effects of the hormone on bone cell activity have been noted [4–14]. In vitro, $1,25(OH)_2D_3$ promotes differentiation and inhibits the growth of various cell lines. It also diminishes the secretion of interleukin 2 from mitogen-stimulated lymphocytes in vitro and alters monocyte and macrophage function.

In the intestine, $1,25(OH)_2D_3$ brings about this effect, at least in part, by a receptor-mediated mechanism that influences the expression of various genes in the nucleus [1–5]. Receptors for the hormone have been characterized with respect to their physical characteristics, ligand-binding properties, and amino acid sequences [6–8]. Protein synthesis is important in bringing about the actions of $1,25(OH)_2D_3$ in the intestine, although contrary views exist [4]. Intestinal lipid metabolism, cyclic nucleotide levels, and the uptake of Ca by Golgi and endoplasmic reticulum are altered by $1,25(OH)_2D_3$ [4]. Extensive work has been performed by us and others concerning the metabolic events that control the tissue levels and metabolism of

[1]Nephrology Research Unit, Departments of Medicine, Biochemistry, and Molecular Biology, Mayo Clinic/Foundation, Rochester, MN 55905, USA

1,25(OH)$_2$D$_3$ [3]. Thermodynamic considerations in the transepithelial movement of Ca have been reviewed by Wasserman and recently discussed by us [4,9]. The transport of Ca across the enterocyte requires energy and sodium ions. The entry of Ca into the enterocyte is down a concentration and electrical gradient and, while it is facilitated by vitamin D, it does not require the expenditure of energy. The energy-requiring step is at the basolateral membrane, where Ca is pumped up a concentration and electrical gradient, most likely by a Ca-pumping ATPase.

Vitamin D-Dependent Calcium Binding Proteins

Physiology and Structure of CaBPs

In the intestine, 1,25(OH)$_2$D$_3$ increases, and sometimes decreases, the synthesis of various proteins and alters the activity of various enzymes [1–5]. In some instances, these changes are related to active intestinal Ca transport in vivo. The most notable of the proteins whose synthesis is altered by 1,25(OH)$_2$D is vitamin D-dependent CaBP [1–5,10–13]; the appearance of the protein in the intestine is temporally related to increases in calcium transport. Careful experiments have shown that CaBP is regulated by vitamin D in intestinal tissue and that it does not act merely as a Ca buffer [12]. Recent work has shown that CaBP plays a role in the diffusion of Ca across the cellular compartment [14]. There is some evidence that CaBP may interact with the plasma membrane Ca pump in order to increase the movement of Ca from within the cellular compartment into the extracellular fluid space; while this is an attractive hypothesis, work from several laboratories, including our own, has shown that this may not be the case [16–17]. Concentrations of CaBP in tissues are regulated by both transcriptional and non-transcriptional mechanisms [18–21]. It is clear that CaBP concentrations in tissues are controlled in large part by transcriptional mechanisms—hence it is likely that 1,25(OH)$_2$D$_3$-specific promoter or enhancer elements are present either proximal (5') to the transcription start site or within the gene itself.

There is considerable information about the structure of CaBPs and their distribution in tissues. As noted in Table 1, CaBP exists in two forms [5,13,18,22]. There is an $\sim$9 kDa CaBP present in the intestine and placenta of mammalian tissues; it is also found in mouse kidney. In addition, an $\sim$28 kDa CaBP is present in the intestine and in other tissues of avian species, and in the brain and distal tubule of mammalian species. The amino acid sequences of porcine, murine, and a truncated form of bovine intestinal CaBP have been determined by Edman degradation [22–27]. The sequence of rat intestinal CaBP has been deduced from the sequence of a cDNA clone [28]. Recently, we determined the sequence of a full-length cDNA clone of bovine intestinal CaBP and demonstrated that the protein encoded by this cDNA was three amino acids longer than that of the truncated protein whose sequence had been determined earlier by Edman degradation [23]. The truncated form arises due to the action of trypsin on a lysine-lysine bond present between amino acids 3 and 4 of the protein. Chick intestinal 28 kDa CaBP has been sequenced by us and by Wasserman using protein sequencing techniques [24,25]. Its amino acid sequence has been derived from the sequence of appropriate cDNA clones [26]. In addition, we have recently determined the sequence of appropriate cDNA clones [26]. In addition, we have recently determined the sequence of rat brain 28-kDa CaBP from the sequence

Table 1. Tissue and species distribution of calbindin-D. (From (5) with permission of the American Physiological Society)

Species and tissue	Approximate molecular weight (kDa)	Cross-reacts with antisera prepared to calbindin-D from
Chicken		
Intestine	28	–
Kidney	28	Chicken intestine, human kidney
Uterus	28	Chicken intestine
Hypothalamus	ND	Chicken intestine
Bone	34	Chicken intestine
Brain	28	Chicken intestine
Pancreas	28	Chicken intestine, human kidney
Blood	ND	Chicken intestine
Parathyroid	ND	Chicken intestine
Adrenal	ND	Chicken intestine
Esophagus	ND	Chicken intestine
Testes	ND	Chicken intestine
Mouse		
Yolk sac	10.05	Rat intestine
Kidney	25 and 10	Human cerebellar, mouse intestine, rat intestine
Intestine	9–10	Rat intestine
Placenta	ND	Rat intestine
Uterus	ND	Rat intestine
Pig		
Intestine	9–13	–
Kidney	12 and 25	Pig intestine
Blood	ND	Pig intestine
Liver	12	Pig intestine
Pancreas	12	Pig intestine
Thyroid	12	Pig intestine
Human		
Intestine	10–28	Chicken intestine, human kidney
Brain	28	Chicken intestine
Kidney	28	Chicken intestine

of appropriate cDNA clones. Others have determined the sequences of the human 27–28 kDa CaBP gene, the chicken 28 kDa CaBP gene, and the rat 9 kDa CaBP gene [29]. All the data concerning the structure of these proteins demonstrates that they are related to other calcium binding proteins of the troponin-C superfamily of proteins.

Biophysical Properties of CaBPs

Recently, several laboratories, including our own, have examined the biophysical properties of CaBPs in order to obtain information on the manner in which they bind Ca and in order to bind insights into how they might act as trigger proteins or facilitate the movement of calcium across cells. The 9 kDa bovine intestinal CaBP binds 2 moles of Ca, whereas the chick intestinal CaBP binds 4 moles of Ca per mole of protein [22]. The 9 kDa and 28 kDa vitamin D-induced CaBPs bind Ca within E-F hand structures. These structures consist of helix-loop-helix structures that were initially described by Kretsinger and his colleagues [22]. The 9 kDa CaBP has two E-F hand structures whereas the 28 kDa CaBP has six. Moffat and colleagues have determined the 3-dimensional x-ray crystal structure of the 9 kDa CaBP.

We examined the mechanism of Ca and lanthanide binding of the 28 kDa CaBP [30]. We demonstrated that the chick intestinal CaBP binds 3 moles of terbium with high affinity, another mole of terbium with relatively high affinity, and several other molecules of terbium with low affinity. Ca binding occurs at two classes of sites; furthermore, the protein undergoes a conformational change upon binding Ca. We have also demonstrated similar conformational changes with human kidney CaBP. Similar Ca^{2+}-dependent conformation changes have been noted with the porcine 9 kDa CaBP. Recently, we examined the Ca binding properties of the rat brain 28 kDa CaBPs in E. coli and purified it and three mutants. We have shown that both the mutants which lack either one or two E-F hands bind Ca in a manner similar to that of the full-length protein. Considerable work, however, needs to be done in defining the precise stoichiometry of Ca binding in the full-length and mutant forms of CaBP. Recently, Forsen and Grundstrom have examined the biophysical properties of mutated forms of the 9 kDa CaBP using NMR and other methods. We have also used NMR techniques in order to examine the NMR characteristics of the 28 kDa CaBP. We have confirmed, by NMR, that the conformation of these CaBPs is controlled by Ca.

References

1. DeLuca HF (1988) The vitamin D story: a collaborative effort of basic science and clinical medicine. FASEB J 2:224–236
2. Minghetti PP, Norman AW (1988) 1,25(OH)$_2$-vitamin D$_3$ receptors: gene regulation and genetic circuitry. FASEB J 2:3043–3053
3. Kumar R (1984) The metabolism of 1,25-dihydroxyvitamin D$_3$. Physiol Rev 64:478–504
4. Kumar R (1986) The metabolism and mechanism of action of 1,25-dihydroxyvitamin D$_3$. Kidney Int 30:793–803
5. Gross MD, Kumar R (1990) Physiology and biochemistry of vitamin D-dependent calcium binding proteins. Am J Physiol 259:F195–F205
6. Pike JW, Sleator NM, Haussler MR (1987) Chicken intestinal receptor for 1,25-dihydroxyvitamin D$_3$. Immunologic characterization and homogeneous isolation of a 60000-dalton protein. J Biol Chem 25:262:1305–1311
7. Baker AR, McDonnell DP, Hughes M, Crisp TM, Mangelsdorf DJ, Haussler MR, Pike JW, Shine J, O'Malley BW (1988) Cloning and expression of full-length cDNA encoding human vitamin D receptor. Proc Natl Acad Sci USA 85:3294–3298
8. Pierce EA, Dame MC, DeLuca HF (1987) Size and charge of the functional 1,25-dihydroxyvitamin D (receptor) in porcine intestine. J Biol Chem 262:17092–17099
9. Wasserman RH, Fullmer CS, Shimura F (1984) Calcium absorption and the molecular effects of vitamin D$_3$. In: Kumar D (ed) Martinus Nijhoff, Hingham, pp 233–257
10. Wasserman RH, Corradino RA, Taylor AN (1968) Vitamin D-dependent calcium-binding protein. Purification and some properties. J Biol Chem 243:3978–3986
11. Response to some physiological and nutritional variables. J Biol Chem 243:3987–3993
12. Bar A, Hurwitz S (1979) Relationship of intestinal and plasma calcium binding protein to intestinal calcium absorption. FEBS Lett 102:79–81
13. Thomasset M, Parkes CO, Cuisinier-Gleizes P (1982) Rat calcium-binding proteins: distribution, development, and vitamin D dependence. Am J Physiol 243:E483–E488

14. Feher JJ, Fullmer CS, Fritzsch GK (1989) Comparison of the enhanced steady-state diffusion of calcium by calbindin-D9K and calmodulin: possible importance in intestinal calcium absorption. Cell Calcium 10:189–203

15. Morgan DW, Welton AF, Heick AE, Christakos S (1986) Specific in vitro activation of Ca, Mg-ATPase by vitamin D-dependent rat renal calcium binding protein (calbindin $D_2$8K). Biochem Biophys Res Commun 138:547–553

16. Walters JR (1989) Calbindin-D9K stimulates the (calcium) pump in rat enterocyte basolateral membranes. Am J Physiol 256:G124–G128

17. Ghijsen WEJM, Van Os CH, Heizmann CW, Murer H (1986) Regulation of duodenal Ca^{2+} pump by calmodulin and vitamin D-dependent Ca^{2+}-binding protein. Am J Physiol 251:G223–G229

18. Christakos S, Gabrielides C, Rhoten WB (1989) Vitamin D-dependent calcium binding proteins: chemistry, distribution, functional considerations, and molecular biology. Endocr Rev 10:3–26

19. Varghese S, Deaven LL, Huang YC, Gill RK, Iacopino AM, Christakos S (1989) Transcriptional regulation and chromosomal assignment of the mammalian calbinding-D28k gene. Mol Cell Endocrinol 3:495–502

20. Clemens TL, McGlade SA, Garrett KP, Craviso GL, Hendy GL (1989) Extracellular calcium modulates vitamin D-dependent calbindin-D28k gene expression in chick kidney cells. Endocrinology 124:1582–1584

21. Dupret JM, Brun P, Perret C, Lomri N, Thomasset M, Cuisinier-Gleizes P (1987) Transcriptional and post-transcriptional regulation of vitamin D-dependent calcium-binding protein gene expression in the rat duodenum by 1,25-dihydroxycholecalciferol. J Biol Chem 262:16553–16557

22. Gross M, Kumar R (1987) The physiology and biochemistry of vitamin D-dependent calcium binding proteins. In: Spelsberg TC, Kumar R (eds) Sterol/steroid hormone action. Martinus Nijhoff, Hingham, pp 371–394

23. Kumar R, Wieben E, Beecher SJ (1989) The molecular cloning of the complementary deoxyribonucleic acid for bovine vitamin D-dependent calcium-binding protein: structure of the full-length protein and evidence for homologies with other calcium-proteins of the troponin-C superfamily of proteins. Mol Cell Endocrinol 3:427–432

24. Tsarbopoulos A, Gross M, Kumar R, Jardine I (1989) Rapid identification of calbindin-D28k cyanogen bromide peptide fragments by plasma desorption mass spectrometry. Biomed Environ Mass Spectrom 18:387–393

25. Fullmer CS, Wasserman RH (1987) Chicken intestinal 28-kilodalton calbindin-D: complete amino acid sequence and structural considerations. Proc Natl Acad Sci USA 84:4772–4776

26. Hunziker W (1986) The 28-kDa vitamin D-dependent calcium-binding protein has a six-domain structure. Proc Natl Acad Sci USA 83:7578–7582

27. Hunziker W, Schrickel S (1988) Rat brain calbindin D28: six domain structure and extensive amino acid homology with chicken calbindin D28. Mol Cell Endocrinol 2:465–473

28. Desplan C, Heidmann O, Lillie JW, Auffray C, Thomasset M (1983) Sequence of rat intestinal vitamin D-dependent calcium-binding protein derived from a cDNA clone. Evolutionary implications. J Biol Chem 258:13502–13505

29. Minghetti PP, Cancela L, Fujisawa Y, Theofan G, Norman AW (1988) Molecular structure of the chicken vitamin D-induced calbindin-D28k gene reveals eleven exons, six Ca^{2+}-binding domains, and numerous promoter regulatory elements. Mol Cell Endocrinol 2:355–367

30. Gross MD, Nelsestuen GL, Kumar R (1987) Observations on the binding of lanthanides and calcium to vitamin D-dependent chick intestinal calcium-binding protein. Implications regarding calcium-binding protein function. J Biol Chem 262:6539–6545

Cystic Diseases of the Kidney

Chair: Jean-Pierre Grünfeld (France)
Eiji Higashihara (Japan)

Control of Renal Cyst Formation and Enlargement

JARED J. GRANTHAM[1]

SUMMARY. Evidence is presented to indicate that renal cysts derived in a collagen matrix in vitro from primary cultures of human cortex and from an established cell line (MDCK) are subject to growth regulation by peptide mitogens (EGF and insulin) and by agents of the adenylyl cyclase signal transduction system. The findings are consonant with recent evidence obtained by direct measurement of fluid transport in liver and kidney cysts of humans with autosomal dominant polycystic kidney disease and support the hypothesis that these potential regulatory mechanisms may participate in the initiation and expansion of cysts.

Introduction and Discussion

Although renal cysts come in different shapes and sizes, recent work leads to the conclusion that when encountered in hereditary and acquired disorders they have certain key elements in common: 1) Cysts evolve from renal tubules; they may arise in fetal kidneys or in otherwise fully mature and well-differentiated renal tubules [1]. 2) Enlargement involves the proliferation of epithelial cells that comprise the wall of the cyst [2], the accumulation of fluid within the cavity formed by the increase in cyst wall area [3], and the remodeling of the extracellular matrix and the interstitium adjacent to the enlarging cysts [4].

We have become accustomed to viewing renal cysts in two general contexts: 1) acquired and 2) hereditary. Acquired cysts develop in renal tubules that have no genetic history of de novo cyst formation, whereas dominant and recessive mutations cause cysts to form with regularity in the renal tubules of susceptible individuals. Acquired cysts can be formed by feeding animals selected chemicals, or they can be formed as a consequence of a severe reduction in the number of functioning nephrons [5]. The maintenance of acquired cysts appears to require the sustained stimulation

---

[1]University of Kansas Medical Center, Kansas City, KS 66103, USA

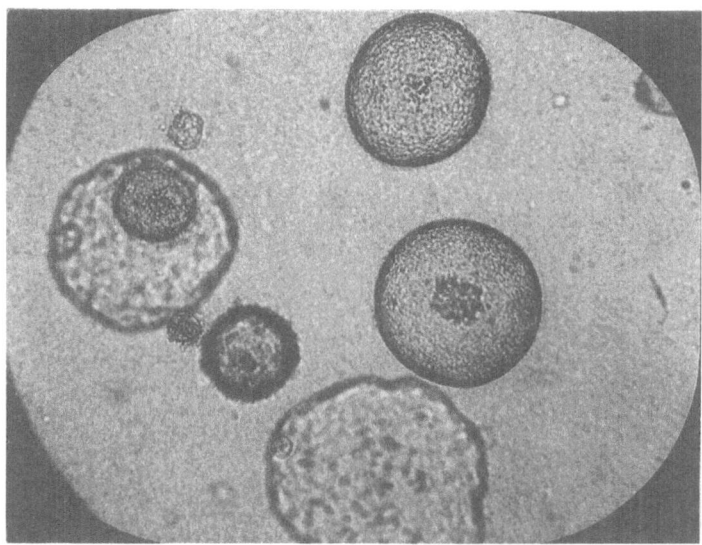

Fig. 1. Madin Darby Canine Kidney (*MDCK*) cysts in hydrated gel of Type 1 collagen. Largest cyst is 367 µm in diameter

of cyst-building forces, since the cysts can be diminished in size by withholding the cystsogen, or by transplanting a functioning kidney [6]. Acquired cystic disease can also be accelerated by increasing the number of inflammatory cells in the kidneys [7].

The highly variable clinical course of autosomal dominant polycystic kidney disease (ADPKD) and autosomal recessive polycystic kidney disease (ARPKD), also suggests that non-genetic factors may have a commanding role in determining the expression of these diseases in the kidneys.

Renal cysts appear to be neoplastic but otherwise differentiated tissue masses that derive from one or more tubule epithelial cells in a segment of renal tubule [8]. Renal cysts are distinguished from solid tumors by the sustained sequestration of fluid within the cavity formed by the orderly expansion of the intact monolayer of epithelial cells. Abnormal proliferation of epithelial cells may be initiated by inherited or acquired factors that interfere with the normal control of cell division. Once cysts are initiated, hormonal, autocrine, or paracrine factors may promote the expansion of both hereditary and acquired cysts by accelerating the rate of cell proliferation and net transepithelial fluid secretion.

In recent studies, my collaborators and I have searched for some of the potential factors that may contribute to the initiation and progressive enlargement of hereditary and acquired cysts [9–14]. We have used two types of in vitro cells to evaluate the roles of mitogens and fluid transport agonists. Madin Darby Canine Kidney (MDCK) cells are a continuous line of epithelial cells that retain certain differentiated features of the distal tubule. When cultured within a matrix of gelled collagen, MDCK cells develop cysts that enlarge progressively [15]. We have examined these cells as a model of cysts with a genetic abberation in the control of cell division (Fig. 1). This *genetic cyst model*

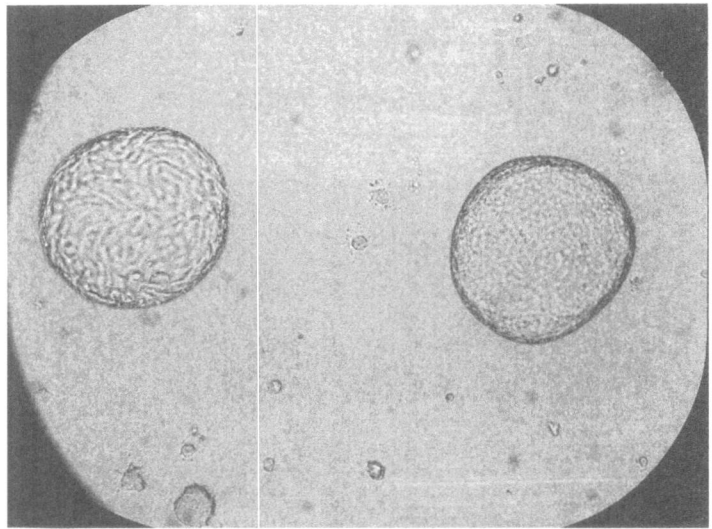

Fig. 2. Normal human kidney (*NHK*) cysts in hydrated gel of Type 1 collagen. Largest cyst is 417 µm in diameter

mimics the autosomal dominant and recessive types of PKD which are caused by mutated DNA. By contrast, we have used primary cultures of human renal cortex to study cyst biogenesis in cells with a normal genetic history with respect to cyst formation. When passaged into a collagen matrix and fed with certain growth factors, human cortex cells form cysts that resemble those observed in the MDCK cell cultures (Fig. 2). We have used the normal human kidney cortex cells (NHK) as an *acquired cyst model*.

Cultures of MDCK and NHK cysts within collagen matrix have been used to assess the impact of exogenous agents on the induction and formation of cysts.

MDCK

In defined medium, MDCK cells embedded in collagen matrix induce cyst formation when they are treated with agonists of the adenylyl cyclase signal transduction pathway [9–14]. Epidermal growth factor (EGF), a renal cell mitogen, does not increase the rate of MDCK cyst formation, but these same cells form cysts when fed with fetal calf serum.

NHK

Only when they are treated with EGF and insulin do NHK cells form cysts [14]. Transferrin and selenium promote cyst growth, but are not essential for cysts to form. Fetal calf serum does not initiate cyst formation. Agonists of the adenylyl cyclase signal transduction pathway also increase the rate of NKH cyst expansion in collagen matrix.

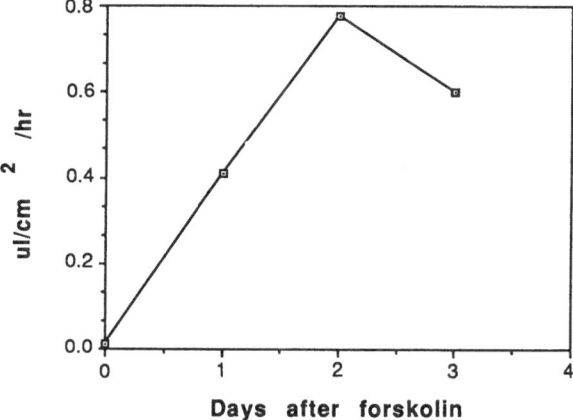

Fig. 3. Effect of forskolin (10^{-5} M) on the rate of net fluid secretion across monolayers of normal human kidney (*NHK*) cells

The formation and expansion of cysts in collagen matrix requires the highly coordinated organization of proliferating cells. Studies of MDCK cells indicate that each cyst derives from a single cell that divides repeatedly, i.e., each cyst represents the clonal growth of a solitary cell [15]. The matrix is critical in determining the type of cyst that will be formed and in determining the polarity of the cells. MDCK cells grown in type 1 collagen have orthodox polarity; however, cysts grown in agarose gels or in suspension culture have reversed polarity, and the Na+K, ATPase is deposited within the apical, rather than within the basolateral plasma membranes [15–17]. The expansion of MDCK cysts in type 1 collagen gel (orthodox polarity) depends in the last analysis on the rate of cell *proliferation* in the cyst wall and on the rate of fluid *secretion* into the cyst cavity. Cyclic AMP agonists stimulate the proliferation of MDCK cells [10,13]. Although the effect of cAMP on the proliferation of NHK cells has not been tested directly, the expansion of the cyst wall area after cAMP stimulation is consistent with stimulation of cell proliferation.

Evaluation of the role of net fluid secretion on the rate of cyst expansion has required a different technical approach. To determine net fluid secretion directly, we grew MDCK and NHK cells on collagen-coated permeable membranes that permitted the collection of fluid which was secreted under a layer of mineral oil directly onto the apical surface of the cells [10,11,13,14]. Monolayers of MDCK cells showed marked stimulation of net fluid secretion when treated with cAMP agonists, but not when treated with EGF and insulin. By contrast, NHK cells revealed marked stimulation of net fluid secretion by EGF and insulin, and the cAMP agonists (Fig. 3). These findings indicate that activation of the adenylyl cyclase signal transduction pathway may promote cyst enlargement by accelerating the rate of net fluid secretion into the cysts. Recent studies indicate that secretin, a hormone that stimulates cyclic AMP production in biliary epithelium, increases the rate of fluid secretion into hepatic and renal cysts of patients with polycystic kidney disease [18].

We have not explicitly determined the extent to which net fluid secretion and cell proliferation are linked in the process of cyst expansion, but simple observation of the increased proliferative response of cells grown on monolayers precludes net fluid accumulation as an explanation for the stimulation of cell growth by cAMP. In addition, cell proliferation can be uncoupled from net fluid secretion by treatment with ouabain [9]. This glycoside, which blocks net fluid secretion, inhibits the enlargement of cysts, but the cells continue to proliferate, leading to solid tumor masses. Such findings would support the view that *cell proliferation* and *fluid secretion* are not obligatorily tied together, and while both protagonists of cyst formation and enlargement appear to be regulated by cAMP, ultimate control of each function may not be conducted through the same effector mechanism.

The foregoing considerations have led to the formulation of an *hypothesis* to explain the progressive enlargement of renal cysts induced by either hereditary or acquired etiologies:

It is hypothesized that cell proliferation and net fluid secretion within established cysts are regulated by a common signal transduction mechanism, the adenylyl cyclase pathway. Mutations in genes which control rate limiting processes in this pathway may alter the sensitivity to surface membrane receptor-mediated agonists, which, at normal levels, may induce cyst formation in hereditary states. In renal tubule cells which lack mutations, autocrine or paracrine mitogens may induce the formation of cysts which expand in response to receptor-mediated cyclase agonists.

References

1. Evan AP, McAteer JA (1990) Cyst cells and cyst walls. In: Gardner KD, Bernstein J (eds) The Cystic Kidney. Kluwer, Highman, pp 21–42
2. Grantham JJ, Geiser JL, Evan AP (1987) Cyst formation and growth in autosomal dominant polycystic kidney disease. Kidney Int 31:1145–1152
3. Grantham JJ (1983) Polycystic kidney disease: A predominance of giant nephrons. Am J Physiol 23:526–529
4. Carone FA, Makino H, Kanwar YS (1988) Basement membrane antigens in renal polycystic disease. Am J Pathol 130:466–471
5. Grantham JJ, Levine E (1985) Acquired cystic disease: Replacing one kidney disease with another. Kidney Int 28:99–105
6. Ishikawa I (1990) Acquired renal cystic disease. In: Gardner KD, Bernstein J (eds) The Cystic Kidney. Kluwer, Highman, pp 351–377
7. Gardner KD Jr, Evan AP, Reed WP (1986) Accelerated renal cyst development in deconditioned germ-free rats. Kidney Int 29:1116–1123
8. Grantham JJ (1990) Polycystic kidney disease: Neoplasia in disguise. Am J Kidney Dis 15:110–116
9. Grantham JJ, Uchic M, Cragoe EJ Jr, Kornhaus J, Grantham JA, Donoso V, Mangoo-Karim R, Evan AP, McAteer J 1989 Chemical modification of cell proliferation and fluid secretion in renal cysts. Kidney Int 35:1379–1389
10. Mangoo-Karim R, Uchic M, Lechene C, Grantham JJ (1989) Renal epithelial cyst formation and enlargement in vitro: Dependence on cAMP. Proc Natl Acad Sci USA 86:6007–6011
11. Mangoo-Karim R, Uchic M, Grant M, Shumate WA, Calvet JA, Park CH, Grantham JJ (1989) Renal epithelial fluid secretion and cyst growth: the role of cyclic AMP. FASEB J 3:2629–2632

12. Grant M, Cragoe EJ, Grantham JJ (1990) Arginine vasopressin stimulates net fluid secretion in a cyst-forming epithelium (MDCK). Kidney Int 37:581
13. Neufeld TJ, Grantham JJ (1990) Epidermal growth factor initiates and cyclic AMP promotes the formation and progressive enlargement of human renal epithelial cysts in vitro. Clin Res 38:444A
14. McAteer JA, Evan AP, Gardner KD (1987) Morphogenetic clonal growth of kidney epithelial cell line MDCK. Anat Rec 217:229-239
16. Wang AZ, Ojakian GE, Nelson WJ (1990) Steps in the morphogenesis of a polarized epithelium 1. Uncoupling the roles of cell-cell and cell-substratum contact in establishing plasma membrane polarity in multicellular epithelial (MDCK) cysts. J Cell Sci 95:137-151
17. Wang AZ, Ojakian GK, Nelson WJ (1990) Steps in the morphogenesis of a polarized epithelium 11. Disassembly and assembly of plasma membrane domains during reversal of epithelial cell polarity in multicellular epithelial (MDCK) cysts. J Cell Sci 95:153-165
18. Everson GT, Emmett M, Brown WR, Redmond P, Thickman D (1990) Functional similarities of hepatic cystic and biliary epithelium: Studies of fluid constituents and in vivo secretion in response to secretin. Hepatology 11:557-656

Inflammatory Mediators in the Progression of Renal Cystic Disease

Kenneth D. Gardner Jr.[1], Janet S. Burnside[1], Lawrence W. Elzinga[2], and Richard M. Locksley[3]

SUMMARY. The possibility that cytokines are present and active in polycystic kidneys was raised by two observations: (i) Endotoxin potentiates cyst formation in the kidneys of germfree rats fed nordihydroguaiaretic acid. (ii) Some cyst fluids are mitogenic for mouse thymocytes. Analyses of fluids from 13 individuals with symptomatic autosomal dominant polycystic kidney disease have detected interleukin-1β, tumor necrosis factor α, interleukin-2, stromelysin, and prostaglandin E$_2$, evidence which not only indicates that interleukin-1β is present but which also supports the likelihood of its biological activity in cyst fluids. The findings provide support for a hypothesis that cytokines participate in the morbidity and/or pathogenesis of autosomal dominant polycystic kidney disease.

Introduction

Two recent, fundamental observations in our laboratory directed our attention to the possibility that cytokines are active in the setting of polycystic kidney disease. One involves the antioxidant nordihydroguaiaretic acid (NDGA), which injures kidney cells [1]. When NDGA is fed to normal rats, cysts form in the animals' kidneys [1]. The effects of NDGA are progressive and evolve over weeks to months. When NDGA is fed to germfree rats, it has little effect on renal morphology unless the rats are exposed to endotoxin. Then, renal cyst formation is dramatic and explosive, even when the animals are maintained under sterile conditions [2]. In this particular model, cysts develop within days after exposure to lipopolysaccharide. The progres-

[1]Department of Medicine, University of New Mexico School of Medicine, Albuquerque, NM 87131, USA
[2]Oregon Health Sciences Center, Portland, OR 97201, USA
[3]University of California, San Francisco, CA 94143, USA

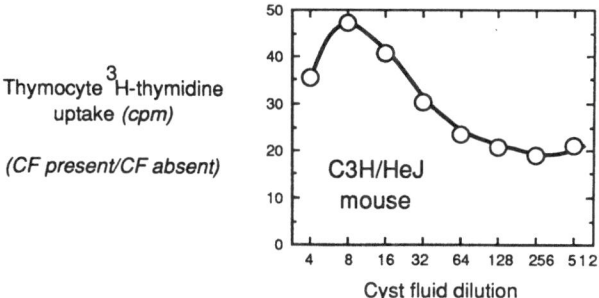

Fig. 1. Mitogenic response of mouse thymocytes to cyst fluid from a polycystic kidney. *Circles* represent means of three determinations. An almost 50-fold increase over baseline thymidine incorporation is evident at the 1:8 dilution. CPM, counts per minute; CF, cyst fluid

sion of the lesion relates directly to the numbers of circulating and infiltrating inflammatory cells.

The second observation is shown in Fig. 1. Fluid drawn from some cysts of human polycystic kidneys induces a proliferative response among thymocytes of the endotoxin-insensitive C3H/HeJ mouse [3]. Such a response is presumptive evidence that cytokine-like substances are present [4,5].

Cytokines are pluripotent proteins [4,5] which are produced by nucleated cells. They act locally and transiently and are present at sites of inflammation and immunologic injury. For example, they may be found in the synovial fluid of acute rheumatoid arthritis and in cerebrospinal fluid during bacterial meningitis. Cytokines mediate the effects of endotoxin [5,6]. Cytokines are mitogenic for mouse thymocytes in comitogen assays [3,7]. One of the best studied cytokines is the monokine, interleukin-1 (IL-1) [5]. IL-1 is relevant to the kidney. It is made by glomerular mesangial cells [8]; it inhibits sodium, glucose, and amino acid transport by renal tubules in vivo [9–11] and it stimulates prostaglandin E_2 (PGE_2) production by papillary collecting duct cells in vitro [12]. IL-1 exists in two forms, IL-1α and IL-1β.

Methods and Results

In order to detect cytokines in cyst fluids we used the enzyme-linked immunoabsorbent assay (ELISA). The sandwich ELISA is highly specific and is a standard technique for the detection of cytokines in biological fluids [13]. An IL-1β-specific commercial ELISA was utilized to assay for IL-1β in most of the 104 aerobic culture-negative fluid samples that had been aspirated from 13 patients with symptomatic autosomal dominant polycystic kidney disease (ADPKD) [14]. Four individuals were female, nine were male. Their ages ranged from 31–54 years. Their renal function, as evaluated by serum creatinines, extended from normal to endstage disease.

Immunoreactive IL-1β concentrations in cyst fluids ranged from 0 to more than 400 pg/ml. The higher concentrations were equal to those that are found in the synovial fluid of rheumatoid arthritics with acute disease [15]. Of 102 fluid samples, roughly one-third contained no IL-1β, one-third contained IL-1β in low concentra-

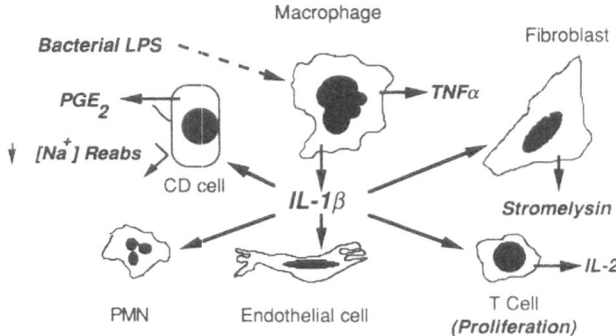

Fig. 2. Cartoon of cellular interactions. Effects of IL-1β on selected target cells are shown in *italics*. All but the reduced reabsorption of sodium by collecting duct cells have been demonstrated in vitro. PMN, polymorphonuclear neutrophils; CD, collecting duct; LPS, lipopolysaccharide (endotoxin)

tions (< 20 pg/ml), and one-third contained IL-1β in relatively high concentrations (> 20 pg/ml). We concluded that immunoreactive IL-1β is present in most cyst fluids of polycystic kidneys.

It remained to be demonstrated that this immunoreactive IL-1β was active biologically. In order to establish bioactivity, we sought evidence of some of the known second-order effects that IL-1 provokes among other cells.

A scheme of IL-1 interactions, as they relate to this study, is shown in Fig. 2. Bacterial lipopolysaccharide (endotoxin) stimulates macrophages to produce and release IL-1 and tumor necrosis factor. Macrophage IL-1, in turn, may stimulate fibroblasts to produce stromelysin [16,17], induce T-cells to proliferate and to produce IL-2 [7], cause endothelial cells and polymorphonuclear leukocytes to become activated [5], and incite cells of the papillary collecting duct to increase their production of PGE₂ [12] and, in vivo, to reduce their reabsorption of sodium [10–11]. The first evidence of bioactivity that we sought was documentation of the proliferative response of T-cells to cyst fluid. We used thymocyte comitogen assays.

In contrast to the sandwich ELISA, thymocyte comitogen assays are not specific [18]. Mouse thymocytes are exposed to fluids suspected of containing mitogenic substances in the presence of a comitogen such as phytohemagglutinin or concanavalin A. Thymidine incorporation is taken as a measure of thymocyte proliferation. The assays are not specific because other cytokines are mitogenic and because IL-1 bioactivity may be inhibited by specific inactivators. The results of these assays, unlike those of the ELISA, represent only presumptive evidence of cytokine presence. We recorded bioassay results in terms of a *stimulation index*: the ratio of counts per minute of tritiated thymidine incorporated by thymocytes in the presence versus the absence of cyst fluid. We defined a *mitogenic fluid* as one with a *stimulation index* greater than unity.

Two-thirds of the cyst fluids were mitogenic (Fig. 3), some provoking upwards of a 50-fold increase in thymocyte proliferation (Fig. 3a). There was no correlation between stimulation indices and IL-1β concentrations. However, most mitogenic

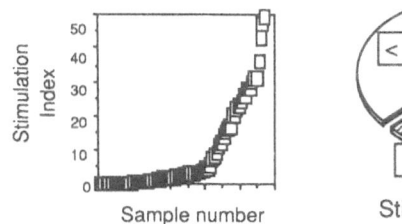 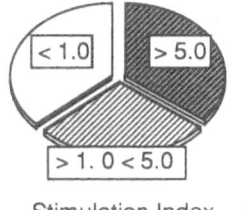

Fig. 3a,b. Mitogenic response to cyst fluids. **a** Range of stimulation indices among 102 tested fluids **b** Responses grouped by degree of response

fluids were fluids that contained immunoreactive IL-1β ($\chi^2 = 3.87$; P < 0.05). Fewer mitogenic fluids had no IL-1β, and IL-1β was present in some non-mitogenic fluids. The observation that a significant majority of fluids that were mitogenic also contained immunoreactive IL-1β implied to us that some, at least, of the immunoreactive IL-1β that we detected by ELISA was active biologically.

We continued to search for evidence which would support bioactivity by performing three additional ELISAs and a radioimmunoassay. We assayed cyst fluids for IL-2, stromelysin, tumor necrosis factor alpha (TNFα), and PGE$_2$, all demonstrated in vitro to be products of specific IL-1β-stimulated cells (Fig. 2). In addition, we tested fluids for bacterial lipopolysaccharide and related the findings to IL-1β concentrations in the same fluids. Finally, we related the concentrations of immunoreactive IL-1β to the concentrations of sodium in the same cyst fluids.

Immunoreactive IL-2 was present in 7 of 23 fluids. Its concentrations were higher in the presence than in the absence of IL-1. They correlated significantly with those of IL-1β (r = 0.65; P < 0.05). This was the result anticipated had thymus-derived cells been present in or near cysts and responded to an IL-1β signal in vivo.

Immunoreactive stromelysin (kindly assayed by MW Lark and LA Walakovits, Merck Sharp and Dohme Research Laboratories, Division of Merck and Co., Inc., Rahway, NJ, USA) was present in 18 of 23 fluids, in concentrations ranging from 0–55 ng/ml. Its mean concentration was higher, but insignificantly so, in IL-1β-containing fluids. While stromelysin concentrations did not correlate directly with those of IL-1β, we found that when fluids were grouped in relation to their IL-1β immunoreactivity, significantly more fluids contained IL-1β and stromelysin together ($\chi^2 = 5.901$; P < 0.05).

Both TNFα (assayed by ELISA) and PGE$_2$ (assayed by radioimmunoassay) were detected in a majority of fluids. While concentrations did not correlate with those of IL-1β, mean concentrations of both TNFα and PGE$_2$ were higher, albeit insignificantly so, in the presence than in the absence of IL-1β.

Bacterial lipopolysaccharide (LPS) was detected in 8 of 41 fluids. The mean concentration of IL-1β was higher in LPS positive fluids, but again the difference was not statistically significant.

The findings, in the form of mean index and concentration differences, are summarized in Fig. 4. Fluids containing immunoreactive IL-1β were more apt to cause T-cells to proliferate. They also were associated with higher mean concentrations of IL-2, stromelysin, TNFα, and PGE$_2$. Finally, the mean concentration of IL-1β was

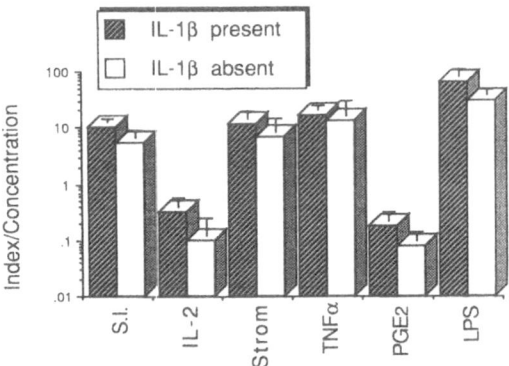

Fig. 4. Mean (±SE) differences (log scale) in index/concentrations between fluids with and fluids without immunoreactive IL-1β. Greater mitogenicity (*S.I.*); and higher concentrations of IL-2, stromelysin, (*strom*) tumor necrosis factor α, (*TNFα*) and PGE$_2$ were found among fluids with IL-1β; a greater mean concentration of IL-1β was recorded among endotoxin-positive (*LPS*) fluids

higher among fluids in which bacterial lipopolysaccharide was detected. Except for the concentration of IL-2 and stromelysin, mean differences between fluids with and without IL-1β were not statistically significant. Means, however, were always greater in IL-1β-containing fluids (Fig. 4), a direction of difference that was predicted by experimental experience (Fig. 2). This is, given its consistency here in six of six independent trials, statistically significant ($P < 0.02$; one tail).

Discussion

We concluded from our observations that IL-1β is present and is biologically active in cyst fluids from polycystic kidneys. The findings raised the question of what role IL-1β and/or other cytokines might play in the morbidity or pathogenesis of ADPKD.

It is not likely that IL-1β is responsible for the salt wasting that is sometimes associated with cystic kidney disease [19]. We found no relationship between the concentrations of sodium and IL-1β. Thus, we found no evidence that intraluminal IL-1β influences sodium concentrations in, and presumably net sodium reabsorption from, cyst fluids. Accordingly, we cannot implicate intraluminal IL-1β activity in the salt wasting of renal cystic disease.

A more likely role for cytokines relates to pain. Of the 13 subjects from whom our fluids came, 11 had painful polycystic kidneys and were undergoing therapeutic cyst aspiration and decompression [14]. We cannot rule out the possibility that cytokines, such as IL-1β and TNFα, are involved in the renal pain of polycystic kidney disease.

A second plausible possibility of a role for cytokines is in the remodeling that characterizes the polycystic kidney. Cystic nephrons are remodeled nephrons. Stromelysin is a metalloproteinase known to participate in the remodeling of joints in rheumatoid arthritis [16,17]. Stromelysin degrades collagen IV and proteoglycan, two components of renal tubular basement membrane, whose abnormalities have long been implicated in the pathogenesis of polycystic kidney disease [20]. Thus, activation of the cytokine cascade in genetically predisposed individuals may account for the dilation of nephrons and the formation of cysts in kidneys which, ultimately, we come to recognize as polycystic kidneys.

Conclusion

This study has shown that cytokines, specifically IL-1β, TNFα, and IL-2, are present in the cyst fluids of polycystic kidneys. The study has provided strong presumptive evidence that the IL-1β in cyst fluid is active biologically. Given the known consequences of cytokine activity at other sites of disease, it must be considered likely that cytokines participate in the morbidity and pathogenesis of autosomal dominant polycystic kidney disease.

References

1. Gardner KD Jr, Evan AP (1984) Cystic kidneys: An enigma evolves. Am J Kidney Dis 3:403–413
2. Gardner KD Jr, Reed WP, Evan AP, Zedalis J, Hylarides MD, Leon AA (1987) Endotoxin provocation of experimental renal cystic disease. Kidney Int 32:329–334
3. Ryan JL, Glode LM, Rosenstreich DL (1979) Lack of responsiveness of C3H/HeJ macrophages to lipopolysaccharide: The cellular basis of LPS-stimulated metabolism. J Immunol 122:932–935
4. Balkwill FR, Burke F (1989) The cytokine network. Immunol Today 10:299–304
5. Fibbe WE, Schaafsma MR, Falkenburg JHF, Willemze R (1989) The biological activities of interleukin-1. Blut 59:147–156
6. Richardson RP, Rhyne CD, Fong Y, Hesse DG, Tracey KY, Marano MA, Lowry SF, Antonacci AC, Calvano SE (1989) Peripheral blood leukocyte kinetics following in vivo lipopolysaccharide (LPS) administration to normal human subjects. Ann Surg 210:239–245
7. Kaye J, Gillis S, Mizel SB, Shevach EM, Malek TR, Dinarello CA, Lachman LB, Janeway CA Jr (1984) Growth of a cloned helper T cell line induced by a monoclonal antibody specific for the antigen receptor: Interleukin 1 is required for the expression of receptors for interleukin 2. J Immunol 133:1339–1345
8. Lovett DH, Ryan JL, Sterzel RB (1983) A thymocyte-activating factor derived from glomerular mesangial cells. J Immunol 130:1796–1801
9. Kohan DE, Schreiner GF (1988) Interleukin 1 modulation of renal epithelial glucose and amino acid transport. Am J Physiol 254:F879–F886
10. Caverzasio J, Rizzoli R, Dayer J-M, Bonjour J-P (1987) Interleukin-1 decreases renal sodium reabsorption: possible mechanism of endotoxin-induced natriuresis. Am J Physiol 252:F943–F946
11. Beasley D, Dinarello CA, Cannon JG (1988) Interleukin-1 induces natriuresis in conscious rats: Role of renal prostaglandins. Kidney Int 33:1059–1065
12. Kohan DE (1989) Interleukin-1 regulation of prostaglandin E_2 synthesis by the papillary collecting duct. J Lab Clin Med 114:717–723

13. Herbelin A, Nguyen AT, Zingraff J, Urena P, Descamps-Latscha B (1990) Influence of uremia and hemodialysis on circulating interleukin-1 and tumor necrosis factor α. Kidney Int 37:116–125
14. Bennett WM, Elzinga L, Golper TA, Barry JM (1987) Reduction of cyst volume for symptomatic management of autosomal dominant polycystic kidney disease. J Urol 137:620–622
15. Smith MD (1989) Cytokines in synovial fluid in rheumatoid arthritis. J Rheumatol 16:706
16. Case JP, Lafyatis R, Remmers EF, Kumkumian GK, Wilder RL (1989) Transin/stromelysin expression in rheumatoid synovium. Am J Pathol 135:1055–1064
17. Teahan J, Harrison R, Izquierdo M, Stein RL (1989) Substrate specificity of human fibroblast stromelysin. Hydrolysis of substance P and its analogues. Biochemistry 28:8497–8501
18. Hurme M (1988) Both interleukin 1 and tumor necrosis factor enhance thymocyte proliferation. Eur J Immunol 18:1303–1306
19. Gardner KD Jr (1988) Cystic kidneys. Kidney Int 33:610–621
20. Carone FA, Hollenberg PF, Makamura S, Punyarit P, Glogowski W, Flouret G (1989) Tubular basement membrane change occurs pari passu with the development of cyst formation. Kidney Int 35:1034–1040

Extrarenal Manifestations of Autosomal Dominant Polycystic Kidney Disease

DOMINIQUE CHAUVEAU, YVES PIRSON[2], DOMINIQUE DROZ, JOSEPH ROSENFELD[3], and JEAN-PIERRE GRÜNFELD[1],

SUMMARY. Among extrarenal manifestations of autosomal dominant polycystic kidney disease (ADPKD), liver abnormalities are the most frequent and intracranial aneurysms, the most severe. Liver cysts develop later than renal cysts, and are more prevalent in females, most particularly in those who have had multiple pregnancies. The treatment of massive polycystic liver is difficult. In very rare families, congenital hepatic fibrosis may be associated with ADPKD. Rupture of an intracranial aneurysm (ICA) is a life-threatening complication. The mean age at rupture is 39 years. This accident may occur in normotensive patients with normal renal function. Routine screening is indicated when there is a positive family history of ICA or when there has been a previous accident of ICA rupture.

Introduction

Extrarenal manifestations in autosomal dominant polycystic kidney disease (ADPKD) encompass both cystic changes, among which liver involvement predominates, and non-cystic changes, including intracranial aneurysms, other cardiovascular lesions, and possible abdominal hernias and colon diverticulosis. Extrarenal involvement may expose ADPKD patients to life-threatening complications, such as rupture of an intracranial aneurysm or severe liver cyst function.

In this review, we will focus mainly on recent data on liver abnormalities, intracranial aneurysms, and mitral-valve prolapse. These manifestations raise not only clinical problems of dealing with their detection and management, but also pathophysiological issues, with regard to the relation between the mechanisms

[1]Département de Néphrologie, Hôpital Necker, 75015 Paris, France
[2]Service de Néphrologie, Cliniques Universitaires Saint-Luc, 1200 Brussels, Belgium
[3]Beilinson Medical Center, Tel Aviv University Medical School, Tel Aviv, Israel

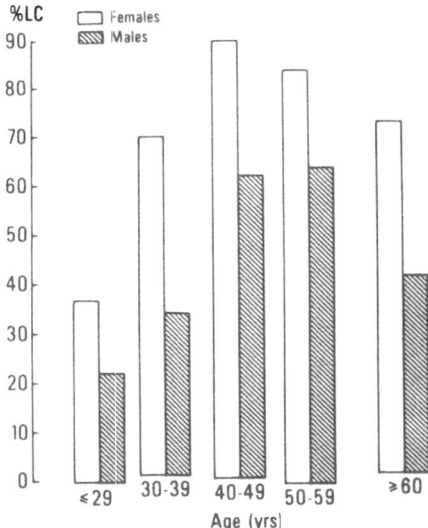

Fig. 1. Prevalence of liver cysts (*LC*) as detected by ultrasonography in 120 non-hemodialyzed ADPKD patients according to age and sex. (From [1] with permission)

involved in renal cyst formation and those implicated in the development of these extrarenal lesions.

Liver Involvement

Liver cysts are frequently found in ADPKD, and their ultrasonographic demonstration may be helpful for diagnosis. The prevalence of liver cysts increases with age and is higher in female patients. In both sexes, liver cysts develop later than kidney cysts. Approximately 70% of ADPKD patients aged 60 years or more have liver cysts detected by ultrasonography [1]. In autopsy series, liver cysts were found in about 90% of cases [1,2]. Liver cysts develop earlier in women than in men (Fig. 1) [1]. Similar findings were reported by Kaehny et al. [3] in patients aged less than 50 years; women had a higher prevalence of, and more numerous liver cysts than men, regardless of age and renal function. Females with liver cysts had had more pregnancies than those without liver cysts. These data suggest that the female hormonal environment may trigger or accelerate the expression and development of the liver cystic process.

   Liver cysts are thought to result from progressive dilatation of von Meyenburg's complexes (or biliary microhamartomas). These complexes are considered to represent the remnants of embryonic bile ductules which were formed in excess and did not involute after failing to establish a connection with canaliculi and interlobular bile ducts [1]. This view has recently been challenged by Ramos et al. [2]. These authors showed that microhamartomas were not observed in young patients and that their number or detectability increased with age. This was in striking contrast to results found by Karhunen [4]. In addition, biliary microhamartomas may contain bile-like material. Ramos et al. indicate that, initially, microhamartomas and microcysts may be connected to biliary canaliculi, whereas later, larger cysts become disconnected. Ramos et al. also suggest that epithelial hyperplasia is crucial in the formation of both liver and kidney cysts [2].

Cystic fluid results from secretion by the biliary-type epithelium of the cyst. The electrolyte composition of hepatic cyst fluid is similar to that of serum. Organic anions normally transported by hepatocytes are not transported into liver cysts. Both IgA and secretory components, and high glutamyltranspeptidase concentrations, are found in cyst fluid. The cyst secretion rate can be stimulated by intravenous administration of secretin, a hormone known to induce secretion by normal biliary epithelium [5]. This suggests that, conversely, somatostatin may decrease the liver cyst fluid formation rate.

The incidence of liver cyst complications has long been underestimated. These complications occur mainly in dialyzed or renal transplanted patients. Liver cyst infections are the most frequent complications (see review in [6]). Cholangiocarcinoma develops in very rare cases, as in other biliary diseases with bile duct proliferation, such as Caroli's disease [1]. Massive polycystic liver, which predominates in women, may be the source of severe discomfort and digestive disorders. The management of such patients is difficult. Cyst fenestration and segmental hepatic resection have recently been advocated [7].

In addition to cysts, other hepatobiliary changes may occasionally be encountered in ADPKD patients. Idiopathic dilatation of intrahepatic [8,9], or extrahepatic (J.P. Grünfeld unpublished cases), biliary tract has been observed. Congenital hepatic fibrosis (diffuse biliary fibroadenomatosis associated with enlarged fibrotic portal spaces), which is responsible for portal hypertension, is the characteristic liver lesion in autosomal recessive polycystic kidney disease (PKD). Rare cases of ADPKD with congenital hepatic fibrosis have, however, been reported. Four families with this association have recently been investigated by Cobben et al. [10]. The liver disease may have a slow rate of progression. Close linkage between the disease allele and DNA markers on the short arm of chromosome 16 has been demonstrated. In these families, the renal lesion is clearly transmitted in an autosomal dominant pattern, whereas congenital hepatic fibrosis has not been found to be vertically transmitted [10]. Several hypotheses have been considered, including the coexistence of the dominant ADPKD mutant gene and of the autosomal recessive PKD mutant gene in these kindreds.

Intracranial Aneurysms

The coexistence of ADPKD and ruptured intracranial aneurysm (ICA) was first reported in 1901 by Borelius (Lund) in a 38-year-old "Kavallerie-Offizier" [11]. In 1904 Dunger first emphasized this association and reported rupture of ICA in a 54-year-old woman with ADPKD whose daughter had died at the age of 26 from a pontine hemorrhage, which may have been due to a ruptured ICA [12]. Dunger therefore probably observed the first ADPKD family with clustering of ICA.

Information on the prevalence and complications of ICA in ADPKD may be found in previous papers [13,14,15]. Cases of subarachnoid hemorrhage have been reported in which no aneurysm was found [13]. Intracranial hemorrhage may occur in patients who are unaware of having ADPKD [16].

Intracranial aneurysms occur in the general population with an incidence of 1.2% to 7.8%. The role of inborn defects in the arterial wall has been put forward, since ICA may be associated with various inherited disorders (type IV Ehlers-Danlos syndrome, Marfan's syndrome, pseudoxanthoma elasticum and ADPKD); a large number of familial cases of ICA, not associated with a recognized inherited disorder have been reported, including eight identical twins who had aneurysms at the same site or at the mirror site [17]. Lozano and Leblanc have analyzed the data from 243 aneurysms in 177 patients from 74 families. They concluded that familial ICAs rupture at a smaller size and when the patient is younger (mean age of 42.3 years versus 51.4 years) than do cases of sporadic aneurysms. There is a similar sex distribution, a similar incidence of multiple aneurysms, and a similar incidence of females over males with multiple aneurysms. Anterior communicating artery aneurysms occur less often in familial than in sporadic cases [17].

It would be of interest to know the epidemiology of ICAs in ADPKD. No large study is so far available. In a Concerted Action of the European Economic Community, we have initiated a cooperative effort on this topic. In a preliminary survey made in France, Belgium and Switzerland, we collected data on 46 patients with ruptured ICA and ADPKD. The age distribution of these patients was similar to that found by Lozano and Leblanc in familial intracranial aneurysms not associated with other inherited defects; the mean age at rupture was 39 years. Approximately 30% of the patients were normotensive and 21 had normal renal function at rupture; only 2 were in end-stage renal failure. Thus, ICA rupture may occur in young patients, and in the absence of hypertension and/or renal function impairment.

Familial clustering of ICA in ADPKD has already been emphasized by others (see [6]). In our study, precise information was available in 37 families: "proven" ICA and "possible" ICA were found in 3 and 7 cases, respectively, i.e., an overall prevalence of 27%. Of note, Torres et al. found a positive family history of ICA in 32% of patients with symptomatic ICA and ADPKD. It should be stressed, however, that a similar positive family history of ICA was detected in 11% of asymptomatic ADPKD patients with negative routine screening for ICA [18].

Intracranial aneurysms are progressive in ADPKD, and a new ICA may develop after successful surgical cure of a rupture accident [19]. We have observed such occurrence in three patients, with the two ICA rupture episodes separated by an interval of from 7–13 years. Madonick et al. (cited in [13]) reported one case in which two episodes of subarachnoid hemorrhage had occurred, with recovery for five years.

The limitations of routine screening for occult ICAs in ADPKD have been extensively discussed by Levey et al. [15]. Using cranial computed tomography and magnetic resonance imaging, Torres et al. recently performed a prospective study in 96 ADPKD patients without central nervous system involvement. They detected no definite ICA [20]. This confirms that routine screening is not rewarding and probably not indicated. In contrast, screening is indicated in the following circumstances: when there is a positive family history of ICA, a previous accident of ICA rupture, and perhaps before major elective surgery, or in high-risk occupations. The best means of screening and the rate of re-screening remain to be determined in ADPKD patients at high risk for ICA.

Mitral Valve Prolapse

Hossack et al. [21] were the first to draw attention to the high prevalence of mitral-valve prolapse in ADPKD patients. Using echocardiography, they studied 163 patients with ADPKD, 130 unaffected family members, and 100 control subjects. In these three groups, the prevalence of mitral-valve prolapse was 26, 14, and 2%, respectively. There was no clear predominance in ADPKD females. A higher prevalence of mitral incompetence, aortic incompetence, tricuspid incompetence and tricuspid valve prolapsus was also found in the ADPKD patients [21]. This association has some clinical implications. As mitral valve prolapse may be complicated by cerebral embolization, this should be considered in the differential diagnosis of cerebrovascular accident in ADPKD patients. In addition, bacterial endocarditis may complicate mitral valve prolapse. Among non-ADPKD patients with this abnormality, those with systolic bruit and leaflet thickening are more prone to develop endocarditis than those without these features. Endocarditis complicating mitral valve prolapse must therefore be considered in ADPKD patients with fever [6].

Of interest, mitral-valve prolapse is a complication of some inherited connective tissue disorders – such as Marfan's syndrome, Ehlers-Danlos syndrome, osteogenesis imperfecta, and the joint hypermobility syndrome – some of which are also diseases predisposing to ICAs (see above). In addition, primary mitral valve prolapse, unassociated with other symptoms of connective tissue disease, can appear as an inherited autosomal dominant trait, a condition also found in familial intracranial aneurysms (see above). Complete concordance in monozygotic twins has been reported. The expression of the diseases is affected by sex, the incidence being higher in females [22]. In three such families, the segregation of the genes encoding the major fibrillar collagens present in valve tissue, collagens I and III, was analyzed by use of restriction enzyme site variants as genetic markers. The primary gene locus for mitral-valve prolapse is not linked to either of the two collagen I loci nor, probably, to the collagen III locus [22].

Other cardiovascular abnormalities, including abdominal aortic aneurysms and annuloaortic ectasia, have been found in ADPKD [6,21]. Dissection of the ascending thoracic aorta has recently been reported in an ADPKD patient after kidney transplantation; the condition required resection and insertion of a teflon graft [23]. This complication again underlines some analogy with Marfan's syndrome. The basic defect predisposing to cardiovascular abnormalities in ADPKD remains, however, unknown. Recent findings by Powell et al., showing that there is a familial tendency to abdominal aortic aneurysm, might be relevant [24]. These authors have shown that genetic variation in the haptoglobin and cholesterol ester protein genes (located on the *long* arm of chromosome 16) appears to influence dilatation of the abdominal aorta. It might be of interest to test this hypothesis in ADPKD patients with intracranial or abdominal aortic aneurysm.

Acknowledgments. We thank Doreen Broneer for her invaluable secretarial assistance, and we thank all the nephrologists who participated in the study on intracranial aneurysms in ADPKD.

References

1. Grünfeld JP, Albouze G, Jungers P, Landais P, Dana A, Droz D, Moynot A, Lafforgue B, Boursztyn E, Franco D (1984) Liver changes and complications in adult polycystic kidney disease. Adv Nephrol 14:1-20
2. Ramos A, Torres VE, Holley KE, Offord KP, Rakela J, Ludwig J (1990) The liver in autosomal dominant polycystic kidney disease. Arch Pathol Lab Med 114:180-184
3. Kaehny WD, Manco-Johnson M, Johnson M, Tangel DJ, Gabow PA (1988) Influence of sex on liver manifestations of autosomal dominant polycystic kidney disease (ADPKD). Kidney Int 33:196
4. Karhunen PJ (1986) Adult polycystic liver disease and biliary microhamartomas (von Meyenburg's complexes). Acta pathol Microbiol Immunol Scand [A] 94:397-400
5. Everson GT, Emmett M, Brown WR, Redmond P, Thickman D (1990) Functional similarities of hepatic cystic and biliary epithelium: Studies of fluid constituents and in vivo secretion in response to secretin. Hepatology 11:557-565
6. Pirson Y, Grünfeld JP (to be published) Autosomal-dominant polycystic kidney disease. In: Cameron JS, Davison AM, Grünfeld JP, Kerr DNS, Ritz E (eds) Oxford Textbook of Clinical Nephrology. Oxford University Press, Oxford
7. Newman KD, Torres VE, Rakela J, Nagorney DM (1990) Treatment of highly symptomatic polycystic liver disease: preliminary experience with a combined hepatic resection fenestration procedure. Ann Surg 212:30-37
8. Terada T, Nakanuma Y (1988) Congenital biliary dilatation in autosomal dominant adult polycystic disease of the liver and kidneys. Arch Pathol Lab Med 112:1113-1116
9. Jordan D, Harpaz N, Thung SN (1989) Caroli's disease and adult polycystic kidney disease: a rarely recognized association. Liver 9:30-35
10. Cobben JM, Breuning MH, Schoots C, ten Kate LP, Zerres K (to be published) Congenital hepatic fibrosis in adult polycystic kidney disease. Kidney Int
11. Borelius J (1901) Zur Genese und klinischen Diagnose der polycystischen Degeneration der Nieren. Nord Med Arkiv I:1-13
12. Dunger R (1904) Zur Lehre von der Cystenniere, mit besonderer Berücksichtigung ihrer Heredität. Beitr Path Anat 35:445-509
13. Brown RAP (1951) Polycystic disease of the kidneys and intracranial aneurysms: The etiology and interrelationship of these conditions: Review of recent literature and report of seven cases in which both conditions coexisted. Glasgow Med J 32:333-348
14. Bigelow NH (1953) The association of polycystic kidneys with intracranial aneurysms and other related disorders. Am J Med Sci 225:485-494
15. Levey AS, Pauker SG, Kassirer JP (1983) Occult intracranial aneurysms in polycystic kidney disease. When is cerebral arteriography indicated? N Engl J Med 308:986-994
16. Ryu SJ (1990) Intracranial hemorrhage in patients with polycystic kidney disease. Stroke 21:291-294
17. Lozano AM, Leblanc R (1987) Familial intracranial aneurysms. J Neurosurg 66:522-528
18. Torres VE, Forbes GS, Wiebers DO, Erickson SB, Smith LH (1987) Value of routine screening for intracranial aneurysms in autosomal dominant polycystic kidney disease. Xth International Congress of Nephrology, London, p 45
19. Chauveau D, Sirieix ME, Schillinger F, Legendre C, Grünfeld JP (1990) Recurrent rupture of intracranial aneurysms in autosomal dominant polycystic disease. Br Med J 301:966-967
20. Torres VE, Wiebers DQ, Forbes GS (1990) Cranial computed tomography and magnetic resonance imaging in autosomal dominant polycystic kidney disease. JASN 1:84-90
21. Hossack KF, Leddy CL, Johnson AM, Schrier RW, Gabow PA (1988) Echocardiographic findings in autosomal dominant polycystic kidney disease. N Engl J Med 319:907-912

22. Wordsworth P, Ogilvie D, Akhras F, Jackson G, Sykes B (1989) Genetic segregation analysis of familial mitral valve prolapse shows no linkage to fibrillar collagen genes. Br Heart J 61:300–306

23. Fitzpatrick PM, Torres VE, Charboneau W, Offord KP, Holley KE, Zincke H (1990) Long-term outcome of renal transplantation in autosomal dominant polycystic kidney disease. Am J Kidney Dis 15:1535–543

24. Powell JT, Bashir A, Dawson S, Vine N, Henney AM, Humphries SE, Greenhalgh RM (1990) Genetic variation on chromosome 16 is associated with abdominal aortic aneurysm. Clin Sci 78:13–16

Malignancy and Cystic Disease

Isao Ishikawa[1]

SUMMARY. The natural history of acquired renal cystic disease (ARCD) has started to become clear over the last 10 years. It is known, for example, that the longer the duration of hemodialysis, the more numerous are the cysts that develop, and that male dialysis patients with the disease tend to reveal more extensive cystic degeneration than do female dialysis patients. In addition, it has been shown that acquired cystic disease regresses after successful renal transplantation. A 10-year prospective study by the present authors has revealed that the incidence of renal cell carcinoma in dialysis patients is one in 249 patient-years. The study also shows that there are two types of renal cell carcinoma in dialysis patients; one occurring in older patients after a short time on hemodialysis and involving fewer renal cysts, and the other, which occurs with extensive cyst formation, in relatively young patients after long-term dialysis. In the latter condition particularly, the development of cysts is closely related to the development of renal malignancy. Thus, there is much circumstantial evidence for a causal relation between acquired renal cystic disease and renal cell carcinoma, however, as yet, there is no direct proof of this via molecular biological and other techniques.

Introduction

Acquired renal cystic disease involves the bilateral development of multiple renal cysts in uremic patients with an initial cyst-unrelated renal disease [1]. Dunnill et al. [2] have pointed out that the major complications of this acquired cystic disease are renal cell carcinoma and hemorrhage due to cyst rupture; the incidence of renal cell carcinoma has been shown, in a previous summary of the literature, to be high [1]. The pathologic investigation by Dunnill et al. [2] indicates that the label acquired

---

[1]Division of Nephrology, Department of Internal Medicine, Kanazawa Medical University, Uchinada, Kahoku, Ishikawa, 92002 Japan

cystic disease of the kidney may encompass a whole spectrum from cyst to adenoma to renal cell carcinoma. Similarly, Hughson et al. report that atypical cysts may be seen in cases of these kidney disorders. These observations suggest that epithelial hyperplasia or proliferation is a likely complication of acquired cystic disease of the kidney [3].

Therefore, we evaluated the incidence of renal cell carcinoma during a 10-year prospective study, and undertook a series of nationwide questionnaire studies on renal malignancy in hemodialysis patients. Moreover, in this paper we review recent developments concerning acquired cystic disease and renal cell carcinoma in dialysis patients.

Natural History of Acquired Renal Cystic Disease

Acquired renal cystic disease is characterized by the bilateral development of multiple cysts in kidneys that are uremic or have sustained nephron loss. This disease appears typically in long-term hemodialysis or in continuous ambulatory peritoneal dialysis (CAPD) patients [1,4]. However, acquired cysts may also appear in native kidneys in predialysis periods or at times of poor graft function [5]. The incidence of acquired cystic disease is 7%–26% in predialysis periods, 35.2%–79.3% in dialysis patients [1,2,6,7], 35% in CAPD patients, [8] and 33% in pediatric dialysis patients [9].

The most important risk factor associated with acquired cystic disease is the duration of uremia or duration of dialysis [1]. The longer either has been present, the more severe the cystic changes that appear in the kidneys. Usually, the original kidney disease causing uremia or chronic renal failure is unrelated to the development of acquired cysts [2], however, every end-stage renal disease has a potential link with cyst formation; even in cases of graft failure where acquired cysts develop in the transplanted kidney, more severe cystic changes may appear in the native kidney [5]. In our study, the incidence of acquired cysts was 43.7% in all dialysis patients and 90% in those on hemodialysis for more than 10 years [1].

A second major variable influencing the onset and proliferation of acquired cysts is the patient's sex [1]. Male patients on dialysis developed more of these acquired cysts and displayed greater kidney enlargement due to cystic changes than did female patients in this study (Fig. 1). In 1979, the mean bilateral kidney volume was 80.5 ± 32.3 ml (mean ± SD) in male patients and 66.4 ± 32.3 ml in female patients after a mean hemodialysis duration of 3.3 years. Ten years later, these values had increased to 207 ± 189.7 ml and 86.3 ± 55.8 ml, respectively [10]. These figures represent a 2.7 ± 1.7-fold enlargement of male kidneys during the 10 year period, but only a slight, statistically insignificant, increase in female kidney size.

Recently, several reports have been published concerning the development of acquired cysts in patients on CAPD [4,8]; they have quoted incidences of acquired cysts [4,8] and renal cell carcinoma [11] in CAPD patients, similar to those mentioned above. However, the exact difference between hemodialysis patients and CAPD patients in severity of acquired cystic disease is not known.

Figure 2 illustrates a third factor affecting the development of acquired cystic disease—successful renal transplantation [12]. During a serial study in recipients with good graft function, the mean volume of bilateral native kidneys of 14 patients subjected to hemodialysis for more than 3 years was found to be 82.1 ± 56.4 ml

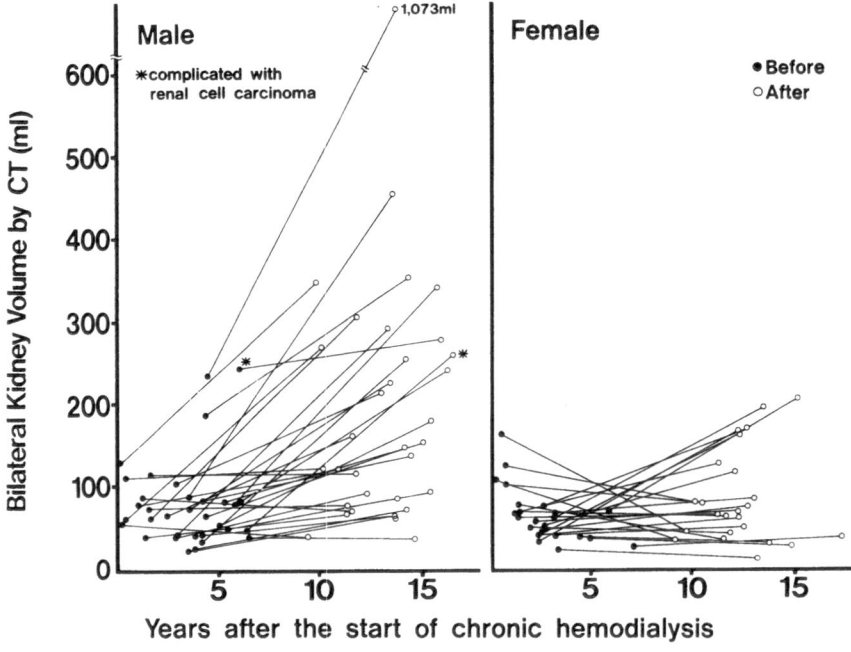

Fig. 1. Ten year follow up study of bilateral kidney volume in hemodialysis patients. The mean kidney volume in male patients after 10 years of follow up increased significantly due to acquired cysts. CT, computerized tomography. From [10] with permission)

prior to kidney transplant; however, this decreased to 42.9 ± 10.8 ml within 1–3 months of surgery, to 35.6 ± 5.9 ml within 1 year, and to 33.8 ± 10.0 ml within 3 years. The rate of kidney shrinkage was greater in patients with more extensive cyst formation (Fig. 2). In another study, the overall incidence of cystic transformation after renal transplantation was calculated to change from 36.1% (base line study) to 42.6% (follow up study) [Ishikawa I, unpublished data]. Thus, the incidence of patients with renal cysts is slightly less in allograft recipients than in hemodialysis patients; however, severity of cystic transformation and change in the kidney volume (as a likely reflection of changes in both cyst size and number) both differ in the two treatment groups. The native kidneys following transplantation are severely atrophic and have only one, or a few visible, cysts, a situation entirely different from that seen in hemodialysis patients.

The mechanism accounting for such rapid regression of acquired cysts after transplantation is not clear; however it may be very important in leading us to an understanding of the pathogenesis of acquired cystic disease. One explanation could be that the disappearance of uremic growth factor after transplantation [12,13] may bring about cyst regression. Another possibility is that the reduction of osmotic load to the remaining glomeruli and/or the improvement of transepithelial sodium movement may cause filtered fluid to diminish, and hence the cysts to reduce in size and number. On the other hand, this regression of acquired cysts is one line of evidence that they are induced "acquired" in nature.

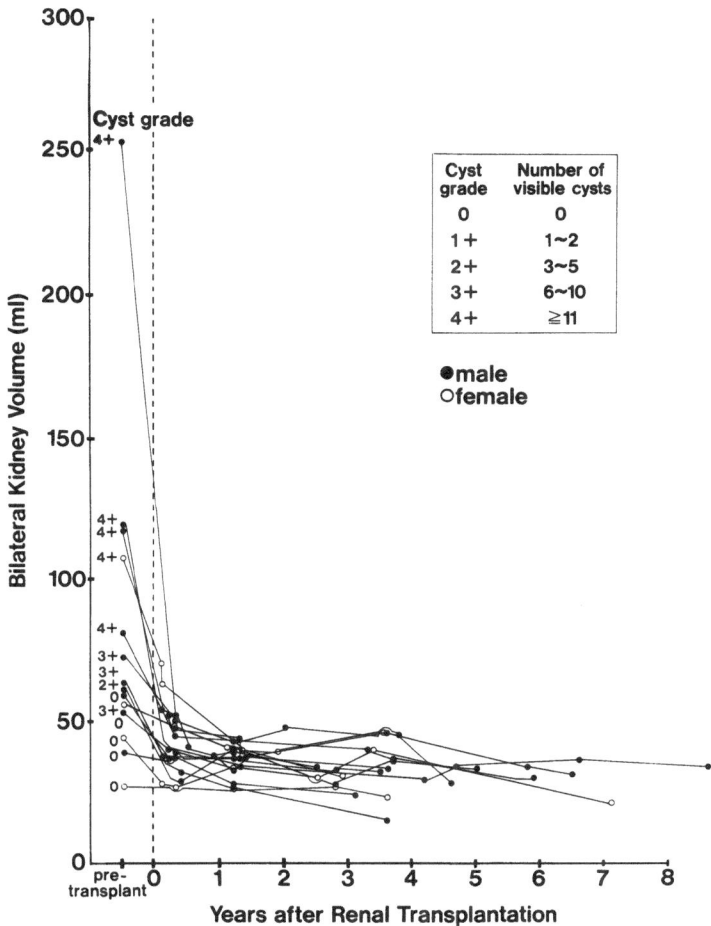

Fig. 2. Volume of native kidneys after renal transplantation. After successful transplantation, mean kidney volume decreases due to the regression of acquired cysts

Characteristics of Renal Cell Carcinoma in Dialysis Patients

It has been suggested that the prevalence of renal cell carcinoma in dialysis patients is 1.4%–2.0% [1], or 7–40 times higher than in the general population. However, some authors [8,11,12] are skeptical of this reported high incidence because the figures were obtained by investigators with high levels of interest in renal cell carcinoma and so may be subject to bias.

In our ten year prospective study of 96 patients begun in 1979, one renal cell carcinoma was detected in 249 patient-years [10]. Over the entire patient-time dialysis period, there were 6 renal cell carcinomas in 1,070 patient-years (1/178 patient-years). The incidence was higher in male patients (1/140 patient-years) than in

Table 1. Renal cell carcinoma in hemodialysis patients (questionnaire studies[a] performed in Japan)

Number of renal cell carcinoma cases	364
male	299(82.1%)
female	65(17.9%)
Mean age (years)	51.2 ± 11.6[b]
Mean duration of hemodialysis (months)	90.8 ± 55.8
Presence of ARCD (%)	276/350(78.9%)
Number of patients with metastases (%)	61/346(17.6%)

[a]results of the past five questionnaires, performed in 1982, 1984, 1986, 1988, and 1990
[b]mean $\pm$ SD
ARCD, acquired renal cystic disease

female patients (1/369 patient-years). This indicates that the incidence of renal cancer in dialysis patients is then 57–134 times higher than the 3–7 per 100000 persons per year seen in the general population. These figures may be applicable only to Japanese patients, since differences in the rates of several cancers have been observed between Japan and the United States. However, the incidence of renal cell carcinoma in Japan is lower than that in the US and Europe, although the incidence of chronic glomerulonephritis is higher in Japan. There are a large number of transplant patients in the US and Europe and many hemodialysis patients in Japan, the latter being screened quite well for renal cell carcinoma.

Table 1 illustrates sex differences in the occurrence of renal cell carcinoma, male cases outweighing female ones by 299 to 65 (82.1% were male patients). Mean age of these patients was 51.2 ± 11.6 years, which is significantly younger than in the general population (64 ± 12 years). One of the other characteristics of renal cell carcinoma as a complication of acquired cysts is that it occurs at higher rates in patients that have been hemodialyzed for longer duration: a survey of the literature reveals a prevalence of 1.5% among all dialysis patients and 5% in those with a greater than 10 year history of dialysis (1). For Japan, questionnaire studies performed by us indicate that the mean duration of hemodialysis was 90.8 ± 55.8 months (Table 1). Thus, it seems at present that there are 2 types of renal cell carcinoma in dialysis patients [15], one afflicting younger people on long-term dialysis and characterized by extensive cystic formation (Figs. 3 and 4), and the other developing in older patients with a short history of dialysis and manifesting few or no cysts. This is illustrated in Fig. 3.

Recently Chung-Park et al. [16] have described renal cell carcinomas in end stage kidney disease before dialysis treatment [16]. In addition, cases of renal malignancy occurring prior to and after dialysis treatment have been collected by the Japanese Society of Dialysis Therapy (1988). This research has shown that malignancy is most common within 1 year before and after the start of dialysis therapy. It may be that a state of immunodeficiency due to uremia causes malignancy, with the treatment modality, whether hemodialysis or CAPD, apparently unrelated to tumor development. There is no relation between the original disease and the incidence of renal cell carcinoma. The incidence of autosomal dominant polycystic kidney disease (ADPKD) was not high, however, and analgesic nephropathy was not evident in our study.

The effect of renal transplantation on the development of renal cell carcinoma in dialysis patients has been investigated previously [Ishikawa I, to be published, 1991].

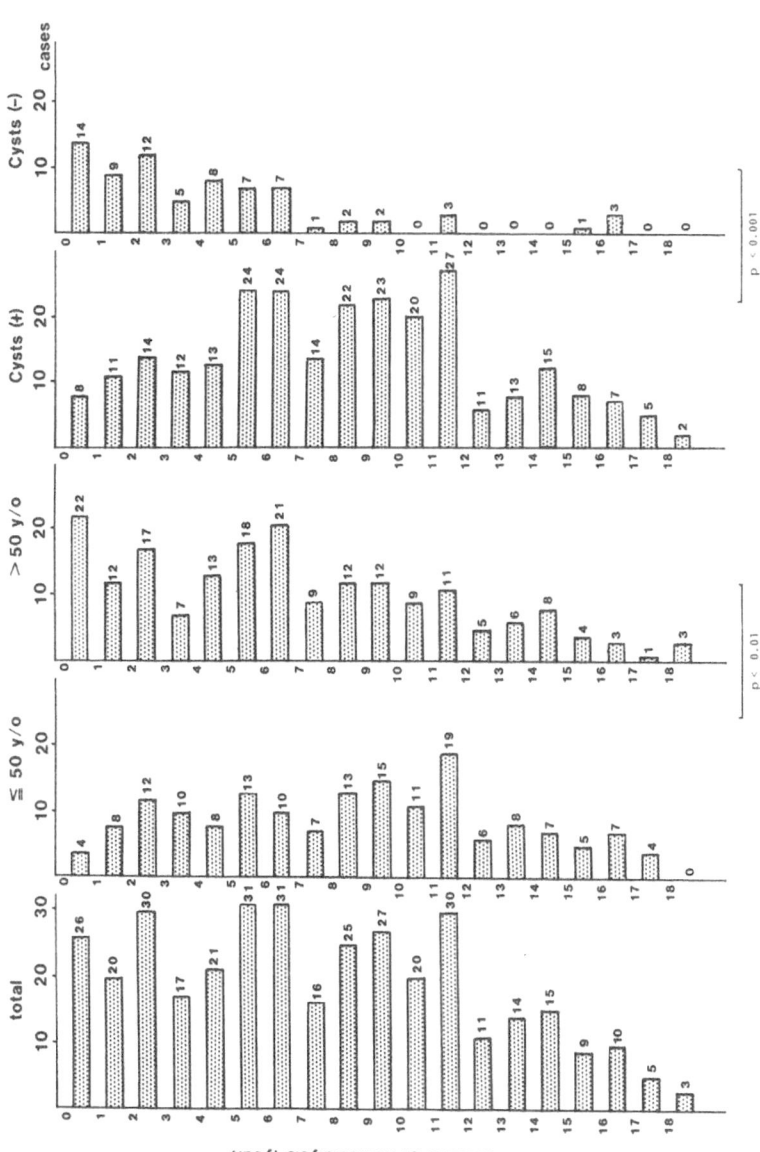

Fig. 3. Patients with renal cell carcinoma ranked (*vertically*) according to duration of hemodialysis (*years*) and (*horizontally*) according to age (*below and above 50 years old* (*y/o*)) as well as according to the *presence* or *absence of cysts* (+) or (−)

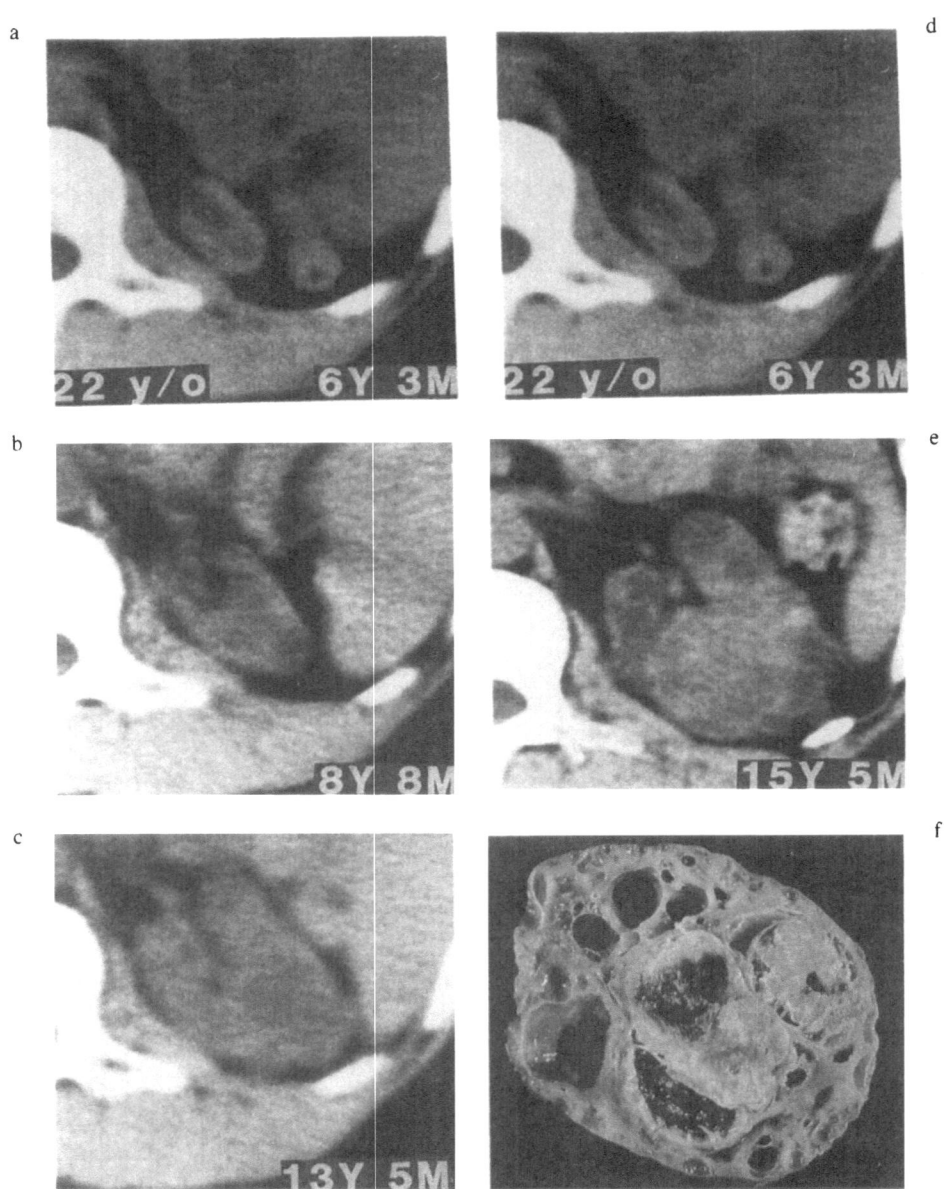

Fig. 4a-f. Development of renal cell carcinoma and acquired renal cysts in long-term hemodialysis patients. The mean kidney size increased over time due to acquired cysts. No trace of renal tumor was noted at 14 years and 4 months of hemodialysis (**d**). A renal tumor 4.5 cm in diameter and surrounded by multiple cysts was seen at 15 years and 5 months (**e**). From [10] with permission)

Acquired cyst regression following transplantation [13] tends to favor the view that the incidence of renal cell carcinoma decreases after such surgery, however, there is no direct evidence for this at present. Rather, Penn and Brunson [17] report a high incidence of renal cell carcinoma after transplantation, especially where cyclosporine is used. These authors list 101 cases with another 16 case reports. We observed one 39 year-old male patient, who was diagnosed as having a 2.4 cm diameter renal cell carcinoma 8 years and 4 months after successful renal transplantation [Ishikawa I, to be published, 1991], but serial CT scans suggested it to have been present before the operation. Therefore, not all renal cell carcinomas diagnosed after transplantation necessarily developed postoperatively, and in fact Noronha et al. point out that there is a low prevalence of metastasizing renal cell carcinomas in transplant recipients [18]. However, a number of case reports do not support this observation [19].

In Japan, as of 1990, 4 cases of renal cell carcinoma have been diagnosed after renal transplantation from 6176 patients, and 364 cases have been diagnosed during hemodialysis from populations of 88553 patients, respectively, undergoing each treatment modality. Since the number of allograft recipients is growing steadily, the question of whether or not the incidence of this cancer decreases after transplantation has become very important.

The biological activity of renal cell carcinomas in dialysis patients is open to question [20]. In a small study, Hughson et al. reported a metastatic rate of 27%, while our own questionnaire survey led us to a figure of 61 patients out of 346 (17.6%) with renal cell carcinoma. Though there are some limitations to questionnaire studies, the following figures were derived: 36 of the 61, 32 male and 4 female patients, displayed extensive acquired cysts, had a mean duration of hemodialysis of 117.1 ± 48.5 months, and a mean age of 55.9 ± 11.1 years; and 20 of the 61 showed no or few cysts, had a mean age of 58.6 ± 37.6 years, and a mean duration of hemodialysis of 50.6 ± 37.6 months. Tumor size was 6.8 ± 3.7 cm in the former group and 7.9 ± 4.5 cm in the latter. The mean duration of hemodialysis is, therefore, significantly longer in cases of metastatic renal cell carcinoma where cystic alteration is extensive than in those cases where there are no or few cysts. It should be noted that reports of metastatic renal cell carcinoma have been increasing recently [21,22].

On the other hand, Hughson et al. describe this tumor as a pathologist's tumor, while other researchers state that they have never seen a metastatic renal cell carcinoma in dialysis patients [8,12,20]; for example, Katz et al. find no such cancer in 353 people undergoing dialysis [8]. Nevertheless, the combination of renal cell carcinoma with acquired renal cystic disease was observed in 276/350 cases (78.9%) in our questionnaire studies.

Evidence for a Causal Relationship Between Acquired Cysts and Renal Cell Carcinoma

Gibson [23] describes four types of relationship between cyst and renal cell carcinoma; (1) chance occurrence of the two diseases together, (2) cystic degeneration or regression or healing of renal cell carcinoma, (3) a tumor originating within a cyst (rare), which we deal with here, and (4) a cyst originating distal to a tumor.

In dialysis patients, there is some circumstantial evidence that a causal link exists between acquired cysts and renal tumors. Extensive cystic transformation often accompanies renal cell carcinoma, and both acquired cystic disease and renal cell carcinoma develop more often in male patients than in female patients. Also, this form of carcinoma occurs in dialysis patients at a relatively younger age than in the general population. Therefore, young male patients with long-term hemodialysis and extensive cystic changes tend to have renal cell carcinoma as a complication [15]. Further support for a causal relation between acquired cysts and renal cell carcinoma is provided by the pathological observation that acquired cystic disease of the kidney often involves a continuum from epithelial hyperplasia to cyst, to atypical cyst, to adenoma and adenocarcinoma [2]. Such pathologic changes have been described by many investigators. Experiments with transgenic mice have proven that epithelial hyperplasia [3] leads directly to cyst and adenoma formation [24].

The origin of renal tumors and of epithelial cells lining the cysts is mainly the proximal tubules; immunohistochemical examination, using lectin [25], together with the study of hippuran excretion have shown that epithelial cells lining cyst walls are derived mainly from proximal tubular cells; Noronha et al. [18] have reported that both cytokeratin and vimentin are stained in microadenomas (therefore, epithelium lining atypical cysts in dialysis patients shows active proliferation). However, there is no direct proof for a causal relationship between acquired cysts and renal tumors, i.e., that acquired cysts cause renal tumors or that cyst walls change to become malignant. It is also probable that the tubular epithelium in acquired cystic kidneys, proliferating either due to ischemia [26] or environmental factors [14], is closely related to the development of renal cell carcinoma, while there is a morphologic gradation from atypical cyst to carcinoma in patients with phacomatosis (atypical cysts and renal cell carcinomas exhibit similar DNA indices and euploidy). In general, it seems evident that acquired cystic kidney demonstrates high proliferative activity that is likely to result in cyst, adenoma, and adenocarcinoma formation.

The mechanisms responsible for the initiation and development of these cysts and tumors have yet to be elucidated; in future investigations we intend to shed light on this area using cytogenetic or molecular biological techniques, such as those used by Vogelstein et al. in their study of chromosomal abnormalities in the progression of colonic polyposis to metastatic adenocarcinoma of the colon [27]. Furthermore, renal cyst growth factor needs to be investigated more thoroughly [28,29].

Screening for Acquired Cysts and Renal Cell Carcinoma

Many, but not all, investigators agree that screening for renal cell carcinoma is necessary. It is also generally agreed that CT scanning is better for this purpose than sonographic examination [30]; however, 60% of cysts are usually smaller than 0.2cm, which is far beyond the detection capability of either of these procedures.

Some conservative investigators point out that patients with end stage renal disease already have a markedly reduced life expectancy and, since the true outcome of acquired cystic disease is not yet known, these investigators are reluctant to apportion resources for screening [31]. Results from our 10 year follow-up and questionnaire studies in Japan lead us to contest this viewpoint; we feel that periodic screening of long-term dialysis patients may be useful for detection of small renal cell carcinomas. Yearly CT screening of patients, especially males, on hemodialysis is highly advisable, and should begin the year treatment starts. The relatively low incidence of renal cell carcinoma in female dialysis patients and in transplant recipients with good graft function suggests that biannual screening would be sufficient in such cases, providing that the prevalence of rapidly growing cancer is proven to be low. The only drawback of screening is, as usual, cost.

References

1. Ishikawa I (1990) Acquired renal cystic disease. In: Gardner KD Jr, Bernstein J (eds) The Cystic Kidney. Kluwer, Dordrecht, pp 351–377
2. Dunnill MS, Millard PR, Oliver D (1977) Acquired cystic disease of the kidneys: A hazard of long-term intermittent maintenance haemodialysis. J Clin Pathol 30:868–877
3. Bernstein J, Evan AP, Gardner KD Jr (1987) Epithelial hyperplasia in human polycystic kidney diseases: Its role in pathogenesis and risk of neoplasia. Am J Pathol 129:92–101
4. Ishikawa I, Moncrief JW, Aguirre F, Brindley BW, Mott CL (1984) Acquired cystic kidney disease in continuous ambulatory peritoneal dialysis patients. In: Maekawa M et al. (eds) Machine free dialysis for patient convenience. ISAO, Cleveland, pp 131–133
5. Ishikawa I, Shikura N, Kitada H, Yuri T, Shinoda A, Nakazawa T (1989) Severity of acquired renal cysts in native kidneys and renal allograft with long-standing poor function. Am J Kidney Dis 14:18–24
6. Grantham JJ, Levine E (1985) Acquired cystic disease: Replacing one kidney disease with another. Kidney Int 28:99–105
7. Gardner KD Jr (1984) Acquired renal cystic disease and renal adenocarcinoma in patients on long-term hemodialysis. New Engl J Med 310:390
8. Katz A, Sombolos K, Oreopoulos DG (1987) Acquired cystic disease of the kidney in association with chronic ambulatory peritoneal dialysis. Am J Kidney Dis 9:426–429
9. Leichter HE, Dietrich R, Salusky IB, Foley J, Cohen AH, Kangarloo H, Fine RN (1988) Acquired cystic kidney disease in children undergoing long-term dialysis. Pediatr Nephrol 2:8–11
10. Ishikawa I, Saito Y, Shikura N, Kitada H, Shinoda A, Suzuki S (1990) Ten-year prospective study on the development of renal cell carcinoma on the development of renal cell carcinoma in dialysis patients. Am J Kidney Dis 16:452–458
11. Fallon B, Williams RD (1989) Renal cancer associated with acquired cystic disease of the kidney and chronic renal failure. Semin Urol 7:228–236
12. Endreny R (1990) Acquired cystic disease. Nephron 55:222
13. Ishikawa I, Yuri T, Kitada H, Shinoda A (1983) Regression of acquired cystic disease of the kidney after successful renal transplantation. Am J Nephrol 3:310–314
14. Grantham JJ (1990) Polycystic kidney disease: Neoplasia in disguise. Am J Kidney Dis 15:110–116
15. Ishikawa I, Shinoda A (1983) Renal adenocarcinoma with or without acquired cysts in chronic hemodialysis patients. Clin Nephrol 20:321–322
16. Chung-Park M, Parveen T, Lam M (1989) Acquired cystic disease of the kidneys and renal cell carcinoma in chronic renal insufficiency without dialysis treatment. Nephron 53:157–161
17. Penn I, Brunson ME (1988) Cancers after cyclosporine therapy. Transplant Proc 20:885–892
18. Noronha IL, Ritz E, Waldherr R, Stein G, Fassbinder W (1989) Renal cell carcinoma in dialysis patients with acquired renal cysts. Nephrol Dial Transplant 4:763–769
19. Ludmerer KM, Kissane JM (1988) Clinicopathologic conference. A new chest mass in a 49-year-old man with a transplanted kidney. Am J Med 84:121–128
20. Miller LR, Soffer O, Nassar VH, Kutner MH (1989) Acquired renal cystic disease in end-stage renal disease: an autopsy study of 155 cases. Am J Nephrol 9:322–328

21. MacDougall ML, Welling LW, Wiegmann TB (1987) Renal adenocarcinoma and acquired cystic disease in chronic hemodialysis patients. Am J Kidney Dis 9:166-171
22. Almirall J, Mallofre C, Campistol JM, Montoliu J, Ribalta T, Revert L (1989) Metastatic renal cell carcinoma in hemodialysis patient with acquired renal cystic disease. Nephron 52:96-97
23. Gibson TE (1954) Interrelationship of renal cysts and tumors: report of 3 cases. J Urol 71:241-252
24. MacKay K, Striker LJ, Pinkert CA, Brinster RL, Striker GE (1987) Glomerulosclerosis and renal cysts in mice transgenic for the early region of SV40. Kidney Int 32:827-837
25. Ishikawa I, Horiguchi T, Shikura N (1989) Lectin peroxidase conjugate reactivity in acquired cystic disease of the kidney. Nephron 51:211-214
26. Cohen EP, Elliott WC (1990) The role of ischemia in acquired cystic kidney disease. Am J Kidney Dis 15:55-60
27. Vogelstein B, Fearon ER, Hamilton SR, Kern SE, Preisinger AC, Leppert M, Nakamura Y, White R, Smits AMM, Bos JL (1988) Genetic alterations during colorectal-tumor development. New Engl J Med 319:525-532
28. Marcus MD, Seline P, Long S, Torrence RJ, Huang JS, Clayman RV (1989) Characterization of a renal cyst growth factor (RCGF). J Urol 141:294A
29. Klotz L, Kulcarni C, Mills G (1989) Analysis of a human renal cell growth factor present in sera of patients with end stage renal disease. J Urol 141:297A
30. Taylor AJ, Cohen EP, Erickson SJ, Olson DL, Foley WD (1989) Renal imaging in long-term dialysis patients: a comparison of CT and sonography. AJR 153:765-767
31. Mindell HJ (1989) Imaging studies for screening native kidneys in long-term dialysis patients. AJR 153:768-769

Continuous Ambulatory Peritoneal Dialysis (CAPD)

Chair: Karl D. Nolph (USA)
Yoshindo Kawaguchi (Japan)

Overview of Continuous Ambulatory Peritoneal Dialysis – 1990

Karl D. Nolph[1]

SUMMARY. As of early 1990, the number of patients maintained on chronic peritoneal dialysis world-wide approached 50,000. In the United States, approximately 80% were on continuous ambulatory peritoneal dialysis (CAPD) while 15% used cycler techniques such as continuous cyclic peritoneal dialysis or nightly peritoneal dialysis. In other countries, the percentage of patients on chronic peritoneal dialysis on CAPD is presumably even higher. Studies from North America, Europe, and Australia-New Zealand all agree that mortalities on CAPD and hemodialysis are not significantly different if populations with similar characteristics are compared. Technique survivals have tended to be lower in CAPD than in hemodialysis, even with population adjustments. Differences in technique survival can, in part, be attributed to the tendency for patients to transfer from CAPD to hemodialysis after severe or frequent peritonitis. However, evidence continues to accumulate from multiple countries that disconnect devices, such as the Y-set, can reduce the rate of peritonitis to less than one episode per 20 patient months. As peritonitis rates decrease, transfer rates decrease and technique survival improves. In some Y-set populations, technique survivals similar to hemodialysis have been reported. Current research interests in CAPD are focused on improved catheters, exit site care, verification that CAPD may preserve GFR better than hemodialysis, manipulation of lymphatic absorption to enhance ultrafiltration, more sophisticated models of peritoneal transport, improved control of calcium and phosphorus without aluminum, and individualization of peritoneal dialysis prescriptions to assure adequacy.

[1]Department of Medicine, University of Missouri, MA436 Health Sciences Center, VA Hospital and Dalton Research Center, Columbia, MO 65212, USA

Demographics

As of early 1990, there were near 50,000 patients world-wide maintained on chronic peritoneal dialysis (A. Holden, Baxter Healthcare, personal communication). In the United States, there were about 19,000 patients on chronic peritoneal dialysis, with approximately 85% of these on continuous ambulatory peritoneal dialysis (CAPD). The other 15% utilized cycler techniques, such as continuous cyclic peritoneal dialysis (CCPD) and nightly peritoneal dialysis.

In an industrial survey of the USA, Europe, Japan, Latin America, South America, and the Far East, the overall population on chronic peritoneal dialysis was found to have grown an average of 13% during calendar year 1989, while the hemodialysis population grew an average of 7% during the same period (A. Holden, Baxter Healthcare, personal communication).

On a worldwide basis, it's estimated that near 13% of dialysis patients are maintained on chronic peritoneal dialysis (mainly CAPD) while 87% are on chronic hemodialysis. This distribution varies markedly from country to country, however. For example, in the United States, the percentage is estimated to be near 17%, while in the United Kingdom, the percentage on chronic peritoneal dialysis is near 45%–50%. In the USA, there are larger PD programs in centers where 39% of the dialysis population is on chronic peritoneal dialysis; also, the percentage of patients on chronic peritoneal dialysis is higher in the midwest than in other sections of the country.

The increasing role of CAPD/CCPD in the United States is reported in the 1989 Annual Data Report of the United States Renal Data System [1]. An increase in the percentage of patients being treated by CAPD/CCPD from 1980 to 1987 is documented. These therapies were used in the 1984 cohort of patients with polycystic kidney disease to a slightly greater extent than in the 1984 cohort with other forms of primary renal disease. This suggests that there are very few patients with polycystic kidney disease that cannot tolerate peritoneal dialysis because of the space occupied by the enlarged kidneys. Near one-third of new end stage renal disease patients in the USA are thought to have diabetic nephropathy and this is reflected in increasing percentages of diabetic patients on all forms of dialysis. In the 1984 cohort, white patients were more likely to be treated with CAPD/CCPD than blacks. Percentages of patients on CAPD/CCPD are much higher in the pediatric population than in the adult population.

Patient Survivals

Numerous comparisons of patient survival on CAPD and hemodialysis have been published [2–6]. All agree that age and the presence or absence of diabetes mellitus are major determinants of mortality on chronic dialysis therapy. Comparisons of CAPD and hemodialysis must be of similar populations or must use statistical tools to correct for the distribution of these and other risk factors. Either by direct comparison of similar populations or by statistical adjustments, mortality rates for CAPD and hemodialysis populations appear to be essentially identical. Some of the reports have suggested even lower mortalities with CAPD in the elderly [5,6]. In the recent report from Australia/New Zealand, lower mortality rates with CAPD were found in diabetics [5].

Technique Survivals – the Impact of Falling Peritonitis Rates

Until recently, most comparisons of technique survivals between CAPD and hemodialysis have shown better results with hemodialysis [3,5,6]. Technique survival refers to percentages of patients, by actuarial analysis, still on dialysis and still on their original dialysis treatment. Death, kidney transplantation, or recovery of renal function are considered losses to risk and not dropout events. A technique failure mainly implies transfer to another mode of dialysis. Many factors may contribute to decisions to transfer, such as development of visual difficulties, severe arthritis, or stroke. Failure to control serum concentrations of nitrogenous metabolites or failure to control edema are rare reasons for transfer (probably less than 2% of patients). Doubtful patients are often given a trial on CAPD, since the training period is short and they can be promptly transferred if things do not go well. Although this can account for CAPD transfers, in part, it allows some doubtful patients to succeed and be offered the benefits of the home therapy. Severe or frequent peritonitis is probably the main reason for the lower technique survival rates with CAPD than with hemodialysis. Registry data from North America and Canada suggest that peritonitis can account for over 30% of transfers from CAPD to hemodialysis [3,7]. However, since those reports were made, peritonitis rates have been decreasing in Europe, Canada, and the United States with the use of disconnect devices such as the Y-set [8,9]. Rates of less than one episode every 20 months are frequently reported. In a population of patients on CAPD for over five years with the Y-set, 49% were still peritonitis-free after five years [4]. Technique survivals similar to those of hemodialysis are reported in such programs. One Italian center using the Y-set has reported technique survivals that are actually better than those on hemodialysis [9]. A multicenter study in the USA has been monitoring technique survivals and has shown improved technique survivals in more recently trained patient cohorts [10].

Peritoneal Membrane Stability

Numerous studies have demonstrated preservation of peritoneal membrane function over many years [4,11,12]. The use of dialysis solutions containing lactate (rather than acetate), the rapid diagnosis and treatment of peritonitis with early catheter removal in refractory cases, and the avoidance of chlorhexidine as an antiseptic have dramatically decreased the incidence of peritoneal sclerosis in countries where it was previously observed [13]. Over time, many patients show some increase in peritoneal permeability and an increased need for more hypertonic exchanges. Such changes may be associated with submesothelial fibrosis, loss of microvilli, and patchy mesothelial denudation [14–16]. Such changes do not seem to progress, however, to advanced peritoneal sclerosis and appear to be compatible with long-term peritoneal dialysis treatment of 10 years or more.

The Manipulation of Ultrafiltration

The major osmotic agent for peritoneal dialysis is still glucose. There was an interest in large molecular weight polymers as potentially slowly-absorbed osmotic agents, but these were found to be absorbed at higher rates than predicted, presumably by convection through subdiaphragmatic lymphatics [17–19]. Solutions containing glucose polymers that are nearly iso-osmotic with plasma are under investigation, but the accumulation of maltose and serum with such solutions mandates additional studies before they are used widely [18].

Net ultrafiltration is reduced substantially by fluid reabsorption through the subdiaphragmatic lymphatics [17]. The addition of agents such as neostigmine and phosphatidylcholine to peritoneal dialysis solution has decreased lymphatic absorption and increased net ultrafiltration [20,21].

Does CAPD Preserve Residual Renal Function Better than Hemodialysis?

In chronic peritoneal dialysis patients, as in chronic hemodialysis patients, residual renal function tends to decline, but there is increasing evidence that residual renal function may be better preserved in patients on chronic peritoneal dialysis [22–25], although additional studies are needed to verify these preliminary observations. There are possible mechanisms to explain such differences, such as (1) the undesirable effects of recurring hypotension and renal ischemia on hemodialysis and (2) the release, during hemodialysis, of cytokines which damage residual renal tissue.

Peritoneal Dialysis Prescriptions to Achieve Adequacy

In our center, we try to provide each patient with at least 40–50 liters of creatinine clearance per week per 1.73 M^2 body surface area. This total clearance represents the sum of dialysis clearance and the residual renal clearance. Patients are classified by the peritoneal equilibration test as high transporters, high average transporters, low average transporters, or low transporters [26]. Although high transporters have high clearances, they also have rapid glucose absorption, early loss of the osmotic gradient for ultrafiltration, and low drainage volumes. They often do better on short cycle techniques, such as nightly intermittent peritoneal dialysis or daytime ambulatory peritoneal dialysis without a nocturnal exchange. Low transporters have poor clearances and good drain volumes. They often need large volume exchanges or more than four exchanges per day to maintain the weekly clearances in the desired range.

The development of edema or an increase in serum creatinine concentration, in our experience, more often reflects the effects of a decline in residual renal function than a change in peritoneal membrane transport. It is important to adjust the peritoneal dialysis prescription to maintain adequate balance of sodium and water and to maintain total clearances in the desirable range as patients lose their residual renal function [27].

The peritoneal dialysis prescription can also be adjusted to provide a targeted weekly urea clearance [28]. The weekly urea clearance is usually normalized to total body water. This urea kinetic modeling approach to CAPD was a major focus of many presentations at the 10th Annual Peritoneal Dialysis Conference in Dallas, Texas, in February of 1990. Based on studies now available and to be published in the Proceedings of this meeting, it would seem desirable to aim for a dietary protein intake of 1.0–1.2 per kg of ideal body weight and a total weekly urea clearance (the sum of dialysis clearance and residual renal function) of at least 1.4 times the volume of total body water. Recommendations for a minimum value for this ratio at the present time range from 1.4 to 2.2. Clinical studies now underway may allow us to target the minimum value recommended more precisely.

CAPD usually provides weekly clearances which are only 50%–60% of those provided by standard three-times-per-week hemodialysis therapy [29]. The peak concentration hypothesis proposes that much higher weekly urea clearances are needed with an intermittent therapy such as hemodialysis in order to maintain the serum urea concentration at all times below or equal to the steady state concentration of CAPD. If hemodialysis therapy three times per week were to provide an overall weekly urea clearance only equal to that of CAPD, the serum urea nitrogen concentration would be above the steady state CAPD value for significant portions of the time, especially on the day before each treatment. If peak concentrations of small molecular weight solutes correlate with uremic symptomatology, then intermittent therapies have an inherent need to provide higher clearances than continuous therapy. This hypothesis has been invoked to explain why lower urea clearances on CAPD appear adequate to alleviate clinical symptoms apparently as well as hemodialysis. It is important to remember that control of serum urea nitrogen concentration alone is not an adequate index of dialysis adequacy; the serum urea nitrogen concentration must be considered in relationship to dietary protein intake and the protein catabolic rate.

Short cycle clearances can be increased 10%–20% using cyclers that incorporate the new tidal peritoneal dialysis approach [30,31]. Tidal peritoneal dialysis cycles frequent volumes, usually of 1000–1500 ml, on top of an indwelling reservoir of 1000–1500 ml. This maintains better solution-membrane contact and delays complete drainage until the end of the total treatment. With complete drainage techniques at the end of every cycle, there are periods during the treatment when very little fluid remains in the peritoneal cavity, resulting in an inherent inefficiency.

There is good evidence that attention to peritoneal dialysis prescriptions and anticipation of changes as residual renal function declines can reduce unnecessary dropout from CAPD programs [27].

Peritoneal Dialysis Access

It is my impression that one of the most important developments in peritoneal catheters has been the permanent bend or "Swan Neck" configuration [32]. At the April 1990 meeting of the American Society for Artificial Internal Organs in Washington, D.C., Dr. Twardowski reviewed experiences with the Missouri Swan Neck Catheter that will be published in the upcoming Transactions. Catheter survivals are better than those reported with other types of catheters and are better than our experiences with other types of catheters at the University of Missouri. Complications, such as exit-cuff extrusion, catheter tip migration, and refractory exit-site infections, seem to have been drastically reduced.

General Comments

I have given brief overviews of the status of chronic peritoneal dialysis worldwide in 1990 and associated areas of interest. Other speakers in this session will address some of these topics in more detail and will address some other areas of interest that I have not mentioned.

Dr. Rippe will update our understanding of the Kinetics of Peritoneal Transport. Dr. Keshaviah will go into more detail on the comparison of the adequacy of CAPD and hemodialysis. Dr. Khanna will expand on the manipulation of lymphatics to control net ultrafiltration. Dr. Maiorca will update the findings with the Y-set. Dr. Gokal will review the current approach to control of serum calcium and serum phosphorus concentrations on CAPD with minimal exposure to aluminum.

References

1. United States Renal Data System 1989 Annual Report, The National Institutes of Health, National Institute of Diabetes and Digestive and Kidney Diseases, August 1989. Bethesda, MD.
2. Nolph KD (1988) Comparison of continuous ambulatory peritoneal dialysis and hemodialysis. Kidney Int 33:S123
3. Nolph KD (1990) Clinical results with peritoneal dialysis – registry experiences. In: Twardowski ZJ, Nolph KD, Khanna R, Stein J (eds) Contemporary issues in nephrology: peritoneal dialysis. Churchill-Livingston, New York, pp 127–144
4. Maiorca R, Cancarini GC, Camerini C, Brunori G, Manili L, Movilli E, Feller P, Mombelloni S (1989) Is CAPD competitive with haemodialysis for long-term treatment of uraemic patients? Nephrol Dial Transpl 4:244–253
5. Disney APS (1989) Twelfth Report of the Australia and New Zealand combined Dialysis and Transplant Registry. Queen Elizabeth Hospital, Woodville, South Australia
6. Maiorca R, Vonesh E, Cancarini GC, Cantaluppi A, Manili L, Brunori G, Camerini C, Feller P, Strada A (1988) A six-year comparison of patient and technique survivals in CAPD and HD. Kidney Int 34:518–524
7. Lindblad AS, Novak JW, Nolph KD (1989) Continuous ambulatory peritoneal dialysis in the USA – final report of the National CAPD Registry 1981-1988. Kluwer, Dordrecht
8. Canadian CAPD Clinical Trials Group (1989) Peritonitis in CAPD: a multi-center randomized clinical trial comparing the Y-connector disinfectant system to standard systems. Perit Dial Int 9:159–163
9. Caballi PL, Viglino G, Goia F, Cottino R, Mariano F, Gandolfo C (1989) CAPD versus hemodialysis: seven years of experience. Adv Perit Dial 5:52–55
10. Holden A, Gaumer G (1987) Best demonstrated practices program promoting CAPD patient retention in the United States. Advances in CAPD. Proceedings of the seventh annual CAPD conference, Kansas City, United States, 3:186–191
11. Krediet RT, Arisz L (1989) Fluid and solute transport across the peritoneum during CAPD. Perit Dial Int 9:15–25
12. Park MS, Lee J, Lee MS, Baick SH, Hwang SD, Lee HB (1989) Peritoneal solute clearances after four years of continuous ambulatory peritoneal dialysis (CAPD). Perit Dial Int 9:75–78
13. An International Cooperative Study Third Report with 40 participating centers (1985) A Survey of ultrafiltration in continuous ambulatory peritoneal dialysis. In: Khanna R, Nolph KD, Prowant B, Twardowski ZJ, Oreopoulos DG (eds) Advances in continuous ambulatory

peritoneal dialysis. Proceedings of the fifth annual CAPD conference, Kansas City, United States. Toronto Press, Toronto, pp 79–86

14. Dobbie JW (1989) Morphology of the peritoneum in CAPD. Blood Purif 7:74
15. Dobbie JW (1989) Monitoring peritoneal histopathology in peritoneal dialysis: the role of a biopsy registry. Dial Transplant 18:319–325, 335
16. Pollock CA, Ibels LS, Eckstein RP, Graham JC, Caterson RJ, Mahony JF, Ross Sheil AG (1989) Peritoneal morphology on maintenance dialysis. Am J Nephrol 9:198–204
17. Mactier RA, Khanna R (1989) Absorption of fluid and solute from the peritoneal cavity: theoretic and therapeutic implications and applications. Trans Am Soc Artif Intern Organs 35:122–131
18. Mistry CD, Gokal R (1989) Alternative osmotic agents. Blood Purif 7:109–114
19. Henderson IS (1989) Composition of peritoneal dialysis solutions: potential hazards. Blood Purification 7:86–94
20. Mactier RA, Khanna R, Moore H, Twardowski ZJ, Nolph KD (1988) Pharmacological reduction of lymphatic absorption from the peritoneal cavity increases net ultrafiltration and solution clearances in peritoneal dialysis. Nephron 50:229–232
21. Mactier RA, Khanna R, Twardowski ZJ (1988) Influence of phosphatidylcholine on lymphatic absorption during peritoneal dialysis in the rat. Perit Dial Int 8:179–186
22. Rottembourg J, Issad B, Gallego JL, Degoulet P, Aime F, Gueffaf B, Legrain M (1982) Evolution of residual renal function in patients undergoing maintenance haemodialysis or continuous ambulatory peritoneal dialysis. Proc Eur Dial Transplant Assoc 19:397–401
23. Rottembourg J, Issad B, Poignet JL, Strippoli P, Balducci A, Slama G, Gahl GM (1983) Residual renal function and control of blood glucose levels in insulin dependent diabetic patients treated by CAPD. In: Keen H, Legrain M (eds) Prevention and treatment of diabetic nephropathy. Lancaster, Boston, pp 339–359
24. Cancarini GC, Brunori G, Camerini C, Brasa S, Manili L, Maiorca R (1986) Renal function recovery and maintenance of residual diuresis in CAPD and hemodialysis. Perit Dial Bull 6:77–79
25. Lysaght M, Vonesh E, Ibels L, Lindholm B, Nolph KD, Pollock C, Prowant B, Farrell P (1989) Decline of residual renal function in hemodialysis and CAPD patients: a risk adjusted growth function analysis. Nephrol Dial Transpl 4:499
26. Twardowski ZJ (1989) Clinical value of standardized equilibration tests in CAPD patients. Blood Purif 7:95–108
27. Twardowski ZJ, Khanna R, Nolph KD (1987) Peritoneal dialysis modifications to avoid CAPD drop-out. Advances in continuous ambulatory peritoneal dialysis. Proceedings of the seventh annual CAPD conference. Kansas City, United States. 3:171–178
28. Lysaght MJ, Pollock CA, Hallet MD, Ibels LS, Farrell PC (1989) The relevance of ureal kinetic modeling to CAPD. Trans Am Soc Artif Intern Organs 35:784–790
29. Keshaviah PR, Nolph KD, Van Stone JC (1989) The peak concentration hypotheses: a urea kinetic approach to comparing the adequacy of CAPD and hemodialysis. Perit Dial Int 9:257–260
30. Twardowski ZJ (1989) New approaches to intermittent peritoneal dialysis therapies. In: Nolph K (ed) Peritoneal dialysis, 3rd edn. Kluwer, Dordrecht, pp 133–151
31. Twardowski ZJ (1990) Dialysis adequacy and new cycler techniques. In: Twardowski ZJ, Nolph KD, Khanna R, Stein JH (eds) Peritoneal dialysis. Churchill-Livingston, New York, pp 67–100
32. Khanna R (1990) Peritoneal dialysis access. In: Twardowski ZJ, Nolph KD, Khanna R, Stein JH (eds) Peritoneal dialysis. Churchill-Livingston, New York, pp 101–126

Understanding the Kinetics of Peritoneal Transport

BENGT RIPPE[1], GUNNAR STELIN[1], and BÖRJE HARALDSSON[1,2]

SUMMARY. In this article we describe the characteristics of peritoneal barrier exchange in terms of a three-pore model of membrane permselectivity. The peritoneal membrane is thus simulated to have a large number of small pores of radius 40–55 Å, a small number of large pores of radius 200–300 Å, and an abundance of transcellular pores of radius 4–5 Å. According to this model, solutes < 25 Å in radius were found to be permeating across the peritoneal membrane mainly by means of diffusion across the small pores, whereas solutes larger than 40 Å were found to reach the peritoneal cavity exclusively by unidirectional convection through the large pores. In addition, water was simulated to be partly transported through the transcellular "ultrapores," which are not accessible to hydrophilic solute permeation. Small solute absorption from the peritoneal cavity was found to occur by diffusion across small pores. However, molecules larger than 30 Å in radius (Mol. weight > 30000) seemed to be absorbed from the peritoneal cavity exclusively via non-size-selective lymphatic drainage. Applying the three-pore model to literature peritoneal equilibration test (PET) data, solute mass transfer area coefficients (PS) appeared to be higher during the first 30 mins of dwell time than subsequently. Reductions in solute PS-values with dwell time are discussed in terms of a progressively increasing impact of interstitial "unstirred layers" on small solute permeation over the course of the cycle.

Introduction

Water and solutes exchanging between the blood and the peritoneal cavity have to permeate at least three serial morphological barriers: 1] the walls of the mesenteric and peritoneal capillaries, 2] the peritoneal interstitium, and 3] the highly permeable mesothelium. In addition, "unstirred layers" in the peritoneal dialysate and/or in the interstitium contribute to the peritoneal barrier characteristics, at least with respect

[1]Dept of Nephrology, Sahlgrenska Hospital, S-413 45 Göteborg, Sweden
[2]Dept of Physiology, University of Göteborg, S-400 33 Göteborg, Sweden

to small solute exchange. Conceivably, however, the capillary walls would be the principal barrier determining transperitoneal fluid and solute exchange, and we have tested the validity of this assumption.

Functional Ultrastructure of Peritoneal Capillary Walls

Peritoneal capillaries belong to the continuous type, as found in, e.g., muscle, heart, and skin. With respect to transcapillary solute exchange, continuous microvascular walls show a bimodal size selectivity. Functionally they behave as membranes having a large number of "small pores" (radius 40–60 Å), accounting for 90%–95% of the total hydraulic conductance (UF-coefficient), and a very small number (1 part per 5000–15000 small pores) of "large pores" (radius 200–300 Å), accounting for 5%–10% of the UF-coefficient [1–2]. Morphologically the small pores correspond to the clefts (slits) between individual endothelial cells. While lipid-soluble species (e.g., O_2 and CO_2) can permeate the endothelial cell membrane proper, the intercellular clefts are the major exchange routes for water and small solutes. These clefts have a complex structure, but small solutes and water can pass from the capillary lumen to the interstitium via tortuous spaces within the clefts, here created by an irregular labyrinth of cell-to-cell adhesion lines [3]. The average cleft width appears to be 200 Å, except for a few "restricted" portions being 70–80 Å in width.

The exact morphological counterpart to the large pores, allowing albumin and larger proteins to filter between plasma and interstitium, has not yet been identified. Large pores may be represented either by interendothelial "gaps," similar to the mentioned clefts but wider, or, less likely, by channels formed by fused plasmalemmal vesicles. Recent evidence strongly indicates that vesicular transport (transcytosis) is not the likely morphological candidate for the large pores [4].

To describe both solute and fluid transfer across vascular walls, capillary physiologists have long proposed the existence of a third exchange route between blood and tissue, namely a transcellular (ultra-small pore) pathway (radius 4–5 Å), accounting for 1%–7% of the total capillary hydraulic conductance [1,5,6]. Hence, the classical two-pore model of vascular permeability may actually be regarded as a "three-pore" model [1].

Two-Pore Model of Peritoneal Exchange

We have tested the hypothesis that the walls of the microvessels in the blood-peritoneal barrier are the major determinants of transperitoneal exchange. Thus, we have determined the blood-peritoneal clearances of several endogenous substances in patients undergoing continuous ambulatory peritoneal dialysis (CAPD), and we have analyzed the data according to current concepts in microvascular physiology.

Measurements were performed in the early phase of 1.36% Dianeal dwells when intraperitoneal (i.p.) solute concentrations were near zero. Transperitoneal "unidirectional" clearances were assessed as transperitoneal mass transfer per time unit (during 10–15 min) as divided by the mean solute concentration gradient through the peritoneal membrane. Data were analyzed according to recent developments of the two-pore theory [2] and according to non-linear solute flux formalism [7], employing current hydrodynamic theories to describe restricted diffusion [6] and reflection coefficients [8] in cylindrical pores.

The first step of a two-pore analysis of membrane transport involves the partitioning of *net* transmembrane filtration flow (J_v) into the separate *partial* volume flows occurring through the small pores (radius 40–60 Å) and the large pores (radius 200–300 Å), respectively. How to do that from J_v, utilizing measured clearances of at least two solutes larger than 50 Å in radius (in order to obtain the large volume flow), has been described previously [2]. Note that regardless of the direction of the net transmembrane fluid transport, there is always blood-peritoneal filtration across large pores, since the "effective" colloid osmotic pressure gradient across these pores is very low (near zero). It is also worth noting that protein transport across large pores is always convective (filtrative) for normal capillary pressures [2,4].

When experimental unidirectional clearance data from patients in CAPD, obtained at a net blood-peritoneal volume flow of 1 ml/min [9], were adapted to the two-pore model of membrane permselectivity as outlined above [10], we obtained a small pore radius (r_s) of 47 ± 1.02 Å ($\pm$SE) and a large pore radius (r_L) of 305 ± 41 Å. The so-called "unrestricted total pore area over unit diffusion path length" ($A_0/\Delta x$) became 45000 ± 2300 cm, while the large pore volume flow was 0.052 ± 0.006 ml/min. The fractional UF-coefficient (L_pS) accounted for by large pores (denoted α_L) was estimated to be 0.055. This "simple" two pore model was found to comply very well with a majority of previously published peritoneal solute flux data obtained in CAPD patients and in animal models [10].

Three-Pore Model of Peritoneal Permselectivity

When modelling fluid transport across microvascular walls, capillary physiologists conventionally take into account a so-called "transcellular" fluid conductive pathway, or "ultra-small pore" pathway, accounting for 1%–5% [6] of L_pS, besides the small and large pores [1,5,6]. Thus, we have extended our analysis to comprise all three fluid conductive pathways existing in microvascular membranes. In this extended analysis we also included the impact of peritoneal lymphatic drainage upon net transperitoneal fluid transfer (J_v). Furthermore, we assumed that the transperitoneal glucose concentration gradient (ΔC_g) generates the major crystalloid osmotic pressure gradient determining the peritoneal fluid shifts (J_v). Partitioning of fluid fluxes between the three sets of pores in this analysis was performed according to:

$$J_{v_n} = \alpha_n \, L_pS \, (\Delta P - \sigma_{prot,n} \, \Delta \pi + \Delta C_g \, R \, T \, \sigma_{g,n}) \qquad (1)$$

Here "n" refers to either small pores (s), large pores (L), or transcellular pores (c). α stands for *fractional*, and L_pS for *total* peritoneal hydraulic conductance (UF-coefficient), while RT is the product of the gas constant and the temperature in degrees Kelvin. σ^3 refers to the osmotic "reflection coefficient" for either total pro-

---

[3] σ denotes the fraction of the *ideal* solute osmotic pressure gradient (exerted across a semipermeable membrane), which is operative across a leaky membrane. σ equals 1 for a semipermeable membrane, from which the molecule is totally reflected; σ equals zero if the membrane is freely permeable to the solute

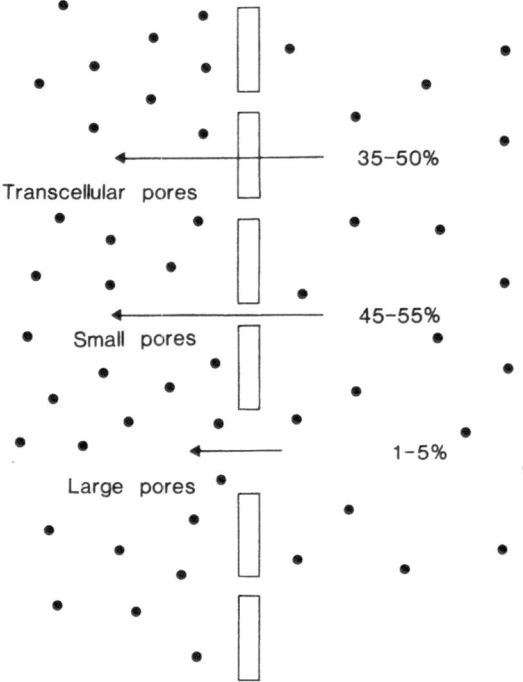

Fig. 1. The partitioning of transperitoneal fluid flows between the different peritoneal pathways, as modelled for a large glucose osmotic gradient across the peritoneal membrane. In this simulation the transcellular pores account for only 1.5% of the total peritoneal ultrafiltration (*UF*)-coefficient

tein (prot) or for glucose (g). ΔP represents the hydrostatic pressure gradient existing between the peritoneal capillaries and the peritoneal fluid and $\Delta \pi$ the transperitoneal colloid osmotic pressure gradient. The difference between the two major "Starling forces," $(\Delta P - \Delta \pi)$, was set to ≈ -12 mmHg, whereas L_pS was set to 0.08 ml/min per mm Hg [10]. Reflection coefficients for glucose and albumin (total protein) were modelled by the Drake and Davis equation [8] using the pore radii determined in our previous two-pore analysis. Thus, the tentative small pore radius was set to 47 Å and the large pore radius to 300 Å. The fractional small pore and large pore L_pS values (α_s and α_L) were set to 0.930 and 0.055, respectively.

We were surprised to find that if α_c was only 0.015–0.02, then approximately *one half* of the peritoneal fluid filtration was found to occur transcellularly, when peritoneal fluid transport was induced by a large glucose osmotic pressure gradient [10]. This is illustrated in Fig. 1. This offers an explanation for the fact that small solute sieving coefficients (Φ), as measured for large glucose induced ultrafiltration rates, are close to 0.5–0.6 during peritoneal dialysis, and not near unity, as predicted by the strict two-pore theory.

The total fluid filtration occurring across the peritoneal membrane ($J_{V_{tot}}$) is obtained by summing up the partial small pore, large pore, and transcellular volume flows (J_{V_S}, J_{V_L} and J_{V_c}, respectively):

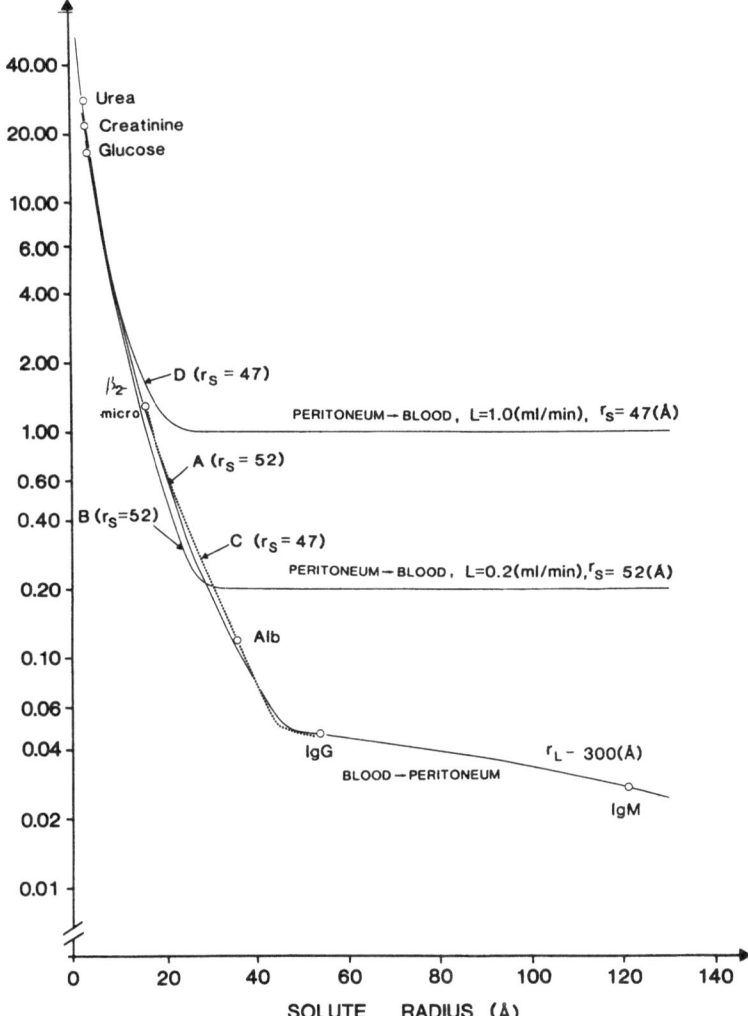

Fig. 2. Semi-log plot of simulated solute clearance as a function of mol. radius, employing the parameters fitting to the data of Rippe et al. [9], as indicated in the figure. Curves *A* and *B* represent clearances simulated for a peritoneal lymph flow of 0.2 ml/min and curves *C* and *D* for a lymph flow of 1.00 ml/min. Curves *A* (r_v = 52) and *C* (r_v = 47) and simulated for transport in the direction from the blood to the peritoneal cavity, whereas curves *B* and *D* show solute clearance vs solute radius for transport occurring in the opposite direction due to transcapillary and lymphatic absorption. (Reprinted from *Kidney International* with permission [10])

$$J_{V_{tot}} = J_{V_S} + J_{V_L} + J_{V_c} \tag{2}$$

Furthermore, the *net* intraperitoneal volume alteration is described by

$$J_V = J_{V_{tot}} - L \tag{3}$$

where L stands for the lymphatic flow from the peritoneal cavity.

For the three-pore model, and for a $J_{V_{tot}}$ of 1.20 ml/min (occurring for a ΔC_g of 34 mmoles/l) and $L = 0.2$ (ml/min) [11], the small pore volume flow (J_{V_S}) is only 0.471 ml/min, using the parameters presented above, and *not* 1.148 (1.20 minus 0.052) ml/min, as would be predicted by the simple two-pore theory. This reduction in calculated volume flow across the small pores causes the small pore radius estimate to increase in the three-pore analysis. In all other respects the two analyses presented are identical.

Figure 2 represents a semi-log plot of "unidirectional" solute clearance (approximately equalling "mass transfer area coefficients" for small solutes) as a function of molecular radius [10]. Curves are simulated to fit experimental data [9] for transport both in the blood-peritoneal (curves A and C) and peritoneal-to-blood direction (curves B and D), and for a peritoneal lymph flow being set to 0.2 ml/min [11] (curves A and B) and to 1 ml/min [12] (curves C and D).

Transport of small solutes seemed to occur by restricted diffusion through "small pores" of radius ≈ 52 Å for $L = 0.2$ (ml/min), or of radius 47 Å for L being set to 1.00 ml/min, whereas the large macromolecules, IgG and IgM, appeared to have reached the peritoneal cavity by unidirectional convection (directed from the blood to the peritoneal cavity) through large pores of radius ≈ 300 Å.

Note the assymmetry of peritoneal transport! According to the model, solutes larger than 30 Å in radius are absorbed from the peritoneal cavity due to non-size-selective convection by lymphatic drainage. Thus, there is no local back transport of large solutes to plasma by direct diffusion across blood capillary walls. Note also the large difference between the unidirectional clearance (mass transfer area coefficient) of urea (29 ml/min) and the blood-peritoneal clearance of albumin (0.1 ml/min), the urea/albumin clearance ratio being near 300! In comparison, the ratio of the *free* diffusion coefficients for urea/albumin is 14. Indeed, transperitoneal transport of albumin must occur by *restricted* and not by free diffusion/convection.

Understanding the Kinetics of Solute Equilibration Between Blood and Peritoneal Cavity

Analyses of transperitoneal solute equilibration, as measured, e.g., in peritoneal equilibration tests (PETs), are complicated by the fact that fluid and solute transport occur simultaneously. Furthermore, only approximately one half of the net volume flow carries solute, namely J_{V_S}. Thus, i.p. solute concentrations are affected by dilution. Setting $L = 0.2$ (ml/min) [11] and employing the assumptions for the three-pore model outlined above, the relationship between J_{V_S} and J_V was previously derived to be approximately [10]:

$$J_{V_S} = 0.649 \, J_V - 0.178 \tag{4}$$

The combined diffusive and convective solute transport, in terms of "unidirectional clearance" (Cl) during a relatively short time period ($t_1 - t_2$), may be obtained as outlined above, i.e., as solute flux divided by the transperitoneal solute concentration, or as

$$Cl = \frac{\overline{V}_D}{t_2 - t_1} \ln \frac{(C_B - C_{D_1})}{(C_B - C_{D_2})} \tag{5}$$

where $\overline{V}_D$ is the mean intraperitoneal (i.p.) volume during the measurement, C_B is the blood concentration of solute and C_{D_1} and C_{D_2} are the i.p. solute concentrations at time t_1 and t_2, respectively (cf [10]).

The solute mass transfer area coefficient (PS) may now be solved from the so-called non-linear flux equation (6) as arranged for "unidirectional" transport, i.e.:

$$PS = J_{V_s} (1 - \sigma_s) \Big/ \ln \left\{ \frac{Cl}{Cl - J_{V_s} (1 - \sigma_s)} \right\} \tag{6}$$

Here the subscript "s" stands for "small pores," and hence, σ_s denotes the small pore solute reflection coefficient (being of the order of 0.02 for small solutes), whereas all other factors have been defined above. Note also that J_{V_s} is the *small pore* volume flow.

We have employed equations 4, 5, and 6 to calculate PS values from PET data previously published [13]. PS was determined sequentially for various time intervals (30–60 min) of the PET cycle, and likewise, sequential values for $\overline{V}_D$ were obtained from an arbitrary function determining the i.p. dialysate volume vs time relationship (cf [14]):

$$V_t = V_o + a_1 (1 - e^{-kt}) - a_2 t \tag{7}$$

Here V_t represents the i.p. dialysate volume as a function of time. V_o is i.p. volume at time zero, and a_1, a_2, and k are some arbitrary coefficients that determine the change occurring in V_t over dwell time [14]. The parameters a_1, a_2, and k were fitted to the average drained volume vs time data published by Twardowski et al. [13] for 22.5 per cent Dianeal in PET tests. The following parameter values were selected: $V_o = (2050 + 300)$ (ml) (instilled volume + residual volume), k = 0.01 (min^{-1}), a_1 = 700 (ml), and a_2 = 1.25 (ml/min). The arithmetic mean value of intraperitoneal volume obtained at t_1 and t_2 in each interval, as calculated according to equation 7, was employed for $\overline{V}_D$.

Figure 3 displays PS values for creatinine, as calculated from published PET data [13] (mean value curve, curve depicting PET data being + 1 SD "above mean" and − 1 SD "below mean," respectively) according to equations 4–7, for 0–30 min, 1–2 h and 3–4 h. Note that PS values for 0–30 min seem to be higher than subsequent values. This may, at least partly, explain why the "initial clearance" data determined by Rippe et al. [9] during the "early" phase (0–30 min) of the dwell are much higher than the average PS values obtained from all the PETs analyzed here for creatinine. Alternatively, our previous investigation [9] comprises a subpopulation of CAPD patients with unusually high solute clearances. However, there are good reasons to believe that the impact of interstitial factors, such as "unstirred fluid layers," may increase with dwell time and lower the "apparent" PS progressively over the dwell.

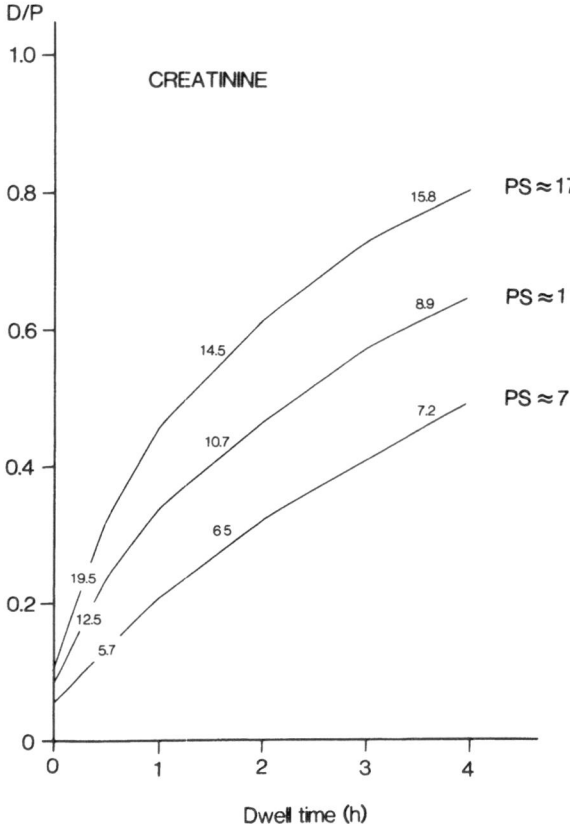

Fig. 3. Dialysate to plasma creatinine concentration ratios (*D/P*), vs dwell time in a population studied by Twardowsky et al. [13] using the "peritoneal equilibration test" as introduced by these authors. PS values calculated according to eqs. 4–7 are indicated in the Fig. for 0–30 min, 60–120 min and 180–240 min, the other calculated results being left out (for didactic reasons). Average approximate PS values calculated for all sequential determinations in each curve are shown *to the right*. Only average D/P vs time curve (*middle curve*) and curves designating D/P vs time relationships being +1 SD "above mean" (*upper curve*) and −1 SD "below mean" (*lower curve*), respectively, are depicted in this figure

This is probably because the large ("stirring") peritoneal ultrafiltrate (UF) flows, existing initially, will gradually "dissipate" with cycle time.

Lymph Flow From the Peritoneal Cavity in CAPD

The parameters determining the intraperitoneal dialysate volume ($V(t)$) vs time curve (cf eq. 7) may be interpreted into meaningful phenomenological coefficients; this is discussed at some length elsewhere [14]. Concerning the parameter a_2 of equation 7, which represents the fluid absorption occurring from the peritoneal cavity to the blood when all major *crystalloid* osmotic concentration gradients have come to equilibrium, it has been most controversial whether a_2 is mainly accounted for by lymphatic drainage or by fluid absorption through the capillary walls [11]. We have shown previously [14] that a_2 can be described by:

$$a_2 = - L_pS (\Delta P - \sigma_{prot} \Delta\pi_{prot}) + L \qquad (8)$$

The numerical value for the expression within the parenthesis is approximately -10 to -11 mmHg. Hence, setting L_pS to 0.08 ml/min per mmHg, as employed above, and a_2 to 1.2–1.3 ml/min, as usually measured for dwell times exceeding 5–6 hours, yields a lymphatic flow (L) of 0.4–0.5 ml/min. Thus, fluid absorption from the peritoneal cavity must occur due to *both* lymphatic flow *and* due to osmotic fluid transport directly into the capillaries [15]. There may, however, be situations when lymphatic absorption is the predominating peritoneal fluid absorptive mechanism. Normally *far from all* of the peritoneal fluid absorption would be lymph flow.

Concluding Remarks

In conclusion, the exchange characteristics of the peritoneal membrane can be adequately described by a three-pore model of membrane selectivity. In this respect the "peritoneal membrane" mimics the continuous capillary wall. Thus, the capillary walls in the peritoneum are likely to be the principal structures determining the blood-peritoneal exchange.

Acknowledgments. This study was supported by grants Nos. 8285 and 8796 from the Swedish Medical Research Council.

References

1. Taylor AE, Granger DN (1984) Exchange of macromolecules across the microcirculation. In: Renkin EM, Michel CC (eds) The cardiovascular system. Am Physiol Soc, pp 467–520 (Handbook of physiology, Sect 2, vol IV)
2. Rippe B, Haraldsson B (1987) Fluid and protein fluxes across small and large pores in the microvasculature. Application of two-pore equations. Acta Physiol Scand 131:411–428
3. Bundgaard M (1984) The three-dimensional organization of tight junctions in a capillary endothelium revealed by serial-section electron microscopy. J Ultrastruct Res 88:1–17
4. Rippe B, Haraldsson B (1987) How are macromolecules transported across the capillary wall? News Physiol Sci 2:135–138
5. Crone C, Levitt DG (1984) Capillary permeability to small solutes. In: Renkin EM, Michel CC (eds) The Cardiovascular System. Am Physiol Soc, pp 411–466 Handbook of physiology, sect 2, vol IV
6. Curry FE (1984) Mechanics and thermodynamics of transcapillary exchange. In: Renkin EM, Michel CC (eds) The Cardiovascular System. Am Physiol Soc, pp 309–374 (Handbook of physiology, sect 2, vol IV)
7. Patlak CS, Goldstein DA, Hoffman JF (1963) The flow of solute and solvent across two-membrane system. J Theor Biol 5:425–442

8. Drake R, Davis E (1978) A corrected equation for the calculation of reflection coefficients. Microvasc Res 15:259

9. Rippe B, Stelin G, Ahlmén J (1981) Basal permeability of the peritoneal membrane during continuous ambulatory peritoneal dialysis (CAPD). In: Gahl GM. Kessel M, Nolph KD (eds) Advances in peritoneal dialysis. Proceedings of the 2nd International Symposium on Peritoneal Dialysis. Excerpta Medica, Amsterdam, pp 5–9

10. Rippe B, Stelin G (1989) Simulations of peritoneal solute transport during CAPD. Application of two-pore formalism. Kidney Int 35:1234–1244

11. Rippe B, Stelin G, Ahlmén J (1986) Lymph flow from the peritoneal cavity in CAPD patients. In: Maher JF, Winchester JF (eds) Frontiers in peritoneal dialysis. Field, Rich, New York, pp 24–30

12. Nolph KD, Mactier RA, Khanna R, Twardowski ZJ, Moore H, McGary T (1987) The kinetics of ultrafiltration during peritoneal dialysis: the role of lymphatics. Kidney Int 32:219

13. Twardowski ZJ, Nolph KD, Khanna R (1987) Peritoneal equilibration test. Perit Dial Bull 7:138–147

14. Stelin G, Rippe B (1990) A phenomenological interpretation of the variation in dialysate volume with dwell time in CAPD. Kidney Int 38:465–472

15. Flessner MF, Dedrick RL, Rippe B (1989) Peritoneal tissue and capillary absorption vs. peritoneal lymphatic transport. (letter). ASAIO Trans 35:178–180

Comparing the Adequacy of Continuous Ambulatory Peritoneal Dialysis (CAPD) and Hemodialysis

Prakash Keshaviah[1] and Karl Nolph[2]

SUMMARY. Inadequate dialysis is easier to define and recognize than adequate dialysis. With hemodialysis, values of the Kt/V urea index < 0.8 (K:clearance, t:treatment time and V:volume of urea distribution), are associated with significant morbidity. For the standard continuous ambulatory peritoneal dialysis (CAPD) regimen (2 L × 4 exchanges/day), the Kt/V for the week is ~ 1.5 or ~ 0.5 for a thrice weekly comparison to hemodialysis. Patients on CAPD do not exhibit the morbidity associated with the same low values of Kt/V in hemodialysis. According to the recently formulated peak concentration, because hemodialysis is an intermittent therapy with peaks and troughs of serum urea concentrations, a higher Kt/V is required to match peak serum urea concentrations to the steady state CAPD concentration. Urea kinetic calculations based on this hypothesis suggest weekly Kt/V values for CAPD < 1.2 may be associated with inadequate dialysis, values > 1.7 being the minimum recommended for adequacy. Pilot clinical studies in 19 patients demonstrate agreement with urea kinetic model predictions concerning the relationship between blood urea nitrogen (BUN), Kt/V and protein catabolic rate. In 74% of the clinical observations there was agreement between assessment of adequacy with Kt/V and a clinical assessment score used at the University of Missouri. Lack of agreement in the remaining observations is being investigated.

Introduction

Adequacy of dialysis eludes a clear-cut definition but inadequate dialysis is more readily defined and recognized. The National Cooperative Dialysis Study (NCDS) [1] established clearly that a high degree of morbidity was evident when the small

---

[1]Baxter Clinical Engineering Laboratory, Renal Division, Baxter Healthcare Corporation, Minneapolis, MN 55404, USA
[2]University of Missouri, Columbia, MO 65212-0001, USA

Table 1. Calculation of Kt/V index for CAPD

	Definition of KT/V
Hemodialysis	K = Urea clearance
	T = Treatment time
	V = Volume of urea distribution determined from urea kinetics
C.A.P.D.	$KT = (V)_{drained} \times (D/P)_{ratio}$
	V = Volume of urea distribution ($\approx$ total body water)
	V estimated from sex, age, height, and weight

Typical KT/V Calculation for CAPD

Regimen: 4 exchanges/day
$V_{dialysate} = 2 \times 4 \; l, \; V_{uf} = 1.5 \; l$
$\therefore \; V_{drained} = 8 + 1.5 = 9.5 \; l$
$D/P = 0.9$
$\therefore \; KT = 0.9 \times 9.5 = 8.55$
$V = 40 \; l \; (B.wt = 70 \; kg)$
$\therefore \; (KT/V)_{day} = 8.55 / 40 = 0.21$
$(KT/V)_{H \; D \; equiv} = 0.21 \times 7 / 3 = 0.49$

marker solute urea was not adequately removed, resulting in high time averaged urea concentrations. Further analysis of this data resulted in the formulation of the Kt/V index [2], K being the dialyzer urea clearance (ml/min), t the treatment time (min) and V the volume of urea distribution (ml), which is commonly considered to be equal to total body water. Analysis of the NCDS and prior literature indicates that the Kt/V urea index provides a good definition of the lower limits of the hemodialysis therapy prescription. At Kt/V levels of $\sim$ 0.5, frank uremic symptoms such as anorexia, nausea, insomnia and pericarditis were noted by Dyck et al. [3]. In the NCDS, Groups II and IV were dialyzed at Kt/V levels of $\sim$ 0.6 and had a high degree of morbidity manifested as medical withdrawals, hospitalizations and death. The underlying medical problems were similar to those observed in the Dyck study. At Kt/V levels of $\sim$0.7, Teschan et al. [4] observed neurobehavioral abnormalities characterized by slowing of the EEG. In both the Dyck and Teschan studies, alleviation of symptoms was noted when Kt/V was increased to $\sim$1.0. In the NCDS, in Groups I and III, the Kt/V was > 0.8 and in these groups a smaller percentage of therapy failures was noted. While none of these short-term studies define the optimal therapy prescription, they clearly delineate inadequate dialysis prescriptions as those with Kt/V < 0.8.

The purpose of this paper is to examine the applicability of the Kt/V urea index to CAPD, a therapy that is different from hemodialysis in several respects. The calculation of the Kt/V index for CAPD is quite different from that for hemodialysis, as shown in Table 1. The sample calculation (based on no residual renal function) indicates that for the typical CAPD regimen of 4 exchanges of 2 L each per day with 1.5 L of ultrafiltration and average peritoneal permeability characteristics, the Kt/V for the average 70 kg patient will be only 0.21 per day or 0.49 for an equivalent thrice weekly schedule comparable to hemodialysis. The additional contributions of residual renal function to the thrice weekly Kt/V index will be approximately 0.08

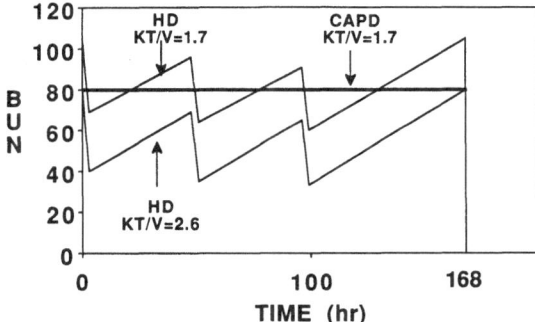

Fig. 1. The weekly blood urea nitrogen (BUN) profile for hemodialysis (HD) and CAPD at the same level of Kt/V = 1.7 and the effect of increasing the Kt/V for hemodialysis from 1.7 to 2.6 to make the peak concentration equal to the steady-state CAPD concentration

for each ml/min of residual urea clearance. So assuming a residual urea clearance of 2 ml/min, the thrice weekly equivalent Kt/V index for CAPD will still be only 0.65, a value similar to that of Groups II and IV of the NCDS. The percentage of patients failing therapy in these groups was of the order of 60%. Such a high degree of morbidity is not commonly observed with the standard CAPD regimen. This, therefore, poses a serious challenge to the validity of the Kt/V index for characterizing the adequacy of CAPD.

Background

As stated earlier, CAPD differs from hemodialysis in several respects. For example, the natural peritoneal membrane has permeability characteristics that are very different from those of conventional cellulosic hemodialysis membranes. The peritoneal membrane is less permeable than cellulosic membranes for small solutes such as urea but is more permeable than cellulosic membranes for larger solutes such as inulin and Beta-2 microglobulin. Those who subscribe to the middle-molecule hypothesis will see in this seeming invalidity of the Kt/V index a reaffirmation of their faith in middle molecules. However, the search for middle molecules, undertaken over more than a decade by well-qualified investigators using sophisticated detection tools, has been unsuccessful.

There is another slightly different hypothesis that can be put forward, based on the differences in permeability of the peritoneal and cellulosic membranes. This hypothesis is that while urea is not toxic per se, it is a surrogate for other toxic solutes that are associated with protein catabolism and urea generation. The relationship between the removal of urea and these toxic catabolites of protein depends on the permeability characteristics of the membrane. As the CAPD membrane is different, the scaling factors between urea removal and these unknown protein catabolites may be different between CAPD and hemodialysis.

While one cannot rule out the above hypotheses based on membrane permeability differences, an alternative hypothesis based on another important difference between CAPD and hemodialysis will be considered. This important difference is that while CAPD is a steady state continuous therapy, hemodialysis is an intermittent therapy characterized by peaks and troughs of serum urea concentrations. Application of the single pool urea kinetic model to these two therapies provides some interesting insights. At the same level of Kt/V, the steady state serum urea concentration with CAPD is almost identical to the time averaged serum urea concentration achieved with hemodialysis. However, because of the intermittent nature of hemodialysis, for approximately half the hours of the week, the serum urea concentration is above this time-averaged correlation (Fig. 1). According to the recently formulated peak concentration hypothesis (5), if the peak concentration is better correlated with uremic toxicity than the mathematically derived abstraction called the time averaged concentration, the hemodialysis Kt/V has to be increased substantially in order to bring the hemodialysis peak concentration down to the steady state CAPD concentration. In other words, serum urea concentration related equivalence between CAPD and hemodialysis is not achieved at the same Kt/V, but may require a higher Kt/V for hemodialysis in order to compensate for the intermittent nature of the therapy. Using the urea kinetic model and the peak concentration hypothesis, Keshaviah et al. [5] have estimated that a Kt/V value of 0.55 for CAPD is equivalent to a value of 1.0 for hemodialysis and that a Kt/V value of approximately 0.4 for CAPD is equivalent to the hemodialysis value of 0.6, a level of Kt/V at which significant morbidity was evident in the NCDS. Converting the Kt/V thrice weekly equivalents to a Kt/V value for the whole week on CAPD, we get a lower bound of 1.2 for inadequate dialysis and a value of 1.7 and above for short-term adequacy. The range from 1.2 to 1.7 represents the transition from inadequate to adequate dialysis according to the peak concentration hypothesis.

Clinical Study

A pilot clinical study in 19 patients was undertaken at the University of Missouri to test the peak concentration hypothesis. The results of this study were presented in some detail at the 10th Annual Conference on Peritoneal Dialysis at Dallas (1990) and will appear in the transactions of the meeting [6]. A brief summary of the results is presented here.

The demographics of the patients studied are presented in Table 2. The patients studied are representative of the typical CAPD population in the United States. The relationship between the steady state serum urea concentration and the weekly Kt/V for urea is shown in Fig. 2. The solid lines represent the theoretical relationship

Table 2. Patient demographics

	Mean	Range
Age (years)	52	(30–75)
Body weight (kg)	71	(44–94)
B.S.A. (M²)	1.81	(1.41–2.21)
Months on dialysis	30	(1–94)
Residual kidney fn. (ml/min) (average of residual urea and creatinine clearances)	2.1	(0–10.1)

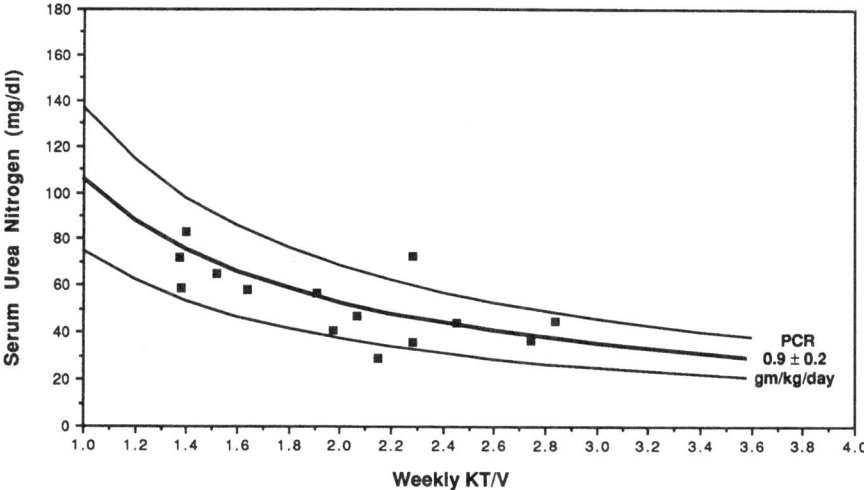

Fig. 2. The steady-state serum urea nitrogen concentration of CAPD (n = 14) plotted against the Kt/V urea with the theoretical relationship derived from urea kinetics for PCR = 0.9 ± 0.2 gm/kg per day superimposed

derived from single pool urea kinetics for a protein catabolic rate (PCR) of 0.9 ± 0.2 gm/kg per day. Of the 19 patients, 14 had a PCR within this range and their data is superimposed on the theoretical predictions of Fig. 2. As is evident from this figure, there is a fairly close match between the experimental measurements and theory. The calculation used for the PCR is based on the relationship of Randerson [7] presented in Table 3. The correlation between the calculated PCR and the dietary protein intake based on a 3 day diet history is shown in Fig. 3. The correlation coefficient for the line of best fit is 0.55, suggesting a fairly strong correlation between the two. A paired t-test revealed no significant difference between the calculated PCR and the dietary protein intake. Three other methods for calculating the PCR in CAPD patients were investigated and yielded similar results to the Randerson formulation.

While the above data confirm the applicability of the urea kinetic model to CAPD, the specific question about CAPD adequacy and Kt/V needs to be addressed. In order to examine this, a clinical assessment score developed at the University of Missouri was used as a clinical indicator of adequacy that could be correlated to the Kt/V measurement. Details of this assessment score are presented in Table 4. With this 12 parameter score, 36 is a perfect score. A score of 23 or less represents inadequate

Table 3. Calculation of PCR for CAPD

PCR (gm/day) = 10.76 (G_{un} + 1.46)

Urea nitrogen generation rate $G_{un\ (mg/min)}$ = ($V_d \times D_{un} + V_u \times U_{un}$)/t

Where V_d and V_u are dialysate and urine volumes respectively (ml), D_{un} and U_{un} are dialysate and urine urea nitrogen concentrations respectively, (mg/dl) and t is the collection time (min)

(Adapted from [7])

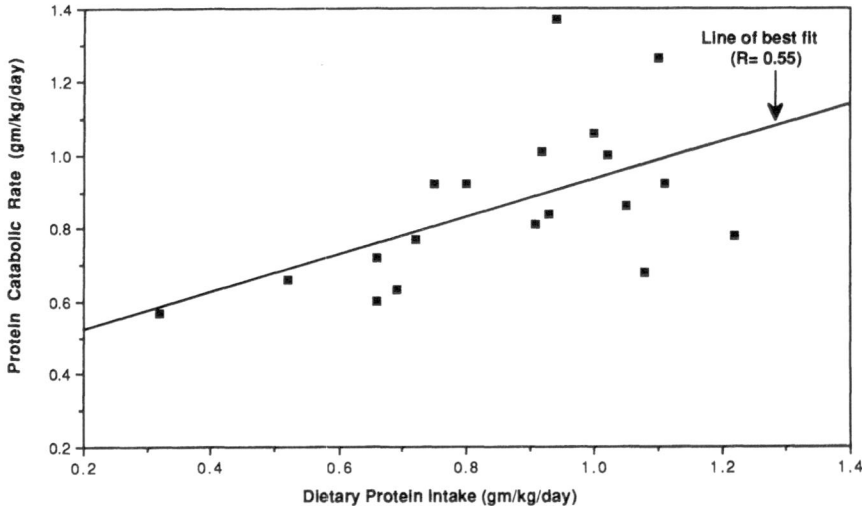

Fig. 3. Correlation between the calculated protein catabolic rate (*PCR*) and the dietary protein intake

therapy, 23–39 is a transitional zone and a score above 29 indicates adequate therapy. The weekly Kt/V ranges derived from the peak concentration hypothesis are < 1.2 connoting inadequate dialysis, 1.2–1.7 being a transition, and > 1.7 being adequate. Figure 4 shows the domains defined by the clinical assessment in conjunction with the weekly Kt/V. There are thus 3 boxes – inadequate, transitional, and adequate dialysis. The clinical measurements of the assessment score and Kt/V are super-

Table 4. Clinical assessment score

	Frequent	Occasional	No problem
Insomnia	1	2	3
Weakness	1	2	3
Dysgeusia	1	2	3
Anorexia	1	2	3
Nausea	1	2	3
Vomiting	1	2	3
Fluid balance	1	2	3
Blood pr. control	1	2	3

	Score 1	Score 2	Score 3
Albumin (gm/dl)	< 3.0	3.0 –3.4	> 3.4
Hct (%)	<20	20–24	>24
Crt. Lean Body Mass (mg/dl per cm ht.)	> 0.10 ↓	0.08–0.10 → (Non-ideal)	< 0.08 ↑ (or ideal)

Inadequate	< 23 points
Marginal	23–29 points
Adequate	29–36 points

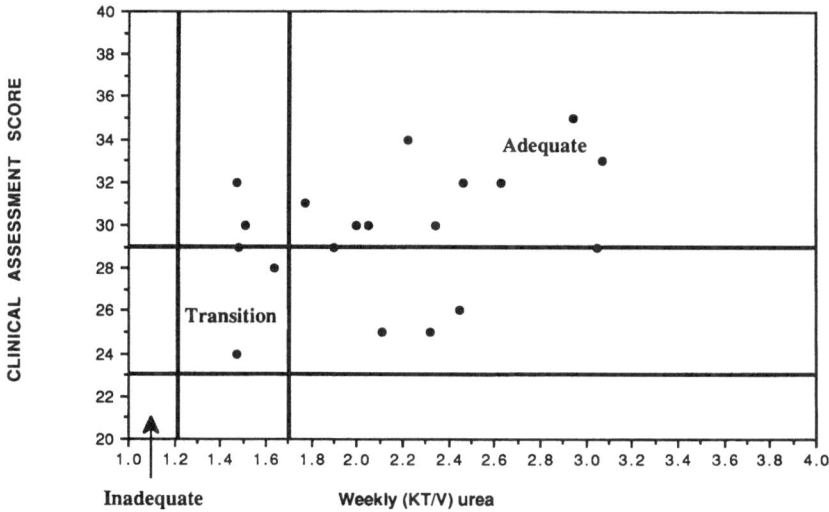

Fig. 4. Plot of the clinical assessment score vs Kt/V urea superimposed on the domains of inadequate, transitional, and adequate dialysis, derived from the intersections of the clinical assessment and Kt/V ranges

imposed on these domains in Fig. 4. Note that none of the patients falls into the inadequate domain. Of the 19 patients, 14 (74%) fall into the appropriate domain boxes. Of the remaining 5, 2 have adequate clinical scores but a low Kt/V (transitional) and 3 have low scores (transition zone) but an adequate Kt/V. It is reasonable to consider the clinical assessment to be the cumulative result of therapy prescription characterized by the Kt/V. Therefore, if a patient is treated with a low Kt/V, it may take several months before the effects of the underdialysis are manifested clinically and measurable as a lower assessment score. Of the two patients with a low Kt/V, one has been on CAPD for only 9 months. It would be interesting to note the time course of the clinical assessment score in this patient. In the 3 patients whose assessment score was low despite an adequate Kt/V, some of the symptoms noted may be unrelated to underdialysis and may have a different etiology. Of the 14 patients who fell into the appropriate domains, 3 were judged to be in the transitional zone by both the clinical assessment and the Kt/V. The therapy prescription in these patients is being increased and the assessment score will be followed to see if it moves upward into the zone of adequacy.

Conclusion

It appears that the urea kinetic model developed for hemodialysis can be applied to CAPD to provide some meaningful insights. The relationship between serum urea concentration, Kt/V and PCR matches the model predictions. The clinical data indicate that patients on CAPD whose Kt/V is much lower than that required for hemodialysis appear to be doing well by clinical assessment criteria. The correlation between clinical assessment and the Kt/V is strong but needs further refinement. The peak concentration hypothesis is an interesting attempt at unifying the comparative bases for adequacy of hemodialysis and CAPD. Its validity has not yet been completely established and awaits further study.

References

1. Lowrie EG, Laird NM, Parker TF, et al. (1981) Effect of the hemodialysis prescription on patient morbidity. N Engl J Med 20:1176-1181
2. Gotch F, Sargent JA (1985) A mechanistic analysis of the National Cooperative Dialysis Study (NCDS). Kidney Int 28:526-534
3. Dyck PJ, Johnson WJ, Lambert EH, O'Brien PC, Daube JR, Oviatt KF (1979) Comparison of symptoms, chemistry, and nerve function to assess adequacy of hemodialysis. Neurology 29:1361-1368
4. Teschan PE, Ginn HE, Bourne JR, Ward JW, Schaffer JD (1983) A prospective study of reduced dialysis. ASAIO J 6:108-122
5. Keshaviah PR, Nolph KD, Van Stone JC (1989) The peak concentration hypothesis: A urea kinetic approach to comparing the adequacy of continuous ambulatory peritoneal dialysis (CAPD) and hemodialysis. Perit Dial Int 9:257-260
6. Keshaviah PR, Nolph KD, Prowant B, Moore H, Ponferrada L, Van Stone J, Twardowski ZJ, Khanna R (1990) Defining Adequacy of CAPD with Urea Kinetics. Adv Perit Dial 6:173-177
7. Randerson DH, Chapman GV, Farrell PC (1981) Amino acid and dietary status in long-term CAPD patients. In: Atkins RC, Farrell PC, Thomson N (eds) Peritoneal dialysis, pp 179-191

Pharmacological Alteration of Ultrafiltration

RAMESH KHANNA, KARL D. NOLPH, and ZBYLUT J. TWARDOWSKI[1]

SUMMARY. Several pharmacological agents have shown a potential for enhancing ultrafiltration in experimental settings during peritoneal dialysis exchanges. Knowledge of ultrafiltration kinetics has improved our understanding of how and at what site these agents are effective in enhancing ultrafiltration. Of all the agents discussed, only phosphatidylcholine, which presumably acts at multiple sites, has shown promise of clinical application. It has several potential advantages. First, phosphatidylcholine is a normal constituent of peritoneal fluid and its addition may help restore and maintain normal peritoneal physiology. Secondly, by reducing intraperitoneal fluid absorption, phosphatidylcholine may decrease dialysate glucose absorption and allow a decrease in the dialysis solution glucose load. Thirdly, studies have indicated that phosphatidylcholine can greatly enhance net ultrafiltration in patients with poor ultrafiltration capacity. Further studies are indicated to clearly define the patients who are likely to benefit from the use of this agent during peritoneal dialysis.

Background

Glucose is an effective osmotic agent for ultrafiltration during peritoneal dialysis. However the use of glucose has been associated with numerous undesirable metabolic effects; this has led to the search for alternative osmotic agents. An average CAPD patient typically absorbs 100–150 grams of glucose per day during the course of CAPD therapy. This inevitable high carbohydrate absorption predisposes to undesirable metabolic problems such as obesity, hypertriglyceridemia, and premature atherosclerosis. In addition, higher doses of insulin required to maintain the blood sugar at normal levels in diabetics may cause hyper-insulinemia, which in healthy persons has been shown to be a risk factor for atherosclerotic heart disease

[1]Department of Medicine, Division of Nephrology, School of Medicine, University of Missouri-Columbia, Columbia, MO 65212, USA

[1,2]. To obviate the undesirable metabolic consequences of glucose absorption, efforts have been made in the past to substitute glucose with alternative osmotic agents such as xylitol [3], amino acids [4], gelatin [5], polyglucose [6], and glycerol [7]. However, none of the agents tried have the favorable therapeutic profile of glucose. Either because of prohibitive cost, or because of an unacceptable toxicity profile, the use of these agents as osmotic agents has been limited. One to two percent amino acid mixtures in the dialysis solution have been used effectively to induce ultrafiltration in nondiabetic CAPD patients [4]. Also, the absorbed amino-acids cause significant increases in the total body nitrogen and transferrin, reduce the inevitable glucose load, and lower serum triglyceride levels. Use of such mixtures in diabetic CAPD patients has the potential to reduce may of the undesirable effects of glucose. However, their effectiveness over long periods has not been established. Furthermore, the high cost of amino-acid mixtures is a major limiting factor. Glycerol-containing dialysis solution has been used successfully in diabetic CAPD patients. This agent was well tolerated by the patients, was non-toxic to the peritoneal membrane, did not cause hepato-toxicity, and did not increase protein losses in the dialysate [7]. Blood sugar was easily controlled with insulin. Some patients did develop signs and symptoms of hyperosmolality. However, glycerol showed no benefits over glucose because it delivered similar total caloric loads and the problem with hyperlipidemia was unaltered. Thus, for now, glucose still remains the least toxic osmotic agent for use in peritoneal dialysis. Also, many non-osmotic pharmacological agents have been shown in experimental settings to enhance net ultrafiltration, by modifying the forces of ultrafiltration kinetics while glucose was still used as the osmotic agent (in concentrations equal to or less than those conventionally used in clinical settings). This concept has lead to the identification of several more pharmacological agents which could be used to enhance ultrafiltration −still using glucose as the osmotic agent while reducing the glucose load per exchange. This review will describe those pharmacological agents known to cause such ultrafiltration enhancement and their mechanisms of action.

Forces That Govern Fluid Transport
Across the Peritoneal Membrane

Under physiological conditions there is a continuous leakage of ultrafiltrate from the capillaries into the peritoneal cavity. The fluid transport across the peritoneum is believed to be governed by the hydrostatic and colloid osmotic pressures in the capillaries and interstitium [8]. The hydrostatic pressure in the capillaries tends to force fluid and its dissolved substances through the capillary pores into the interstitial spaces, particularly from the proximal capillaries. This process is aided by the colloidal pressure and the relatively low hydrostatic pressure in the interstitial spaces. Under physiological conditions, in the tissues around the peritoneal cavity, the net hydrostatic pressure across the capillary membrane is greater than the net colloid osmotic pressure of plasma and interstitial proteins, causing net transmembrane pressure to favor ultrafiltration from the capillary lumen into the surrounding interstitium. This outward net driving pressure causes continuous leakage of ultrafiltrate out of the capillaries. It is this ultrafiltrate that becomes interstitital free fluid.

Lymph is derived from this interstitial fluid. The exact proportions of this fluid reabsorbed in lymphatics, distal capillaries, and venules in the peritoneum are unknown. Small amounts of this fluid constantly enter the peritoneal cavity, probably to lubricate the mesothelial surface of the organs that protrude into the cavity. Turnover is maintained by the continuous uptake of this fluid by the subdiaphragmatic lymphatics.

Kinetics of Ultrafiltration During Peritoneal Dialysis

During peritoneal dialysis, in order to induce ultrafiltration, glucose is added to dialysis solution at concentrations that greatly exceed the plasma concentration. This concentration difference creates a large driving force for ultrafiltration to occur from the interstitium and the capillary blood. When 2 liters of dialysis solution containing glucose are introduced into the peritoneal cavity during peritoneal dialysis, the forces that normally are operative across the capillary are modified in favor of enhanced ultrafiltration into the peritoneal cavity. For example, the net osmotic pressure difference across the peritoneum contributed by glucose when using dialysis fluid containing 4.25% dextrose is 210 mosm/kg H_2O (3990 mm Hg). Because of the relatively low reflection coefficient for glucose across the peritoneal membrane, this potential osmotic force is not fully manifested. Glucose is fairly rapidly absorbed across the peritoneal membrane into the capillaries. Therefore, transcapillary ultrafiltration is maximum at time zero and decreases exponentially as the dialysate glucose concentration is dissipated by a combination of dilution due to ultrafiltration and transperitoneal glucose absorption. As osmotic and solute equilibrium is approached, transcapillary ultrafiltration rate becomes equal to reabsorption rate and peak ultrafiltration volume is observed.

Fluid and solute absorption from the peritoneal cavity may occur by way of distal capillaries, venules, or lymphatics. The driving force for capillary and venular uptake is the net sum of hydrostatic and osmotic pressure gradients across the membrane. Peritoneal lymphatics continuously absorb intraperitoneal fluid by convective flow, mainly via the specialized end lymphatics located on the under surface of the diaphragm [9–12]. The physiologic role of the peritoneal lymphatics is to act as a one-way pathway for returning excess intraperitoneal fluid and proteins to the systemic circulation. Under normal conditions, there is a balance between the rate of ultrafiltration and lymph drainage, which allows for only a small volume of isosmotic fluid to be maintained within the peritoneal cavity.

The measured net ultrafiltration volume at the end of each exchange equals the dialysate drain volume minus the infusion volume, but physiologically this represents the difference between cumulative net transcapillary ultrafiltration into the peritoneal cavity and the total lymphatic drainage out of the peritoneal cavity over the dwell time. The term "net transcapillary ultrafiltration" refers to the total net influx of fluid from the peritoneal capillaries and interstitium into the peritoneal cavity in response to the osmotic pressure of the dialysis solution. The resultant net influx of fluid would equal measured net ultrafiltration if it were not for the constant drainage via the peritoneal lymphatics. Depending on the glucose concentration used and the peritoneal membrane transport rates, peak intraperitoneal volume is observed at about 2–6 h into the dwell, when the lymph flow rate equals the transcapillary ultrafiltration rate. From then on, the intraperitoneal volume will start decreasing when the lymph flow rate (which is nearly constant) exceeds the transcapillary ultrafiltration rate (which declines due to the gradual dissipation of the glucose osmotic gradient). Glucose equilibrium is achieved after peak volume, perhaps as late as 6–8 h after the infusion. Transcapillary ultrafiltration, though at a very low rate, continues beyond osmolar equilibrium. The likely reasons for the continued ultrafiltration are two-fold: persistent glucose disequilibrium even though osmotic equilibrium is achieved, and the sum effect of Starling's forces, favoring movement of fluid out of the capillary. Any persistent glucose gradient can still generate a net osmotic pressure since the reflection coefficient for glucose is greater than that for electrolytes and urea. Equilibrium is achieved before glucose equilibrium, in part because of electrolyte sieving and the low electrolyte content of ultrafiltrate. Hydrostatic pressure in peritoneal capillaries may also contribute to continued transcapillary ultrafiltration in the presence of osmotic equilibrium and even total equilibrium for all solutes.

Studies done in CAPD patients have shown that a 2 liter volume of 2.5% dextrose dialysis solution, when infused and permitted to dwell for 4 hours in the peritoneal cavity, causes about 500–800 ml of cumulative net transcapillary ultrafiltration [13]. During the same period, cumulative absorption from the sub-diaphragmatic lymphatics would be about 350 ml. Thus, the net measured ultrafiltration would be appreciably reduced to 150–450 ml. In short-dwell exchanges, net transcapillary ultrafiltration exceeds lymphatic absorption, so the reduction in the dialysate drain volume due to lymphatic drainage is relative minor.

Pharmacological Enhancement of Ultrafiltration

There are a number of potential sites where pharmacological agents could act to enhance ultrafiltration during peritoneal dialysis (Table 1). The agents can be divided into those which primarily act to enhance transcapillary ultrafiltration and those which mainly reduce lymphatic absorption.

Drugs that Enhance Transcapillary Ultrafiltration

Theoretically transcapillary ultrafiltration can be enhanced by drugs which either modify the forces acting across the peritoneal membrane or alter membrane mass transfer area coefficients.

Modification of Forces Across Peritoneal Membrane

Increasing the capillary hydrostatic pressure, lowering the capillary oncotic pressure, or reducing the interstitial hydrostatic pressure, singly or in combination, could accentuate the balance of forces which, under physiological conditions, favor ultrafiltration out of capillary lumen. In experimental settings, except for dopamine, vasoactive agents in general have failed to increase capillary hydrostatic pressure at the peritoneal level [14–20]. The capillary hydrostatic pressure in the body is not easily altered, due to the phenomenon of capillary flow autoregulation (the systemic arterial pressure can be changed over a wide range, and the blood flow and perfusion

Table 1. Potential sites where pharmacological agents could act to enhance ultrafiltration during peritoneal dialysis

A. Drugs that enhance transcapillary ultrafiltration	
1. Modification of forces across peritoneal membrane	2. Alter resistance sites
a. Raise capillary hydrostatic pressure	a. Increase hydraulic permeability
Dopamine	Secretin
L-epinephrine	Puromycine
b. Lower capillary oncotic pressure	Amphotericin B
Hypoproteinemia	Verapamil
c. Reduce interstitial hydrostatic pressure	$1,25(OH)_2D_3$
???	b. Reduce stagnant fluid film layer
d. Generate osmotic pressure gradient	(surfactants)
	Chlorpromazine
	Docusate sodium
	Phosphatidylcholine
	Furosemide

B. Drugs that reduce lymph flow	C. Drugs that improve mechanics of flow
Close stomata:	Reduce/dissolve fibrin heparin
Neostigmine	Heparin
Phosphatidylcholine	Streptokinase
	Urokinase
	Lessen catheter compression laxatives

pressures through the tissue capillaries will remain almost unaltered). Supportive evidence for the autoregulation is seen in the settings of hypotension and hypothermia, in which peritoneal transport rates of solutes and water are only modestly decreased. Vasodilator and vasopressor therapies in these situations do not significantly alter the peritoneal transport rates [14,15]. L-norepinephrine decreases solute clearances without change in ultrafiltration [21,22]. Administration of intravenous or intraperitoneal dopamine during a peritoneal dialysis exchange increases both solute and water transport. This is unaffected by the simultaneous administration of propranolol, is decreased by phentolamine, and is abolished by haloperidol, a dopamine receptor competitor [22,23]. Since the predominant effect of dopamine at the microcirulatory level is shown to be venular constriction, in contrast to L-epinephrine [24], the augmented ultrafiltration probably results from an increased net capillary hydrostatic pressure [21]. Neither dopamine nor L-norepinephrine have been found clinically usable because of their widespread unwanted actions elsewhere in the body.

Hypoproteinemia results in a lowered oncotic pressure and contributes to the generation of ascites in certain disease conditions. In those CAPD patients who are severely malnourished with very low plasma protein and albumin concentrations, enhanced ultrafiltration rates have been observed. Such a phenomenon, however, is unlikely to provide a therapeutic role in the manipulation of ultrafiltration in clinical situations.

There is as yet no practical method to lower interstitial fluid pressure during a peritoneal dialysis exchange. This approach, therefore, is clinically not used in CAPD patients.

Osmotic pressure generation with alternative non-glucose osmotic agents has had limited success; as discussed above an agent with a therapeutic profile comparable to glucose has not been found.

Thus, in experimental settings, several pharmacological agents have been shown to enhance transcapillary ultrafiltration by modifying forces which function across the peritoneal membrane under physiological conditions. But clinically useful agents other than non-glucose osmotic agents have not been, as yet, identified.

Agents that Modify the Membrane Resistance Sites

Major increases in membrane permeability, such as those which occur with peritonitis, may enhance glucose uptake, cause rapid loss of the osmotic gradient, and decrease net ultrafiltration. Investigators have searched for agents that increase hydraulic permeability without major changes in glucose absorption. Theoretically, this could be made possible by increasing the number or size of very tiny pores available for water transport.

Solutes and fluid must cross resistance sites in moving from peritoneal capillaries into the peritoneal dialysis solution [25]. These sites include stagnant fluid films in the capillary, the endothelial cell layer, the capillary endothelial basement membrane, the interstitium, the mesothelial cell layer, and the stagnant fluid films in the peritoneal cavity. Modification in one or more sites is referred to as alteration in hydraulic permeability.

The hydraulic permeability of rabbit mesentery has been significantly altered with the gastrointestinal hormone, secretin, and the aminonucleoside, puromycin, when applied from the vascular side only [26]. These agents significantly augment osmotically induced water flux. Amphotericin B, when applied from the serosal side, presumably by creating channels in biological membranes for solute and water, increases ultrafiltration rate more than 70% compared to control without changing the osmotic gradient [27]. Because of the short half life and/or serious toxic side effects, these agents have not found clinical application in peritoneal dialysis.

The calcium channel blocker, Verapamil, after a few months of therapy in CAPD patients with reduced ultrafiltration capacity, has been shown to cause significant increases in the drainage volume [28]. In addition, when verapamil was used in these patients for up to 6 months, they showed a progressive decrease in intracellular calcium, secretory product interferon-Y and interleukin-1 in the peritoneal lymphocytes and macrophages. Based on these observations, the authors proposed that increases in the concentrations of lymphokines in the peritoneal cavity probably stimulate fibroblastic proliferation, resulting in peritoneal structural and functional alterations with a change in peritoneal hydraulic permeability. Verapamil presumably reverses these trends.

The stagnant dialysis fluid films in the peritoneal cavity and the resistance site overlying the mesothelial cell layer have been modified by drugs with surfactant properties. The peritoneal effluent in CAPD patients was reported to contain a phospholipid surface active material, identified on thin layer chromatography as positively charged phosphatidylcholine [29]. Peritoneal physiology may be altered in CAPD patients by the constant removal of phosphatidylcholine and other phospholipids in the dialysis effluent [29]. Phospholipid concentrations in the dialysate effluent are significantly reduced after long-term CAPD and during peritonitis [30]. The prominence of intracellular synthetic organelles in the mesothelium from CAPD patients may reflect increased production of phosphatidylcholine in an attempt to compensate for constant losses in the dialysate [30,31]. The poor ultrafiltration capacity in such patients is greatly improved with the addition of 50 mg/l of phos-phatidylcholine to the infused dialysis solution, despite the likelihood of co-existing alterations in the integrity, and perhaps in the surface anionic charge of the mesothelium [31–33]. The observed net increase in the ultrafiltration and solute clearances with the addition of phosphatidylcholine to the infused dialysis solution has been attributed to its surface tension lowering properties [26,30]. It is believed that surfactants increase ultrafiltration by narrowing the stagnant dialysate layers over the mesothelium and by creating a water repellent lining on the surface of the peritoneum. Since glucose absorption from the dialysate does not increase during exchanges with phosphatidylcholine [30,34], it is proposed that the thinning of fluid films over the mesothelium causes unidirectional enhancement of peritoneal trans-port from the peritoneal microcirculation to the dialysis solution. Since the original studies of Di Paolo et al. [30], several recent studies have either confirmed [35,36] or refuted [37,38] the observation of enhanced ultrafiltration, with the use of either oral or intraperitoneal phosphatidylcholine administration. Our studies in rats [36] have confirmed enhanced ultrafiltration with phosphatidylcholine, but we have pro-posed an additional mechanism for its action, which will be discussed more in the section on reduced lymphatic absorption from the peritoneal cavity (see below).

Intraperitoneal chlorpromazine (2 mg/l dialysis solution), another surfactant, was reported to increase ultrafiltration and solute clearance rates more than 50% in 12 patients on CAPD [39]. These changes were unaccompanied by any changes in the dialysate osmolality or protein concentration. This agent was also shown to lower dialysate surface tension in vitro and was hence postulated to alter the thickness of the stagnant fluid films and to enhance water flux across the peritoneum.

Agents that Reduce Lymph Flow From the Peritoneal Cavity

We have previously shown that cumulative lymphatic absorption from the peritoneal cavity significantly reduces net ultrafiltration and solute clearances during long-dwell exchanges in man [13] and rat [40]. Most lymphatic drainage from the peritoneal cavity occurs by convective transport via the subdiaphragmatic stomata [9–12]. Fixed contraction of these stomata, which has been observed with intraperitoneal infusion of cholinergic drugs [41], also ought to reduce lymphatic absorption of intraperitoneal fluid [12,42]. Neostigmine, a quaternary ammonium carbamyl ester anticholinesterase agent, has been used therapeutically in myasthenia gravis and paralytic ileus [43]; it was shown to enhance net ultrafiltration in rats dur-ing a peritoneal dialysis exchange using 2.5% dextrose dialysis solution [44]. The enhancement of ultrafiltration was achieved by a reduction in cumulatiave lymphatic absorption, and was achieved without an increase in total capillary ultrafiltration during the dwell time. Likewise, solute clearances were augmented with neostig-mine, primarily due to the increase in dialysate drain volume without a change in dialysate to serum solute ratios. Despite the impressive ultrafiltration enhancement during glucose ultrafiltration, neostigmine, because of its cumulative systemic toxic-ity, is clinically unusable for the long-term peritoneal dialysis patient. The effect of phosphatidylcholine in enhancing ultrafiltration during a peritoneal dialysis exchange in the rat was shown to be similar to that of neostigmine [44]. Besides the surfactant properties discussed earlier, based on our rat studies, phosphatidylcholine causes reduction of lymph flow during a peritoneal dialysis exchange in the rat. This lymph flow reducing property of phosphatidylcholine may be related to one of the following two mechanisms: 1) It has a cholingeric effect when taken systemically. This cholinergic effect [45–50] has been the biochemical basis of its reported beneficial effects when large doses were given to patients with tardive dyskinesia [51–53], Friedreich's ataxia [54], Alzheimer's disease [55], and memory and mood disorders [56–59]. Our rat studies suggest that, similarly to neostigmine, the cholinergic effects of phosphatidylcholine, when given intraperitoneally, cause the subdiaphragmatic stomata to contract and reduce lymph flow. The uptake of Indian ink by the lymphatics of rats who received dialysis exchanges without phosphatidylcholine, and the lack of uptake in rats treated with phosphatidylcholine are supportive of this hypothesis [36]. 2) Alternatively, another presumptive mode of action of phosphatidylcholine relates to its charge effect. The high density anionic charges on the lymphatic endothelium and, to a lesser extent, the microvilli and intercellular clefts of the subdiaphragmatic mesothelium, may play a role in the resorption of intraperitoneal fluid into the interstitium or lymphatics by a mechanism of charges repelling one another in such a way as to favor open stoma [60]. Positively charged choline may bind to and negate the surface anionic charge thereby reducing the functional patency of the intercellular channels between mesothelial and endothelial cells [36]. This hypothesis is supported by the observation that the cationic dye, alcian blue, abolishes the effect of phosphatidylcholine on isolated membranes in vitro [61]. The optimal conditions necessary for phosphatidylcholine (PC) to be effective are unclear at this time. Is it effective only when PC is deficient in phospholipid content? What concentration in the dialysis solution is required for it to be clinically useful? Is oral administration as effective as ip administration? These are some of the questions that need to be answered before it would prove to be clinically usable.

Drugs that Improve Mechanics of Flow

Mechanical problems resulting in slow drainage are often associated with build up of a residual volume. This may enhance reabsorption and/or dilute infused glucose concentrations and thereby decease daily net ultrafiltration.

Use of heparin in the dialysis solution improves drainage and reduces residual volume in patients who are prone to form fibrin, especially during peritonitis. Intraperitoneal heparin, up to a dose of 5000 units/2 l dialysis solution, causes very little activity in the plasma [62]. A slightly higher concentration of antithrombin in dialysate at the end of 4 hour dwell time is sufficient to inhibit fibrin formation in heparinized dialysis solution [63]. Despite the lack of evidence for other mechanisms of action for heparin at the membrane level, some believe it enhances ultrafiltration due to a charge effect.

Constipation frequently leads to poor drainage. Laxatives, by relieving constipation, improve drainage simply by reducing external pressure on the intraperitoneal segment of the catheter.

References

1. Stout RW (1979) Diabetes and atherosclerosis – The role of insulin. Diabetologia 16:141
2. Zavaroni A, Bonora E, Pagliara M, Dall'Aglio E, Luchetti L, Buonanno G, Bonati PA, Bergonzani M, Gnudi L, Passeri M, Reaven G (1989) Risk factor for coronary artery

disease in healthy persons with hyperinsulemia and normal glucose tolerance. N Engl J Med 320:702–706

3. Bazzato G, Coli U, Landini S (1982) Xylitol and low doses of insulin: New perspectives for diabetic uremic patients on CAPD. Perit Dial Bull 2:161

4. Williams FP, Marliss EB, Anderson GH, et al. (1982) Amino acids absorption following intraperitoneal administration in CAPD patients. Perit Dial Bull 2:124

5. Twardowski ZJ, Khanna R, Nolph KD (1986) Osmotic agents and ultrafiltration in peritoneal dialysis. Nephron 42:93

6. Mistry CD, Mallick NP, Gokal R (1986) The use of large molecular weight glucose polymer as an osmotic agent in CAPD. In: Khanna R, Nolph KD, Prowant BF, Twardowski ZJ, Oreopoulos DG (eds) Advances in continuous ambulatory peritoneal dialysis. Peritoneal Dialysis Bulletin, Toronto, pp 7–11

7. Matthys E, Dolkart R, Lameire N (1987) Extended use of a glycerol containing dialysate in the treatment of diabetic CAPD patients. Perit Dial Bull 7:10

8. Guyton AC (1981) The lymphatic system, interstitial fluid dynamics, edema, and pulmonary fluid. Textbook of medical physiology, 6th edn. Saunders, Philadelphia, pp 370–380

9. Courtice FC, Simmonds WJ (1954) Physiological significance of lymph drainage of the serous cavities and lungs. Physiol Rev 34:419–448

10. Von Recklinghausen F (1863) Zur Fettresorption. Arch Patholog Anat Physiol Klin Med 26:172

11. Khanna R, Mactier R, Twardowski ZJ, Nolph KD (1986) Peritoneal cavity lymphatics. Perit Dial Bull 6:113–121

12. Raybuck HE, Allen L, Harms WS (1960) Absorption of serum from the peritoneal cavity. Am J Physiol 119:1021–1024

13. Mactier RA, Khanna R, Twardowski ZJ, Nolph KD (1987) Contribution of lymphatic absorption to loss of ultrafiltration and solute clearances in CAPD. J Clin Invest 80:1311–1316

14. Patton JF, Doolittle WH, Hamlet MP (1974) Peritoneal clearance of urea and potassium following experimental hypothermia. J Appl Physiol 36:403–406

15. Greene JA, Lapco L, Weller JM (1970) Effect of drug therapy of hemorrhagic hypotension on kinetics of peritoneal dialysis in the dog. Nephron 7:178–183

16. Surdiel LG, Castillo D, Martin-Malo A (1985) Effect of verapamil and prostaglandin E_1 on peritoneal membrane transport (abstract). Proc Eur Dial Transplant Assoc, p 95

17. Nolph KD, Ghods AJ, Van Stone J, et al. (1976) The effects of intraperitoneal vasodilator on peritoneal clearances. Trans Am Soc Artif Intern Organs 22:586–594

18. Wideroe TE, Smeby LC, Dahl K, et al. (1988) Definitions of differences and changes in peritoneal membrane transport properties. Kidney Int 33:S107–113

19. Grzegorzewska A, Grala T, Alexiewicz J (1984) Effect of intraperitoneal administration of furosemide and sodium nitroprusside on the elimination of water, sodium and potassium during peritoneal dialysis. Pol Arch Med Wewn 71:281–291

20. Panasiuk E (1985) Effect of sodium nitroprusside, furosemide and dopamine on the efficiency of peritoneal dialysis. Pol Arch Med Wewn 74:316–326

21. Hirszel P, Lasrich M, Maher JF (1979) Divergent effects of catecholamines on peritoneal mass transport. Trans Am Soc Artif Intern Organs 25:110

22. Hirszel P, Lasrich M, Maher JF (1979) Augmentation of peritoneal mass transport by dopamine: Comparison with norepinephrine and evaluation of pharmacologic mechanisms. J Lab Clin Med 94:747

23. Chan MK, Varghese Z, Baillod RA, et al. (1980) Peritoneal dialysis: effect of intraperitoneal dopamine. Dial Transplant 9:380

24. Goldberg LI (1972) Cardiovascular and renal actions of dopamine; potential clinical applications. Pharmacol Rev 24:1

25. Nolph KD, Miller F, Rubin J, et al. (1980) New directions in peritoneal dialysis concepts and applications. Kidney Int 18:S111–S116

26. Maher JF, Hirszel P, Lasrich M (1979) The effects of gastrointestinal hormones on transport by peritoneal dialysis. Kidney Int 16:130
27. Maher JF, Hirszel P, Bennett RR, et al. (1984) Amphotericin B selectively increases peritoneal ultrafiltration. Am J Kidney Dis 4:285–288
28. Lamperi S, Carozzi S, Nasini MG (1987) Calcium antagonists improve ultrafiltration in patients on continuous ambulatory peritoneal dialysis. Trans Am Soc Artif Intern Organs 33:657–663
29. Grahame GR, Torchia MG, Dankewich KA, et al. (1985) Surface-active material in peritoneal effluent of CAPD patients. Perit Dial Bull 5:109
30. DiPaolo N, Buoncristiani U, Capotundo L, et al. (1986) Phosphatidylcholine and peritoneal transport during peritoneal dialysis. Nephron 44:365
31. Dobbie JW, Zaki M, Wilson L (1981) Ultrastructural studies on the peritoneum with special reference to chronic ambulatory peritoneal dialysis. Scott Med 26:213–223
32. Di Paolo N, Sacchi G, De Mia M, et al. (1986) Morphology of the peritoneal membrane during peritoneal dialysis. Nephron 44:204–211
33. Verger C, Brunschvigg O, Le Carpentier Y, et al. (1981) Structural and ultrastructural peritoneal membrane changes and permeability alterations during CAPD. Proc Eur Dial Transplant Assoc 18:199–203
34. Breborowicz A, Sombolos K, Rodela H, et al. (1987) Mechanism of phosphatidylcholine action during peritoneal dialysis. Nephron 7:6
35. Chan H, Abraham G, Oreopoulos DG (1989) Oral lecithin improves ultrafiltration in patients on peritoneal dialysis. Perit Dial Int 9:203–205
36. Mactier RA, Khanna R, Twardowski ZJ, Moore H, Nolph KD (1988) Influence of phosphatidylcholine on lymphatic absorption during peritoneal dialysis in the rat. Perit Dial Int 8:179–186
37. De Vecchi A, Castelnovo C, Guerra L, et al. (1989) Phosphatidylcholine administration in continuous ambulatory peritoneal dialysis (CAPD) patients with reduced ultrafiltration. Perit Dial Int 9:207–210
38. Di Paolo B, Chakrabarti, Maher JF (1989) Phosphatidylcholine does not affect peritoneal transport of intact rabbits. Perit Dial Int 9:211–213
39. Indraprasit S, Sooksriwongse C (1985) Effect of chlorpromazine on peritoneal clearances. Nephron 40:341–343
40. Nolph KD, Mactier RA, Khanna R, et al. (1987) Kinetics of peritoneal ultrafiltration: the role of lymphatics. Kidney Int 32:219–226
41. Tsilibary EC, Wissig SL (1983) Lymphatic absorption from the peritoneal cavity: regulation of patency of mesothelial stomata. Microvasc Res 25:22–39
42. Lill SR, Parsons RH, Bohac I (1979) Permeability of the diaphragm and fluid resorption from the peritoneal cavity in the rat. Gastroenterology 76:997–1001
43. Koelle GB (1975) Anticholinesterase agents. In: Goodman LS, Gilman A (eds) The pharmacological basis of therapeutics, 5th edn. Macmillan, New York, pp 445–466
44. Mactier RA, Khanna R, Moore H, Twardowski ZJ, Nolph KD (1988) Pharmacological reduction of lymphatic absorption from the peritoneal cavity increases net ultrafiltration and solute clearances in peritoneal dialysis. Nephron 50:229–232
45. Cohen EL, Wurtman RJ (1975) Brain acetylcholine: Increase after systemic choline administration. Life Sci 16:1095–2000
46. Hambrich DR, Chippendale TJ (1977) Regulation of acetylcholine synthesis in nervous tissue. Life Sci 20:1465–1478
47. Hirsch MJ, Ulus IH, Wurtman RJ (1976) Elevation of brain and adrenal acetylcholine levels and of adrenal tyrosine hydroxylase activity following administration of choline via stomach tube. Neurosci Abstr 1:765
48. Cohen EL, Wurtman RJ (1976) Brain acetylcholine: control by dietary choline. Science 191:561–562

49. Morley BJ, Robinson GR, Brown GB, et al. (1977) Effect of dietary choline on nicotinic acetylcholine receptors in brain. Nature 266:848–859
50. Ulus IH, Wurtman RJ (1976) Choline administration: activation of tyrosine hydroxylase in dopaminergic neurons of rat brain. Science 194:1060–1061
51. Fann WE, Lake CR, Gerber CT, et al. (1974) Cholinergic suppression of tardive dyskinesia. Psychopharmacologia 37:101–107
52. Growdon JH, Gelenberg AJ, Doller J, et al. (1978) Lecithin can suppress tardive dyskinesia. N Engl J Med 297:524–527
53. Jackson IV, Davis LG, Cohen RK, et al. (1981) Lecithin administration in tardive dyskinesia: Clinical and biomedical correlates. Biol Psychiatry 16:85–89
54. Pentland B, Martyn CN, Steer CR, et al. (1981) Lecithin treatment in Friedreich's ataxia. Br Med J [Clin Res] 282:1197–1198
55. Etienne P, Gauthier S, Dastoor D, et al. (1979) Alzheimer's disease: clinical effect of lecithin treatment. In: Barbeau A (ed) Nutrition and the brain. Raven, New York, pp 389–396
56. Drachman DA, Sahakian BJ (1979) Effects of cholinergic agents on human learning and memory. In: Barbeau A (ed) Nutrition and the brain. Raven, New York, pp 351–366
57. Sitaram N, Weingartner H, Christian Gillin J (1979) Choline chloride and arecoline: Effects on memory and sleep in man. In: Barbeau A (ed) Nutrition and the brain. Raven, New York, pp 367–376
58. Harris CM, Davis JM, Janowsky DS (1979) Use of cholinergic drugs in mental illness. In: Barbeau A (ed) Nutrition and the brain. Raven, New York, pp 397–408
59. Tamminga CA, Nutt JG (1979) Cholinergic influences on affect. In: Barbeau A (ed) Nutrition and the brain. Raven, New York, pp 409–416
60. Leak LV (1986) Distribution of cell surface charges on mesothelium and lymphatic endothelium. Microvasc Res 31:18–30
61. Breborowicz A, Sombolos K, Rodela H, Oreopoulos DG (1987) Mechanism of phosphatidylcholine action during peritoneal dialysis. Perit Dial Bull 7:6–9
62. Gries E, Paar D, Graben N, Bock KD (1986) Intraperitoneal fibrin formation and its inhibition in CAPD. Clin Nephrology 26:209–212

The Impact of the Y-System and Low Peritonitis Rate on CAPD Results

R. Maiorca, G.C. Cancarini, L. Manili, C. Camerini, and G. Brunori

SUMMARY. The impact of peritonitis rate on continuous ambulatory peritoneal dialysis (CAPD) results was evaluated in 288 patients. Of these 288 patients 186 used a Y-connector with an in-line disinfectant (Y-system) from the same firm; 142 patients used this system from the beginning of their first treatment. The Y-system was confirmed to be an effective means of preventing peritonitis episodes, with 50% of patients being peritonitis-free after 3 and a half years (5 months for the standard set). A minority of patients had had 2 (7%) or 3 or more (9%) peritonitis episodes after a follow-up of 290 patient-years (19% and 33% after 77 patient-years, on the standard set).

Peritoneal function (ultrafiltration volume and peritoneal equilibration tests), peripheral neural function (motor nerve conduction velocity), and several laboratory data (blood urea nitrogen (BUN), serum creatinine, hemoglobin, total proteins, albumin, transferrin, pseudocholinesterase, cholesterol, triglycerides), some of them indicative of nutritional status, did not appear to be affected by peritonitis frequency. Serum beta-2m also was not influenced by the rate of peritonitis.

An influence of peritonitis frequency on patient survival was seen only after excluding patients who died before having a peritonitis episode. In the entire population, causes other than peritonitis were of major importance for patient survival. Peritonitis almost completely accounted for the greater drop-out rate from the CAPD technique than from the hemodialysis (HD) technique. A low rate of peritonitis, such as that obtained with the Y-system, appears to be important for improving CAPD results.

Introduction

As is well known, the Y-system consists of a Y-shaped connector filled with a disinfectant during the dwell-time and flushed before filling the peritoneal cavity [1].

Institute of Nephrology, University of Brescia, 25100, Brescia, Italy, and Division of Nephrology, Spedali Civili, 25100, Brescia, Italy

This system, suggested by Buoncristiani et al. some years ago [2], has been shown in controlled studies [1,3] to reduce peritonitis frequency better than any other method [4]. In this paper, the results obtained in a single institution with a large experience of the Y-system are analyzed in order to evaluate the impact of the low peritonitis rate on CAPD results.

Patients and Methods

Overall CAPD experience at the Institute of Nephrology of the University of Brescia includes 288 patients, in part new patients and in part patients coming from other treatments, using other connection systems. Of these 288 patients, 186 were put on Y-solution transfer sets purchased from one firm. Of these, 142 were new patients. For these 186 patients, in 3479 patient-months, we had 104 peritonitis episodes, with an incidence of 1 every 33.4 patient-months. All our experience with the standard set was in the first years of our use of CAPD, because after the good results obtained with the Y-set, all our patients were put on this connector. However, the peritonitis incidence recently reported in the literature with standard sets [4] is the same as our former results.

Routine methods were used for biochemical tests, and radio-immunoassay (RIA) was used for β2-microglobulin. Motor nerve conduction velocity was measured on the external sciatic popliteal nerve.

Statistics: patient and method survivals were calculated and compared according to Peto et al. [5,6]. Analysis of variance and multiple regression analysis were done with Statworks from Cricket Software.

Results

Peritonitis Frequency on Y and Standard Connectors

Peritonitis incidence has changed over the years, from a minimum of 1 episode every 23 patient-months to 1 every 64 patient-months, with the usual incidence being over 30. In our experience the 50% patient probability of remaining peritonitis free was 5 months on the standard set and 3 and half years on the Y-system. On the standard set, the probability of having the second and the third peritonitis episode was about the same as for the first (50% after 6 months), whereas on the Y-system, the 50% probability of having the second episode after the first was 1.5 years and, for the third episode, was 6 months (Fig. 1). Actually, for our 142 patients who had begun on the Y-system, after a follow-up of 290 patient-years, only 9% had had three or more peritonitis episodes, a figure to be compared to the 33% for the standard set after a follow-up of 77 patient-years.

Patient and Technique Survival

To better evaluate the impact of the low peritonitis rate on CAPD results we examined our entire group of 288 patients, treated from the start of our experience by CAPD. These were in large part new patients, but also included patients switched from other

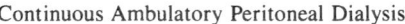

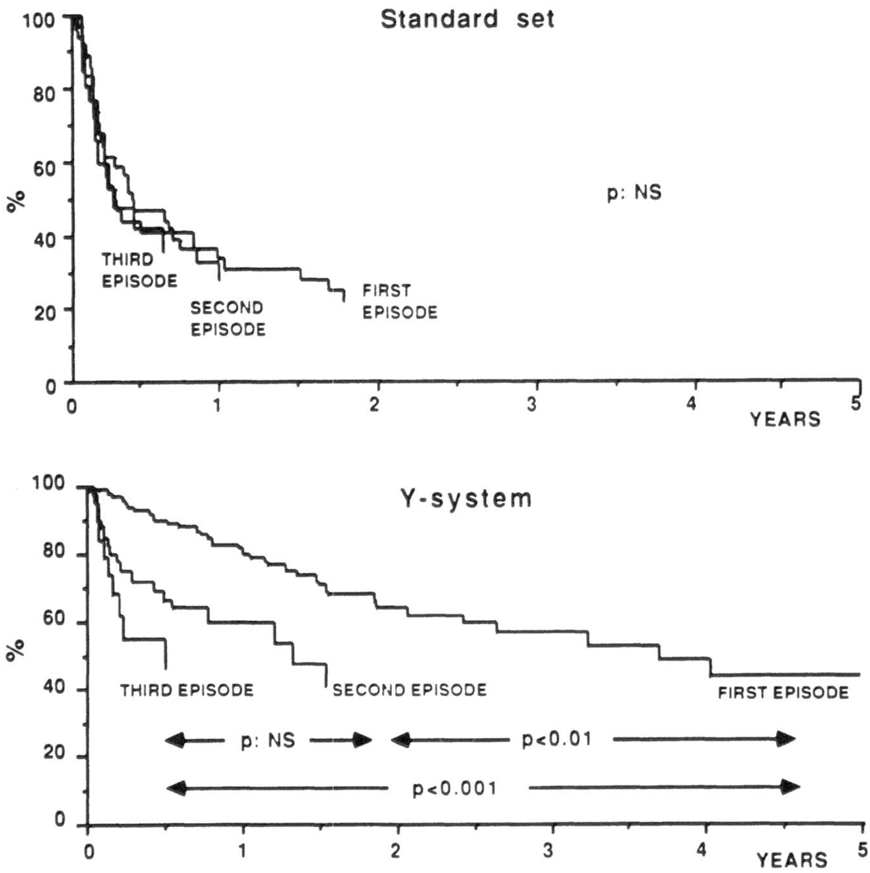

Fig. 1. Probability of remaining peritonitis-free for new patients on the Standard-set (*upper panel*) and the Y-system (*lower panel*)

treatments, and put on standard and on the Y-set; this last Y-set included Y-connectors and solutions of two different brands. Patients were divided into 4 groups, one with no peritonitis episodes; one with fewer than 0.5; one group with up to 1; and one group with more than 1 peritonitis episode per year. Number and mean age of

Table 1. Groups of patients according to peritonitis rate

Group	Peritonitis rate (episode/year)	Number of patients	Mean age at start (M±SD)	Months on CAPD (M±SD)
1	No. episodes	131	61 ± 13	16 ± 15
2	<0.5	33	60 ± 11	61 ± 25
3	0.5–1	53	61 ± 14	43 ± 24
4	>1	71	60 ± 16	25 ± 23

Table 2. Causes of death in patients divided according to peritonitis rate. Events/100 patients per year

Cause of death	Group 1	Group 2	Group 3	Group 4
Cardiac	10.11	3.59	1.57	6.04
Vascular	3.93	2.39	1.57	1.34
Infectious	1.68	0	1.57	1.34
Peritonitis	0	0	2.09	3.36
Cachexia	1.12	0.60	0.52	0.67
Dementia	1.12	0.60	0	0.67
Malignancy	3.37	0	1.05	1.34
Liver diseases	0	0.60	0.52	2.63
Other	1.12	1.20	0.53	1.34

patients and follow-up for each group are given in Table 1. Table 2 shows the incidence of every cause of death in the groups with different rates of peritonitis. Those patients who were more seriously ill died from their associated illnesses in the first months of treatment, before they arrived at a first peritonitis episode. The mortality rate was maximal for patients with cardio-vascular disease and malignancy. In this group and in the one with a very low peritonitis rate, which included the great majority of patients treated with the Y-system, there were no deaths because of peritonitis. In the groups with high peritonitis rates, death was due to cardio-vascular causes, liver disease, and other causes as well as to peritonitis. Among the liver disease patients, the percentages with cirrhosis, were 5%, 9%, 7%, and 13%, for the four groups, respectively. Finally, there was no relationship between other infections or cachexia-dementia or other causes of death and the peritonitis rate.

Excluding patients who had no peritonitis episodes, life table analysis of patient survival showed different survival curves for the three groups of patients with different peritonitis rates (Fig. 2). The difference was significantly different only between the groups with very low and very high peritonitis rates. Patients with more than 1

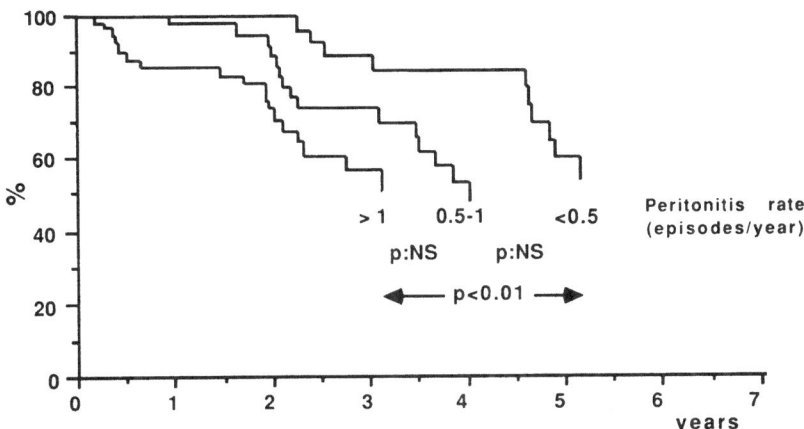

Fig. 2. Patient survival, according to peritonitis rate

Table 3. Causes for drop-out of patients divided according to peritonitis rate. Events/100 patients per year

Cause of CAPD failure	Group 1	Group 2	Group 3	Group 4
Poor compliance	1.68	0	0	1.34
Inadequate ultrafiltration	1.68	0	0	0
Poor biochemical control	1.12	0.60	0	0.67
Patient choice	3.37	0	0.52	0
Catheter/abdominal wall related	0.56	0.60	0.52	0.67
Clinical	1.12	0	0	4.03
Peritonitis	0	0	2.09	6.04
Other	0.56	0	0	0

peritonitis episode per year seem to have a definitely greater probability of death than patients with fewer than 0.5 episodes per year.

In the same patients, causes of drop-out were examined according to peritonitis rate (Table 3). A large number of drop-outs were in the first group, patients who changed methods before having a peritonitis episode. The causes were poor compliance, inadequate ultrafiltration (UF) or biochemical control, and, less important, other clinical reasons (metabolic, others). In the groups with more than 0.5 peritonitis episodes per year, peritonitis and other problems related to the catheter and to the abdominal well were the most frequent causes for leaving the method, with a low incidence of other causes.

True *technique survivals*, obtained by treating those patients who had died, had transplants, or had recovered renal function as lost to follow-up in the analysis, were high for patients with up to 1 peritonitis episode per patient-year, but were significantly worse for patients with more than 1 peritonitis episode per patient-year. The difference was statistically significant only between patients with fewer than 0.5 episodes per year and patients with more than 1 episode per year (Fig. 3).

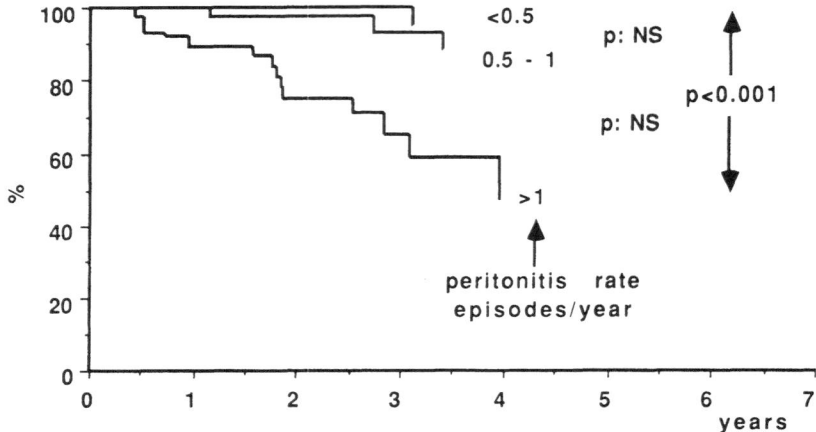

Fig. 3. True technique survival (only CAPD failure considered as final event), according to peritonitis rate

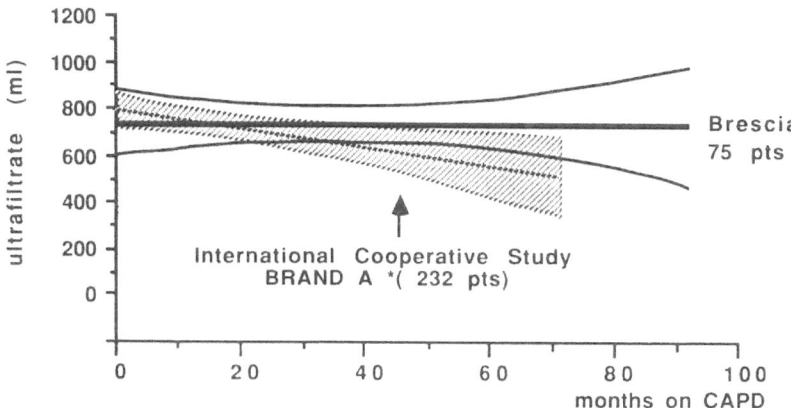

Fig. 4. Trend of ultrafiltration volume over time on CAPD. Comparison between the results of the International Cooperative Study and data of our center

Peritoneal Function

Of our CAPD Y-patients 71 were studied with peritoneal equilibration tests, performed with 2 liters 4.25% glucose and a dwell-time of 4 hours. Mean CAPD duration was 25 months, with a mean number of 0.8 peritonitis episodes during this time.

We found no relationship between glucose absorption, or creatinine transfer, or drainage volume and the number of peritonitis episodes, incidence of peritonitis episodes, or time on CAPD.

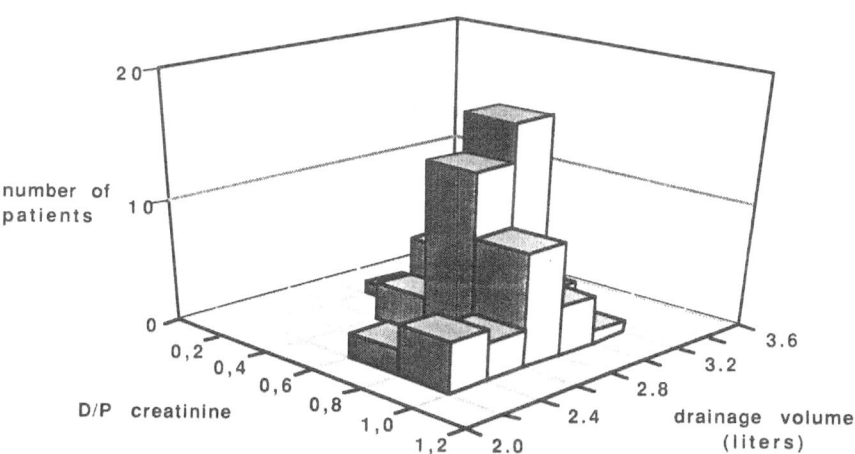

Fig. 5. Seventy-one patients on CAPD. (D/P) creatinine and drainage volume after a 4-hour dwell with 4.25% glucose, two liter bag

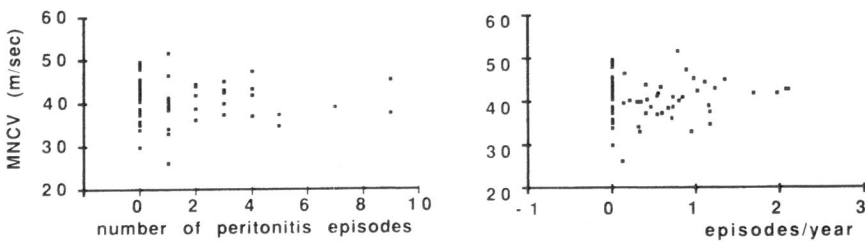

Fig. 6. Motor nerve conduction velocity (*MNCV*) versus number of peritonitis episodes and peritonitis rate

In the International Cooperative Study published in 1984 [7] the relationship between ultrafiltrate volume with 4.25% glucose bags and time on CAPD was investigated in a large number of patients. In that study, the ultrafiltered volume appeared to become smaller as time on treatment lengthened. Such a negative relationship was not apparent in our patients, all on the Y-system, who were followed up until more than 90 months of treatment (Fig. 4). In our series only a very few cases had low, but still sufficient, drainage volumes or low solute transfer (Fig. 5). In no cases were the two indexes of peritoneal function associated, as has been seen in the severe peritoneal malfunction which evolves in sclerosing encapsulating peritonitis. Actually, in the 142 new patients put on the Y-set, we have so far observed only 1 patient with inadequate ultrafiltration and 2 patients with poor biochemical control. In our overall experience with 288 patients, we have had 3 cases (1%) with inadequate ultrafiltration and 4 cases (1.4%) with poor biochemical control. In no case have we had sclerosing encapsulating peritonitis.

Metabolic and Nutritional Data

The influence of peritonitis rate on some biochemical tests was investigated in 108 unselected patients with a mean age of 63 ± 13 years, who had been on CAPD for 28 ± 25 months (range 4-100). In the analysis of variance, we found no relationship between incidence of peritonitis and BUN, serum creatinine, hemoglobin, serum

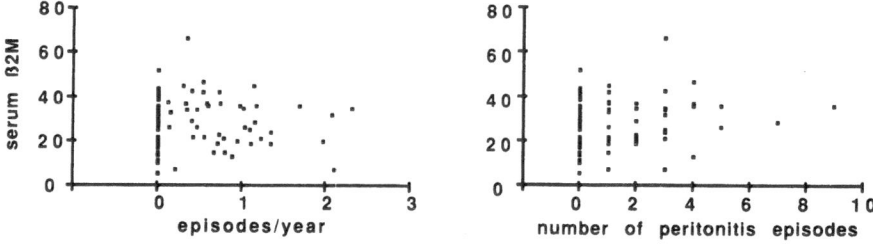

Fig. 7. Serum β2-microglobulin (*Serum β2M*) concentration versus peritonitis rate and number of peritonitis episodes

Table 4. Multiple regression analysis of variables that might affect serum β2-microglobulin concentration

Independent variables:	P
Age	0.338
Time of CAPD	0.830
Number of peritonitis episodes	0.593
Peritonitis rate	0.487
Residual urinary volume	<0.001

protein levels (total proteins), albumin, transferrin, pseudocholinesterases, cholesterol, or triglycerides.

Conduction velocity in a motor nerve, the external sciatic-popliteal nerve, did not change as a function of the number of peritonitis episodes or as a function of their frequency (Fig. 6). We also found no relationship between number and frequency of peritonitis episodes and serum level of beta-2 microglobulin (Fig. 7). The only independent variable that clearly influenced the serum beta-2m level in CAPD was the residual urinary volume (Table 4, Fig. 8), that is, the residual renal function.

Discussion

The peritonitis free survival curve was much better with the Y-system than with the standard set for the first two peritonitis episodes, but the intervals between the second and the third peritonitis episodes were the same for the standard and the Y-set. Interpretation of these data is difficult. One possible explanation might be that after the first episodes some changes, such as non-apparent tunnel infections, or intra-catheter bacterial slime, or other changes, also immunological factors, intervene to make new peritonitis episodes more likely. Another possibility is that the Y-system

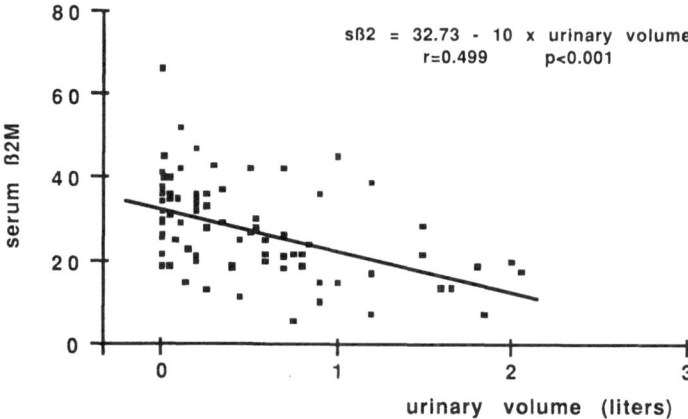

Fig. 8. Relationship between residual urinary volume (*r*) and serum β2-microglobulin (*Serum β2M*) concentration

reveals one population of patients for whom the Y-system is ineffective. As mentioned above, the Y-system cannot prevent hematogenic peritonitis, or peritonitis from bowel infections or from exit-site or tunnel infections. From the clinical point of view it is important to realize that the Y-system becomes of little help when three or more peritonitis episodes follow. In these patients, who are only a minority of the population on the Y-system (9% in our experience with 142 patients with a follow-up of 3479 patient-months), substitution of the catheter or a change to hemodialysis might be taken into consideration. Also, methods that might re-establish the preventive efficacy of the Y-system, for instance fibrinolytic, or other treatment, should be tested.

The impact of the peritonitis rate on patient survival is difficult to assess because of the interference caused by the frequent cardiovascular and neoplastic deaths which occurred even before the appearance of the first peritonitis episode. Excluding the first group of patients who did not have any peritonitis episodes, we can see that patient mortality increased with peritonitis frequency. Patients in the different peritonitis rate groups had the same mean age, so the differences in survival were not due to patient age at the beginning of CAPD. Since cardiac and liver disease are, with peritonitis, the main causes of death in the higher peritonitis rate group, the question arises whether cardiac and hepatic patients are more prone to peritonitis or whether high peritonitis frequency can worsen the prognosis for these patients. Presumably, both statements are right. A high peritonitis rate does not cause an increased death rate from cachexia: so the increased loss of proteins during peritonitis seems to be without consequence for patient survival.

Obviously, the peritonitis rate influences method survival, but a high percentage of drop-outs happen before the appearance of the first peritonitis episode, due to patient choice, or poor compliance, or inadequate peritoneal function, or due to clinical reasons. It is interesting to note, as we documented in a multicenter study (accepted for publication on Pent. Dial. Intern.) of 480 patients on CAPD and 373 on HD, that if we exclude peritonitis as a cause for dropping-out, the relative risk of leaving CAPD is lowered from 1.8 to 1.1, very close to that for hemodialysis, set at 1.

Peritonitis frequency does not affect peritoneal function; this was also assessed by Stablein et al. [9], for the large series of the National Institutes of Health (NIH) Registry. In our patients there was seldom need to change method because of inadequate peritoneal function, and in no case was there an association of low solute transport with low ultrafiltration. Contrary to what was observed in the International Cooperative Study [7], in our patients there was no trend to reduced peritoneal ultrafiltration volume with time. The good prognosis for long term function in CAPD patients on the Y-system is supported by the absence, in our patients, of cases of sclerosing encapsulating peritonitis.

The lack of any relationship between incidence of peritonitis and some protein indexes seems to point out that, within the limits of our experience and of such an evaluation, the peritonitis rate does not significantly affect nutritional status. Also, as shown before, the percentage of deaths due to malnutrition did not differ between CAPD and HD. In former studies [10,11] we showed that protein levels remained stable on CAPD for 4 years and more. As regards the relationship between peritonitis and beta-2M serum levels, our observations seem to indicate that a high peritonitis rate is not a sufficient stimulus to persistently increase the synthesis of this molecule, which is so deeply involved in uremic amyloidosis.

Conclusions

Our experience with the Y-system is largely reassuring, in that it shows that this method can avoid some important side-effects of CAPD. Under our conditions, peritoneal function, neuropathy, nutritional status, and beta-2m levels do not appear to be affected by peritonitis frequency. An influence of peritonitis rate on patient survival can be seen only after excluding patients who died before having a peritonitis episode; in the entire population, causes other than peritonitis are of major importance for patient survival. Peritonitis almost completely accounts for the greater drop-out rate from the CAPD technique than from the HD technique. A low peritonitis rate, such as that obtained with the Y-system, appears to be important for improving CAPD results.

References

1. Maiorca R, Cantaluppi A, Cancarini GC, et al. (1983) Prospective controlled trial of a Y-connector and disinfectant to prevent peritonitis in continuous ambulatory peritoneal dialysis. Lancet II:642–644
2. Buoncristiani U, Bianchi P, Cozzari M, et al. (1980) A new safe simple connection system for CAPD. Int J Nephrol Urol Androl 1:50–53
3. Canadian CAPD Clinical Trials Group (1989) Peritonitis in continuous ambulatory peritoneal dialysis. Randomized clinical trial comparing the Y connector disinfectant system to standard systems. Perit Dial Int 9:159–164
4. Maiorca R, Cancarini GC, Camerini C (1989) Prevention of peritonitis during CAPD: special precautions and use of connection systems. In: Andreucci VE (ed) Vascular and peritoneal access for dialysis. Kluwer Academic, Boston, pp 333–355
5. Peto R, Pike MC, Armitage P, et al. (1976) Design and analysis of randomized clinical trials requiring prolonged observation of each patient. Part 1. Br J Cancer 34:585–621
6. Peto R, Pike MC, Armitage P, et al. (1977) Design and analysis of randomized clinical trials requiring prolonged observation of each patient. Part 2. Br J Cancer 35:1–39
7. A survey of ultrafiltration in continuous ambulatory peritoneal dialysis. An international cooperative study. Second Report. (1984) Perit Dial Bull 4:137–142
8. Dasgupta MK, Ulan RA, Bettcher KB, et al. (1986) Effect of exit site and peritonitis on the distribution of biofilm encased adherent bacterial microcolonies (BABM) on Tenckhoff catheters in patients undergoing continuous ambulatory peritoneal dialysis. In: Khanna R, Nolph KD, Prowant B, Twardowski Z, Oreopoulos DG (eds) Advances in continuous ambulatory peritoneal dialysis 1986. Peritoneal Dialysis Bulletin, Toronto, pp 102–109
9. Stablein DM, Nolph KD, Lindblad AS (1989) Timing and characteristics of multiple peritonitis episodes: a report on the National CAPD Registry. Am J Kidney Dis 14:44–49
10. Maiorca R, Cancarini G, Manili L, et al. (1988) CAPD is a first class treatment: results of an eight-year experience with a comparison of patient and method survival in CAPD and hemodialysis. Clin Nephrol 30:S3–S7
11. Maiorca R, Cancarini GC, Camerini C, et al. (1989) Is CAPD competitive with Haemodialysis for long-term treatment of uraemic patients? Nephrol Dial Trans 4:244–253

Calcium, Phosphorus, Aluminum, and Bone Disease in Continuous Ambulatory Peritoneal Dialysis (CAPD) Patients

R. Gokal and A. Hutchison[1]

SUMMARY. In patients on continuous ambulatory peritoneal dialysis (CAPD), factors that influence calcium balance include calcium intake and net dialysis mass transfer; the latter is positive into the patient, when a current dialysate calcium content of 1.75 mmol/l in dialysis fluid containing 1.36% glucose is used. However, if calcium salts are to be used as phosphate binders, then the risk of hypercalcemia is markedly increased; this can be avoided by lowering the dialysate calcium to 1.25 mmol/l. Using calcium carbonate at meal times, both as a calcium supplement and as an oral phosphate binder, high normal ionized calcium levels are readily achieved. Appropriate dietary phosphate binding in the gut is also achieved (1000 mg phosphate intake and 300 mg dialysate clearance, results in need to bind 700 mg in the gut), while serum phosphate levels are maintained at around 1.5 mmol/l. With this sort of control, serum parathyroid hormone (PTH) levels decline, with significant improvement in the high turnover hyperparathyroid bone disease (osteitis fibrosa) as well as in vitamin D osteomalacia. The pathogenesis of the recently described non-aluminum aplastic bone disease is unknown, but may be related to "severe" PTH reduction and hypercalcemia. The major source of aluminum intoxication is the use of aluminum containing phosphate binders; this can now be totally avoided, thus reducing the risk considerably.

Introduction

Renal osteodystrophy is a virtually universal complication of renal failure. It encompasses the histological lesions of osteitis fibrosa and mild hyperparathyroidism (high bone turnover), and the histological lesions of osteomalacia, aplastic bone disease and mixed lesions (low bone turnover). The pathogenetic mechanisms for the above are complex, but include the interrelationship between calcium and phosphate,

---

[1]Manchester Royal Infirmary, Manchester, M13 9WL, UK

parathyroid hormone (PTH), vitamin D, and aluminum metabolism. The use of CAPD in the management of end stage renal failure further affects these interrelationships in a variable manner. Over the last ten years the use of CAPD has increased dramatically [1], and considerable knowledge has been gained in this area, enabling the development of a rational approach to the prevention and treatment of renal osteodystrophy during CAPD [2].

Calcium and Phosphate Metabolism

Using a dialysate calcium content of 1.75 mmol/l and a glucose concentration of 1.36%, there is net mass calcium transfer into the patient. However, the reported literature shows a wide disparity in calcium balances. Calcium balance was positive (84–300 mg/day) in two studies where ionized calcium levels were not measured [3,4], while Delmez et al. [5] showed that the transfer of calcium was not only dependent on the ionized serum calcium level but also on the ultrafiltration rate and volume. Thus, a 1.36% glucose solution resulted in a 10 mg calcium uptake into the patient but hypertonic 3.86% glucose solution led to a net loss of 20 mg of calcium. A negative balance resulted from the use of dialysate calcium of 1.5 mmol/l [6] but a positive balance resulted when a level of 2.0 mmol/l was used [7]. In reality, while there is this conflict, total serum and ionized calcium levels are readily normalized upon commencing CAPD in new patients [2]. However, in order to suppress PTH overactivity, the desired ionized calcium level appears to be at the upper limit of normal [8], and to achieve this, a high intake of calcium may be necessary. This factor has to be balanced with the risk of hypercalcemia resulting from high oral calcium intake and the use of 1.75 mmol/l dialysate calcium. This approach does need considerable modification in view of the need to lower serum phosphate levels and the danger of using aluminum free phosphate binders.

While the hyperphosphatemia of renal failure is rapidly improved by CAPD, serum phosphate fails to normalize on CAPD therapy. The obligatory intake of phosphate is about 1000 mg/day, with only 300 mg removed through dialysis. This leaves about 700 mg to be bound and removed fecally [5]. Assuming 50% gut absorption, a considerable phosphate load would result, which would lead to hyperphosphatemia. This condition plays a key role in the development of secondary hyperparathyroidism. The need for an appropriate and effective phosphate binding agent is paramount.

Calcium Carbonate as Phosphate Binder and Low Dialysate Calcium

Hyperphosphatemia has been traditionally managed with aluminum-containing phosphate binders such as aluminum hydroxide. Although these agents are effective as phosphate binders, they lead to an accumulation of aluminum in the body; over a prolonged period of time this can result in vitamin D refractory osteomalacia, microcytic anemia, and dialysis encephalopathy [9]. Hence, there is continued interest in developing alternative but effective non-toxic phosphate binders.

In 1966 Clarkson et al. [10] reported that high calcium carbonate intake resulted not only in a positive calcium balance, but also in reduced gastrointestinal absorption of phosphate. Subsequent reports have shown calcium carbonate to be an effective phosphate binder. However, hypercalcemia, with the risk of metastatic calcification, is the most common side effect [11,12]. Additional problems occur with compliance, gastrointestinal symptoms, and preparation and timing of administration.

If calcium carbonate is to be used as the sole phosphate binder, then in order to achieve fecal phosphate excretion of 700 mg, as Sheikh et al. [13] have shown, 6.25 gm calcium carbonate (2500 mg elemental calcium) is required. Assuming 25% calcium absorption, a considerable amount of calcium would be taken in and hypercalcemia would result. An attractive way to reduce this risk would be to adjust and lower dialysate calcium. Martis et al. [14] have calculated, on theoretical grounds, that a dialysate concentration of 1.25 mmol/l would allow the use of oral calcium carbonate without the risk of hypercalcemia. Our own experience in Manchester, in a group of new CAPD patients using this low calcium dialysis fluid, shows that effective phosphate binding can be achieved (serum levels of about 1.5 mmol/l readily achieved) with the use of a mean daily dose of 10 gm calcium carbonate (Calcichew) given at meal times. No significant hypercalcemia resulted and there was a concomitant decrease in PTH [15]. Similar results have been reported by Hercz et al. [16] who used 1 mmol/l calcium solution in hypercalcemia CAPD patients who had low turnover aplastic bone disease.

Current evidence would suggest that a lower dialysate calcium is essential if the large doses of calcium carbonate needed for phosphate binding are to be used in place of aluminum hydroxide.

Vitamin D and Parathyroid Hormone

The levels of 1,25 dihydroxyvitamin D3 are generally reported to be low in CAPD patients, but levels of 25 hydroxyvitamin D3 are usually normal at the start of therapy, then decline with time [17] or remain stable [7]. This discrepancy may be related to the amount of sunlight exposure [18] and availability of adequate amounts of parent vitamin D [7]. The role of routine vitamin D supplementation is not clear and the danger of hypercalcemia and hyperphosphatemia does mean that this therapy should be based on clinical indications of hypocalcemia and hyperparathyroid bone disease. The intraperitoneal route of administration has evoked some interest; this route raised ionized calcium levels with PTH suppression greater than that obtained with an increased dialysate calcium of 2 mmol/l [7]. In addition, Carozzi et al. [19] have shown that low dialysate calcium level and 1,25 dihydroxyvitamin D3 given intraperitoneally can enhance peritoneal macrophage and antimicrobial function in CAPD.

Even though CAPD removes substantial quantities of PTH (mainly in the form of carboxyterminal fragments), interpreting the results on CAPD has been difficult. The steady decline in PTH with time in some reports [17,18] has not been confirmed by others [6]. However, suppression of high PTH activity may only be brought about by high normal serum ionized calcium levels, in conjunction with normal phosphate levels, suggesting a higher set point than expected for calcium regulated PTH secretion [8].

Recently, Hercz et al. [16] described a non aluminum aplastic bone lesion. In these patients, who were hypercalcemic, PTH levels were "low" (2–3 × normal); on correction of the hypercalcemia with low dialysate calcium the PTH levels rose. This phenomenon raises the question of the role of "low" serum PTH levels in the pathogenesis of the aplastic bone disease. It would be interesting to see further studies in this area. This also raises the issue of how low the PTH level can fall before the aplastic lesion is manifest.

Aluminum Metabolism

Oral ingestion of aluminum containing phosphate binders is the main source of aluminum in CAPD patients, now that manufacturers are able to produce fluids with levels well below 10 µg/l. After 2–3 years on CAPD a significant elevation of serum aluminum (30–40 µg/l) was found in patients who had intermittent aluminum exposure [17]; however those with no aluminum exposure at all were able to maintain levels within the normal range [20].

Although the number of cases of aluminum related osteomalacia (low turnover aplastic bone disease) is small in patients on CAPD [16], this may well increase with prolonged use of aluminum containing phosphate binders. However, now that calcium salts are becoming the major form of phosphate binders (used in conjunction with low dialysate calcium solution) the problem of aluminum related toxicity should diminish into oblivion.

The problems of assessing the total tissue load of aluminum are enormous. Channon et al. [21] showed a good correlation between bone aluminum content and total dose of aluminum prescribed, but showed a poorer correlation between bone aluminum and serum aluminum levels; the latter almost certainly reflect recent exposure to aluminum. The desferrioxamine test has not proven to be a reliable indicator, either of tissue stores or of the development of osteomalacia [22]. In practical terms serum aluminum levels of >50 µg/l (in the absence of recent aluminum exposure) may be cause for concern; levels of >100 µg/l need action which may necessitate therapy with desferrioxamine, which is given intravenously or intraperitoneally [23]. The ultimate diagnostic tool for tissue load may reside in bone histology and bone content of aluminum. For those patients with aluminum toxicity, the use of desferrioxamine has caused a significant rise in hemoglobin and has increased the effectiveness of recombinant human erythropoietin therapy.

Avoidance of aluminum as a phosphate binder appears to be of paramount importance. This is now possible; caution should be exercised in the use of calcium citrate as a phosphate binder. This compound does enhance aluminum absorption and should be avoided.

Renal Bone Disease

There have not been enough studies done on sufficiently large numbers of patients, observed for sufficient lengths of time, to enable firm conclusions to be drawn on the aforementioned interrelationships and on the measures to be used on renal osteodystrophy in CAPD patients. Some reports support the view that careful management can prevent or ameliorate symptomatic hyperparathyroid bone disease [17,18,24], while other reports show no change [25,26], or even deterioration [6,27,28]. These conflicting reports reflect the heterogeneity of patients and their management. However, several recent studies have shown improved control of renal osteodystrophy under CAPD as compared to the control under hemodialysis [29–31].

The major concern of late has been a report on the fairly high incidence of the new histological entity of aplastic, or low turnover, bone disease unrelated to aluminum (Hercz et al. [16]). In a cross-sectional study of both hemodialysis and CAPD patients ($n-260$), nearly 50% of the biopsies showed an aplastic histopathological change; of these, roughly a third had less than 5% aluminum staining. Interestingly, PTH levels were significantly lower in these patients when compared to levels in those patients with normal or high bone turnover. When the patients with less than 5% aluminum staining were switched to a low dialysate calcium the PTH levels increased, escaping the seemingly suppressant effect of an elevated dialysate calcium. These findings raise interesting questions, not only about the pathogenesis of this entity, but also about its significance, its management, and the level of PTH to aim for–should that be important. These are important issues which will be answered only with long term careful observation, now that aluminum can be eliminated as a source of histological aluminum-related osteomalacia.

Overall, it seems that parathyroid bone disease can be ameliorated on CAPD, as can vitamin D related osteomalacia.

In conclusion, it seems that when serum PTH declines with time there is a concomitant improvement in osteitis fibrosa. Suppression of PTH is unlikely, unless a high serum ionized calcium level is achieved together with a normal phosphate level. Non-aluminum related osteomalacia at the start of CAPD invariably improves. Aluminum related aplastic bone disease remains a potential problem, which needs to be minimized by avoiding aluminum containing phosphate binders; however, this disease can be treated with desferrioxamine. There is still considerable debate about the role of vitamin D therapy in the prevention of renal osteodystrophy. What seems to be crucial is the need for maintaining high normal serum ionized calcium levels and normal phosphate levels; this can be only achieved by low calcium concentration in the peritoneal dialysis fluid, coupled with high oral intake of calcium carbonate; in this setting vitamin D analogues may be useful in healing bone, but a role for prophylactic vitamin D cannot be justified. The newly emerging non-aluminum related aplastic bone disease is interesting; its pathogenesis is unclear, as is its significance. Further understanding of this entity may well modify our approach to managing CAPD patients with renal bone disease. Recommendations for managing patients are included in Table 1.

Table 1. Recommendations for managing ROD in CAPD patients

1. Dietary phosphate reduction within 1–1.2 g/kg protein intake
2. Use of $CaCO_3$ (with meals) as phosphate binder–serum phosphate 1.5 mmol/l
3. Serum ionized Ca–upper limit of normal
4. Use of low dialysate Ca (1.25 mmol/l) to achieve 2 and 3
5. Routine vit D unnecessary; based on overt bone disease
6. Monitor PTH. How low PTH?–to avoid aplastic bone disease
7. Monitor aluminum–bone biopsy, serum levels persistently 100 μg/l–use DFO

ROD, renal osteodystrophy; DFO, desferrioxamine

Acknowledgments. Our sincere thanks to Kerry Hulme for typing the manuscript.

References

1. Gokal R (1987) Continuous ambulatory peritoneal dialysis (CAPD) – 10 years on. Q J Med 63:465–472
2. Gokal R (1988) Renal osteodystrophy and aluminum bone disease in CAPD patients. Clin Nephrol 30(Suppl 1):564–567
3. Blumenkrantz M, Kopple J, Moran J, Coburn JW (1982) Metabolic balance studies and dietary protein requirements in patients undergoing CAPD. Kidney Int 21:849–864
4. Parker A, Nolph KD (1980) Magnesium and calcium transfer during CAPD. Trans Am Soc Artif Intern Organs 26:194–196
5. Delmez JA, Slatopolsky E, Martin KJ, Gearing BJ, Harter HR (1982) Minerals, Vitamin D and parathyroid hormone in CAPD. Kidney Int 21:362–367
6. Digenis G, Khanna R, Pierratos A, Meema H, Rabinovich S, Petit J, Oreopoulos D (1983) Renal osteodystrophy in patients managed by CAPD for more than 3 years. Perit Dial Bull 3:81–86
7. Delmez JA, Dougan S, Gearing BK, Rothstein M, Windus D, Rapp N, Slatopolsky E (1987) The effects of intraperitoneal calcitriol on calcium and parathyroid hormone. Kidney Int 31:795–799
8. Slatopolsky E, Martin KJ, Morrissey JJ, Hruska KA (1985) Parathyroid hormone alterations in chronic renal failure. In: Robinson RR (ed) Nephrology, vol II. Springer, New York, pp 1292–1304
9. Wills MR, Savory J (1983) Aluminum poisoning: Dialysis encephalopathy, osteomalacia and anaemia. Lancet II:29–34
10. Clarkson EM, McDonald SJ, deWardener HE (1966) The effect of a high intake of calcium carbonate in normal subjects and patients with chronic renal failure. Clin Sci 30:425–438
11. Stein HD, Yudis M, Sirota RA (1987) Calcium carbonate as a phosphate binder. N Engl J Med 315:609–610
12. Slatopolsky E, Weerts C, Lopex-Hilker S, Norwood K, Zinc M, Winders D, Delmez J (1986) Calcium carbonate as a phosphate binder in patients with chronic renal failure undergoing dialysis. N Engl J Med 315:157–161
13. Sheikh MS, Maguire JA, Emmett M (1989) Reduction of dietary phosphorus absorption by phosphate binders. A theoretical in vitro and in vivo study. J Clin Invest 83:66–73
14. Martis L, Serkes KD, Nolph KD (1989) Calcium carbonate as a phosphate binder: is there a need to adjust peritoneal dialysate calcium concentrations for patients using $CaCo_3$? Perit Dial Int 9:325–328
15. Hutchison A, Gokal R (to be published) Low calcium dialysis fluid and oral calcium carbonate in CAPD. Nephrol Dial Transpl
16. Hercz G, Pei Y, Manueal A (1990) Aplastic osteodystrophy without aluminum in dialysis patients (abstract). Kidney Int 37:449
17. Gokal R, Ramos JM, Ellis HA, Parkinson I, Sweetaman V, Dewar J, Ward MK, Kerr D (1983) Histological renal osteodystrophy and 25 hydroxycholecalciferol and aluminum levels in patients on CAPD. Kidney Int 23:15–21
18. Cassidy M, Owen JP, Ellis HA, Dewar J, Robinson CJ, Wilkinson R, Ward MK, Kerr DNS (1985) Renal osteodystrophy and metastatic calcification in long term CAPD. Q J Med 213:29–48
19. Carozzi S, Nassini M, Schelotto C, Cavelgia P, Santoni O, Barocci S, Versace F, Cantaluppi A, Salit M, Lamperi S (1989) Ca# and function in CAPD. In: Khanna et al. (eds) Peritoneal dialysis bull, Toronto pp 103–110

20. Gokal R (to be published) Peritoneal Dialysis. In: Davidson et al. (eds) Oxford Textbook of Nephrology. Oxford University Press, Oxford

21. Channon SM, Arfeen S, Ward MK (1988) Long term accumulation of aluminium in patients with renal failure. Trace Elements in Medicine 5:154–157

22. Millinar DS, Nebeker H, OHS, Sherrard D, Andrers D, Alfrey AC, Coburn J (1984) Desferrioxamine infusion tests for diagnosis of aluminium osteomalacia. Kidney Int 30:944–948

24. Rahman R, Heaton A, Goodship T, Rodger R, Tapson J, Sellars L, Ellis H, Wilkinson R, Ward MK (1987) Renal osteodystrophy in patients on CAPD: A five year study. Perit Dial Bull 7:1–4

25. Delmez J, Fallon MD, Bergfeld MA, Gearing BK, Dougan CS, Teitelbaum S (1986) CAPD and Bone. Kidney Int 30:379–384

26. Nilsson P, Danielsson BG, Grefberg N, Wide L (1985) Secondary hyperparathyroidism in diabetic and non diabetic patients in long term CAPD. Scand J Urol Nephrol 19:59–65

27. Kurtz SB (1985) Clinical parameters of renal bone disease: a comparison of CAPD and haemodialysis. Dial Transplant 14:30–36

28. Bucciante G, Biachi ML, Valenti G (1984) Progress of renal osteodystrophy during CAPD. Clin Nephrol 6:279–283

29. Shusterman NH, Wasserstein AG, Morrison G, Audet P, Fallon M, Kaplan F (1987) Controlled study of renal osteodystrophy in patients undergoing dialysis. Improved response to CAPD compared with hemodialysis. Am J Med 82:1148–1156

30. Zuccelli P, Catizone L, Casanova S, Fusarole L, Fabri L, Ferran G (1984) Renal osteodystrophy in CAPD patients. Min Electrol Metab 10:326–332

31. Ramsey M, Tapson J, Ward MK (1989) Comparison of renal osteodystrophy between hemodialysis and CAPD (abstract). Perit Dial Int 9(Suppl 1):208

Autacoids and the Kidney

Chair: Raymond Ardaillou (France)
Keishi Abe (Japan)

Oxidant Mechanisms in Glomerulonephritis

SUDHIR V. SHAH[1]

SUMMARY. Several lines of evidence derived from both in vitro and in vivo studies suggest an important role for reactive oxygen metabolites and glomerular pathophysiology. Both leukocytes and glomeruli have been shown to increase the generation of reactive oxygen metabolites in response to a wide variety of stimuli. Reactive oxygen metabolites generated enzymatically or by stimulated neutrophils have been shown to affect several biological processes of potential importance in glomerular injury, including glomerular basement degradation, eicosanoid synthesis, cyclic nucleotide metabolism, and glomerular ADPase activity. Scavengers of reactive oxygen metabolites have been shown to reduce proteinuria in several leukocyte-dependent and leukocyte-independent models of glomerular disease. Taken together, these studies suggest an important role of reactive oxygen metabolites in glomerular disease.

Introduction

Despite extensive investigation, the mechanisms that ultimately cause the functional and morphological changes in glomerular diseases (one of the commonest causes of end stage renal disease), remain poorly understood. A large body of evidence accumulated over the last decade indicates that partially reduced oxygen metabolites are important mediators of ischemic, toxic, and immune-mediated tissue injury [1–3]. In this review, I will introduce the term reactive oxygen metabolites, and then present the available evidence in support of the role of reactive oxygen metabolites in glomerular disease.

Oxygen normally accepts four electrons and is converted directly to water. However, partial reduction of oxygen can and does occur in biological systems, leading to

[1]Tulane University School of Medicine, Department of Medicine, Section of Nephrology, New Orleans, LA 70112, USA

the generation of partially reduced and potentially toxic reactive oxygen metabolites. Thus, when oxygen accepts one electron, superoxide anion, a free radical is generated.

$$O_2 \xrightarrow{e^-} O_2^- \xrightarrow{e^-} H_2O_2 \xrightarrow{e^-} HO\cdot \xrightarrow{e^-} H_2O$$

When oxygen accepts two electrons either directly or by the dismutation of superoxide, hydrogen peroxide is formed. Further reduction of oxygen leads to the generation of highly reactive hydroxyl radical. These oxygen metabolites, including the free radical species, superoxide and hydroxyl radical, and other metabolites such as hydrogen peroxide and hypohalous acids (derived from myeloperoxidase-hydrogen peroxide-halide system) are often collectively referred to as reactive oxygen metabolites.

Several human and experimental glomerulonephritides are characterized by the infiltration of glomeruli by neutrophils and/or monocytes. The importance of leukocytes as mediators of glomerular injury has been delineated in experiments in which selective depletion of neutrophils or monocytes led to amelioration of the glomerular injury. In many other common forms of glomerular diseases (for example, minimal change disease, membranous nephropathy) leukocytes do not play an important role in the glomerular injury. Evidence in support of the role of reactive oxygen metabolites in leukocyte-dependent and leukocyte-independent glomerular disease will be considered separately.

Role of Reactive Oxygen Metabolites in Leukocyte-Dependent Glomerular Disease

Although glomerular injury has been attributed to the release of enzymes from leukocytes, studies from other tissues and recent studies related to glomerular injury indicate that neutrophil-derived reactive oxygen metabolites are also important in tissue injury. Neutrophils and monocytes/macrophages exhibit a burst of oxidative metabolism (respiratory burst) with marked increase in oxygen uptake and the generation of reactive oxygen metabolites in response to plasma membrane perturbation by a variety of soluble and particulate stimuli [3]. Phagocytosis, per se, is not essential to trigger the oxidative burst; pertubation of the plasma membrane appears to be the critical event. Of particular interest is the demonstration that several immune reactants such as serum treated zymosan, a C_3b receptor stimulus, heat aggregated IgG, an Fc receptor stimulus, immune complexes, and complement components, have all

Table 1. Potential sources of reactive oxygen metabolites

Cells	Stimuli
Neutrophils Monocytes	A wide variety of soluble and particulate stimuli, including immune complexes, complement components, and ANCA
Glomeruli Mesangial Cells	Phorbol myristate acetate, zymosan, trypsin, chymotrypsin, PAF, immune complexes, MAC, TNF, and Adriamycin

PAF, platelet aggregation factor; MAC, membrane attack complex; TNF, tumor necrosis factor; ANCA, antineutrophil cytoplasmic autoantibodies

Autacoids and the Kidney

Table 2. Effect of reactive oxygen metabolites on biological processes relevant to glomerular pathophysiology

Reactive oxygen metabolites generated enzymatically or by stimulated neutrophils:
  • Increase glomerular eicosanoid synthesis [1]
  • Increase glomerular cyclic AMP content [6]
  • Participate in GBM degradation [5]
  • Reduce glomerular ADPase activity [14]

been shown to trigger the oxidative burst [3]. Of interest, in a recent study it was shown that antineutrophil cytoplasmic autoantibodies (ANCA), which are present in the circulation of most patients with pauci-immune necrotizing vasculitis and pauci-immune crescentic glomerulonephritis, significantly increased the generation of superoxide by neutrophils [4]. Thus, stimulated neutrophils or monocytes are potential sources of reactive oxygen metabolites in leukocyte-dependent glomerular injury.

Superoxide and hydrogen peroxide appear to be the primary species generated; these may then play a role in the generation of additional and more reactive oxidants, including the hydroxyl radical and hypochlorous acid. The direct interaction between superoxide and hydrogen peroxide is rather slow and it has been postulated that in biological systems a trace metal, such as iron, participates in the reaction commonly referred to as the metal-catalyzed Haber-Weiss reaction. This reaction may be summarized as follows:

$$Fe^3 + O_2^- \rightarrow Fe^2 + O_2$$
$$\underline{Fe^2 + H_2O_2 \rightarrow Fe^3 + OH^- + HO\cdot}$$
$$O_2^- + H_2O_2 \rightarrow O_2 + OH^- + HO\cdot$$

It must be pointed out that while several studies have clearly documented the generation of a potent oxidizing species in the presence of a metal, the possibility that the oxidant may not be hydroxyl radical has been recently raised. Additional reactive oxygen metabolites can be formed, as a result of the metabolism of hydrogen peroxide by neutrophil- and macrophage-derived myeloperoxidase (MPO), to produce high reactive toxic products, including hypochlorous acid.

$$H_2O_2 + Cl^- \xrightarrow{MPO} HOCl + H^+$$

Other hypohalous acids may also be generated, for example, generation of hypobromous acid by eosinophils has recently been reported. Human neutrophils have also

Table 3. In vivo evidence for the role of reactive oxygen metabolites in neutrophil dependent glomerular injury

Scavengers of reactive oxygen metabolites reduce proteinuria in:
  • Neutrophil-dependent glomerular injury induced by phorbol myristate acetate and cobra venom factor [8]
  • Complement and neutrophil-dependent heterologous phase of anti-GBM antibody disease [12,13]
Infusion of myleo-peroxidase-hydrogen peroxide causes significant proteinuria, endothelial cell swelling, and marked cell foot process effacement. Four to ten days later a marked proliferative glomerular lesion develops [9]

Table 4. In vivo evidence for the role of reactive oxygen metabolites in neutrophil independent glomerular injury

Scavengers of reactive oxygen metabolites reduce proteinuria in:
- Puromycin aminonucleoside model of minimal change disease [20–22]
- Passive Heymann nephritis model of membranous nephropathy [18]
- Cationized gamma globulin-induced immune complex glomerulonephritis [19]

been reported to generate long-lived oxidants (half-life approximately 18 hours) with characteristics similar to N-chloramines.

It is generally accepted that leukocytes cause proteinuria (a hallmark of glomerular diseases) by damaging the glomerular basement membrane (GBM) which serves as the major ultrafiltration barrier to restrict the entry of proteins into the urinary space. Recently, the degradation of the GBM by stimulated neutrophils was shown to be due to the activation of a latent metalloenzyme (most likely gelatinase) by hypochlorous acid or a similar oxidant generated by the myeloperoxidase-hydrogen peroxide-halide system [5]. In addition, several recent studies have shown that oxidants could contribute to GBM damage by increasing its susceptibility to proteolytic damage and by inactivating the alpha-1-proteinase inhibitor (the primary regulator of neutrophil elastase) thus allowing the released elastase to more readily inflict damage to the extracellular matrix. Prevention of proteinuria by catalase in neutrophil-dependent glomerulonephritides suggests that the oxidative mechanism for GBM degradation described above may be quite relevant to leukocyte-dependent glomerular injury.

While the critical role played by leukocytes in proteinuria is generally accepted, infiltrating leukocytes in proliferative glomerulonephritides may also modulate the inflammatory response and glomerular function by altering glomerular metabolism. Reactive oxygen metabolites generated by the xanthine-xanthine oxidase system or by stimulated neutrophils have been shown to increase cyclic AMP content [1,6] and to enhance the synthesis of prostaglandin E_2 (PGE$_2$), prostaglandin $F_{2\alpha}$ (PGF$_{2\alpha}$), 6 ketoPGF$_{1\alpha}$ (the stable metabolite of prostacyclin), and TXB$_2$ (the stable metabolite of thromboxane) by glomeruli [1]. Thus, by affecting glomerular cyclic nucleotides and/or eicosanoid synthesis, reactive oxygen metabolites may play an important modulatory role in glomerular pathophysiology. In addition, reactive oxygen metabolites affect biological pathophysiology in other tissues relevant to glomerular pathophysiology. For example, several interactions between reactive oxygen metabolites and platelets (which have been postulated to be important in the development of local glomerular injury) have recently been described, infusion of myeloperoxidase-hydrogen peroxide in the renal artery caused glomerular injury that was associated with marked influx of platelets in the glomerular capillaries [7].

Support for the role of reactive oxygen metabolites generated by neutrophils in glomerular injury has been recently obtained from several in vivo studies. Infusion of phorbol myristate acetate (PMA) (a well known potent activator of leukocytes) or infusion of cobra venom factor in the renal artery caused significant proteinuria which was prevented by catalase (which destroys hydrogen peroxide) and neutrophil depletion [1,8]. These studies indicate that hydrogen peroxide and/or its metabolites generated by the neutrophils can cause proteinuria. Johnson et al. reasoned that hydrogen peroxide-mediated injury may involve the myeloperoxidase-hydrogen peroxide-halide system [7]. They demonstrated that infusion of myeloperoxidase followed by infusion of hydrogen peroxide in a chloride-containing solution into the renal artery in rats results in significant proteinuria [9] and four to ten days later, results in the development of a marked proliferative glomerular lesion [7]. In addition, halogenation (as measured by the incorporation of [125I]) in glomeruli and GBM was demonstrated in an in situ model of neutrophil-mediated immune complex glomerulonephritis [10]. These studies indicate the activation of myeloperoxidase-hydrogen peroxide-halide in a model of neutrophil-mediated immune complex glomerulonephritis, and indicate that the myeloperoxidase-hydrogen peroxide-halide system is capable of inducing glomerular injury that results in proteinuria.

In addition to increased glomerular permeability, the other common manifestation of glomerular disease is an alteration in glomerular function. Rehan et al. observed that PMA infusion or infusion of cobra venom factor reduced the whole kidney glomerular filtration rate (GFR) by about 50%–90% but catalase (in doses that reduced the proteinuria) did not prevent the fall in GFR [8]. In contrast, Yoshioka et al. have reported that unilateral infusion of PMA led to a fall in the single nephron GFR and evoked a profound constrictive response in the glomerular microcirculation which was prevented by neutrophil depletion or pre-treatment with catalase [11].

One of the best characterized models of complement- and neutrophil-dependent glomerular injury is the heterologous phase of anti-GBM antibody disease. In this model of neutrophil-dependent glomerular injury, treatment with catalase markedly reduced the proteinuria, whereas superoxide dismutase had no protective effect [12]. In another study, dimethylthiourea, a potent hydroxyl radical scavenger, or deferoxamine, an iron chelator, significantly attenuated proteinuria in the complement- and neutrophil-dependent heterologous phase of anti-GBM antibody disease in rabbits [13]. Although the role of iron is not completely understood, the protective effect of iron chelators has been generally taken as evidence for the participation of hydroxyl radical in tissue injury, because iron is critical in the generation of hydroxyl radical (via the Haber-Weiss reaction). Taken together, the studies with PMA, cobra venom factor, and studies in the heterologous phase of anti-GBM antibody disease, demonstrate that reactive oxygen metabolites generated by activated neutrophils play an important role in altering glomerular permeability.

It has been suggested that glomerular ADPase is of major importance in preventing intra-glomerular thrombus formation in experimental glomerulonephritis [14]. These membrane associated enzymes are apparently highly susceptible to reactive oxygen metabolites [15]. Recently it was shown that there is a marked decrease in the activity of these enzymes in two models of glomerulonephritis (anti-GBM and anti-Thy1) which are characterized by the influx of polymorphonuclear neutrophils [14]. Additionally, scavengers of oxygen metabolites prevented the decrease in glomerular ADPase, suggesting a role of reactive oxygen metabolites in the reduction of glomerular ADPase activity [14].

Neutrophil-Independent Glomerular Injury

In proliferative glomerulonephritis, the infiltrating neutrophils and monocytes are potential sources for reactive oxygen metabolites. But what about the non-proliferative glomerulonephritides? Because of the presence of phagocyte-like cells in the glomerulus (particularly mesangial cells) it was postulated that glomerular cells, like other phagocytic cells, would also generate reactive oxygen metabolites in response to a plasma membrane perturbation. In response to PMA, rat glomeruli showed a marked chemiluminescence response, a sensitive measure of the generation of reactive oxygen metabolites by phagocytic cells [16]. In a subsequent study, chymotrypsin or trypsin were shown to markedly increase light emission from the glomeruli. Neutral proteases from infiltrating leukocytes and/or from renal tissue have been shown to be released in glomerular diseases; these results which show the generation of chemiluminescence in response to neutral proteases suggest a potential mechanism for the production of reactive oxygen metabolites in glomerular diseases. In addition to these studies with freshly isolated glomeruli, several investigators have demonstrated the ability of mesangial cells to generate superoxide and hydrogen peroxide in response to a variety of stimuli, including opsonized zymosan, immune complexes, membrane attack complex, and platelet activating factor [1,17]. Thus, the ability of glomerular cells to generate reactive oxygen metabolites in response to plasma membrane perturbation appears to be well established. In addition, as described below, enhanced intracellular generation of reactive oxygen metabolites (for example, hypoxanthine-xanthine oxidase) may also be relevant to glomerular pathophysiology.

The ability of glomerular cells to generate reactive oxygen metabolites suggests that reactive oxygen metabolites may be important mediators of glomerular injury in glomerular diseases that lack infiltrating leukocytes. Passive Heymann nephritis, induced by a single intravenous injection of anti-Fx1A, is a complement-dependent and neutrophil-independent model of glomerular disease that resembles membranous nephropathy in humans. Shah reported that superoxide dismutase or catalase (native or polyethylene glycol-coupled) did not affect the anti-Fx1A-induced proteinuria. In contrast, scavengers of hydroxyl radical, and an iron chelator, deferoxamine, markedly reduced the proteinuria [18]. The protective effects of both the hydroxyl radical scavengers and an iron chelator suggest a role of the hydroxyl radical in passive Heymann nephritis. Similarly, Sedor et al. have reported that two hydroxyl radical scavengers significantly reduced the proteinuria in cationized gamma globulin-induced immune complex glomerulonephritis, a complement- and neutrophil-independent model of membranous nephropathy [19]. Taken together, these studies suggest an important role for hydroxyl radical in animal models of membranous nephropathy.

A single intravenous injection of puromycin aminonucleoside (PAN) results in marked proteinuria and glomerular morphological changes that are similar to minimal change disease in humans. Recently, Diamond et al. postulated that the glomerular injury associated with PAN was mediated by oxygen free radical generation, since hypoxanthine, an intermediate metabolite of PAN, can serve as a substrate for superoxide anion production via the xanthine oxidase system [20]. They reported that allopurinol (an inhibitor of xanthine oxidase) and superoxide dismutase were protective in PAN-induced nephrotic syndrome, suggesting a role for xanthine oxidase generated superoxide anion in this model of minimal change disease [20]. Beaman et al. confirmed the protective effect of superoxide dismutase and, in addition, reported that proteinuria was significantly reduced in rats receiving polyethylene glycol (PEG)-catalase, suggesting a role for both hydrogen peroxide and superoxide anion in this model of glomerular disease [21]. Superoxide anion and hydrogen peroxide may interact (with iron as catalyst) to generate the hydroxyl radical. Several studies have, in fact, shown that enhanced generation of hydrogen peroxide and superoxide anion is accompanied by enhanced generation by hydroxyl radical (or a similar highly oxidizing species). Thakur et al. reported the protective effect of two hydroxyl radical scavengers and an iron chelator, implicating hydroxyl radical in PAN-induced nephrotic syndrome [22].

Conclusions

Reactive oxygen metabolites have been implicated in the development of tissue injury in an increasing number of diseases. While it is currently popular to incriminate oxygen metabolites as ultimate injurious agents, given the complexity and multifaceted nature of inflammation, the cooperative and sometimes complex interaction between different injurious mechanisms appears much more likely. The interaction between proteases and oxidants in the degradation of GBM is just one example of this. Nonetheless, the existence of a sufficient body of in vitro and in vivo information allows us to postulate that reactive oxygen metabolites appear to be important mediators in glomerular pathophysiology.

References

1. Baud L, Aradillou R (1986) Reactive oxygen species: production and role in the kidney. Am J Physiol 251:F765–F776
2. Cross CE, Halliwell B, Borish ET, Pryor WA, Ames BN, Saul RL, McCord JM, Harman D (1987) Davis Conference: Oxygen radicals and human disease. Ann Intern Med 107:526–545
3. Fantone JC, Ward PA (1982) Role of oxygen-derived free radicals and metabolites in leukocyte-dependent inflammatory reactions. Am J Pathol 107:397–418
4. Falk FJ, Terrell RS, Charles LA, Jennette JC (1990) Anti-neutrophil cytoplasmic autoantibodies induce neutrophils to degranulate and produce oxygen radicals in vitro. Proc Natl Acad Sci USA 87:4115–4119
5. Shah SV, Baricos WH, Basci A (1987) Degradation of human glomerular basement membrane by stimulated neutrophils: Activation of metalloproteinase/s by reactive oxygen metabolites. J Clin Invest 79:25–31
6. Basci A, Wallin JD, Shah SV (1987) Effect of stimulated neutrophils on cyclic nucleotide content in isolated rat glomeruli. Am J Physiol 252:F429–F436
7. Johnson RJ, Guggenheim SJ, Klebanoff SJ, Ochi RF, Wass A, Baker P, Schulze M, Couser WG (1988) Morphologic correlates of glomerular oxidant injury induced by the myeloperoxidase-hydrogen peroxide-halide system of the neutrophil. Lab Invest 5:294–301
8. Rehan A, Wiggins RC, Kunkel RG, Till GO, Johnson KJ (1986) Glomerular injury and proteinuria in rats after intrarenal injection of cobra venom factor. Am J Pathol 123:57–66
9. Johnson RJ, Couser WG, Chi EY, Adler S, Klebanoff SJ (1987) New mechanism for glomerular injury. Myeloperoxidase hydrogen peroxide-halide system. J Clin Invest 79:1379–1387
10. Johnson RJ, Klebanoff SJ, Ochi RF, Adler S, Baker P, Sparks L, Couser WG (1987) Participation of the myeloperoxidase-H_2O_2-halide system in immune complex nephritis. Kidney Int 32:342–349

11. Yoshioka T, Badr KR, Ichikawa I (1988) Reactive oxygen species (ROS) mediate the reduction in ultrafiltration coefficient (Kf) and increase in efferent arteriolar resistance induced by activated polymorphonuclear leukocytes (PMN) (abstract). Kidney Int 33:369
12. Rehan A, Johnson KJ, Wiggins RC, Kunkel RG, Ward PA (1984) Evidence for the role of oxygen radicals in acute nephrotoxic nephritis. Lab Invest 51:396–403
13. Boyce NW, Holdsworth SR (1986) Hydroxyl radical mediation of immune renal injury by desferrioxamine. Kidney Int 30:813–817
14. Poelstra K, Hardonk MJ, Koudstaal J, Bakker WW (1990) Intraglomerular platelet aggregation and experimental glomerulonephritis. Kidney Int 37:1500–1508
15. Bakker WW, Baller JFW, Hardonk MJ (1987) Decrease of glomerular ATP-ase activity induced by adriamycin is mediated by oxygen free radical species (abstract). Kidney Int 31:1045–1046
16. Shah SV (1981) Light emission by isolated rat glomeruli in response to phorbol myristate acetate. J Lab Clin Med 98:46–57
17. Adler S, Baker PJ, Johnson RJ, Ochi RF, Pritzl P, Couser WG (1986) Complement membrane attack complex stimulates production of reactive oxygen metabolites by cultured rat mesangial cells. J Clin Invest 77:762–767
18. Shah SV (1988) Evidence suggesting a role for hydroxyl radical in passive Heymann nephritis in rats. Am J Physiol 254:F337–F344
19. Sedor J, Emancipator S, Rahman M (1987) Hydroxyl radical (OH) scavengers ameliorate proteinuria in immune complex glomerulonephritis (IC-GN) (abstract). Proceedings of the Xth international congress of nephrology July 26–31, 1987. p 404
20. Diamond JR, Bonventre JV, Karnovsky MJ (1986) A role for oxygen free radicals in aminonucleoside necrosis. Kidney Int 29:478–483
21. Beaman M, Birtwistle R, Howie AJ, Michael J, Adu D (1987) The role of superoxide anion and hydrogen peroxide in glomerular injury induced by puromycin aminonucleoside in rats. Clin Sci 73:329–332
22. Thakur V, Walker PD, Shah SV (1988) Evidence suggesting a role for hydroxyl radical in puromycin aminonucleoside-induced proteinuria in rats. Kidney Int 34:494–499

Mechanisms of the Biological Effects of Eicosanoids in the Glomerulus

Paolo Menè, Anna Taranta, Francesco Pugliese,
Giulio A. Cinotti[1], and Angela D'Agostino[2]

SUMMARY. Human glomerular mesangial cells respond to stimulation by vasoconstrictor eicosanoids, such as thromboxane A_2 (TxA_2), with a rapid and sustained elevation of cytosolic Ca^{2+} ($[Ca^{2+}]_i$), followed by enhanced Na^+/H^+ exchange activity. These early ionic signals are accompanied by immediate and persistent membrane depolarization, triggered by enhanced Cl^- conductance. Depolarization is independent of extracellular Na^+, while the amplitude of the $[Ca^{2+}]_i$ transient is regulated by transmembrane Na^+ gradients via a Na^+/Ca^{2+} exchanger. The exchanger is, in turn, activated by a TxA_2 mimetic, suggesting its homeostatic role in controlling $[Ca^{2+}]_i$ of activated cells. Enhanced cycling of intracellular ions is followed within three hours of stimulation with a TxA_2 mimetic by complex changes in the pattern of cellular proteins, with enhanced expression of membrane and cytosolic proteins of approximate MW 38–53 Kda and 125–200 Kda, in the presence or absence of serum, respectively. Regulation of human mesangial cell function and structure by vasoconstrictor eicosanoids in culture may reflect a critical role of these compounds in renal pathophysiology.

Introduction

Glomerular cells metabolize arachidonic acid (AA) to a vast group of biologically active eicosanoids, i.e., 20 C atom unsaturated lipids [1,2]. Only recently, along with some of their biologic effects functional receptors for eicosanoids have been described in cultured cells of glomerular origin [3–5]. Eicosanoids can therefore be regarded as glomerular autacoids, or compounds with a site of action on the same cells, or cells contiguous to those that produce them. The implications of these obser-

[1]Cattedra di Nefrologia Medica, 2a Clinica Medica, Policlinico Umberto I, Viale del Policlinico, 00161 Rome, Italy
[2]Istituto di Istologia ed Embriologia generale, University "La Sapienza," 00161 Rome, Italy

vations are several-fold: first, glomerular eicosanoids may participate in the autocrine and paracrine regulation of intrinsic glomerular cells; second, eicosanoids could mediate cell-to-cell communication between glomerular cells and blood-borne cells; and third, enhanced AA metabolism in renal inflammation may contribute to functional changes of glomerular cells [1,6].

We have undertaken an investigation of the intracellular mechanisms which lead to responses of glomerular cells to eicosanoids. Employing cultured human mesangial cells, we have demonstrated that two families of receptors for eicosanoids can be distinguished, on the basis of their coupling with intracellular signalling mechanisms. A first group of receptors is linked to a phospholipase C, and mediates contraction of smooth muscle-like mesangial cells [4,5]. Typical responses to thromboxane A_2 (TxA$_2$), prostaglandin $F_{2\alpha}$ (PGF$_{2\alpha}$), and leukotrienes C_4/D_4 (LTC$_4$, LTD$_4$) include phosphoinositide breakdown, accumulation of water-soluble inositol phosphates, and the release of intracellularly stored Ca^{2+} [4,5]. These agents also activate Na^+/H^+ exchange, which results in cytosolic alkalinization in the absence of HCO_3^- [4,7]. Since Na^+/H^+ exchange is promoted by a number of activators of protein kinase C, it is possible that vasoconstrictor eicosanoids also enhance translocation of this cytosolic enzyme to the plasma membrane [8]. These signals trigger modest proliferation of G_0/G_1-arrested cells, while they modulate proliferation initiated by peptide growth factors [9]. Vasodilator eicosanoids such as PGI$_2$ — or prostacyclin — and PGE$_2$ activate adenylate cyclase, thus leading to enhanced formation of cyclic adenosine 3,5-monophosphate (cAMP) [3,10]. Stimulation of this pathway leads to relaxation of the cells, refractoriness to contractile stimuli, and a substantial inhibition of mitogen-stimulated proliferation [9,10]. Some overlap exists between these signalling mechanisms, with certain PGs capable of activating both vasoconstrictor and vasodilator receptors, such as is the case with PGE$_2$ [5]. Discrete receptors appear to exist for the various eicosanoids, although competitive binding and displacement have been shown, consistent with most other biologic systems sensitive to eicosanoids [5].

Phospholipase C activation is only one early step in the complex cellular responses of cultured human mesangial cells to the vasoconstrictor eicosanoid, TxA$_2$. In the present study, we briefly review both the early effects of TxA$_2$ on ion transport mechanisms, and later functional changes, revealed by regulation of the cellular synthesis of protein.

Materials and Methods

Cell Culture

Human mesangial cells were cultured from glomerular explants isolated by sequential sieving from histologically normal nephrectomy specimens. Cells were characterized and grown as described [5,11]. Culture medium was RPMI 1640 supplemented with 17% fetal bovine serum (FBS, Gibco, Paisley, U.K.), 5 ug/ml human recombinant insulin (Novo, Copenhagen, Denmark), and 10 ug/ml ceftriaxone (Roche, Basel, Switzerland). Confluent monolayers from four independent cell lines in passages 2–15 were used.

Measurement of Cytosolic Free Ca²⁺ ([Ca²⁺]ᵢ)

$[Ca^{2+}]_i$ was measured by a modification of previously described fluorimetric techniques [4,5]. Confluent monolayers on plastic Aclar coverslips (Allied Engineered Plastics, IL) were grown for 24 h in serum-free RPMI 1640 medium and were then loaded with 1 uM fura-2 (Molecular Probes, Eugene, OR) for 40 min at 37°C [12]. The cells were then incubated for a further 20 min in fluoroprobe-free medium, and were then placed on ice until assayed. Measurements were performed at 37°C in Krebs-Hensleit-based solutions buffered with 20 mM HEPES. Whenever appropriate, Na^+ was replaced isoosmotically with choline chloride or n-methyl-D-glucamine chloride. The coverslips were inserted into thermostatically controlled quartz cuvettes in a Perkin-Elmer LS5B spectrofluorometer fitted with stirring equipment. Ca^{2+}-dependent fluorescence was measured with excitation/emission wavelengths set at 339/500 nm, respectively. The recordings were calibrated with standard formulae by saturation of $[Ca^{2+}]_i$ with 15–40 uM ionomycin, followed by chelation to minimal fluorescence with 7.5 mM EGTA + 60 mM Tris base [12,13].

Measurement of Membrane Potential (Eₘ)

E_m was measured in bis-(1,3-diethylthiobarbiturate)-trimethineoxonol (bisoxonol, Molecular Probes, Eugene, Ore.)-equilibrated suspensions [14]. Confluent monolayers grown in 750 ml tissue culture flasks (Becton & Dickinson, Lincoln Park, N.J.) were released by brief trypsinization (3 min, 0.05% trypsin + 0.02% Na-ethylenediamine-tetraacetate, GIBCO, Paisley, United Kingdom), followed by gentle scraping in serum-free RPMI 1640 supplemented with neutralizing amounts of soybean trypsin inhibitor (1:3 trypsin/inhibitor, w/w, Fluka, Buchs, Switzerland). The cells were spun for 10 min at 900 g and the pellet was resuspended in the appropriate experimental solutions at a final density of 2×10^6 cells/ml. Bisoxonol was then added to 1 ml of the cell suspension under continuous stirring in the fluorometer, to a final concentration of 0.2 uM. Equilibration of bisoxonol was achieved within 2–5 min, as indicated by stable fluorescence readings at 540/580 nm excitation/emission wavelengths. Slits were 5/10 nm, respectively. Calibration of E_m-dependent fluorescence was performed in the presence of the monovalent cation ionophore, gramicidin D, 0.2 uM. Its addition determined rapid hyperpolarization of the cells, reflected by a downward shift of fluorescence. Graded additions of extracellular Na^+ progressively depolarized the cells, as revealed by a linear increase of fluorescence in the range of calculated E_m values between -50 and 0 mV. E_m in the presence of gramicidin D was calculated by the equation $E_m = -59 \log [K^+ + Na^+]_i / [K^+ + Na^+]_e$, assuming $[K^+ + Na^+] = 140$ mM [15,16]. The fluorescence readings at various imposed E_m were employed to draw a standard curve, to which recordings from experiments on aliquots of the same cell preparation were normalized. Choline (as the Cl salt) was employed for replacement of Na^+ in Na^+-free experiments, while gluconate (as the Na^+, K^+, and Ca^{2+} salts) was employed for Cl^- replacement.

Metabolic Labelling and Fluorography of Cellular Proteins

Confluent monolayers were grown in 250 or 750 ml tissue culture flasks in the continuous presence of FBS, or in the absence of FBS, for 72 h after reaching con-

fluence. The monolayers were incubated for 1 h in methionine-free Dulbecco's modified minimal essential medium (DMEM), followed by labelling with 15 uCi/ml [^{35}S]-
methionine in methionine-free DMEM for 4 h. At the end of labelling, monolayers
were scraped off the flasks in 20 ml total Ca^{2+}, Mg^{2+}-free phosphate buffer saline
(PBS) supplemented with 3 mM ethylenediaminotetraacetic acid (EDTA). Cells
were spun at 500 g for 10 min, resuspended in 1 ml 10 mM Tris-HCl solution containing 2 mM polymethylsulfonate, and homogenized with 10 strokes of a Teflon
pestle. Cell homogenates were spun at 3000 g for 20 min to eliminate nuclei, then at
12000 g for 30 min to discard mitochondria. The resulting supernatant was run at
100000 g for 60 min, to yield a membrane protein pellet and a cytosolic protein
supernatant. Aliquots of the two preparations were TCA-precipitated for total protein
assay, by a modification of Lowry's technique [17], and counted for total radioactivity by liquid scintillation spectrometry. The remaining sample material was subjected to sodium dodecylsulfate gel electrophoresis (SDS-PAGE) with a modification
of Laemmli's technique [18], followed by fluorography.

Results

Short-Term Effects of TxA_2

Stimulation of human mesangial cells with the TxA_2 mimetic, U-46619 (Upjohn,
Kalamazoo, Mich.), induces a rapid, partially reversible increase of $[Ca^{2+}]_i$. These

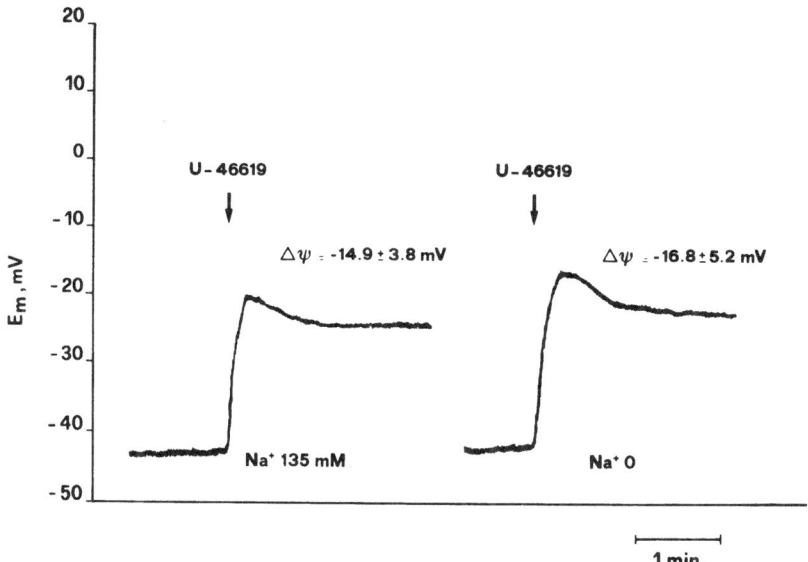

Fig. 1. Effects of the TxA_2 mimetic U-46619, 1 uM, on membrane potential (E_m) of cultured
human mesangial cells bathed in 135 mM Na^+ solution (*left*), or Na^+-free, choline chloride
solution (*right*). Mean depolarization in mV $\pm$ SE from $n=5$ experiments on *top of each graph*

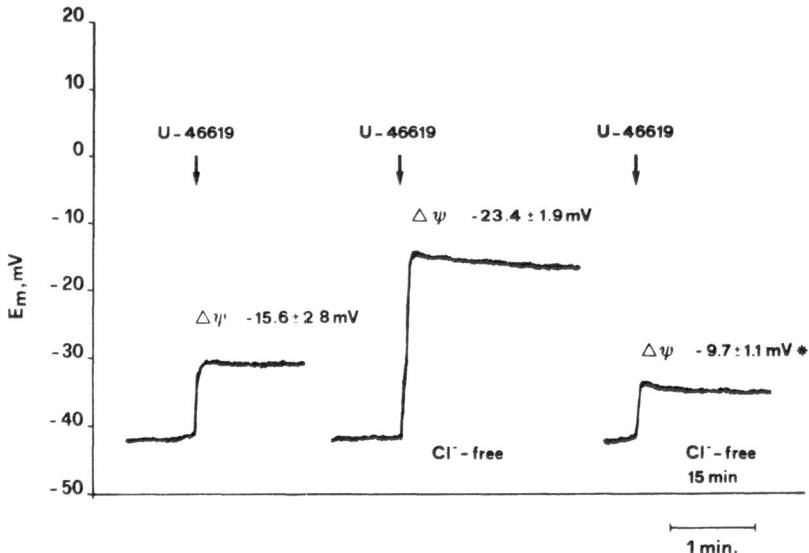

Fig. 2. Effects of 1 uM U-46619 on membrane potential (E_m) of cultured human mesangial cells. *Left*, 135 mM Na⁺ solution; *middle*, acute exposure to Cl⁻-free solution; *right*, cells preincubated for 15 min in Cl⁻-free solution. Mean depolarization in mV ± SE from $n = 5-8$ experiments on *top of each graph*. *P < 0.05 vs Cl⁻ solution, one-way analysis of variance

effects are paralleled by transient cytosolic acidification and followed by enhanced Na⁺/H⁺ antiport activity, unmasked by HCO_3^- removal from the bathing solution [7]. We asked whether enhanced ion fluxes, i.e., Ca^{2+} and Na⁺ entry, result in, or are to any extent related to, perturbation of E_m. Cells loaded with the lipophilic anion, bisoxonol, were rapidly depolarized by application of U-46619, as revealed by an immediate increase of fluorescence due to internalization of the dye (Fig. 1). Depolarization was dose-dependent, persistent both in Na⁺-containing and Na⁺-free solutions, and was therefore unrelated to Na⁺ influx (Fig. 1). Since Ca^{2+} influx would not account for the observed large changes of E_m, we turned to Cl⁻ as the major anion potentially responsible for depolarization. Acute isoosmotic replacement of Cl⁻ with gluconate, which by itself did not depolarize the cells, magnified the depolarizing response to U-46619, presumably by facilitated efflux of Cl⁻ (Fig. 2). Conversely, cells incubated in Cl⁻-free solution for 15 min at 37°C displayed marked inhibition of depolarization, consistent with Cl⁻ depletion. This indicates that TxA_2, in a manner similar to that of arginine vasopressin (AVP, not shown), enhances a Cl⁻ conductance in human mesangial cells, thus leading to depolarization of the plasma membrane. In turn, depolarization is possibly responsible for the opening of voltage-gated Ca^{2+} channels, thus contributing to the rise of $[Ca^{2+}]_i$ brought upon by the eicosanoid.

Other pathways of Ca^{2+} influx exist, however, in these cells. We have recently obtained evidence for a Na⁺/Ca^{2+} exchange mechanism in cultured human mesangial

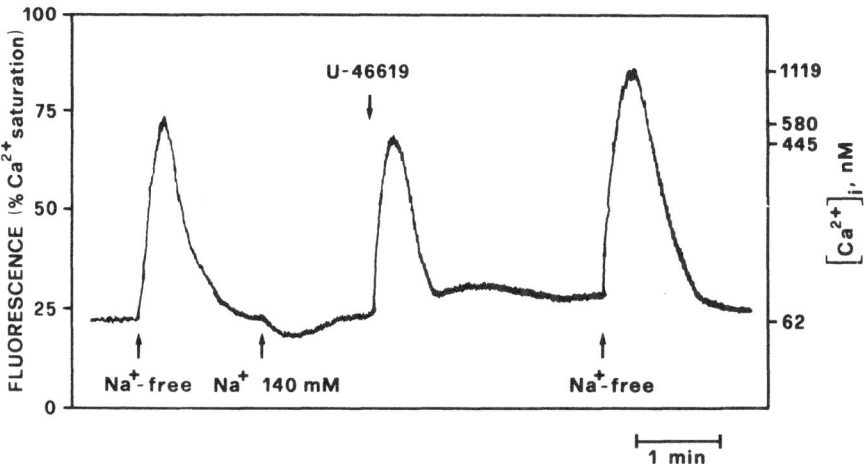

Fig. 3. Effects of rapid Na$^+$ removal (Na$^+$-free) on [Ca^{2+}]$_i$ of fura-2-loaded monolayers of cultured human mesangial cells. Note enhancement of the effects of repeated Na$^+$ removal, following stimulation of the same monolayer with 1 uM U-46619. Continuous fluorescence monitoring representative of $n=6$ experiments

cells. As shown in Fig. 3, abrupt withdrawal of extracellular Na$^+$, by replacing the bathing solution with isoosmotic choline or n-methyl-D-glucamine chloride solutions, stimulates a rapid rise of [Ca^{2+}]$_i$, resulting from Ca^{2+} influx. Evidence for this pathway includes suppression of the [Ca^{2+}]$_i$ response in EGTA-containing solutions, lack of sensitivity to blockers of voltage-operated Ca^{2+} channels, inhibition by amiloride, enhancement by Na$^+$-loading the cells with ouabain, and the action of the Na$^+$ ionophores, monensin and gramicidin [19]. Following the initial influx of Ca^{2+}, exposure of the cells to 1 uM U-46619 in Na$^+$ solution markedly enhanced the [Ca^{2+}]$_i$ response to a second removal of Na$^+$ in the same monolayer. In $n=5$ experiments, U-46619 increased the peak [Ca^{2+}]$_i$ response to Na$^+$ removal from 1009±142 to 1442±247 nM (P <0.05 by unpaired analysis of variance). Conversely, the amplitude of the [Ca^{2+}]$_i$ spike in response to 1 uM U-46619 was significantly enhanced in Na$^+$-free solutions, from 688±220 to 1152±123 nM (P <0.01 by unpaired analysis of variance, $n=5$). This implies that (1) Na$^+$/Ca^{2+} exchange contributes to the efflux of Ca^{2+} upon stimulation of mesangial cells by vasoconstrictor eicosanoids, and (2) activation of this exchanger by TxA$_2$ may serve homeostatic functions, modulating the amplitude of the [Ca^{2+}]$_i$ transient.

Long-Term Effects of TxA$_2$

Activation of these early signals translates into later functional changes. We and others have previously described the antagonism between adenylate cyclase-and phospholipase C-transduced eicosanoids on the contraction and proliferation of mesangial cells [9,10]. We have now undertaken a study of the effects of TxA$_2$ on

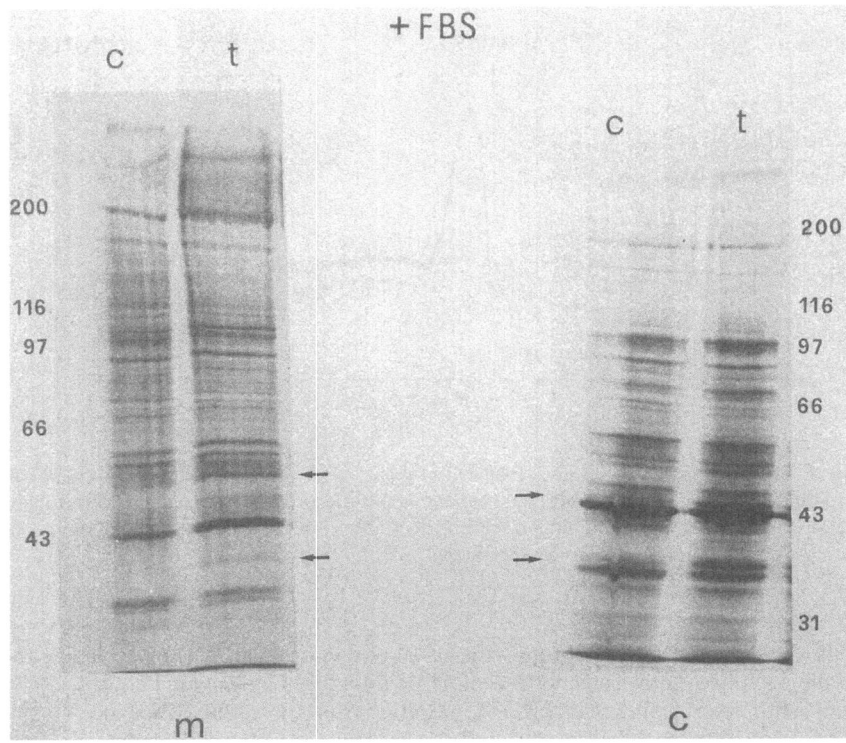

Fig. 4. Effects of U-46619 on protein synthesis of cultured human mesangial cells proliferating in response to 17% fetal bovine serum (*FBS*). SDS-PAGE of membrane-associated (*m*) and cytosolic (*c*) [^{35}S]-methionine-labelled proteins, 24-h incubation with 1 uM U-46619 (*t*) vs control (*c*). Representative fluorography of $n=4$ experiments

protein synthesis of confluent monolayers of human mesangial cells. Both types of cells maintained in the presence of FBS, i.e., cycling cells, and quiescent cells after 72 h in the absence of FBS, responded to acute (4 h) and chronic (24 h) exposure to 1 µM U-46619 with typical changes of the pattern of protein synthesis. Despite a modest, non-significant reduction of total [^{35}S]-methionine incorporation into cell proteins during 24-h incubations with U-46619 (membrane proteins $-6\pm13\%$ and $-136\pm 113\%$, cytosolic proteins $-11\pm20\%$ and $-57\pm55\%$, w/ and w/FBS, respectively; % of control $\pm$ SE, $n=4$), increased expression of membrane and cytosolic proteins of approximate MW 38–53 Kda in the presence of FBS (Fig. 4), as well as membrane proteins of MW 125–200 Kda in the absence of FBS, indicated specific induction of multiple transcripts by TxA$_2$. While identification of such proteins is in progress, these results are consistent with modulation of mesangial cell phenotype by TxA$_2$, with possible differentiation and expression of specialized functions.

Discussion

Human mesangial cells respond to stimulation by vasoconstrictor eicosanoids with multiple functional changes, reflecting activation of specific receptors. We herein report that a TxA_2 mimetic acutely depolarizes the cells, presumably by promoting a Cl^- current. The process is independent of extracellular Na^+, and may lead to initiation of Ca^{2+} influx, with resulting sustained elevations of $[Ca^{2+}]_i$. Similar findings have been reported with fluorimetric and electrophysiological techniques in rat mesangial cells exposed to peptide vasoconstrictors [15,20,21]. In turn, the Ca^{2+} signalling pathway is markedly altered by removal of extracellular Na^+, which magnifies the stimulatory effects of the TxA_2 mimetic, as well as the effects of other vasoconstrictors (not shown). Na^+ removal unmasks the presence of a mechanism linking Ca^{2+} and Na^+ fluxes, namely a Na^+/Ca^{2+} exchanger. This transporter is acutely activated by TxA_2, as revealed by the larger amplitude of the $[Ca^{2+}]_i$ spike in cells prestimulated by U-46619. This activation may result from (i) synergism with TxA_2- promoted discharge of Ca^{2+} from internal stores, (ii) Na^+-loading via Na^+/H^+ exchange, with resulting increased Na^+ export via Na^+/Ca^{2+} exchange, or (iii) Ca^{2+} or protein kinase C direct effects on the exchanger. In general, enhancement of the antiporter by phospholipase C agonists may represent a homeostatic mechanism modulating the $[Ca^{2+}]_i$ surges. Evidence for such Na^+/Ca^{2+} exchange mechanisms has been presented for several smooth muscle cell lines, although differences exist in their regulation and sensitivity to vasoconstrictors [22–24]. The presence of a Na^+/Ca^{2+} exchanger in cultured mesangial cells strengthens the belief that these cells structurally and functionally resemble smooth muscle [25]. From these experiments, one may conclude that vasoconstrictor eicosanoids promote a resetting of ion balance across the plasma membrane, taking place within seconds to a few minutes. The process is followed by functional changes including contraction, interference with cell proliferation, and complex alterations of protein synthesis. This last aspect is particularly interesting, in view of the stimulation of specific protein synthesis, even though total protein synthesis is substantially unchanged, both in the presence and in the absence of FBS. This phenomenon is consistent with a substantial lack of stimulation or inhibition of cell growth, previously described by us in quiescent and cycling cells, respectively [9]. On the other hand, stimulation of certain protein products points to structural modifications of the cells, which may acquire a differentiated phenotype upon exposure to vasoconstrictor eicosanoids. Clearly, further work is required in order to identify the proteins induced by TxA_2, as well as their location and function. This may lead to significant progress in our understanding of the pathophysiologic role of eicosanoids in the kidney.

Acknowledgments. We are indebted to Ms. Stefania De Grossi, Ms. Tiziana Menna and Mr. Salvatore Greci for expert technical assistance. These studies were partially funded by grants from the Ministry of Education of Italy (quota 40% and 60%).

References

1. Dunn MJ (1983) Renal prostaglandins. In: Dunn MJ (ed) Renal Endocrinology. Williams and Wilkins, Baltimore, pp 1–74

2. Ardaillou N, Hagege J, Nivez MP, Ardaillou R, Schlondorff D (1985) Vasoconstrictor-evoked prostaglandin synthesis in cultured human mesangial cells. Am J Physiol 248 (Renal Fluid Electrolyte Physiol 17):F240–F246

3. Friedlander G, Chansel D, Sraer J, Bens M, Ardaillou R (1983) PGE_2 binding sites and PG-stimulated cyclic AMP accumulation in rat isolated glomeruli and glomerular cultured cells. Mol Cell Endocrinol 30:201–214

4. Simonson MS, Menè P, Dubyak GR, Dunn MJ (1988) Identification and transmembrane signaling of leukotriene D_4 receptors in human mesangial cells. Am J Physiol 255:C771–C7805

5. Menè P, Dubyak GR, Abboud HE, Scarpa A, Dunn MJ (1988) Phospholipase C activation by prostaglandins and thromboxane A_2 in cultured mesangial cells. Am J Physiol 255:F1059–F1069

6. Menè P, Cinotti GA (1989) Paracrine and autocrine functions of glomerular mesangial cells. J Endocrinol Invest 12:497–509

7. Menè P, Dubyak GR, Scarpa A, Dunn MJ (1991) Regulation of cytosolic pH of cultured mesangial cells by prostaglandin $F_{2\alpha}$ and thromboxane A_2. Am J Physiol 260 (Cell Physiol 29)

8. Nishizuka Y (1986) Studies and perspectives of protein kinase C. Science 233:305–312

9. Menè P, Abboud HE, Dunn MJ (1990) Regulation of human mesangial cell growth in culture by thromboxane A_2 and prostacyclin. Kidney Int 38:232–239

10. Menè P, Dunn MJ (1988) Eicosanoids and control of mesangial cell contraction. Circ Res 62:916–925

11. Striker GE, Killen PD, Farin FM (1980) Human glomerular cells in vitro: isolation and characterization. Transplant Proc 12:88–99

12. Grynkiewicz G, Poenie M, Tsien RY (1985) A new generation of Ca^{2+} indicators with greatly improved fluorescence properties. J Biol Chem 260:3440–3450

13. Cobbold PH, Rink TJ (1987) Fluorescence and bioluminescence measurement of cytoplasmic free calcium. Biochem J 248:313–328

14. Waggoner AS (1979) The use of cyanine dyes for the determination of membrane potentials in cells, organelles, and vesicles. Methods Enzymol 55:689–695

15. Kremer SG, Breuer WV, Skorecki KL (1989) Vasoconstrictor hormones depolarize renal glomerular mesangial cells by activating chloride channels. J Cell Physiol 138:97–105

16. Rink TJ, Montecucco C, Hesketh TR, Tsien RY (1980) Lymphocyte membrane potential assessed with fluorescent probes. Biochim Biophys Acta 595:15–30

17. Markwell MK, Haas SM, Bieber LL, Tolbert NE (1978) A modification of the Lowry procedure to simplify protein determination in membrane and lipoprotein samples. Anal Biochem 87:206–210

18. Laemmli UK (1970) Cleavage of structural proteins during the assembly of the head of bacteriophage T4. Nature 227:680–685

19. Menè P, Pugliese F, Cinotti GA (1990) Na^+/Ca^{2+} exchange in cultured human mesangial cells (abstract). Kidney Int 37:210

20. Okuda T, Yamashita N, Kurokawa K (1986) Angiotensin II and vasopressin stimulate calcium-activated chloride conductance in rat mesangial cells. J Clin Invest 78:1443–1448

21. Okuda T, Kojima I, Ogata E, Kurokawa K (1989) Ambient Cl^- ions modify rat mesangial cell contraction by modulating cell inositol trisphosphate and Ca^{2+} via enhanced prostaglandin E_2. J Clin Invest 84:1866–1872

22. Vigne P, Breittmayer J-P, Duval D, Frelin C, Ladzunski M (1988) The Na^+/Ca^{2+} antiporter in aortic smooth muscle cells. Characterization and demonstration of an activation by phorbol esters. J Biol Chem 263:8078–8083

23. Smith JB, Zheng T, Smith L (1989) Relationship between cytosolic free Ca^{2+} and Na^+/Ca^{2+} exchange in aortic muscle cells. Am J Physiol 256 (Cell Physiol 25):C147–C154
24. Aaronson PI, Benham CD (1989) Alterations in $[Ca^{2+}]_i$ mediated by sodium-calcium exchange in smooth muscle cells isolated from the guinea-pig ureter. J Physiol (Lond) 416:1–18
25. Menè P, Simonson MS, Dunn MJ (1989) Physiology of the mesangial cell. Physiol Rev 69:1347–1424

The Functional Significance of Lipoxygenase Products of Arachidonic Acid in the Glomerular Microcirculation

Kamal F. Badr and Kihito Takahashi[1]

SUMMARY. Intrarenal administration of Lipoxin A_4 (LXA_4) results in vasodilatory responses, but reduces the ultrafiltration coefficient, K_f. Lipoxin A_4 competes for the ^3H-Leukotriene D_4 (LTD_4) binding to rat mesangial cells and stimulates inositol trisphosphate ($INsP_3$) formation from these cells. Reversal of stereochemical orientation of the polar substituents at C5 and C6 from S,R to R,S in both LTD_4 and LXA_4 abolishes both homologous and heterologous competition for ^3H-LTD_4 binding to mesangial cells and leads to total loss of biologic activity. Taken together, these data provided evidence for the involvement of a common recognition site mediating the actions of these two eicosanoids on mesangial cells. Cyclooxygenase inhibition reversed the vasodilatory action of LXA_4, suggesting that LXA_4-mediated increases in RPF were due to the secondary release of vasodilatory cyclooxygenase products. Intrarenal arterial administration of other lipoxins, LXB_4 and 7-cis, 11-trans LXA_4, induced vasoconstriction. Administration of the last named lipoxin which has a configuration at C5 and C6 identical with that of LTD_4, resulted in systemic and renal effects similar to those of LTD_4, suggesting that these actions resulted from activation of LTD_4 receptor-coupled responses.

Introduction

The functional significance of lipoxygenase metabolites of arachidonic acid in glomerular inflammation has been increasingly recognized. We have previously shown that intrarenal arterial infusion of Leukotriene D_4 (LTD_4) resulted in vasoconstriction [1], while that of Lipoxin A_4 (LXA_4) induced vasodilatory responses [2]. However, interestingly, both compounds reduced the glomerular capillary ultrafiltration coefficient, K_f, which is currently considered to result from the con-

[1]Division of Nephrology, Vanderbilt University School of Medicine, Nashville, TN 37232, USA

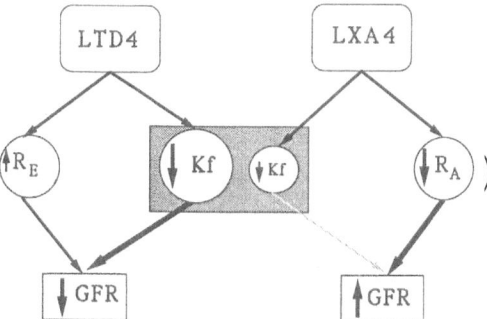

Fig. 1. Summary of LTD$_4$ and LXA$_4$-induced changes in glomerular dynamics. LTD$_4$ reduces GFR as a result of combined reductions in glomerular plasma flow [induced mainly by an increase in efferent arteriolar resistance (R$_E$)] and ultrafiltration coefficient, K$_f$. On the other hand, LXA$_4$ reduces selectively afferent (R$_A$), but not efferent arterial resistance, thereby leading to increases in glomerular plasma flow and net transcapillary hydraulic pressure difference. This results in an increase in GFR, an effect partially offset by a simultaneous fall in K$_f$

certed contractile action of smooth muscle-containing glomerular mesangial cells; this action thereby reduces the total glomerular capillary surface area available for filtration [3] (Fig. 1). Recently, we have characterized the binding of LTD$_4$ to rat mesangial cells and its intracellular signal transduction pathways [4]. Because LTD$_4$ and LXA$_4$ share a common orientation of polar substitutes at the C5 and C6 positions (5S, 6R), and this stereochemical configuration is an absolute requirement for the biological activity of these eicosanoids [5], we investigated whether LXA$_4$-induced falls in K$_f$ were in part due to its action on the mesangial cell LTD$_4$ receptors. In addition, we

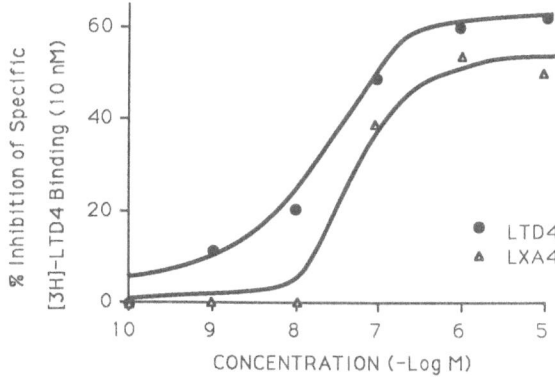

Fig. 2. Percent inhibition of ^{3}H-LTD$_4$ (10 nM) binding to rat glomerular mesangial cells by LTD$_4$ (●) and LXA$_4$ (△). Each point represents the mean of four experiments performed in duplicate. (From [5])

investigated the mechanism of LXA_4-induced vasodilatation, and, in view of expanding interest in other lipoxins, the effects of LXB_4 and a newly discovered biologically active isomer of LXA_4, 7-cis, 11-trans LXA_4, [6] on the renal vasculature.

Methods

All micropuncture studies were performed on Inactin-anesthetized male Munich-Wistar rats, weighing 200-230 g, which were prepared for micropuncture according to protocols previously described [1]. A 30-gauge needle was placed at the root of the left renal artery; through this were infused all the compounds tested in this study. Homologous rat plasma was administered i.v. to maintain euvolemia. Studies of ^3H-LTD_4 binding were performed routinely at $4°C$ on mesangial cells grown to confluence in 24-well cluster dishes. The formation of $InsP_3$ in ^3H-inositol labelled mesangial cells, in response to either LTD_4 or LXA_4, was measured by separating ^3H-$InsP_3$ by anion-exchange column chromatography by Berridge's method [7].

Results and Discussion

Intrarenal arterial administration of LXA_4 (0.75 µg/kg/min) induced significant increases in single nephron glomerular filtration rate (SNGFR) and plasma flow (Q_A) from 38.4 ± 1.7 to 45.5 ± 3.0 nl/min (P<0.05) and from 95 ± 6 to 127 ± 9 nl/min (P<0.05), respectively. The increase in Q_A was due to a selective fall in preglomerular resistance (R_A) from 2.55 ± 0.16 to 1.75 ± 0.20 10^{10} dyn.s.cm^{-5} (P<0.05), while postglomerular resistance (R_E) was unchanged: from 1.70 ± 0.22 to 1.50 ± 0.08 10^{10} dyn.s.cm^{-5}. The constancy of R_E coupled with the increase in Q_A, leads to an increase in the ultrafiltration pressure difference, ΔP. These increases in Q_A and ΔP were jointly responsible for the observed increase in SNGFR. However, the latter effect was partially offset by a concomittant significant reduction in K_f, which fell from 0.060 ± 0.013 to 0.033 ± 0.005 nl/(s.mmHg) (P<0.05).

To investigate the mechanism of the LXA_4-mediated fall in K_f, we performed competitive binding inhibition studies. Competitive binding inhibition showed that the addition of unlabelled LXA_4 competed with ^3H-LTD_4 in binding to mesangial cells. Half-maximal inhibition of binding by LXA_4 was at 100 nM compared to 10 nM for the homoligand. This degree of ^3H-LTD_4 binding inhibition was equivalent to that seen with LTE_4, and several orders of magnitude greater than that of the biologically inactive 5R, 6S isomers of LTD_4 and LXA_4 (Fig. 2). Furthermore, five seconds after addition of LXA_4 (1, 10, 50 and 100 nM) to mesangial cells labelled with ^3H-inositol, low but significant increases [$46 \pm 14\%$ (P<0.05), $50 \pm 21\%$ (P<0.05), $44 \pm 22\%$ (P<0.05), and $45 \pm 26\%$ (P<0.05), respectively] were observed in radioactive counts (cpm). These increases, corresponding to inositol trisphosphate ($InsP_3$) formation by these cells, were noted to be more than those in vehicle-treated samples. Incubation of mesangial cells with the LTD_4 receptor antagonist, SKF 104353 (100 nm) abolished the LXA_4-induced stimulation of ^3H-$InsP_3$ formation in these cells. Addition of 10 and 50 nM LTD_4 to these cells was associated with $146 \pm 20\%$ (P<0.01) and $106 \pm 13\%$ (P<0.005) increases, respectively, in ^3H-$InsP_3$ counts compared to the controls; values significantly greater than

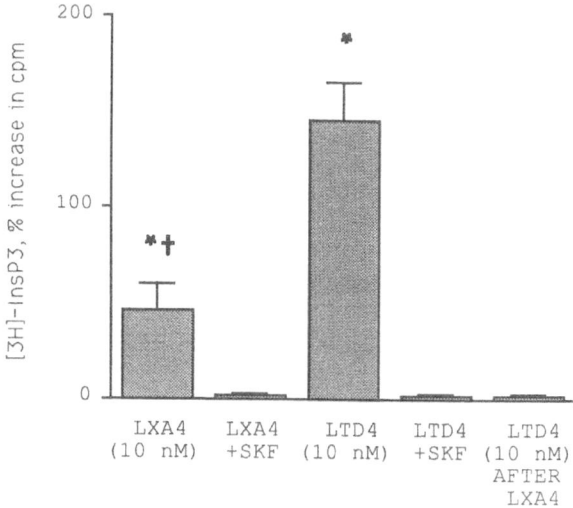

Fig. 3. InsP$_3$ formation in rat mesangial cells in response to LXA$_4$ and LTD$_4$ and its complete abolition in the presence of 100-fold concentration of SKF 104353 (SKF). The *far right column* depicts the abrogation of LTD$_4$-induced stimulation of InsP$_3$ formation by preexposure of the cells to 100 nM LXA$_4$ for 10 min. *, P < 0.01 versus vehicle-stimulated controls. †, P < 0.05 versus LTD$_4$ alone. (From [5])

those for LXA$_4$ (P < 0.05). Incubation of mesangial cells with SKF 104353 in a concentration 100-fold that of the ligand, followed by addition of LTD$_4$, was associated with total abrogation of the LTD$_4$-induced stimulation of ^{3}H-InsP$_3$ formation in these cells. And similarly, preincubation of these cells with LXA$_4$ (100 nM) for 10 min before adding 10 nM LTD$_4$ completely prevented LTD$_4$-induced InsP$_3$ generation (Fig. 3). Taken together, these data provide evidence for the involvement of a common recognition site which mediates the actions of these two eicosanoids on mesangial cells.

Intrarenal arterial infusion of LTD$_4$ (0.5, 7.0, 14.0 and 20.0 μg/kg/min) was associated with dose-dependent reductions in GFR and RPF. Mean percent falls in GFR/RPF during LTD$_4$ infusion were 27/24, 25/40, 70/65, 73/70 at the doses above, respectively. However, administration of these doses of LTD$_4$ in the presence of LXA$_4$ (1.0 μg/kg/min) was associated with marked blunting of LTD$_4$-induced reduction in GFR, but no such blunting occurred in RPF. Mean percent falls in GFR/RPF during LTD$_4$ infusion in the presence of LXA$_4$ were 9/20, 11/37, 42/51, and 50/68 at the doses above, respectively. The relative protection given by LXA$_4$ against the GFR-depressant action of LTD$_4$, despite the absence of any modification of the potent vasoconstrictor actions of LTD$_4$, is interpreted as LXA$_4$-mediated prevention of the LTD$_4$-induced fall in K$_f$. These data support our in vitro finding, which showed competition by LXA$_4$ for LTD$_4$ receptors on mesangial cells.

To elucidate the mechanism for LXA$_4$-induced vasodilatation, we investigated the effect of cyclooxygenase inhibition in vivo on the renal action of LXA$_4$, in the light of lipoxin-induced prostaglandin release from bronchial and vascular tissues [8,9]. In non-cyclooxygenase-inhibited rats, LXA_4, infused into the left renal artery at 1.0 and 2.0 μg/kg per min led to dose-dependent increases in RPF and GFR. In the presence of the cyclooxygenase inhibitor, ibuprofen (20 mg/kg i.v.), these responses were reversed. Thus, these data suggested that LXA_4-mediated increases in RPF were due to the secondary release of vasodilatory cyclooxygenase products.

To investigate the effects of lipoxin B_4 and 7-cis, 11-trans LXA_4 on renal functions, we performed clearance studies by infusing these compounds into the left renal artery. The infusion of lipoxin B_4 (2.0 μg/kg per min) had no effect on systemic arterial pressure and hematocrit, whereas this compound induced a mild but significant decrease in GFR and RPF. The GFR decreased from 0.75 to 0.67 ml/min ($P < 0.05$) and the RPF decreased from 4.20 to 3.66 ml/min ($P < 0.05$). Filtration fraction was unchanged, due to the similar magnitude of GFR and RPF reductions. While modest in magnitude, these changes were notable in that they were opposite in nature to those observed in response to LXA_4. The infusion of 7-cis, 11-trans LXA_4 (1.0 μg/kg per min) induced an increase in hematocrit and in systemic arterial pressure, as well as inducing dramatic reductions in GFR and RPF, which were similar to those induced by Leukotrien C_4 and D_4 [1,10].

Because of the identical configuration, at C5 and C6 of 7-cis, 11-trans LXA_4 and LTD_4, it is reasonable to postulate that the systemic and renal action of 7-cis, 11-trans LXA_4 results from the activation of LTD_4 receptor coupled responses. The mechanism for the activity of LXB_4 remains unclear. In view of previous reports suggesting the secondary release of other eicosanoids by lipoxins in vitro [8,9], possible mechanisms could include interactions with other eicosanoids.

References

1. Badr KF, Brenner BM, Ichikawa II (1987) Effects of leukotriene D_4 on glomerular dynamics in the rat. Am J Physiol 22:F239–F243
2. Badr KF, Serhan CN, Nicolaou KC, Samuelsson B (1987) The action of lipoxin-A on glomerular microcirculatory dynamics in the rat. Biochem Biophys Res Commun 145:408–414
3. Harris RC, Hoover RL, Jacobson HR, Badr KF (1988) Evidence for glomerular actions of epidermal growth factor in the rat. J Clin Invest 82:1028–1039
4. Badr KF, Mong S, Hoover RL, Schwarzberg M, Ebert J, Jacobson HR, Harris RC (1989) Leukotriene D_4 binding and signal transduction in rat glomerular mesangial cells. Am J Physiol 26:F280–F287
5. Badr KF, Deboer DK, Schwarzberg M, Serhan CN (1989) Lipoxin A_4 antagonizes cellular and in vivo actions of leukotriene D_4 in rat glomerular mesangial cells: Evidence for competition at a common receptor. Proc Natl Acad Sci USA 86:3438–3442
6. Nicolaou KC, Marron BE, Veale CA, Webber SE, Dahlen SE, Samuelsson B, Serhan CN (1989) Identification of a novel 7-cis-11-trans-lipoxin A_4 generated by human neutrophils: total synthesis, spasmogenic activities and comparison with other geometric isomers of lipoxins A_4 and B_4. Biochem Biophys Acta 1003:44–53
7. Berridge MJ (1984) Inositol trisphosphate and diacylglycerol as second messengers. Biochem J 220:345–360
8. Dahlen SE, Frazen L, Raud J, Serhan CN, Westlung P, Wikstrom E, Bjorck T, Matsuda H, Webber SE, Veale CA, Puustinen T, Haeggstrom J, Nicolaou KC, Samuelsson B (1988) Actions of lipoxin A_4 and released compounds in smooth muscle preparations and on the

microcirculation in vivo. In: Wong WY-K, Serhan CN (eds) Lipoxins: Biosynthesis, Chemistry and Biological activities. Plenum, New York, pp 107–130

9. Brezinski ME, Gimbrone MA JR, Nicolaou KC, Serhan CN (1989) Lipoxins stimulate prostacyclin generation by human endothelial cells. FEBS Lett 245:162–172

10. Badr KF, Baylis C, Peffer JM, Peffer MA, Soberman RJ, Lewis RA, Austen KF, Corey EJ, Brenner BM (1984) Renal and systemic hemodynamic responses to intravenous infusion of leukotriene C_4 in the rat. Circ Res 54:492–499

Activation by Adenosine of Cultured Mesangial Cells: Receptors Involved and Intracellular Mechanisms

Ana Olivera, Manuela Tomás[1], and José M. López-Novoa[2]

SUMMARY. We studied the effects of the adenosine (ADO) analogues R-PIA (A1 agonist) and NECA (A2 agonist) on cAMP production and calcium inflow in cultured rat mesangial cells (MC). NECA, 10^{-6} M overstimulated cAMP content, and this effect was inhibited by the selective A_1 antagonist PD115199 (AT_2, 10^{-6} M). R-PIA 10^{-6} M, decreased cAMP content in forskolin-stimulated MC and this effect was blocked by the selective A_2 antagonist PD116948 (AT_2, 10^{-6} M). In addition, 10^{-6} M R-PIA + 10^{-6} M AT_2 increased ^{45}Ca-uptake after 30 s of stimulation, whereas 10^{-6} M NECA + 10^{-6} M AT_1 mediated a reduction in ^{45}Ca uptake in MC. Adenosine 10^{-4} M induced an increase in cAMP levels in forskolin-stimulated MC and an increase in ^{45}Ca^{2+} uptake. Neither AT_2 nor AT_1 affected ADO-induced cAMP production in forskolin-stimulated MC, but this effect was inhibited by 10^{-4} M theophylline. ADO-induced ^{45}Ca^{2+} uptake stimulation was inhibited by AT_2, unlike the effect shown with R-PIA. This effect was also inhibited by AT_1. These data demonstrate in a functional way the existence of A_1 and A_2 type receptors in cultured rat mesangial cells. Activation of the A_1-type stimulates calcium entry and inhibits cAMP generation. In contrast, activation of the A_2-type stimulates cAMP generation and inhibits calcium entry. Adenosine stimulates both cAMP generation and calcium uptake, but these actions do not seem to be mediated by the A_1 or A_2 receptors present in mesangial cells.

Introduction

Adenosine (ADO) has been shown to mediate a large number of physiological responses in cells from different tissues. Two specific cell surface receptors for

---

[1]Fundación Jimenez Diaz, Consejo Superior de Investigaciones Cientificas, Madrid, Spain
[2]Department of Physiology and Pharmacology, Faculty of Medicine, University of Salamanca, Avenida del Campo Charro s/n, 37007-Salamanca, Spain

adenosine have been classically described, on the basis of their ability to stimulate (A_2 ADO receptor) or inhibit (A_1 ADO receptor) membrane adenylate cyclase [1,2]. Synthesis of ADO derivatives with differential effects on adenylate cyclase activity has been developed in recent years. This has permitted a characterization of ADO receptor subtypes by additional pharmacological criteria [3]. Although A_1 or A_2 ADO receptors have been characterized, in most cells, some investigators have suggested the existence of a third ADO receptor, in order to explain some ADO-induced effects that cannot be attributed to activation of A_1 or A_2 subtypes [4–6].

Adenosine and the Kidney

In the kidney, ADO produces a wide range of responses, including a transient reduction of renal blood flow and a persistent decrement of glomerular filtration rate [7–9], inhibition of renin secretion [10,11], and some direct effect on renal tubules [12]. The two receptors defined for ADO have been identified in several renal structures and cells [12–14].

Freissmuth et al. described both A_1 and A_2 ADO receptors in rat isolated glomeruli [13], but the distribution of these receptors in the different glomerular cell types remains to be elucidated. We have previously demonstrated that ADO is able to contract rat mesangial cells in culture, probably through an A_1 ADO receptor [15]. Another set of experiments performed in our laboratory also suggests the existence of a functional A_2 receptor. Preincubation of MC with 10^{-6} M NECA, a potent A_2 agonist, partially blocked Angiotensin II-induced MC contraction (data not shown). Although all these data seem to indicate the existence of both A_1 and A_2 receptors in MC, we performed a further characterization of ADO receptors in these cells.

Functional Identification of A_1 and A_2 Receptors by the Effects of Adenosine Agonist on cAMP Levels

We studied the effects of the ADO analogues R-PIA and NECA on cAMP production. Mesangial cells were prestimulated for 5 min with 5 μM forskolin to augment cyclase activity. This methodological approach is frequently used to make agonist-induced effects, especially the inhibitory ones, on adenylate cyclase more evident.

After 2 minutes of incubation, 10^{-6} M NECA overstimulated intracellular cAMP content, whereas 10^{-6} M R-PIA decreased cAMP content in forskolin-stimulated MC (Fig. 1). The stimulation induced by NECA was inhibited only in the presence of the selective A_2 antagonist PD115199 [19] (AT_2, 10^{-6} M), whereas the inhibition of cAMP production was blocked in the presence of the A_1 antagonist PD115948 [20] (AT_1, 10^{-6} M) (Fig. 1). The contrasting effects of the agonists on cAMP content, the inhibition of these effects by the respective antagonists, and the direction of the change suggest that A_1 and A_2-like ADO receptors, linked by adenylate cyclase exist in MC.

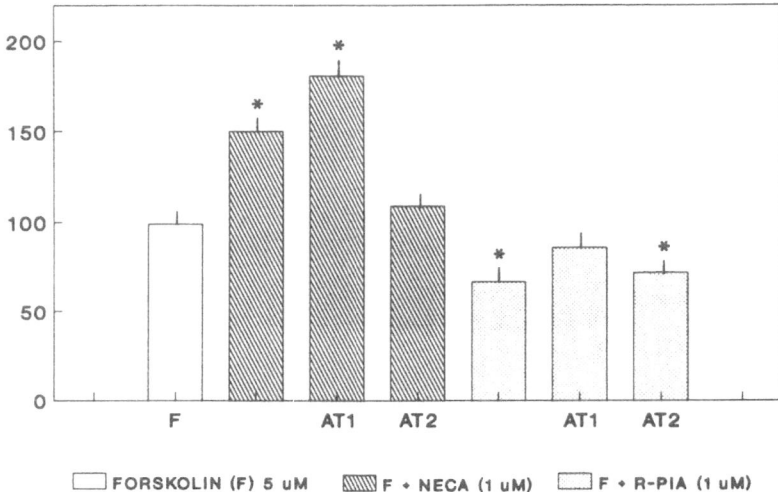

Fig. 1. Effect of the ADO agonists NECA (A_2) and R-PIA (A_1) and the selective antagonists PD 116948 (AT_1, 1 μM) and PD 115199 (AT_2, 1 μM) on cAMP intracellular content in Forskolin-pre-stimulated mesangial cells after 2 min of incubation. cAMP was extracted from the cells with ethanol, samples were dried and cAMP was determined by a specific RIA. Data are mean ± SEM of at least 12 determinations. *Asterisks* represent significant differences ($P < 0.05$) with respect to F-treated MC. RIA, radio-immunoassay

Effects of the Agonists on $^{45}Ca^{2+}$ Uptake

Adenylate cyclase is not the only effector system that has been described to be modulated by ADO receptors. For instance, ADO can modify calcium currents in several cell types [21–23]. As mesangial cell contraction induced by ADO seems to be dependent on extracellular calcium [15], we also decided to study the effect of preferential activation of A_1 or A_2 receptors on ^{45}Ca uptake in these cells.

The A_1 agonist R-PIA (10^{-6} M) increased ^{45}Ca-uptake after 30 s of stimulation, whereas the potent A_2 agonist NECA (10^{-6} M) mediated a reduction in ^{45}Ca uptake that did not reach statistical significance (Fig. 2). Since ADO agonists, specially NECA, are not absolutely selective for one or another kind of ADO receptor [3], we tried to further characterize NECA's actions by blocking the opposite receptors with the selective ADO antagonists PD116948 (A_1, 10^{-6} M) and PD115199 (AT_2, 10^{-6} M). Blockade of the A_2 receptor with AT_2 potentiated the increase of $^{45}Ca^{2+}$-uptake induced by the preferential activation of the A_1 receptor by R-PIA. On the other hand, blockade of the A_1 receptor with AT_1 potentiated the tendency of NECA to decrease $^{45}Ca^{2+}$ uptake in MC (Fig. 2).

Thus we can identify two subtypes of ADO receptors in MC, with opposite effects on cAMP production and on $^{45}Ca^{2+}$ uptake, i.e., and R-PIA-activable ADO receptor that mediates a reduction of cAMP levels and an increase in $^{45}Ca^{2+}$ uptake, which can then be defined as an A_1-like receptor, and a NECA-activable ADO receptor that

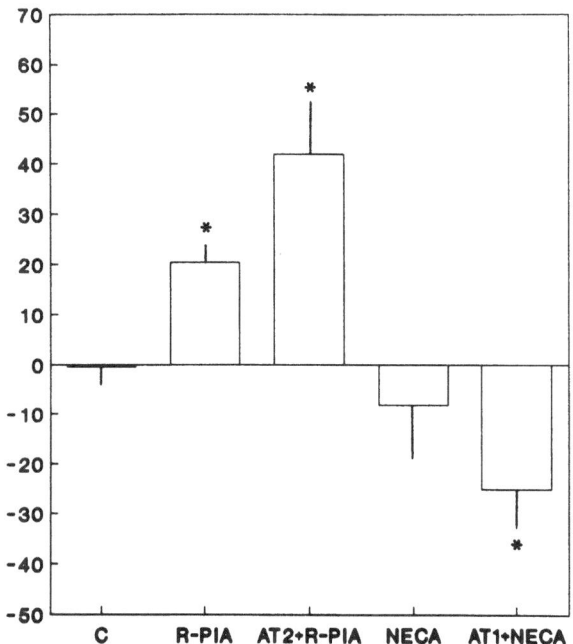

45-Calcium uptake (Δ%)

Fig. 2. Effect of the ADO agonists NECA (A_2, 1 μM) and R-PIA (A_2, 1 μM) alone or together with the selective antagonists of the opposite receptors PD 116948 (AT_1, 1 μM) and PD 115199 (AT_2, 1 μM) on ^{45}Ca uptake by mesangial cells. When corresponded, cells were preincubated with the antagonists for 10 min, and were then incubated in the presence of the isotope and the agonists for 30 s. Intracellular ^{45}Ca content was measured by liquid scintillation counting. Data are mean ± SEM of at least 12 determinations. *Asterisks* represent significant differences ($P < 0.05$) with respect to basal uptake

produces an increase in cAMP levels and a decrease on ^{45}Ca^{2+} uptake, which can then be defined as an A_2-like ADO receptor.

Effects of Adenosine on cAMP Production and on ^{45}Ca^{2+} Uptake: Possibility of a Third Adenosine Receptor

Once we had defined A_1 and A_2-like ADO receptors in MC, we studied the effects of ADO both on cAMP levels and on ^{45}Ca^{2+} uptake, and on ^{45}Ca^{2+} uptake, and we tried to characterize the receptor involved in these responses.

Adenosine 10^{-4} M induced, as did NECA, an increase in cAMP levels in forskolin-stimulated MC (Fig. 3) and, as did R-PIA, an increase in ^{45}Ca^{2+} uptake (Fig. 4). To characterize the receptor involved in ADO responses we studied the effects of the selective antagonists on the actions of ADO.

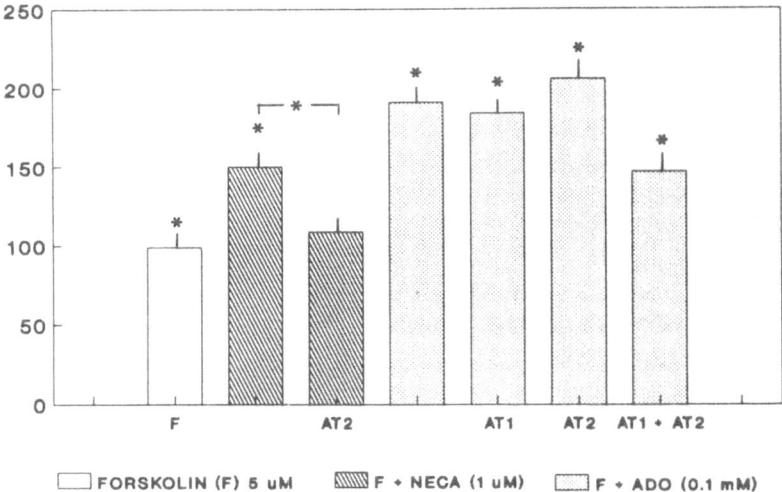

Fig. 3. Effect of the selective antagonists PD 116948 (AT_1, 1 μM) and PD 115199 (AT_2, 1 μM) on the 10^{-4} M adenosine-induced increase in cAMP intracellular content in forskolin-prestimulated mesangial cells (*MC*) after 2 min of incubation. Data of NECA and NECA + AT_2 are also shown for comparison. Methods as in Fig. 1. Data are mean ± SEM of at least 12 determinations. *Asterisks* represent significant differences ($P < 0.05$) with respect to f-treated MC

Effects on cAMP

Comparing the effect of ADO with the effects of the analogues on cAMP production, it would seem very likely that ADO action on cAMP production was mediated through the activation of an A_2 receptor. If this is right, blockade of the A_2 receptor should inhibit the ADO-induced stimulatory effect, as was observed with NECA. However, neither A_2 nor A_1 selective ADO antagonists affected the ADO-induced increase in cAMP content in forskolin-stimulated MC, and only the combination of A_1 and A_2 antagonists partially inhibited this increase (Fig. 3). The effects of ADO are mediated by a surface receptor, since 10^{-4} M theophylline (THEO) inhibited the increase in cAMP induced by ADO within 5 min of incubation (C: 11.4 ± 2.8, THEO: 13.1 ± 2.7; ADO: 25.32 ± 5.4, $P < 0.05$ with respect to the control of cAMP content; THEO+ ADO: 15.07 ± 2.7, NS), but these results do not support the involvement of a receptor such as that activated by NECA.

Effects on $^{45}Ca^{2+}$ Uptake

The comparison of the effect of ADO and its analogues on $^{45}Ca^{2+}$ uptake would lead us to the conclusion that an A_1 receptor should be involved in the ADO-mediated stimulation of $^{45}Ca^{2+}$ uptake. However, the relatively selective antagonist A_2, instead of potentiating the effect of ADO, as we had observed with R-PIA, completely inhibited the $^{45}Ca^{2+}$ uptake stimulated by ADO (Fig. 4). This effect was also inhibited

45-Calcium uptake (dpm/mg x 10³)

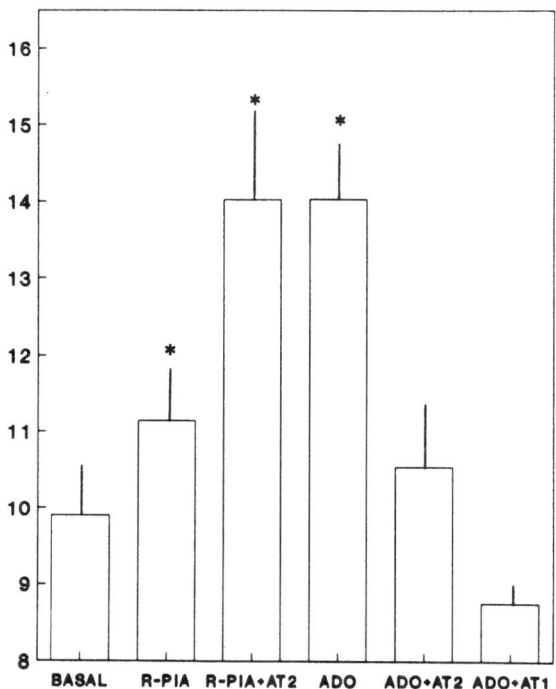

Fig. 4. Effect of the selective antagonists PD 116948 (AT_1, 1 μM) and PD 115199 (AT_2, 1 μM) on the 10^{-4} M adenosine-induced increase in ^{45}Ca uptake after 30 min of incubation. Data of R-PIA and R-PIA + AT_2 are also shown for comparison. Methods as in Fig. 3. Data are mean ± SEM of at least 12 determinations. *Asterisks* represent significant differences ($P < 0.05$) with respect to basal uptake

by the A_1 antagonist. So we have to discard again the involvement of a typical A_1 ADO receptor for explaining the effects of ADO on ^{45}Ca^{2+} uptake.

Considering all the effects which ADO has on cAMP formation and on ^{45}Ca^{2+}, we should suggest either that 1) a third receptor for ADO exists, whose functional activity does not fit the pharmacological criteria usually accepted, or that 2) simultaneous occupation of A_1 or A_2 receptors by ADO synergizes both the A_2-mediated cAMP response and the A_1-mediated calcium influx response.

Some investigators have found actions of ADO that cannot be explained as a result of the activation of either of the described A_1 or A_2 ADO receptors [4–6,24], and the existence of another kind of ADO receptor with different binding [6] and pharmacological [4] properties to those of A_1 and A_2 receptors has been suggested. Our results could well be more evidence for the existence of a third kind of receptor for ADO. However, it is also possible that a synergism between A_1 and A_2 receptors occurs in the activator responses when both are equally occupied by ADO. In this regard, we have demonstrated that simultaneous addition of R-PIA and NECA to the cells enhanced R-PIA-induced stimulation of calcium entry, and accelerated NECA-induced stimulation of cAMP production (results not shown). An effect similar to this has been found in parathyroid acinar cells in which occupation of α and β adrenergic receptors by norepinephrine evoked a secretory response greater than the sum of the responses elicited by each adrenergic receptor separately [25].

For these reasons, we think that occupation of A_1 and A_2 sites in high proportion may induce a conformational or aggregatory receptor state that makes possible a special coupling to transduction systems different from that produced by activation of each receptor individually. Another possibility may be that when both receptors are equally occupied, there exists a synergism in the cross talk between the cAMP and Ca^{2+} messenger systems which potentiate calcium entry and cAMP production, respectively, and mask negative responses. Cyclic AMP has been shown to phosphorylate calcium channels [26] and to stimulate calcium entry [27]. In addition, Ca^{2+} has also been shown to activate adenylate cyclase in some cells [28].

It is worth noting that the effects of the high affinity antagonists on cAMP and on $^{45}Ca^{2+}$ uptake differ, i.e., both of them failed to inhibit ADO-induced increases in cAMP, whereas both of them completely inhibited ADO-induced stimulation of $^{45}Ca^{2+}$ uptake. This could be interpreted as a different coupling effectiveness to the transduction systems of each second messenger. The distortion induced by the selective antagonists in the binding of ADO can affect in a distinct way the coupling to calcium channels and to adenylate cyclase, because of the different threshold of each effector. Another explanation could be a model in which simultaneous activation of both receptors changes their spatial conformation, creating a pore for calcium as a part of the molecule. The antagonists A_1 and A_2 would not displace ADO binding (they do not modify the increase of cAMP levels), but would occupy main domains for the functionality of the pore (they inhibit calcium uptake).

Conclusions

The experiments shown above demonstrate in a functional way the existence of A_1 and A_2 type receptors in cultured rat mesangial cells. These receptors have contrasting effects on cAMP generation and calcium uptake. Activation of the A_1-type stimulates calcium entry and inhibits calcium entry. Adenosine stimulates both cAMP generation and calcium uptake, but these effects do not seem to be mediated by the A_1 or A_2 receptors present in mesangial cells. All these results may implicate a very complex regulation of adenosine metabolism in glomeruli or in the mesangium and also a complex role for adenosine in mesangial cells.

References

1. Londos C, Cooper DMF, Wolff J (1980) Subclasses of external adenosine receptors. Proc Natl Acad Sci USA 77:2551–2554
2. Shimizu H (1983) Adenosine receptors associated with the adenylate cyclase system. In: Daly JW, Kuroda Y, Phillis JW, Shimizu H, Ui M (eds) Physiology and pharmacology of adenosine derivates. Raven, New York, pp 31–40

3. Bruns RF, Daly JW, Snyder SH (1983) Adenosine receptor binding: structure-activity analysis generates extremely potent xanthine antagonists. Proc Natl Acad Sci USA 80:2077–2080

4. Belloni FL, Belardinelli L, Halperin C, Hintze TH (1989) An unusual receptor mediates adenosine-induced SA nodal bradycardia in dogs. Am J Physiol 256:H1553–H1564

5. Arend LJ, Burnatowska-Hledin MA, Spielman WS (1988) Adenosine receptor-mediated calcium mobilization in cortical collecting tubule cells. Am J Physiol 255:C581–C588

6. Chin JH, Delorenzo RJ (1986) A new class of adenosine receptors in brain. Characterization by 2-chloro[^{3}H]-adenosine binding. Biochem Pharmacol 35:847–856

7. Hall JE, Granger JP (1986) Renal hemodynamics and arterial pressure during chronic intrarenal adenosine infusion in conscious dogs. Am J Physiol 250:F32–F39

8. Osswald H, Spielman WS, Knox FG (1978) Mechanisms of adenosine-mediated decreases in glomerular filtration rate in dogs. Circ Res 43:465–469

9. Churchill PC, Bidani A (1987) Renal effects of selective adenosine receptor agonists in anesthetized rats. Am J Physiol 252:F299–F303

10. Arend L, Haramati A, Thompson CI, Spielman W (1987) Adenosine-induced decrease in renin release: dissociation from hemodynamic effects. Am J Physiol 247:F447–F452

11. Tagawa H, Vander AJ (1970) Effect of adenosine compounds on renal function and renin secretion in dogs. Circ Res 26:327–338

12. Arend LJ, Sonnenburg WK, Smith WL, Spielman WS (1987) A$_1$ and A$_2$ adenosine receptors in rabbit cortical collecting tubule cells. J Clin Invest 79:710–714

13. Freissmuth M, Hausleithner V, Tuisl E, Nanoff C, Schutz W (1987) Glomeruli and microvessels of the rabbit kidney contain both A$_1$ and A$_2$ adenosine receptors. Naunyn Schmiedebergs Arch Pharmacol 335:438–444

14. Palacios JM, Fastbom J, Wiederhold KH, Probst A (1987) Visualization of adenosine A1 receptors in the human and the guinea-pig kidney. Eur J Pharmacol 138:273–276

15. Olivera A, Lamas S, Rodriguez-Puyol D, Lopez-Novoa JM (1989) Adenosine induces mesangial cell contraction by an A$_1$-type receptor. Kidney Int 35:1300–1305

16. Fredholm BB, Jonzon B, Lindstrom K (1983) Adenosine receptor mediated increases and decreases in cyclic AMP in hippocampal slices treated with forskolin. Acta Physiol Scand 117:461–463

17. Jonzon B, Nilson J, Fredholm BB (1985) Adenosine receptor-mediated changes in cyclic AMP production and DNA synthesis in cultured arterial smooth muscle cells. J Cell Physiol 124:451–456

18. Darfler FJ, Maham LC, Koachman AM, Insel PA (1982) Stimulation by Forskolin of intact S49 Lymphoma cells involves the nucleotide regulatory protein of adenylate cyclase. J Biol Chem 257:11901–11907

19. Bruns RF, Fergus JH, Badger EW, Bristol JA, Santay LA, Hays SJ (1987) PD 115,199: an antagonist ligand for adenosine A$_2$ receptors. Naunyn Schmiedebergs Arch Pharmacol 335:64–69

20. Haleen SJ, Steffen RP, Hamilton HW (1987) PD 116,948, a highly selective A$_1$ adenosine receptor antagonist. Life Sci 40:555–561

21. Cerbai E, Klöckner U, Isenberg G (1988) Ca-antagonistic effects of adenosine in guinea pig atrial cells. Am J Physiol 255:H872–H878

22. Fenton RA, Bruttig SP, Rubio R, Berne RM (1982) Effect of adenosine on calcium uptake by intact and cultured vascular smooth muscle. Am J Physiol 242:H797–H804

23. Ramagopal MV, Mustafa SJ (1988) Effect of adenosine and its analogues on calcium influx in coronary artery. Am J Physiol 255:H1492–H1498

24. Ribeiro JA, Sebastiao AM (1986) Adenosine receptors and calcium: basis for proposing a third (A$_3$) adenosine receptor. Prog Neurobiol 26:179–209

25. McKinney JS, Desole MS, Rubin RP (1989) Convergence of cAMP and phosphoinositide pathways during rat parotid secretion. Am J Physiol 257:C651–C657
26. Nunoki K, Florio V, Catteral WA (1989) Activation of purified calcium channels by stoichiometric protein phosphorylation. Proc Natl Acad Sci USA 86:6816–6820
27. Bourdeau JE, Eby BK (1990) Cyclic AMP-stimulated rise in rabbit connecting tubules: role of peritubular Ca. Am J Physiol 258:F751–F755
28. Alkon DL, Rasmussen H (1988) A spatial-temporal model of cell activation. Science 239:998–1005

Interactions Between Glomerular Autacoids

RAYMOND ARDAILLOU, LAURENT BAUD, NICOLE ARDAILLOU, and
DOMINIQUE CHANSEL[1]

SUMMARY. Cell-cell interaction occurs in glomeruli via locally formed messengers acting in the vicinity of their sites of synthesis (autacoids). One autacoid from a given cell may act on a second autacoid at the stage of its synthesis or at successive steps of its cellular mode of action: by binding to receptors, by formation of second messengers, or by action on final biological effects. Various examples of modified synthesis are presented. Hydrogen peroxide (H_2O_2) produced by macrophages increases prostaglandin synthesis in glomerular cells; macrophages coincubated with glomeruli produce more prostaglandins than could be expected from the amounts synthesized separately by both preparations. The latter effect is due to the stimulation of macrophages by hydroperoxyeicosatetraenoic acids (HPETEs) of glomerular origin and is associated with the binding of stimulated macrophages to glomeruli. Macrophages also release interleukin-1 and tumor necrosis factor (TNF) which increase ecto 5′-nucleotidase expression and PGE_2 production in mesangial cells, PGE_2 in turn limiting TNF production. Alternatively, autacoids interact at the stage of their cellular effects. For example, H_2O_2 reduces the number of TNF receptors via inhibition of their synthesis and cyclic GMP-producing agonists inhibit angiotensin II (AII)-stimulated intracellular calcium concentration. PGE_2 inhibits LTD_4- or TNF-induced cell proliferation and AII-stimulated mesangial cell contraction. PGE_2-stimulated renin synthesis by mesangial cells is inhibited by 12-HETE. These different examples indicate that: Interaction between glomerular resident cells and blood-borne cells is bidirectional; regulatory loops occur frequently; final effects may imply cascade reactions, and autacoids often act synergistically. Any therapeutical approach will have to take into consideration the multiplicity of autacoids and their interactions.

Introduction

Autacoids are mediators which act at or near their sites of synthesis. Glomerular autacoids may originate from the resident glomerular cells or bone marrow-derived

[1]INSERM U64, Hôpital Tenon, 4 rue de la Chine, 75020 Paris Cedex 20, France

cells including monocyte-macrophages, polymorphonuclear leukocytes, and platelets invading the glomerular capillaries. Autacoids are not specific to the glomerulus and belong to a variety of chemical species, essentially reactive oxygen species, metabolites of arachidonic acid (prostaglandins and products of lipoxygenase), bioactive phospholipids such as platelet activating factor, cytokines and growth factors, proteolytic enzymes, products of local autocrine and paracrine systems such as angiotensin II, endothelin, bradykinin, adenosine, and finally, the recently discovered endothelium-derived relaxing factor identified as nitric oxide. These various autacoids interact in different ways and behave as messengers between two cells. Schematically, one autacoid from a given cell may act on the synthesis of a second autacoid in another cell or modify the mode of action of a second autacoid in its target cells. In the latter hypothesis, the effect may occur at different steps of the cellular mode of action: binding to receptors, formation of second messengers, or during final biological events. We should like, in this short review, to give examples of these different processes of interaction and to draw some general conclusions about the mechanism of glomerular injury and its therapeutic approach.

Interactions Between Two Autacoids at the Stage of Synthesis

The most studied of these interactions have been those between macrophages and isolated glomeruli or macrophages and mesangial cells. Macrophages are known to be the source of a variety of mediators, particularly metabolites of arachidonic acid, reactive oxygen species and cytokines [1]. The role of macrophages in both human and experimental glomerulonephritis has been advanced for the following reasons: Circulating monocytes infiltrate the glomerulus. They migrate into the subendothelial area, the mesangial matrix and the urinary space and undergo transformation into macrophages [2]; a close temporal relationship has been observed between macrophage accumulation and proteinuria [3]; monocyte depletion, as well as administration of a macrophage antiserum, [4] inhibits the progression of glomerular injury.

We have demonstrated in several studies [5,6] that during interaction between glomerular and bone marrow-derived cells, changes occur in arachidonate (C20:4) metabolism. We investigated the conversion of ^{3}H C20:4 into hydroxyeicosatetraenoic acids (HETE) and prostaglandins (PG) by isolated glomeruli and macrophages from rats, separately and in combination. As demonstrated by high performance liquid chromatography (HPLC), glomeruli converted C20:4 predominantly to lipoxygenase products, mainly 12-HETE, and to a lesser extent, to PG, mainly PGE_2 and $PGF_{2\alpha}$. Resident macrophages converted C20:4 to equivalent amounts of HETE and PG, mainly 12-HETE and 6 keto-$PGF_{1\alpha}$. When macrophages and glomeruli were studied in combination, a striking interaction was detected in both pathways of C20:4 metabolism. Production of 6 keto-$PGF_{1\alpha}$ was stimulated and considerable amounts of PGD_2, TXB_2 and hydroxyheptadecatrienoic acid (HHT), another product of thromboxane synthetase activity, were also produced (Fig. 1). Total 12-HETE production was unchanged. When a lipid extract of glomeruli, containing oxygenated metabolites of C20:4, was added to macrophages, there was stimulation of both the lipoxygenase (12- and 15-HETE) and cyclooxygenase (TXB_2 and 6 keto-$PGF_{1\alpha}$) production. Similar results were obtained by direct addition to macrophages of 12-

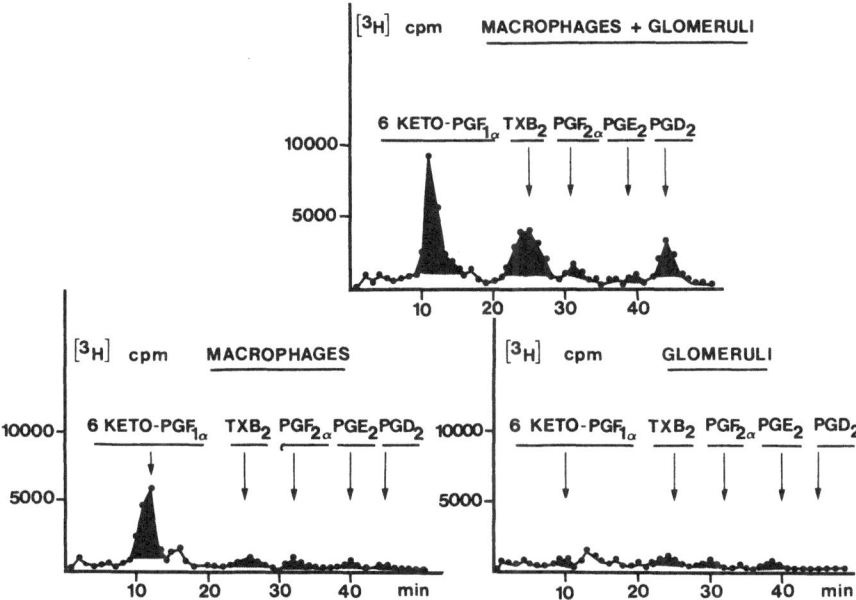

Fig. 1. High performance liquid chromatography profile of cyclooxygenase products synthesized by macrophages and glomeruli, alone and in combination. (From [5] with permission)

HPETE, which suggests that this metabolite was the agent present in the lipidic glomerular extract which was responsible for macrophage activation. When, in contrast, a lipid extract from macrophages was added to glomeruli, 12-HETE production by glomeruli was almost completely abolished. Thus, the unchanged total 12-HETE production obtained by coincubated glomeruli and macrophages resulted from its increased production by macrophages and its decreased production by glomeruli. We have also evaluated, in vitro, the role of lipoxygenase products of glomeruli origin in the attachment of rat macrophages to glomeruli [6]. We found that ^{3}H-uridine labeled macrophages bound to isolated glomeruli. Binding was related to the glomerular protein and macrophage concentrations, temperature, and time of incubation, and was a saturable process. Macrophage adherence depended on glomerular lipoxygenase activity, but not on glomerular cyclooxygenase activity, since preincubation of glomeruli with nordihydroguaiaretic acid inhibited this phenomenon. Preincubation with indomethacin was ineffective.

Macrophages also release reactive oxygen species which may stimulate arachidonic acid metabolism in isolated glomeruli. Indeed, rat glomeruli incubated in the presence of enzymatically generated superoxide anion (O_2^-) synthesized PGE_2, $PGF_{2\alpha}$, 6 keto-$PGF_{1\alpha}$, and TXB_2 in greater amounts than under control conditions [7]. Inhibition of this effect by catalase and the direct stimulatory effect of H_2O_2 itself suggested that H_2O_2 was the by-product responsible. The increase in PG synthesis in response to H_2O_2 was due to activation of glomerular phospholipase. The same stimulatory effect of H_2O_2 on PGE_2 synthesis has also been found in rat cultured mesangial cells [8]. As in the glomeruli, catalase was inhibitory. We have also shown that rat cultured mesangial cells produced H_2O_2 and O_2^- in response to particulate (opsonized zymosan) or soluble (platelet activating factor) stimuli [9]. Therefore, reactive oxygen species released either by infiltrating inflammatory cells or by resident glomerular cells may modulate immune-inflammatory events within the glomerulus and modify the glomerular microcirculation via PG synthesis. Because PGE_2 and PGI_2 stimulate adenylate cyclase and endogenous cyclic AMP production in murine [10] as well as in human [11] glomerular cells, the effect of reactive oxygen species on glomerular cyclic AMP has also been studied. Shah demonstrated that enzymatically produced O_2^- and H_2O_2 stimulated cyclic AMP synthesis in glomeruli and that this effect was suppressed in the presence of cyclooxygenase inhibitors, which confirmed its dependence on PG synthesis [12].

Macrophages are the source of a number of cytokines, particularly interleukin-1 (IL-1) and tumor necrosis factor (TNF). We have demonstrated that human recombinant TNFα stimulated the production of PG by cultured rat mesangial cells [13]. This effect was demonstrable from 6 hours, was dose-dependent, and affected the synthesis of PGE_2, $PGF_{2\alpha}$ and 6 keto-$PGF_{1\alpha}$ (Fig. 2). It required both RNA and protein synthesis but was not associated with a modification of cell proliferation, at least in cycling cells. TNF also stimulated cyclic AMP levels in mesangial cells. Indomethacin suppressed the effect of TNF on PG but only reduced that effect on cyclic AMP, indicating that PG production mediates, only in part, the increase in cyclic AMP. In the presence of indomethacin, TNF was mitogenic, which confirms that in this system, as in others, [14] PGE_2 production inhibits cell proliferation. TNFα also increased PGE_2 synthesis in human mesangial cells. IL-1 exhibited a similar effect both in rat [15] and human [16] mesangial cells. Using a L-929 fibroblast lytic assay, we showed that TNF was also synthesized by rat mesangial cells [17]. TNF biological activity was detectable only when mesangial cells were exposed to bacterial lipopolysaccharide for periods longer than one hour. PGE_2 produced in the presence of TNF in turn regulated TNF synthesis in a negative feed-back manner. Indeed, lipopolysaccharide caused a dose-dependent increase of PGE_2 synthesis by mesangial cells; treatment with indomethacin promoted suppression of PGE_2 production together with an increase of TNF synthesis. Addition of PGE_2 or 8 bromo-cyclic AMP induced similar dose-dependent reductions of TNF synthesis. Thus the inhibitory effect of PGE_2 probably required, in part, the accumulation of cyclic AMP. These events provide an example of a loop between two autacoids, with TNF stimulating the synthesis of PGE_2 and PGE_2 in turn limiting that of TNF.

We have been interested in the effect of cytokines on ecto 5'-nucleotidase expression in mesangial cells and thereby on their role in the control of local adenosine production. First, we demonstrated that a macrophage-conditioned medium produced a dose-dependent increase of mesangial ecto 5'-nucleotidase activity. A similar effect was observed in cocultures of rat mesangial cells and peritoneal macrophages [18]. The effect of the macrophage-conditioned medium was apparent after 24h and increased with time. Stimulation of ecto 5'-nucleotidase activity by the macrophage-conditioned medium was inhibited by cycloheximide, which, together with the necessary lag-time suggested that protein synthesis was required. Because the macrophage-conditioned medium contained high concentrations of IL-1 and TNF, we investigated whether or not these cytokines were responsible for this effect. We found that IL-1β and TNFα stimulated mesangial cell 5'-nucleotidase activity in a

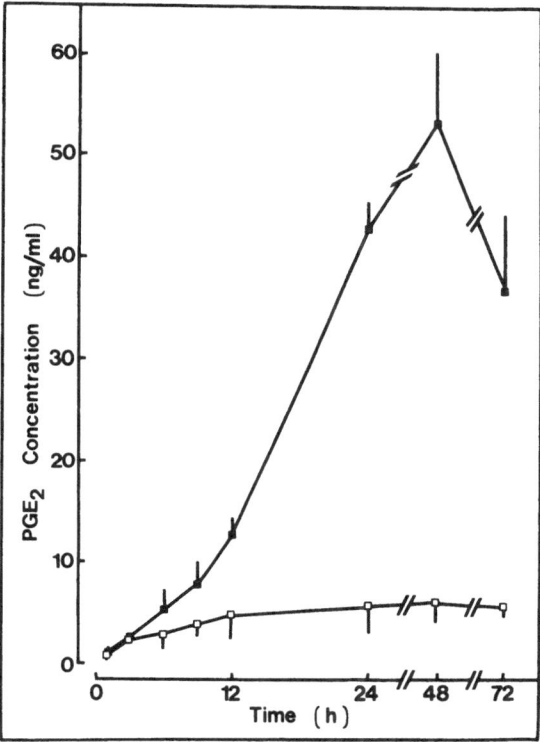

Fig. 2. Time-course of PGE$_2$ release from rat mesangial cells incubated without, (unfilled squares) and with, (filled squares) 100 ng/ml TNF. (From [13] with permission)

dose-dependent manner after a treatment of 24h. Maximum increases reached 4.5 times and 1.7 times basal values for IL-1β (20 U/ml) and TNFα (25 ng/ml), respectively. The effect of both cytokines was additive. Stimulation of 5′-nucleotidase by IL-1β and TNFα was specific, as had been observed with the macrophage-conditioned medium, since the activity of another ectoenzyme, Mg^{2+}-ATPase, was unchanged. Cycloheximide suppressed the cytokine-dependent increase of 5′-nucleotidase activity. Cyclooxygenase inhibitors such as indomethacin and ibuprofen inhibited approximately 50% of the effects of both cytokines. Their inhibitory effect was abolished in the presence of PGE$_2$. In addition, PGE$_2$ itself produced a dose-related (0.1 - 10 μM) increase of 5′-nucleotidase activity with a maximum of 2.2 times basal values. PGE$_2$ operated likely via cyclic AMP synthesis since 8-bromo cyclic AMP, a permeant analogue of cyclic AMP, was also active [19]. Taken together, these results indicate that IL-1, essentially, and TNFα, to a lesser extent, regulate 5′-nucleotidase expression in the plasma membrane of cultured mesangial cells and that their effect depends in part on PGE$_2$ synthesis. The enzyme 5′-nucleotidase plays a key role in the synthesis of adenosine from nucleotides. Therefore, factors controlling its expression may influence the local production of

adenosine, which displays both powerful vasoactive and antiinflammatory properties. The effect of IL-1 on adenosine is an example of a cascade reaction, implying
successively, PGE_2, cyclic AMP, and adenosine.

The role of platelets in glomerular injury has also been advanced, essentially
because they represent the main site of synthesis of thromboxane which is considered
to be a noxious agent in the development of glomerular injury. We have shown that
platelets could be activated by saturated fatty acids of glomerular origin [20].
Initially, we demonstrated that when a tracer dose of ^3H C20:4 was added to a mixture of human glomeruli and platelets, a striking increase in ^3H TXB_2 production was
observed. It was verified, by aspirin pretreatment, that platelets were responsible for
the excess of TXB_2 generated and that the stimulus was of glomerular origin. When
TXB_2 generated from endogenous C20:4 was measured by radioimmunoassay in
coincubated cells, a dramatic increase of this metabolite was detected. We found that
the factors responsible for this stimulation were present in the lipidic extract of
glomeruli and corresponded to saturated and monounsaturated fatty acids (C14:0,
C16:0, C18:0, and C18:1). An exogenous supply of the same synthetic acids produced the same stimulatory effect. The question of whether this glomerulus-platelet
interaction also occurs in vivo cannot be answered easily. It is possible that injured
glomerular cells with membrane disturbances may release these fatty acids together
with the procoagulant factor which plays a role in the formation of thrombi. We also
found this procoagulant factor in the glomerular supernatant in vitro.

Interactions at the stage of synthesis may also correspond to a sharing of substrate
between two cell types. This process has been described between polymorphonuclear
leukocytes and platelets. For example, 12-HETE synthesized by platelets is further
hydroxylated in leukocytes into 12,20 diHETE or 5,12 diHETE by the ω-lipoxy-
genase and the 5 lipoxygenase present in the latter cell type [21]. It is also admitted
that endothelial cells utilize platelet endoperoxides to produce PGI_2 [22]. Such interactions may also occur within the glomerular capillaries.

Interactions Between Two Autacoids at the Stage of Binding to Surface Receptors or Second Messenger Formation

Many agents induce the simultaneous production of cytokines and reactive oxygen
species by macrophages and mesangial glomerular cells. This led us to examine
whether cell sensitivity to TNF might also be regulated by reactive oxygen species
[23]. When L-929 fibroblasts, which represent a TNF-sensitized murine cell
line, were exposed simultaneously to TNF and H_2O_2 (100 to 500 μM), the cytotoxic activity of TNF was inhibited by up to 67%. This inhibition was also effective when the cells were pretreated with H_2O_2, but not when TNF alone was preex-
posed to H_2O_2. These data suggest that H_2O_2 altered the cell sensitivity to TNF
without modifying the activity of the TNF molecule. Maximum loss of cell sensitivity to TNF occurred after 30 min preexposure to 500 μM H_2O_2; complete
restoration of TNF sensitivity was obtained within 12h following H_2O_2 removal.
Restoration required protein synthesis, as demonstrated by the suppressive effect of
actinomycin D. The inhibitory effect of H_2O_2 was suppressed by catalase, but was
unaffected by the scavengers of hydroxyl radical (OH·) and hypochlorous acid

(O Cl⁻), suggesting that H_2O_2 itself, and not one of its metabolites, was responsible for this inhibition. Binding experiments of ^{125}I-TNF to L-929 fibroblasts revealed that the mechanism whereby H_2O_2 affected cell sensitivity to TNF involved the reduction, by about 50%, of the density of TNF receptors. There was no change in TNF affinity for its receptors. Moreover, H_2O_2 did not affect the rate of degradation of TNF, and only slightly increased the degree of internalization of ^{125}I-TNF receptors. Therefore the effectiveness of H_2O_2 appears to be mediated at the TNF receptor level. Another example of interaction between two autacoids at the receptor level is the demonstration by Badr et al. [24] that lipoxin A_4 (LXA_4) antagonizes the in vivo and cellular actions of leukotriene D_4 (LTD_4) in rat glomerular mesangial cells, via competition at a common receptor. Evidence was obtained from the inhibition of binding of [³H] LTD_4 to mesangial cells in the presence of LXA_4, the prevention – by LXA_4 – of LTD_4-induced inositol trisphosphate generation, and the blockade of LXA_4-induced inositol trisphosphate stimulation by a LTD_4 receptor antagonist.

It is also possible for an autacoid to modify the effect of a second autacoid at the stage of the production of its second messenger. An example is the control that cyclic GMP-producing mediators exert on the effects of such vasoconstrictory agents as angiotensin II, or endothelin, on vascular smooth muscle cells. It has been shown that endothelial cells released a relaxing factor different from the other well known vasodilatory agents, PGI_2 and adenosine. This factor was named endothelium-derived relaxing factor; it has been identified as nitric oxide. It originates from L-arginine and stimulates the soluble guanylate cyclase of the adjacent smooth muscle cells [25]. Thus, it could counteract the vasoconstriction induced by angiotensin II or endothelin by decreasing the intracellular concentration of calcium, via stimulation of cyclic GMP production. This hypothesis would be in accordance with the demonstration by Hassid [26] that atrial natriuretic factor, another activator of guanylate cyclase, is an endogenous antagonist of calcium-mediated processes.

Interactions Between Two Autacoids at the Stage of Biological Effect

Finally, one autacoid may act on the target cell of a second autacoid at the stage of biological effect. For example, PGE_2 inhibits LTD_4- or TNF-induced cell proliferation and AII-stimulated mesangial cell contraction. We have shown that LTC_4 and LTD_4 promoted the proliferation of human glomerular epithelial cells [27] and of fibroblasts [14]. Human glomerular epithelial cells synthesize little PG, whereas fibroblasts produce large amounts of PGE_2. We demonstrated that, in the latter cell line, the mitogenic effect of sulfidopeptide leukotrienes was apparent only in the presence of cyclooxygenase inhibitors. Under these conditions, LTD_4 promoted proliferation of growing cells as well as of quiescent cells. Interestingly, LTD_4 and LTC_4 did not modify PGE_2 production by fibroblasts, thus showing no evidence for a negative feed-back loop. Similarly, the mitogenic effect of TNF on rat mesangial cells occurred only when PGE_2 synthesis was inhibited [28]; the mitogenic effect of IL-1 was suppressed in the presence of PGE_2 [29]. These latter examples are associated with negative feed-back loops, since both cytokine stimulate the synthesis of PGE_2 in mesangial cells [13,19].

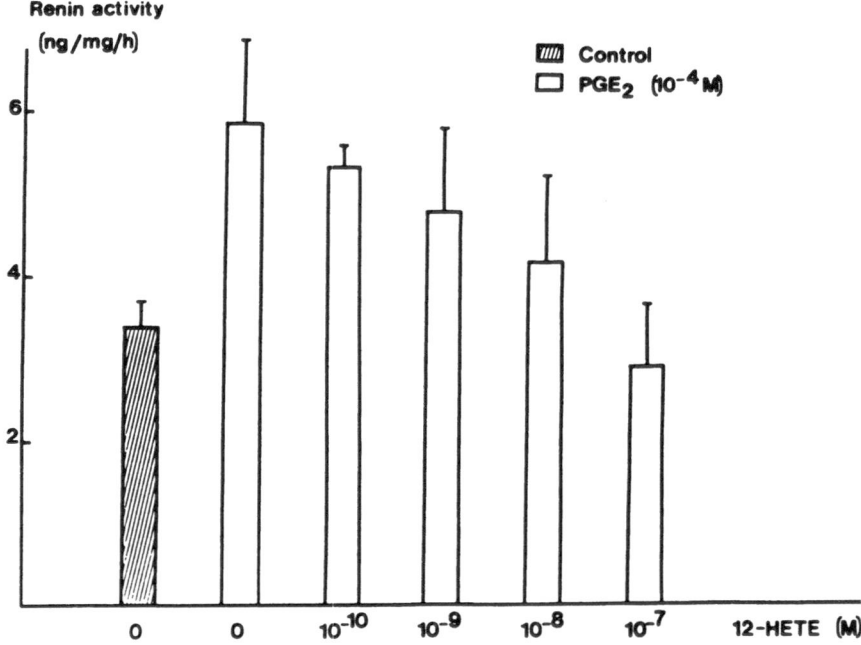

Fig. 3. Effect of increasing doses of 12-HETE on PGE$_2$-simulated renin activity produced by human cultured mesangial cells. (From [11] with permission)

AII can be considered as a glomerular autacoid which is generated locally by juxtaglomerular or glomerular renin and the converting enzyme of the vascular endothelial cells. AII stimulated PG synthesis by isolated glomeruli [30] and murine [31] or human [32] mesangial cells. In the human mesangial cell preparation, threshold stimulation was observed at around 10 pM AII. Schlondorff et al. [28] have proposed that AII preferentially, but not exclusively, stimulates a phosphatidylinositol specific phospholipase C. This results in the formation of diacylglycerol which could serve as an intermediate in the release of arachidonic acid. Phospholipase A$_2$ activation could also occur as a consequence of the increase in intracellular calcium concentration and of the phosphorylation of lipocortin by a diacylglycerol-sensitive protein kinase C. The arachidonate released in response to AII is tightly coupled to cyclooxygenase and thus transformed into PG. AII, after binding to specific receptors, also produces contraction of isolated glomeruli via contraction of mesangial cells. Scharschmidt et al. [33] have demonstrated that glomerular vasoreactivity has great sensitivity to AII with a threshold dose of 0.01 pM. The maximum surface area decrease was 20% and occurred at 0.1 nM AII. These authors showed that the dose-effect curve was displaced toward the left (lower concentrations of AII) in the presence of indomethacin and towards the right (higher concentrations of AII) in the presence of arachidonic acid or PGE$_2$. The mechanism of the inhibitory effect of PGE$_2$ is mediated by cyclic AMP. PGE$_2$ stimulates adenylate cyclase activity and increases the cellular content in cyclic AMP, which in turn activates protein kinase A. Activation of protein kinase A produces phosphorylation of myosin light chain kinase and, as a consequence, decreases its affinity for the calcium-calmodulin complex, resulting in inhibition of cell contraction. In this schema, PGE_2 acts as a self-induced inhibitor of AII.

Mediators other than PGE_2 may also act to modulate the effects of autacoids at the stage of their biological effects. We have demonstrated that the stimulatory effect of PGE_2 on renin production by human mesangial cells was inhibited by 12-hydroxy-eicosatetraenoic acid (12-HETE) between 0.1 and 100 nM [11]. Extracellular and intracellular renin were affected similarly. The effects of 15-hydroxyeicosatetraenoic acid (15-HETE), 12-hydroperoxyeicosatetraenoic acid (12-HPETE), and 15-hydro-peroxyeicosatetraenoic acid (15-HPETE) were the same as those of 12-HETE (Fig. 3). We hypothesized that in this system, as in others [34], the lipoxygenase products inhibited diacylglycerol kinase, which could result in an increase of diacylglycerol concentration and stimulation of protein kinase C. Such stimulation has been shown to be associated with the inhibition of renin production [35].

Conclusions

It is possible to draw general conclusions from these various examples of interaction between glomerular autacoids. First, it is clear that interactions are not only represented by the effects which autacoids from blood-borne cells have on glomerular resident cells. The reverse also occurs frequently. In addition, there are interactions between different types of blood cells and between different types of glomerular cells. In particular, the role of mesangial cells, which are proinflammatory cells, has now been extensively demonstrated. These cells, in addition to their smooth muscle cell-like properties, possess many characteristics resembling those of macrophages. Therefore, they release a variety of autacoids which act both on the other glomerular resident cells and on the circulating blood cells they can attract in the glomeruli. A second conclusion is that of the frequency of cross-talks between different pathways. PGs play a major role in these cross-talks as agents of regulatory feed-back loops. In particular, PGs inhibit vasoconstriction and cell proliferation which are often promoted by the same compounds. Cross-talks between pathways may also result in synergy between the effects of both autacoids. This has been well demonstrated between cytokines, particularly between IL-1 and TNF. Finally, the most characteristic feature of these interactions between autacoids is their complexity. This complexity has several consequences: A single autacoid is not responsible for a pathological effect. Therefore the question is: What kinds of autacoids exist, how do they interact, and what is the sequence of the reactions? The answer to the last question is essential for a therapeutic approach. Autacoids have several cellular sources, but what their relative parts are and what cells must be the targets for drugs, have still to be established. The mechanism of the toxicity of autacoids is, for the most part, unknown. In the cascade of reactions between the response of the initial mediator to glomerular injury and the production of the agents which cause proteinuria, the main event—which must be the target of treatment—is still often unknown. A given autacoid may be blocked either at the stage of its synthesis by synthesis inhibitors, or at the stage of its effects by antagonists. Ideal drugs should be specific to an autacoid, devoid of toxicity, easily administrable, and efficient, both extra- and intracellularly.

References

1. Takemura R, Werb Z (1984) Secretory products of macrophages and their physiological functions. Am J Physiol 246: C1–C9
2. Holdsworth SR, Neale TJ, Wilson CB (1980) The participation of macrophages and monocytes in experimental immune complex glomerulonephritis. Clin Immunol Immunopathol 15: 510–524
3. Schreiner GF, Cotran RS, Pardo V, Unanue ER (1978) A mononuclear cell component in experimental immunological glomerulonephritis. J Exp Med 147: 369–384
4. Holdsworth SR, Neale TJ, Wilson CB (1981) Abrogation of macrophage-dependent injury in experimental glomerulonephritis in the rabbit. Use of an antimacrophage serum. J Clin Invest 68: 686–698
5. Sraer J, Baud L, Bens M, Podjarny E, Schlondorff D, Ardaillou R (1984) Glomeruli cooperate with macrophages in converting arachidonic acid to prostaglandins and hydroxyeicosatetraenoic acids. Prostaglandins Leukotrienes Med 13: 67–74
6. Baud L, Sraer J, Delarue F, Bens M, Balavoine F, Schlondorff D, Ardaillou R, Sraer JD (1985) Lipoxygenase products mediate the attachment of rat macrophages to glomeruli in vitro. Kidney Int 27: 855–863
7. Baud L, Nivez MP, Chansel D, Ardaillou R (1981) Stimulation by oxygen radicals of prostaglandin production by rat renal glomeruli. Kidney Int 20: 332–339
8. Sedor JR, Abboud HE (1985) Hydrogen peroxide stimulates PGE_2 synthesis by cultured rat mesangial cells (Abstract). Kidney Int 29: 291
9. Baud L, Hagege J, Sraer J, Rondeau E, Perez J, Ardaillou R (1983) Reactive oxygen production by cultured rat glomerular mesangial cells during phagocytosis is associated with stimulation of lipoxygenase activity. J Exp Med 158: 1836–1852
10. Friedlander G, Chansel D, Sraer J, Bens M, Ardaillou F (1983) PGE_2 binding sites and PG-stimulated cyclic AMP accumulation in rat isolated glomeruli and glomerular cultured cells. Mol Cell Endocrinol 30: 201–214
11. Chansel D, Béa ML, Ardaillou R (1989) Modulation of renin synthesis by lipoxygenase products in cultured human mesangial cells. Mol Cell Endocrinol. 62: 263–271
12. Shah SV (1984) Effect of enzymatically generated reactive oxygen metabolites on the cyclic nucleotide content in isolated rat glomeruli. J Clin Invest 74: 393–401
13. Baud L, Perez J, Friedlander G, Ardaillou R (1988) Tumor necrosis factor stimulates prostaglandin production and cyclic AMP levels in rat cultured mesangial cells. FEBS Lett 239: 50–54
14. Baud L, Perez J, Denis M, Ardaillou R (1987) Modulation of fibroblast proliferation by sulfidopeptide leukotrienes: effect of indomethacin. J Immunol 138:1190–1195
15. Lovett DH, Resch K, Gemsa D (1987) Interleukin 1 and the glomerular mesangium II Monokine stimulation of mesangial cell prostanoid secretion. Am J Pathol 129: 543–551
16. Topley N, Floege J, Wessel K, Hass R, Radeke AH, Kaever V, Resh K (1989) Prostaglandin E_2 production is synergistically increased in cultured human glomerular mesangial cells by combinations of IL-1 and tumor necrosis factor α. J Immunol 143: 1989–1995
17. Baud L, Oudinet JP, Bens M, Noe L, Peraldi MN, Rondeau E, Etienne J, Ardaillou R (1989) Production of tumor necrosis factor by rat mesangial cells in response to bacterial lipopolysaccharide. Kidney Int 35: 1111–1118
18. Stefanovic V, Savic V, Vlahovic P, Ardaillou N, Ardaillou R (1989) Macrophages selectively stimulate ecto 5′-nucleotidase activity of cultured mesangial cells. Kidney Int 36: 249–256
19. Savic V, Stefanovic V, Ardaillou N, Ardaillou R (1990) Induction of ecto 5′-nucleotidase of rat cultured mesangial cells by interleukin 1β and tumour necrosis factor α. Immunology 70:321–326

20. Sraer J, Wolf C, Oudinet JP, Bens M, Ardaillou R, Sraer JD (1987) Human glomeruli release fatty acids which stimulate thromboxane synthesis in platelets. Kidney Int 32: 62–68

21. Marcus AJ, Broekman MJ, Safier LB, Ullman HL, Islam N (1982) Formation of leukotrienes and other hydroxyacids during platelet-neutrophil interactions in vitro. Biochem Biophys Res Commun 109: 130–137

22. Schafer AI, Crawford DD, Gimbrone MA (1984) Unidirectional transfer of prostacyclin endoperoxides between platelets and endothelial cells. J Clin Invest 73: 1105–1112

23. Baud L, Affres H, Perez J, Ardaillou R (1990) Reduction in tumor necrosis factor binding and cytotoxicity by hydrogen peroxide. J Immunol 145:556–560

24. Badr KF, DeBoer DK, Schwartzberg M, Serhan CN (1989) Lipoxin A_4 antagonizes cellular and in vivo actions of leukotriene D_4 in rat glomerular mesangial cells: Evidence for competition at a common receptor. Proc Natl Acad Sci USA 86: 3438–3442

25. Förstermann U, Mulsch A, Bohme E, Basse R (1986) Stimulation of soluble guanylate cyclase by an acetylcholine-induced endothelium-derived factor from rabbit and canine arteries. Circ Res 58: 531–538

26. Hassid A (1986) Atriopeptin II decreases cytosolic free Ca in cultured vascular smooth muscle cells. Am J Physiol 251: C681–C686

27. Baud L, Sraer J, Perez J, Nivez MP, Ardaillou R (1985) Leukotriene C_4 binds to human glomerular epithelial cells and promotes their proliferation in vitro. J Clin Invest 73: 374–377

28. Perez J, Baud L, Ardaillou R (1989) Tumor necrosis factor stimulates prostaglandin, cyclic AMP and DNA synthesis by cultured rat mesangial cells. Kidney Int 35: 318 (Abstr.)

29. Stahl RAK, Thaiss F, Kahf S, Shaw A, Schoeppe W (1989) Cyclooxygenase inhibition enhances rat interleukin 1β-induced proliferation of rat mesangial cells in culture (abstract). Kidney Int. 35: 320

30. Schlondorff D, Rocznick S, Satriano JA, Folkert WW (1980) Prostaglandin synthesis by isolated rat renal glomeruli: effect of angiotensin II. Am J Physiol 239: F486–F495

31. Sraer J, Foidart J, Chansel D, Mahieu P, Ardaillou R (1980) Prostaglandin synthesis by rat isolated glomeruli and glomerular cultured cells. Int J Biochem 12: 203–207

32. Ardaillou N, Nivez MP, Schlondorff D, Ardaillou R (1985) Vasoconstrictor-evoked prostaglandin synthesis in cultured human mesangial cells. Am J Physiol 248: F240–F246

33. Scharschmidt LA, Lianos E, Dunn MJ (1983) Arachidonate metabolites and the control of glomerular function. Fed Proc 42: 3058–3063

34. Setty YBN, Graeber JE, Stuart J (1987) The mitogenic effect of 15- and 12-hydroxyeicosatetraenoic acid on endothelial cells may be mediated via diacylglycerol kinase inhibition. J Biol Chem 262: 17613–17622

35. Kurtz A, Pfeilschifter J, Hutter A, Bührle C, Nobiling R, Taugner R, Hackenthal E, Bauer C (1986) Role of protein kinase C in inhibition of renin caused by vasoconstrictors. Am J Physiol 250: C563–C571

Ion Channels of the Kidney

Chair: Rainer Greger (FRG)
Mamoru Fujimoto (Japan)

Ion Channels in the Mammalian Nephron

R. Greger, E. Schlatter, M. Bleich[1], and H. Gögelein[2]

Summary. After the initial description of ion channels by patch clamp analysis in cultured cell lines derived from renal epithelia some 7 years ago, much progress has been made in the application of this technique to primary cultures of renal cells of defined origin, and to intact and even to in vitro perfused renal tubules. The present brief overview will focus mostly on data derived from intact tubules; the emphasis will be on the most recent data on ion channel regulation. Comparison to data obtained from cultured cells reveals that there are distinct differences between various preparations. Furthermore, in patch clamp experiments, several types of ion channels have been found which are probably not relevant for the normal function of the intact tubule cell. Conversely, some of the conductance properties of the intact cell are not recovered by corresponding ion channels in patch clamp experiments. Much further work and new methods will be required to reconstitute the conductance properties of the intact tubule from the findings in single ion channels.

Ion Channel Properties of Renal Epithelia

The renal tubules possess various K^+ channels, non-selective cation channels, Cl^- channels and Na^+ channels. In the following we will address only some of these channels and we refer the reader to recent, more general reviews on this topic [1–7].

Patch Clamp Studies in Cell Cultures of Renal Origin

The easiest way to study tubule cells by the patch clamp technique is to use established cell lines such as Mardin-Darby Canine Kidney (MDCK) cells, opossum

[1]Albert-Ludwigs-Universität Freiburg, Hermann-Herder-Straße 7, D 7800 Freiburg, Federal Republic of Germany
[2]Pharma-Forschung, Hoechst AG, D 6230 Frankfurt/Main 80, Federal Republic of Germany

kidney cells, etc. One example will be discussed in this volume by Ohno-Shosaku. These kinds of studies have been very helpful in the detailed description of the properties of several types of channels [3] and in the study of hormonal control of the maxi K$^+$-channel [2].

Primary cell cultures offer the advantage that they resemble the properties of native tissue more closely than do cultured cell lines. In cultures from the proximal tubule, several types of K$^+$-channels and non-selective cation channels have been reported [8–10]. Some of this work will be discussed in this volume by Poujeol. A recent review of ion channels in the proximal tubule by one of the authors of this study [11] reveals that most of the channels reported in these studies (except for the maxi K$^+$-channel) correspond well with those found in the isolated perfused proximal tubule [12].

In cultures of thick ascending limb cells maxi K$^+$-channels have been found [13] and described in much detail, regarding inhibitors [14–16]. As will be shown below, this type of K$^+$-channel is *not* responsible for K$^+$ recycling across the luminal membrane. It appears to be activated by cell volume increase [17]; this will be discussed by Guggino in this volume. In the isolated thick ascending limb segment other K$^+$-channels have been found [18,19], (also c.f. below).

Primary cultures of collecting ducts obtained from collecting duct-"anlagen" have been examined in much detail [20,21]. Nonselective cation channels with small to intermediate conductance, and small and large K$^+$ channels have been found, but the Na$^+$-channel, which has been described in much detail in studies with isolated collecting ducts [22], could not be identified at the single channel level. The authors conclude that the Na$^+$ channel might have a conductance of $<$5pS in their preparation and might therefore be difficult to detect in single channel studies [21]. In primary cultures of inner medullary collecting duct a non-selective cation channel with intermediate conductance has been found. This channel was claimed to be sensitive to amiloride with a reasonable K$_D$ [23]. It should be noted, however, that the amiloride inhibition was only deduced from unpaired observations. In intercalated cells from cortical collecting duct, excision activated Cl$^-$ channels [24] with a large conductance of around 300 pS have been found [24a].

Patch Clamp Analysis of Single Channel Properties of Isolated Nephron Segments

Several approaches have been developed to study the single channel properties of isolated tubules. In one approach the tubule is cut open and the luminal cell membrane becomes accessible to the patch pipette [25]. In another approach the tubules are treated with the collagenase, the basement membrane is destroyed, and the basolateral membrane can be studied [26,27]. We have developed a method in which the tubule segment is perfused in vitro [28,29]. The free end of the tubule is then accessible to the patch electrode which can then be pressed against the lateral membrane of the free end of the tubule, hence enabling one to study the properties of the basolateral membrane. Alternatively, the patch pipette is inserted into the lumen and a recording is made from the luminal membrane. The free tubule end can be immobilized by another suction pipette which is attached to one edge. With this technique we have studied rabbit, rat, and mouse tubule segments of the proximal nephron [30–32], the thick ascending limb of the loop of Henle [18,33,34], and the cortical collecting duct [35]. In our experience mouse and rat tubules are more suited for this method, because they are easier to tear at one end and the lumen of this end can be held wide open. The disadvantage of this method is its complexity. It is rather difficult to insert the patch pipette into the lumen without touching any structure before pressing the pipette against the luminal surface of the cell to be studied. Furthermore, only lateral membranes of the torn end can be studied; it is tacitly assumed that the properties of these lateral membranes resemble those of the basolateral membrane of the remainder of the tubule. In our experience, this assumption seems to be correct. The advantages of this method can be summarized as follows: The tubule lumen perfusate is under experimental control. The tubule is in exactly the same state as that from which we have other pertinent information on its function and properties. Another relevant methodological detail is the fact that all our experiments, unlike those in most other studies, were carried out at $37°C$.

Properties and Regulation of Ion Channels in the Proximal Tubule

This issue has been reviewed recently [11,12]. In the luminal membrane of rabbit and mouse proximal tubule a K^+ channel with 33–63 pS was found. This channel was found in cell attached patches, indicating that it is present on cells with physiologically low cytosolic Ca^{2+} activities. It is highly selective for K^+ over Na^+. This channel requires further examination. In the luminal membrane of S_3-segments of the rabbit a Na^+ channel with around 12 pS conductance was found in cell attached and in cell excised patches [31]. This channel could be inhibited from the cytosolic side by high concentrations of amiloride. We have argued that the right shift in the dose response curve was due to the fact that amiloride had to cross the membrane and to enter the patch pipette before it inhibited this channel from its binding site on the outside mouth of the channel.

In the basolateral (c.f. lateral, above) membrane two types of K^+ channels have been found in rabbit S_2 and S_3 segments. Both were of intermediate conductance (36 and 46 pS, respectively) [36]. The larger channel was seen more frequently. It had flicker type kinetics with burst appearance. It was present in cell attached patches, and it was shown to be Ca^{2+} independent in excised patches. In fact, it was perfectly activated in seemingly Ca^{2+} free solutions. This channel showed an increasing open state probability with increasing depolarization of the clamp voltage. With respect to its conductance and Ca^{2+} insensitivity, this channel is comparable to the K^+ channel present in the luminal membrane of the thick ascending limb of rabbit [19] and rat [18] (also c.f. below).

In addition to these K^+ channels we found a non-selective cation channel in the basolateral membrane of rabbit S_2 and S_3 segments. We have seen this channel in cell attached and in cell excised patches. With identical solutions on both sides the channel had a linear current voltage relation with a mean conductance of 24 pS. This channel was Ca^{2+} sensitive and it required some 10^{-5} mol/l Ca^{2+} for its activation [37]. It was non-selective in the sense that it did not discriminate between Na^+ and K^+ [11]. It was inhibited reversibly by stilbenes such as 4-acetamido-4'-isothiocyanostilbene-2,2' disulfonic acid (SITS) and by diphenylamino-2-carboxylate. This type of channel has been found in many other preparations of the thick ascending limb, collecting duct-"anlagen," and the cortical collecting duct [18,21,35,38], and it cannot be entirely excluded that it is the same channel as that found in cultures of inner medullary collecting duct [23]. We still have no firm information on the function of this channel in the intact cell.

Properties and Regulation of Ion Channels in the Thick Ascending Limb of the Loop of Henle

The luminal membrane of this nephron segment contains a K^+ conductance through which K^+ recycles into the lumen. A few years ago it was speculated that this conductance corresponded to a Ca^{2+} sensitive maxi K^+ channel [39]. This was, however, highly unlikely since this type of channel required rather high cytosolic Ca^{2+} activity to become activated [13]. These data were obtained in cell cultures of chicken kidney cells and, later, in cell cultures from rabbit thick ascending limb. More recently, we and others have reexamined this issue and have tested the properties of the luminal membrane of thick ascending limbs of rabbit [19] and rat [18]. In cell attached patches we did not find the above maxi K^+ channel but found, rather, an intermediate conductance (60 pS) K^+ channel [18,33,34]. The most intriguing properties of this channel are its control by cytosolic pH, Ca^{2+} and ATP. An example of this channel is shown in Fig. 1. It is apparent from this figure that the open probability of this channel is reduced markedly when cytosolic pH falls just slightly below the normal value. The sensitivity towards cytosolilc pH is very steep. Comparable observations have been made in the diluting segment of amphibian kidney [40], reinforcing the similarity of the thick ascending limb and other diluting segments. Figure 1 shows that this channel in the thick ascending limb has a Ca^{2+} sensitivity which is opposite to that found for the maxi K^+ channel. Low Ca^{2+} increases, and high Ca^{2+} reduces, the open state probability. This effect is not very marked for physiological cytosolic Ca^{2+} activities [41]. A comparable Ca^{2+} effect has been noted in the basolateral K^+ channel of the rectal gland of *Squalus acanthias* [42]. Ca^{2+} insensitivity of a K^+ channel in the luminal membrane of the rabbit thick ascending limb has been noted in another study [19]. Inhibition of K^+ channels by ATP was first noted in the pancreas [43], and is now known to occur in a variety of K^+ channels in skeletal and heart muscle [44,45]. Recently, ATP inhibition was also reported for a Ca^{2+} activated K^+ channel in the amphibian diluting segment and in respiratory cells [46,47]. It is likely that the ATP sensitivity of K^+ channels and non-selective cation channels [38,48] is much more common than is recognized at this stage. Unlike the maxi K^+ channel, this smaller K^+ channel is not inhibited by charybdotoxin [34]. This fits well with the finding that charybdotoxin, when added to the luminal perfusate, has no effect on the equivalent short circuit current in isolated in vitro perfused rabbit thick ascending limb segments (unpublished work). The sensitivities of this kind of K^+ channel to other blockers are summarized in Table 1. None of the blockers used is characteristic in a qualitative sense for this type of channel, and none of the known toxins (apamin, dendrotoxin, or charybdotoxin) inhibits. In our study we found no other type of channel in the luminal membrane, even in the presence of high Ca^{2+} on the cytosolic side. Hence, we believe that more but increased cytosolic Ca^{2+} is necessary for the activation of the maxi K^+ channel in our preparation of the thick ascending limb.

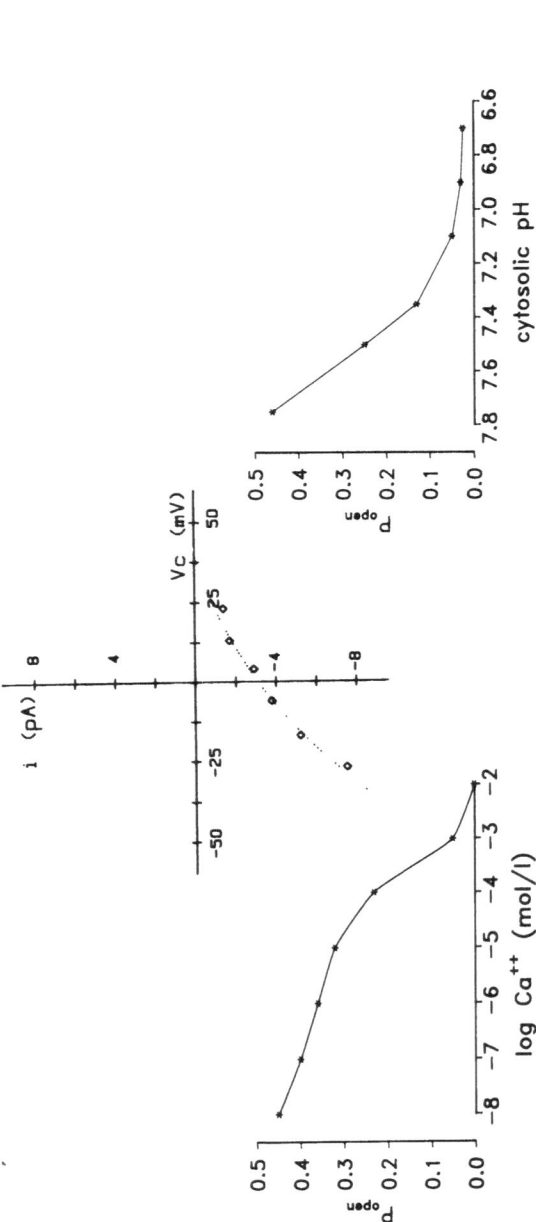

Fig. 1. K⁺-channel in the luminal membrane of a rat thick ascending limb. Excised inside/out patch. Pipette KCl, Bath NaCl. The current-voltage (i/V_c) relation was fitted by the Goldman-Hodgkin-Katz equation. The conductance at 0 mV clamp voltage was around 60 pS. *Lower left panel:* The open state probability (p_open) of this channel is plotted against the cytosolic Ca²⁺ activity. Clamp voltage 0 mV. Note that p_open was reduced with increasing Ca²⁺. *Lower right panel:* The open state probability of this channel as a function of the cytosolic pH. Note that p_open is reduced sharply with acid pH

Table 1. Inhibitors of the K^+ channel of the luminal membrane of rat thick ascending limb. The concentrations refer to half maximal inhibition (IC_{50} in mmol/l)

Substance	Side of action	IC_{50}	Type of block
H^+	cytosolic	pH 7.4	P_0 reduced
Ba^{2+}	cytosolic	0.1	P_0 reduced
Ca^{2+}	cytosolic	0.1	P_0 reduced
Mg^{2+}	cytosolic	5.0	P_0 reduced
Rb^+	both sides	>50, estimate	P_0 reduced
Cs^+	both sides	<50, estimate	P_0 reduced
NH_4^+	both sides	<50, estimate	P_0 reduced
Choline	both sides	~50	current amplitude reduced
TEA	outside	<1	P_0 reduced
	cytosolic side	>10	Current amplitude reduced
lidocain	both sides	10	flicker block
quinine	both sides	0.01	flicker block
quinidine	both sides	0.01	flicker block
verapamil	both sides	0.01	flicker block
diltiazem	both sides	0.1	flicker block

TEA, tetraethylammonium

In the basolateral (cf lateral above) membrane Cl^- channels of intermediate conductance were found in cell attached patches [33]. These channels had a mean conductance of 41 pS for positive and 31 pS for negative clamp voltages in excised patches with identical NaCl solutions on both sides of the channel. The open state probability was increased with depolarization of the clamp voltage. These channels were inhibited reversibly by the Cl^- channel blocker 5-nitro-2-(3-phenylpropyl-amino)-benzoate (NPPB). An example of this kind of channel is shown in Fig. 2. It has been shown that this channel is a weak outward rectifier [24]. The effect of NPPB was entirely reversible. As in other Cl^- channels, NPPB induced a flicker type block [49,50]. In another study [51], a similar channel was noted in the basolateral membrane of collagenase treated non perfused mouse thick ascending limb segments; it was reported that this channel was found more frequently after pretreatment with forskolin and 8-Br-cAMP.

We [33] and others [26] have found a non-selective cation channel with a mean conductance of 20–30 pS in the basolateral membrane of the thick ascending limb of rat and mouse. This channel requires high cytosolic Ca^{2+} activity to become activated. It is apparently inhibited by ATP [38]. As in the case of the proximal tubule, we have no firm indication of the physiological role of this channel (c.f. above).

Properties and Regulation of Ion Channels in the Distal Tubule

Recently, using distal convoluted tubules from rabbit kidneys treated with collagenase, K^+ channels were found in the basolateral membrane [27]. These channels had conductances in the range of 50 and 60 pS; they were inhibited by Ba^{2+}. Apart from the finding that the open state probability was not strongly altered with varying clamp voltages, little is known at this stage about these two types of K^+ channels.

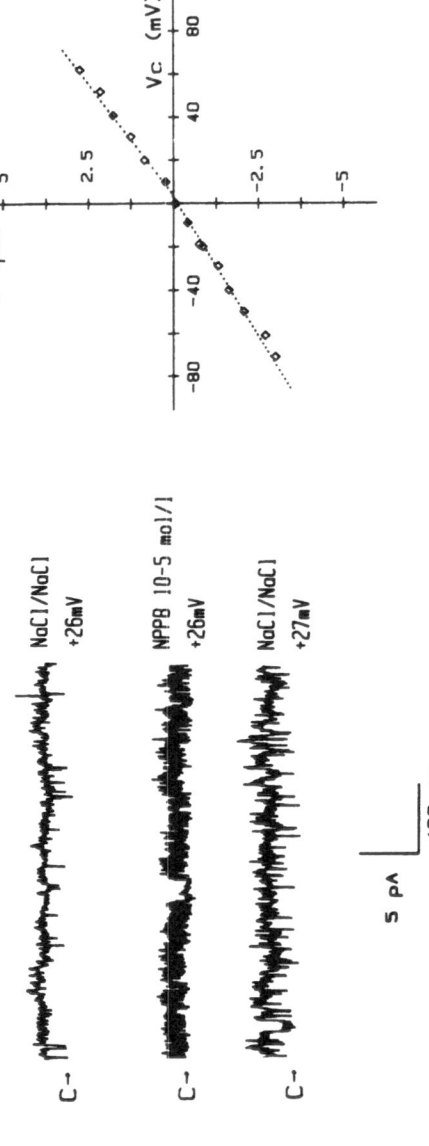

Fig. 2. Cl⁻ channels in the basolateral membrane of a rat thick ascending limb. Excised inside/out patch. Pipette and bath NaCl. *Left panel:* Typical recording and effect of 5-nitro-2-(3-phenylpropylamino)-benzoate (*NPPB*). $C\rightarrow$ denotes the closed state of this channel. Note the flicker block induced by NPPB. *Right panel:* Current-voltage relationship (i/V_c) of this channel

Properties and Regulation of Ion Channels in the Collecting Duct

Amiloride sensitive Na$^+$ channels in the luminal membrane of isolated cortical collecting ducts of Na$^+$ deprived rats have been reported previously [52,53]. These channels were localized in the principal cell; they had a small conductance of 5 pS. They were not directly regulated by cytosolic Ca^{2+}, but they showed increased open state probability with alkaline versus acid pH on the cytosolic side [53]. On the basis of the voltage dependent block of these Na$^+$ channels by impermeant ions, a model for this channel has recently been proposed [54]. This channel is permeable for H$^+$, Li$^+$, and Na$^+$, but is impermeable for K$^+$, guanidinium ions, and tetraethylammonium. Comparable channels have been found in pilot experiments in the luminal membrane of isolated in vitro perfused rat cortical collecting ducts [35]. It is not quite clear whether the Na$^+$ channel of this membrane can also occur with an even smaller conductance. This might explain the difficulty of finding this channel (reported in several studies [21], [25], and found in our own unpublished work). One alternative approach to dealing with this problem is the use of whole cell patch clamp analysis. This approach has been used recently [55], and an amiloride sensitive conductance increased by low Na$^+$ diet has been identified.

Besides these Na$^+$ channels, K$^+$ channels have been found in several studies in the luminal membrane of cortical collecting ducts of rabbit [25] and rat [35,56,57]. The channel found in the rabbit had an intermediate conductance and was Ca^{2+} dependent [25]. In the rat [35,57] the Ca^{2+} dependent channel belongs to the maxi K$^+$ channel family. Much knowledge has recently been gained concerning the properties of this channel. It seems unlikely that the channel is responsible for K$^+$ secretion in this nephron segment. We found this channel only very rarely in cell attached patches when the cells were depolarized by high extracellular K$^+$ concentrations. The finding that this channel coexists with Na$^+$ channels in the same cell membrane indicates that the channel is also localized in the principal cell [35]. The same channel has also been observed in cultures of collecting duct-"anlagen" [20]. We and others have found yet another K$^+$ channel in the same cell membrane. This channel had a small to intermediate conductance of some 20–35 pS. It was Ca^{2+} independent and may be controlled by cytosolic pH. A recording of this K$^+$ channel is shown in Fig. 3. In this figure the small and the large K$^+$ channel were present in the same membrane patch. It is highly likely that K$^+$ secretion occurs via this small conductance K$^+$ channel. This small channel has also been noted in experiments with collecting duct-"anlagen" [21]. Much more work is needed to characterize this channel in more detail.

A few Cl$^-$ channels were noted in our studies on the luminal membrane of the rat cortical collecting duct [35]. Again, this matches well with previous studies in collecting duct-"anlagen" [21]. This Cl$^-$ channel had an intermediate conductance of 20–60 pS and was inhibited by NPPB. We have no indication of the function of this channel, nor do we know whether it occurs in intercalated or in principal cells.

Conclusion

The present short review indicates that our knowledge of ion channels in renal tubules is still far from complete. The problems are manifold: 1) Several cell membranes have not been looked at with sufficient thoroughness. One such example is the lumi-

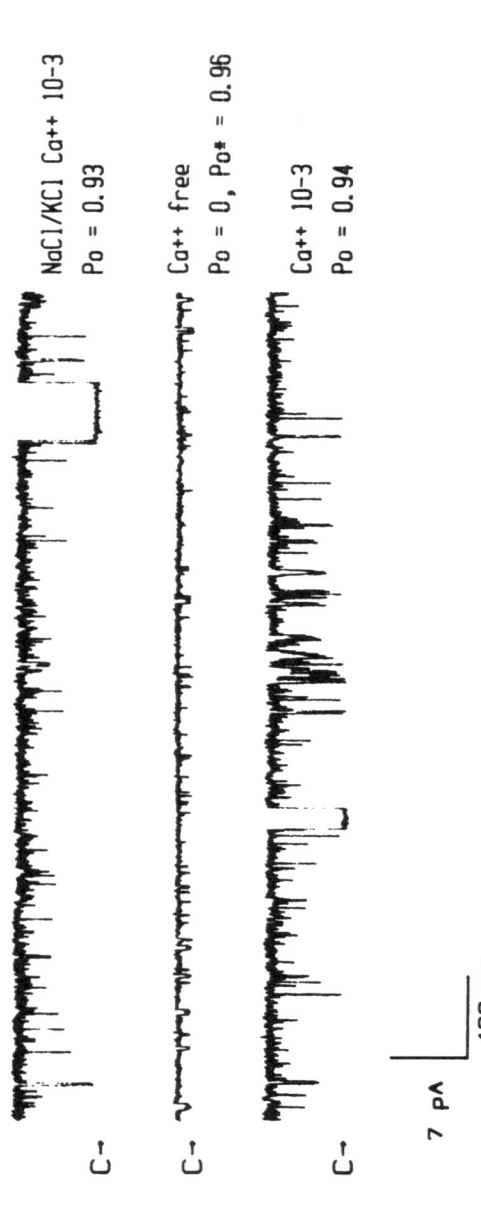

Fig. 3. Coexisting small and large K[+]-channels in the luminal membrane of a rat cortical collecting duct. Inside/out patch. Pipette NaCl, bath KCl. Typical traces at 0 mV clamp voltage. $C\rightarrow$ indicates the zero current level. Note that the large (maxi) K[+]-channel is inhibited in Ca[2+]-free solution (*middle trace*). Now the small K[+]-channel, which, upon close inspection, is also hidden in the *upper* and *lower trace*, becomes clearly apparent. P_0 and P_0* denote the open state probability of the large and small K[+]-channel, respectively

nal membrane of the proximal tubule. Other nephron segments are entirely empty spots on our map. 2) Analysis of the basolateral membrane is complicated by the fact that pretreatment with collagenase is required. Analysis of the properties of the lateral membrane at the torn end of the tubule makes the assumption that this membrane has properties identical with those of the basolateral membrane. 3) Several channels, such as the non-selective cation channel and the maxi K^+ channel, have been found in many excised patches of several nephron segments. These channels probably do not function in the normal cell and are activated under circumstances which are, so far, not clearly understood. 4) Other channels, which we know are present in a given membrane, are difficult to demonstrate by single channel analysis. One such example is the Na^+ channel in the collecting duct. Another example is the Ca^{2+}-channel in the luminal membrane of the thick ascending limb. 5) Culture techniques have made an important contribution to our current understanding of single channel properties in renal epithelia. Unfortunately, only with much caution can such data be extrapolated to the intact tubule. 6) The method of single channel analysis has an "analytical window" through which we view the conductance properties of a given membrane. With a time resolution in the 1 kHz range, only channels with open states lasting for around 1 ms will be detectable. Furthermore, the noise band of current traces filtered at 1 kHz is usually of the order of 0.3–0.5 pA. Any channel with a conductance <5 pS will have a current amplitude of <0.5 pA if the driving force is as high as 100 mV, and will therefore be difficult to detect. 7) That ion channels which operate on the cell are inactivated by the excision procedure cannot be excluded. These channels could therefore only be described in cell attached and possibly in whole cell recordings. Much more work and probably new techniques will be required to provide us with a more complete understanding of the function of ion channels in renal tubules.

Acknowledgments. This work was supported by Deutsche Forschungsgemeinschaft Gr 480/10 Schl 277/2-1.

References

1. Greger R, Gögelein H (1987) K^+ conductive pathways in the nephron. Kidney Int 31:1055–1064
2. Lang F, Friedrich F, Schobersberger W, Jungwirth A, Ritter M, Steidl M, Weiss H, Wöll E, Tschernko E, Paulmichl R, Hallbrucker C (1990) Ion channels in Mardin-Darby canine kidney cells. Renal Physiol Biochem 13:82–93
3. Kolb HA (1990) Ion channels in opossum kidney cells. Renal Physiol Biochem 131:26–36
4. Gögelein H (1988) Chloride channels in epithelia. Biochim Biophys Acta 947:521–547
5. Hunter M, Kawahara K, Giebisch G (1988) Calcium-activated epthelial potassium channels. Min Electrol Metab 14:48–57
6. Garty H, Benos DJ (1988) Characteristics and regulatory mechanisms of the amiloride-blockade Na^+ channel. Physiol Rev 68:309–373
7. Hunter M (1990) Patch clamp studies of the amphibian nephron. Renal Physiol Biochem 13:94–111
8. Parent L, Cardinal J, Sauve R (1988) Single-channel analysis of a K channel at basolateral membrane of rabbit proximal convoluted tubule. Am J Physiol 254:F105–F113

9. Merot J, Bidet M, Le Maout S, Tauc M, Poujeol P (1989) Two types of K⁺ channels in the apical membrane of rabbit proximal tubule in primary culture. Biochim Biophys Acta 978:134–144

10. Merot J, Bidet M, Gachot B, Le Maout S, Tauc M, Poujeol P (1988) Patch clamp study on primary culture of isolated proximal convoluted tubules. Pflugers Arch 51:61

11. Gögelein H (1990) Ion channels in mammalian proximal renal tubule. Renal Physiol Biochem 13:8–25

12. Gögelein H, Greger R (1988) Patch clamp analysis of ionic channels in renal proximal tubules. In: Davison AM (ed) Proceedings of the Xth international congress of nephrology. Baillere Tindall, London, pp 159–178

13. Guggino SE, Guggino WB, Green N, Sacktor B (1987) Ca²⁺-activated K⁺ channels in cultured medullary thick ascending limb cells. Am J Physiol 252:C121–C127

14. Cornejo M, Guggino SE, Sastre A, Guggino WB (1989) Isomeric yohimbine alkaloids block calcium-activated K⁺ channels in medullary thick ascending limb cells of rabbit kidney. J Mem Biol 107:25–33

15. Cornejo M, Guggino SE, Guggino WB (1987) Modification of Ca²⁺-activated K⁺ channels in cultured medullary thick ascending limb cells by N-bromoacetamide. J Membr Biol 99:147–155

16. Cornejo M, Guggino SE, Guggino WB (1989) Ca²⁺-activated K⁺ channels from cultured renal medullary thick ascending limb cells: effects of pH. J Membr Biol 110:49–55

17. Taniguchi J, Guggino WB (1989) Membrane stretch: a physiological stimulator of Ca²⁺-activated K⁺ channels in thick ascending limb. Am J Physiol 257:F347–F352

18. Bleich M, Schlatter E, Greger R (1990) The luminal K⁺ channel of the thick ascending limb of Henle's loop. Pflugers Arch 415:449–460

19. Wang W, White S, Geibel J, Giebisch G (1990) A potassium channel in the apical membrane of rabbit thick ascending limb of Henle's loop. Am J Physiol 258:F244–F253

20. Gitter AH, Beyenbach KW, Christine CW, Gross P, Minuth WW, Frömter E (1987) High-conductance of K⁺ channel in apical membranes of principal cells cultured from rabbit renal cortical collecting duct anlagen. Pflugers Arch 408:282–290

21. Laskowski FH, Christine CHW, Gitter AH, Beyenbach KW, Gross P, Frömter E (1990) Cation channels in the apical membrane of collecting duct principal cell epithelium in culture. Renal Physiol Biochem 13:70–81

22. Palmer LG, Frindt G (1986) Epithelial sodium channels: characterization by using the patch-clamp technique. Fed Proc 45:2708–2712

23. Light DB, McCann FV, Keller TM, Stanton BA (1988) Amiloride-sensitive cation channel in apical membrane of inner medullary collecting duct. Am J Physiol 255:F278–F286

24. Kunzelmann K, Pavenstädt H, Greger R (1989) Properties and regulation of chloride channels in cystic fibrosis and normal airway cells. Pflugers Arch 415:172–182

24a. Light DB, Schweibert EM, Fejes-Toth G, Naray-Fejes-Toth A, Karlson KH, McCann F, Stanton B (1990) Chloride channels in the apical membrane of cortical collecting duct cells. Am J Physiol 268:F273–F280

25. Hunter M, Lopes AG, Boulpaep E, Giebisch GH (1986) Regulation of single potassium ion channels from apical membrane of rabbit collecting tubule. Am J Physiol 251:F725–F733

26. Teulon J, Paulais M, Bouthier M (1987) A Ca²⁺-activated cation-selective channel in the basolateral membrane of the cortical thick ascending limb of Henle's loop of the mouse. Biochim Biophys Acta 905:125–132

27. Taniguchi J, Yoshitomi K, Imai M (1989) K⁺ channel currents in basolateral membrane of distal convoluted tubule of rabbit kidney. Am J Physiol 256:F246–F254

28. Burg M, Grantham J, Abramow M, Orloff J (1966) Preparation and study of fragments of single rabbit nephrons. Am J Physiol 210(6):1293–1298

29. Greger R, Hampel W (1981) A modified system for in vitro perfusion of isolated renal tubules. Pflugers Arch 389:175–176
30. Gögelein H, Greger R (1984) Single channel recordings from basolateral and apical membranes of renal proximal tubules. Pflugers Arch 401:424–426
31. Gögelein H, Greger R (1986) Na⁺ selective channels in the apical membrane of rabbit late proximal tubule (pars recta). Pflugers Arch 406:198–203
32. Gögelein H, Greger R, Schlatter E (1987) Potassium channels in the basolateral membrane of the rectal gland of *Squalus acanthias*. Regulation and inhibitors. Pflugers Arch 409:107–113
33. Greger R, Bleich M, Schlatter E (1990) Ion channels in the thick ascending limb of Henle's loop. Renal Physiol Biochem 13:37–50
34. Greger R, Bleich M, Schlatter E (to be published) Ion channel regulation in the thick ascending limb of the loop of Henle. Kidney Int
35. Schlatter E, Bleich M, Greger R (1989) Properties of the luminal K⁺-channel of isolated perfused cortical collecting ducts (CCT) of the rat (abstract). Proc Am Soc Nephrol 22nd annual meeting, Washington DC, 374A
36. Gögelein H, Greger R (1987) Properties of single K⁺ channels in the basolateral membrane of rabbit proximal straight tubules. Pflugers Arch 410:288–295
37. Gögelein H, Greger R (1986) A voltage dependent ionic channel in the basolateral membrane of late proximal tubules of the rabbit kidney. Pflugers Arch 407:S142–S148
38. Paulais M, Teulon J (1989) A cation channel in the thick ascending limb of Henle's loop of the mouse kidney: inhibition by adenine nucleotides. J Physiol 413:315–327
39. Guggino SE, Suarez-Isla BA, Guggino WB, Sacktor B (1985) Forskolin and antidiuretic hormone stimulate a Ca²⁺-activated K⁺ channel in cultured kidney cells. Am J Physiol 249:F448–F455
40. Hunter M, Oberleithner H, Henderson RM, Giebisch G (1988) Whole-cell potassium currents in single early distal tubule cells. Am J Physiol 255:F699–F703
41. Nitschke R, Fröbe U, Greger R (1991 in press) ADH increases cytosolic Ca²⁺-activity in isolated perfused rabbit thick ascending limb via a V1 receptor. Pflugers Arch
42. Greger R, Gögelein H, Schlatter E (1987) Potassium channels in the basolateral membrane of the rectal gland of the dogfish (*Squalus acanthias*). Pflugers Arch 409:100–106
43. Cook DL, Hales CN (1984) Intracellular ATP directly blocks K⁺ channels in pancreatic B-cells. Nature 311:271–273
44. Stanfield PR (1987) Nucleotides such as ATP may control the activity of ion channels. Trends Neurosci 10:335–339
45. Noma A (1983) ATP-regulated K⁺ channels in cardiac muscle. Nature 305:147–148
46. Hunter M, Giebisch G (1988) Calcium-activated K-channels of amphibiuma early distal tubule: inhibition by ATP. Pflugers Arch 412:331–333
47. Kunzelmann K, Pavenstädt H, Greger R (1989) Characterization of potassium channels in respiratory cells II. Inhibitors and Regulation. Pflugers Arch 414:297–303
48. Petersen OH, Gallacher DV (1988) Electrophysiology of the pancreatic and salivary acinar cells. Annu Rev Physiol 50:65–80
49. Hayslett JP, Gögelein H, Kunzelmann K, Greger R (1987) Characteristics of apical chloride channels in human colon cells (HT₂₉). Pflugers Arch 410:487–494
50. Dreinhöfer J, Gögelein H, Greger R (1988) Blocking kinetics of Cl⁻ channels in colonic carcinoma cells (HT₂₉) as revealed by 5-nitro-2-(3-phenylpropylamino)-benzoic acid (NPPB). Biochim Biophys Acta 959:135–142
51. Paulais M, Teulon J (1990) cAMP-activated chloride channel in the basolateral membrane of the thick ascending limb of the mouse kidney. J Membr Biol 113:253–260
52. Palmer LG, Frindt G (1986) Amiloride-sensitive Na channels from the apical membrane of the rat cortical collecting tubule. Proc Natl Acad Sci USA 83:2767–2770
53. Palmer LG, Frindt G (1987) Effects of cell Ca and pH on Na channels from rat cortical collecting tubule. Am J Physiol 253:F333–F339

54. Palmer LG (1990) Epithelial Na channels: the nature of the conducting pore. Renal Physiol Biochem 13:51–58
55. Frindt G, Sackin H, Palmer LG (1990) Whole-cell currents in rat cortical collecting tubule: low-Na diet increases amiloride-sensitive conductance. Am J Physiol 258:F562– F565
56. Frindt G, Palmer LG (1987) Ca-activated K channels in apical membrane of mammalian CCT, and their role in K secretion. Am J Physiol 252:F458–F467
57. Frindt G, Palmer G (1989) Low-conductance K channels in the apical membrane of the rat cortical collecting tubule. Am J Physiol 256:F143–F151

Single Sodium Channels in the Apical Membrane of Proximal Tubule Cells in Culture

EMILE L. BOULPAEP and ROSEMARIE DRAKE-BAUMANN[1]

SUMMARY. Isolated proximal tubule cells of Ambystoma kidney were grown in primary cultures to confluence. Using the patch clamp technique single Na$^+$ channels were found in the apical membrane of the proximal tubule cells. In control conditions in the cell attached configuration these Na$^+$ channels showed a single channel conductance of 3 to 4 pS (referred to symmetrical 100 mM Na) and were highly selective. In the presence of 10 μM amiloride added to the pipette solution there was an increased number of transitions without complete block, and the single channel conductance, referred to symmetrical 100 mM Na, increased to 10–13 pS. In control conditions the probability of opening increased with hyperpolarization of the membrane patch. In the presence of amiloride open probability decreased with hyperpolarization. Analysis of open and closed time constants revealed a single open and closed time constant in control conditions, but multiple time constants after the addition of amiloride. It is concluded that the apical membrane of the amphibian proximal tubule has a subtype of Na$^+$ channels whose properties differ, qualitatively and quantitatively, from other epithelial sodium channels.

Introduction

Multiple transport systems account for the translocation of sodium from the ultrafiltrate in the lumen of the proximal tubule to the cytoplasm of the cell. In isolated tubule preparations of Ambystoma [1], the following Na transporters have been identified at the level of the apical cell membrane: rheogenic Na$^+$/glucose symport [2] Na$^+$/aminoacids symport [2], electroneutral Na$^+$/lactate$^-$ symport [3], and electroneutral Na$^+$-H$^+$ antiport [4]. No evidence has been found for Na$^+$/K$^+$/2Cl$^-$ symport [5,6] or Na$^+$/Cl$^-$ symport [5,6]. In the presence of ultrafiltrate-like solutions, a major

---

[1]Department of Cellular and Molecular Physiology, Yale University School of Medicine, 333 Cedar Street, New Haven, CT 06510, USA

moiety of Na uptake from lumen to cell is mediated by Na^+/substrate cotransport [2]. However, in the absence of Na^+/substrate symport and of Na^+-H^+ antiport, apical Na entry was detected from changes in intracellular Na activity measured with ion-selective microelectrodes, indicating the presence of conductive Na channels at the luminal membrane [5]. Following preferential reabsorption of organic substrates and HCO_3^- in early proximal tubule, Na channels may thus contribute appreciably to Na entry at the end of the proximal tubule.

In rabbit, late proximal tubule Na channels have been reported by patch-clamping of the microvillar surface [7], but baseline tracings were too noisy to record channel activity at normal resting potentials. Moreover, the effect of amiloride was examined only from the cytoplasmic side of the membrane patch [7].

Patch clamping of the apical surface of dissected proximal tubules is not readily feasible, in view of the presence of numerous tall microvilli. Confluent monolayers of epithelial cells offer free access to the apical membrane. We have developed primary cultures of salamander proximal tubule cells and have characterized the ultrastructural and electrophysiological properties as representative of proximal tubule function in situ [8].

Typical epithelial sodium channels have been described by patch-clamping of apical membranes in models of Na^+ absorbing "tight" epithelia such as A6 cells [9,10] and rat cortical collecting tubules [11-14]. The present study attempts, first, to identify the presence of Na^+ channels in apical membranes of cultured salamander proximal tubule cells using the patch clamp technique, and second, to establish whether these channels have properties identical to classical epithelial sodium channels.

Procedure

Confluent cultures of Ambystoma proximal tubule cells grown for two to three weeks on permeable supports were used. All patch clamp recordings were performed on the apical cell membrane in the cell-attached configuration. Patch pipettes were filled either with a control solution containing Na^+ 100 mM, K^+ 2.44 mM, Mg^{2+} 1 mM, Ca^{2+} 0.9 mM, Cl^- 89.68 mM, HCO_3^- 10 mM, HPO_4^{2-} 0.56 mM, $H_2PO_4^-$ 0.14 mM, SO_4^{2-} 0.5 mM, pyruvate$^-$ 4.3 mM, and glucose 1.9 mM, or with a low chloride solution containing Na^+ 100 mM, K^+ 2.44 mM, Ca^{2+} 1.8 mM, Cl^- 6.0 mM, and cyclamate$^-$ 95 mM. In addition, each solution was buffered with 10 mM Hepes acid titrated to pH 7.45 with NaOH. The bath contained the culture medium with an electrolyte composition similar to the pipette control solution.

Proximal Tubule Apical Na^+ Channels

With symmetrical control 100 mM Na^+ solutions in pipette and bath, spontaneous activity of inward currents of small amplitude was noted at the resting membrane potential, i.e., when the clamp voltage of the pipette V_{pip} was held at 0 mV (Fig. 1). Channel openings and closings lasted for intervals ranging from about 10 ms–1 second.

Hyperpolarization of the membrane patch with more negative values of -V_{pip} enhanced the amplitude of the inward current. At depolarized membrane patch

Control

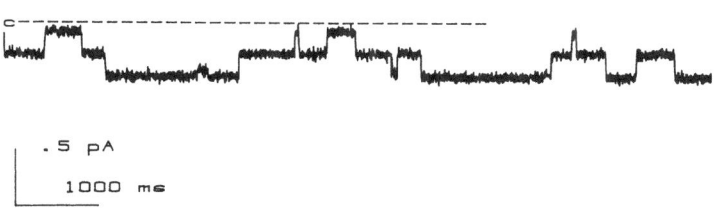

.5 pA

1000 ms

Amiloride 10 μM

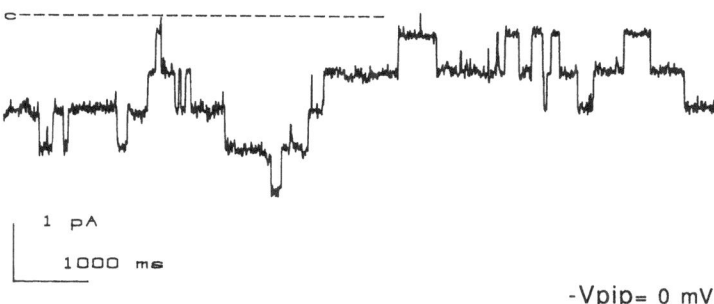

1 pA

1000 ms

-Vpip= 0 mV

Fig. 1. Patch clamp recordings of apical sodium channels from cultured Ambystoma proximal tubule cells. Single channel currents were recorded in cell-attached configuration with 100 mM Na⁺ in the pipette solution and bath. *Upper tracings* are the control condition. At least two channels are present in the patch. *Lower tracings* are obtained in the presence of 10 μM amiloride. At least four channels are present in the patch. Both recordings were obtained at resting membrane potential, i.e. $-V_{pip} = 0$ mV. Note the different current scale for the two records

potentials ($-V_{pip} = +$) outward currents could not be resolved. Often multiple channels per patch were observed, up to 7 channels in a single patch. The top part of Fig. 1 shows a patch with at least two channels.

Using current amplitude histograms of the current measured at different pipette potentials, single channel current amplitudes were plotted against -V_{pip} potentials of +40 to −100 mV. The experimental current-voltage relations were adequately fitted by theoretical Goldman curves predicted for a perfectly selective Na⁺ channel under the asymmetric Na concentrations prevailing across the membrane patch. The theoretical curves extrapolated to a reversal potential of +93 mV, assuming a membrane potential of −50 mV (Drake-Baumann R. et al., to be published) [8] and a E_{rev} for Na⁺ of + 43 mV calculated from an intracellular Na activity of 19 mM. Single channel conductance g_{Na}^* for a symmetrical 100 mM Na⁺ concentration, as obtained from the Goldman equation, ranged from 3–4 pS.

Single channel conductance for Na⁺ in the Ambystoma proximal tubule compares closely with the conductance of classical epithelial Na⁺ channels, e.g., the apical Na channel in rat cortical collecting tubule [11] and the low conductance highly selective channel of A6 cells [15–18]. However, the g_{Na}^* of Na⁺ channels in the amphibian proximal tubule is less than the values reported for Na⁺ channels in mammalian proximal tubules, such as rabbit straight proximal segments [7] and rat proximal tubules [19]. Our Na channels also have a lower conductance than the high conductance non-selective Na⁺ channel in A6 cells [15,16,20], and the Na⁺ channel in LLC PK1 cells [21].

Amiloride Effect on Proximal Tubule Apical Na⁺ Channels

When the pipette solution contained 100 mM Na⁺ and 10 μM amiloride and the bath contained 100 mM Na⁺, the spontaneous activity of inward currents at the resting membrane potential exhibited no closure of the channel, but exhibited frequent brief interruptions, as shown in the lower part of Fig. 1. In the example of Fig. 1, the patch contained at least 4 channels and it is clear that 10 μM amiloride did not suppress the single channel currents, but altered its kinetics. At hyperpolarized potentials the frequency of interruptions was even more pronounced.

Current amplitude histograms were obtained and single channel currents were plotted against $-V_{pip}$ potentials of +70 to −100 mV. These current-voltage relations were adequately fitted by theoretical Goldman curves predicted for a perfectly selective Na⁺ channel; which also extrapolated to the theoretical reversal potential of +93 mV. Thus, amiloride does not alter the high selectivity of the Na⁺ channel. However, a striking observation is that, in the presence of amiloride, single channel conductance g_{Na}^* for a symmetrical 100 mM Na⁺ concentration, as obtained from the Goldman fits, rose to values of 10–13 pS/channel. Note the difference in current amplitude scale in the upper and lower portion of Fig. 1.

There is no precedent in the literature for the higher single channel conductance in amiloride treated patches. It is known that A6 cells exhibit both unselective high conductance (7–10 pS) channels and highly selective low conductance (4–5pS) channels [9]. Several arguments plead against the existence of two populations of channels in the amphibian apical membrane. First, in control conditions, high conductance channels were never observed. Second, in amiloride-treated membranes, low conductance channels were never seen. Third, there is no indication for the occurrence of highly selective as well as unselective channels, since the current-voltage relationships of both control and amiloride-treated channels extrapolated well to a reversal potential predicted for an ideal high Na⁺ selectivity. We conclude that the amphibian proximal tubule Na⁺ channel is an isoform of the classical epithelial channel with a qualitatively different amiloride response.

Voltage-Dependence of Channel Activity

The open probability was studied on recordings obtained from single-channel and multi-channel patches. Open probability was calculated as the product nP_o, where n = number of channels and P_o is the single channel open probability. To permit com-

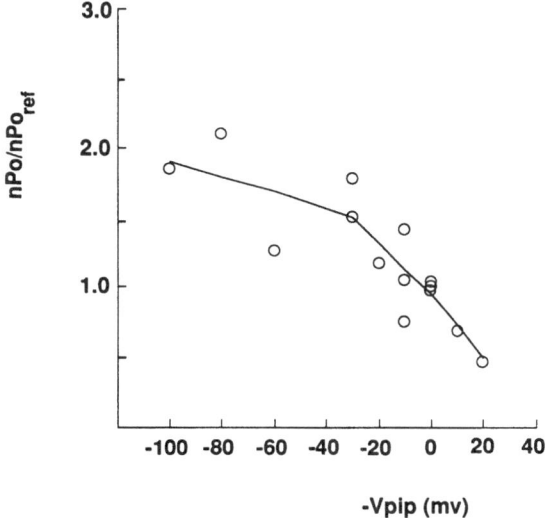

Fig. 2. Normalized open probability nP_o/nP_{oref} values in spontaneously active channels, at various pipette potentials where the normal resting potential at $-V_{pip} = 0$ mV is the reference potential

parison of the open probability from patches containing a different number of channels n, the nP_o values were normalized to a reference value nP_{oref} which was the value of P_o at the resting potential when $-V_{pip} = 0$. Fig. 2 shows the ratio nP_o/nP_{oref} for a spontaneously active Na$^+$ channel in the 100 mM Na control conditions. There was a moderate rise in open probability with hyperpolarization of the patch membrane. The data in Fig. 2 were fitted by Lowess fits, indicating a maximum rate of voltage dependence in the range of $-V_{pip} + 20$ mV to -30 mV. From fitting the data of Fig. 2 to a Boltzmann equation it was possible to conclude that the gating charge for the opening for the Na$^+$ channel did not appreciably depart from 1.

There is conflicting evidence in the literature regarding the voltage dependence of epithelial Na$^+$ channels. The voltage dependence in Fig. 2 is of the same shape and sign as in the apical Na$^+$ channel of the rat cortical collecting tubule [14]. However, in the highly selective Na$^+$ channels of A6 cells there appears to be no clear voltage-dependence [17], whereas the non-selective Na$^+$ channels in A6 cells [9] appear to have a voltage dependence of a sign opposite to our proximal tubule Na$^+$ channels.

The voltage dependence of Ambystoma apical Na$^+$ channels was drastically different in the presence of amiloride. Fig. 3 illustrates that the addition of 10 µM amiloride reversed the sign of the voltage dependence. In Fig. 3 hyperpolarization of the patch pipette reduced the nP_o/nP_{oref} of the sodium channel, as opposed to the increase of nP_o/nP_{oref} seen above in the absence of amiloride. The curve in Fig. 3 is a Lowess fit and shows the highest sensitivity of open probability to potential in the range of $-V_{pip} = 0$ to -60 mV. Alternatively, fitting the data to a Boltzmann equation showed that the gating charge for the voltage dependence of amiloride block does not differ from 1.

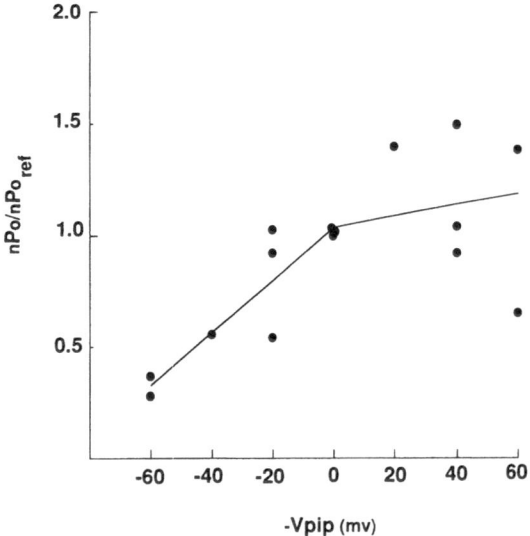

Fig. 3. Normalized open probability nP_o/nP_{oref} values in the presence of 10 μM amiloride, at various pipette potentials where the normal resting membrane potential at $-V_{pip} = 0$ mV is the reference potential

Voltage-dependent amiloride block of Na channels is well known to exist in A6 cells [20], in inner medullary collecting duct, [22] and "tight" epithelia [23]. The voltage dependence of amiloride blocking is thought to result from the position of the amiloride binding site in the channel, such that the cationic guanidinium group of amiloride senses the transmembrane electrical field.

Kinetics of Single Channels

Using a threshold analysis program [24] open and closed time durations were tabulated. From histograms of dwell time distributions plotted on a logarithmically binned time axis, a number of open and closed time components could be resolved, using the maximum likelihood method to fit a probability density function [25].

In control conditions, at a holding potential of $-V_{pip} = -60$ mV, only a single open time constant $\tau_{ol} = 312$ ms was calculated, as well as a single closed time constant of $\tau_{cl} = 289$ ms. However, in the presence of 10 μM amiloride at a holding potential of $-V_{pip} = -60$ mV, two open time constants τ_o were noted: flickery openings with a $\tau_{ol} = 0.3$ ms and longer openings with a time constant of $\tau_{o2} = 152$ ms. The longer time constant was, however, much shorter than the open time constant in control conditions. Examination of the closed time events during amiloride inhibition revealed four time constants τ_c. These were a rapid flickery block with time constants $\tau_{cl} = 0.32$ ms and $\tau_{c2} = 3.7$ ms; a third time constant $\tau_{c3} = 113$ ms was shorter than that of the single closed time constant observed in control channels; a fourth component, $\tau_{c4} = 813$ ms resulted from long closures or a blocked state condition.

Physiological Role of Proximal Tubule Na⁺-Channels

Na^+ entry from apical bath to cell through conductive channels is not inhibited by amiloride in isolated perfused Ambystoma proximal tubules [5]. The present study reports responses to amiloride which are qualitatively and quantitatively different from other epithelial channels. Although flickering and the addition of several closed time constants was induced by amiloride in the amphibian proximal tubule, the time-averaged mean open probability was not significantly reduced after amiloride. This observation, when combined with the increased single channel conductance of amiloride-treated channels, most likely explains why macroscopic membrane conductance and transmembrane conductive fluxes are not inhibited by amiloride in intact proximal tubules.

The relative contribution of Na^+ uptake derived from the activity of Na^+ channels, as opposed to other Na^+ transporters, is an important issue in the overall regulation of proximal sodium handling. Two properties may converge to achieve powerful regulation. First, rheogenic symporters, such as rheogenic Na^+/glucose symport [2], induce a depolarization of the apical membrane as Na^+ ions enter the cell. Second, the present study shows that the probability of opening of Na^+ channels is very dependent on potential. It is therefore likely that regulatory feedback results from the interaction of these two properties. As long as glucose or other organic substrates are present, the apical membrane potential depolarizes as a result of rheogenic symport activity and the Na^+ channels should be closed. However, in the absence of these organic substrates, the apical membrane should hyperpolarize and the Na^+ channels should open.

Acknowledgments. This work was supported by grants DK-13844 and DK-17433 from the National Institute of Diabetes and Digestive and Kidney Diseases.

References

1. Sackin H, Boulpaep EL (1981) Isolated perfused salamander proximal tubule: methods, electrophysiology and transport. Am J Physiol 241:F39–F52
2. Morgunov N, Boulpaep EL (1987) Electrochemical analysis of renal Na⁺-glucose cotransport in salamander proximal tubules. Am J Physiol 252:F154–F169
3. Siebens AW, Boron WF (1987) Effect of electroneutral luminal and basolateral lactate transport on intracellular pH in salamander proximal tubules. J Gen Physiol 90:799–831
4. Boron WF, Boulpaep EL (1983) Intracellular pH regulation in the renal proximal tubule of the salamender: Na-H exchange. J Gen Physiol 81:29–52
5. Abdulnour-Nakhoul S, Boulpaep EL (1986) Apical membrane transport mechanisms for Na entry in Ambystoma kidney proximal tubule. Kidney Int 29:403
6. Abdulnour-Nakhoul S, Boulpaep EL (1988) Chloride transport mechanisms linked to sodium in Ambystoma proximal tubule. Kidney Int 33:423
7. Gogelein H, Greger R (1986) Na⁺ selective channels in the apical membrane of rabbit late proximal tubules. Pflugers Arch 406:198–203
8. Drake-Baumann R, Maunsbach A, Boulpaep EL (to be published) Primary cultures of Ambystoma proximal tubule cells: ultrastructure and electrophysiology. Am J Physiol
9. Eaton DC, Hamilton KL (1988) The amiloride-blockable sodium channel of epithelial tissue. In: Toshio Narahashi (ed) Ion channels vol 1. Plenum, New York, pp, 151–282

10. Garty H, Benos DJ (1988) Characteristics and regulatory mechanisms of the amiloride-blockable Na⁺ channel. Physiol Rev 68:309–373

11. Palmer LG, Frindt G (1986) Amiloride-sensitive Na channels from apical membrane of the rat cortical collecting tubule. Proc Natl Acad Sci USA 83:2767–2770

12. Palmer LG, Frindt G (1987) Effect of cell Ca and pH on Na channels from rat cortical collecting tubule. Am J Physiol 253:F333–F339

13. Palmer LG (1987) Ion selectivity of epithelial Na channels. J Membr Biol 96:97–106

14. Palmer LG, Frindt G (1988) Conductance and gating of epithelial Na channels from rat cortical collecting tubule. J Gen Physiol 92:121–138

15. Sariban-Sohraby S, LaTorre R, Burg M, Olans L, Benos D (1984) Amiloride-sensitive epithelial Na⁺ channels reconstituted into planar lipid bilayer membranes. Nature 308:80–82

16. Olans L, Sariban-Sohraby S, Benos DJ (1984) Saturation behavior of single amiloride-sensitive Na⁺ channels in planar lipid bilayers. Biophys J 46:831–835

17. Hamilton KL, Eaton DC (1986) Single channel recordings from two types of amiloride sensitive epithelial Na⁺ channels. Membr Biochem 6:149–171

18. Hamilton KL, Eaton DC (1986) Regulation of single sodium channels in renal tissue: a role in sodium homeostasis. Fed Proc 45:2713–2717

19. Marom S, Dagan D, Winaver J, Palti Y (1989) Brush-border membrane cation conducting channels from rat kidney proximal tubules. Am J Physiol 257:F328–F335

20. Hamilton KL, Eaton DC (1985) Single-channel recordings from amiloride-sensitive epithelial sodium channel. Am J Physiol 249:C200–C207

21. Moran A, Moran N (1984) Amiloride-sensitive channels from LLC-PK1 apical membranes. Fed Proc 43A:447

22. Light DB, McCann FV, Keller TM, Stanton BA (1988) Amiloride-sensitive cation channel in apical membrane of inner medullary collecting duct. Am J Physiol 255:F278–F286

23. Palmer LG (1984) Voltage-dependent block by amiloride and other monovalent cations of apical Na channels in the toad urinary bladder. J Membr Biol 80:153–165

24. Colquhoun D, Sigworth F (1983) Fitting and statistical analysis of single-channel records. In: Sackmann B, Neher E (eds) Single Channel Recording. Plenum, New York, pp 191–264

25. Sigworth FJ, Sine SM (1987) Data transformations for improved display and fitting of single-channels dwell time histograms. Biophys J 52:1047–1054

Regulation of K+ Channels in Proximal Tubules: Studies in Opossum Kidney Cells

Takako Ohno-Shosaku, Takahiro Kubota, Yoshiaki Mori, Jun Yamaguchi, and Mamoru Fujimoto[1]

SUMMARY. Using the patch clamp technique, we examined the properties of an inwardly rectifying K+ (K_{in}) channel, which contributes greatly to an overall K+ conductance in opossum kidney (OK) cells. The K_{in} channel was sensitive to Ba^{2+} and quinine, less sensitive to tolbutamide, and insensitive to tetraethylammonium (TEA). Experiments with inside-out patches demonstrated that the activity of K_{in} channels was regulated by intracellular Mg^{2+} and ATP. The K_{in} channel was inactivated by Mg^{2+} and reactivated by Mg-ATP, via a process requiring hydrolysis of ATP. The inactivation/reactivation of the K_{in} channel is suggested to be due to a dephosphorylation/phosphorylation of the channel protein. Intracellular pH also influenced the activity of K_{in} channels. The activity was low at acid pH and high at alkaline pH, presenting a sigmoidal pH-dependence with a half-maximum activation at pH 7.5. The pH-effects could be attributed to a combination of two different processes: one, a simple binding of H+ to the channel protein, and the other, a H+-induced inactivation of the channel, probably due to a dephosphorylation of the channel protein. These results suggest that under physiological conditions the K+ conductance of OK cell membranes is controlled by intracellular Mg^{2+}, ATP, and pH.

Introduction

Electrophysiological studies with conventional microelectrodes have demonstrated the presence of K+ conductive pathways in the basolateral membrane of proximal tubules [1]. The evidence so far suggests that the properties of the K+ conductance are subject to regulation, although the precise mechanisms are still unknown. The purpose of this study is to detect the intracellular factors regulating the K+ conductance, using the patch clamp technique, which enables us to examine the direct effects of intracellular factors on single K+ channels.

---

[1]Department of Physiology, Osaka Medical College, Takatsuki, Osaka, 569 Japan

Cultured opossum kidney (OK) cells [2] have been used as a model system for proximal tubular epithelia [3,4], since they retain some physiological functions of proximal tubules [5,6]. We have already found an inwardly rectifying K⁺ channel in this cell line [7], which contributes largely to the overall K⁺ conductance. In the following pages, the activity of the K⁺ channel, controlled by intracellular Mg^{2+}, ATP, and pH, will be demonstrated. Some of the results have been reported previously [7,8].

Materials and Methods

Cell Culture

OK cells were cultured in Dulbecco's modified Eagle's medium, supplemented with 10% fetal bovine serum, at 37°C in 5% CO_2. For patch-clamp experiments, the cells were harvested from confluent monolayers with trypsin, and were then incubated in the above culture medium for 4–8 hours before use. All experiments were performed at room temperature.

Electrical Recordings

Patch-clamp experiments were performed according to the method of Hamill et al. [9]. Electrical measurements and data analysis were made as described previously [8]. The composition of the solutions used in this study is given in Table 1. Patch pipettes were filled with either a 3 mM adenosine triphosphate (ATP) solution for whole-cell and outside-out patch experiments, or a K-rich solution for inside-out patch experiments. The pH values of ATP-free and 3 mM ATP solutions were adjusted to the desired levels with KOH or HCl, while the free Ca^{2+} concentration was held constant at either 10^{-8} M in ATP-free solutions or 3×10^{-7} M in 3 mM ATP solutions. The free Ca^{2+} concentration was calculated using the absolute values of the stability constants of ethylene bis(oxyethylenenitrilo)tetra-acetic acid (EGTA) for binding of Ca^{2+}, Mg^{2+}, and H^+ [10]. Values for the potential represent the voltages at the cytoplasmic side of the membrane with respect to the extracellular side. Currents flowing from the cytoplasmic side to the extracellular side were defined as outward and are shown as upward deflections in the figures.

Table 1. Compositions of bath solutions (in mM)

	NaCl	KCl	MgCl₂	CaCl₂	EGTA	HEPES	KOH	Na₂ATP	Glucose
Na-rich solution	140	5	1	2		10			10
K-rich solution		145	1			10			
Mg²⁺-, ATP-free solution		115		3	10	5	30		
ATP-free solution		115	1	3	10	5	30		
1 mM ATP solution		115	2	3	10	5	30	1	
3 mM ATP solution		115	4	3	10	5	30	3	

The pH was adjusted to 7.3 with KOH, NaOH or HCl. HEPES, hydroxyethylpiperazine ethanesulfonic acid

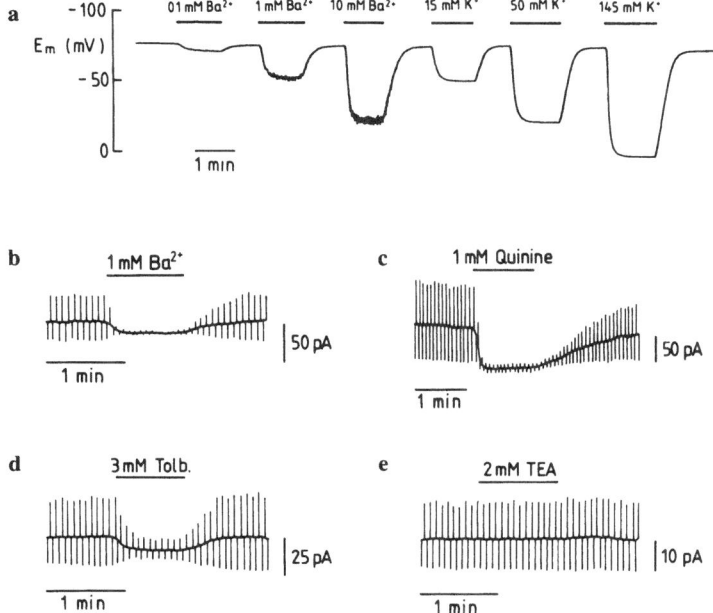

Fig. 1a-e. Whole-cell recordings of OK cells at the current-clamp mode (**a**) or the voltage-clamp mode (**b-e**). The bath contained a Na-rich solution with or without K⁺ channel inhibitor, or a solution with the indicated K⁺ concentration, which was made by replacing an appropriate amount of NaCl with KCl in a Na-rich solution. **a** The current was clamped at zero. **b-e** The membrane potential was clamped at -70 mV, and positive and negative voltage pulses of 10 mV were alternately applied to the membrane. The amplitude of the current deflection induced by a voltage pulse reflects a membrane conductance. Tolb., tolbutamide; TEA, tetraethylammonium

Results and Discussion

Whole-Cell Recordings

The electrical properties of the cell membranes were examined using the whole-cell configuration. The membrane potential was measured at the current-clamp mode, and the membrane conductance was measured by applying voltage pulses at the voltage-clamp mode. In a Na-rich solution the membrane potential was -69.4 ± 1.5 mV ($n=16$). Ba^{2+}, a K⁺ channel blocker, depolarized the membrane in a dose-dependent manner (Fig. 1a). The membrane potential was greatly affected by changes in K⁺ concentration of the bath solution, indicating a K⁺-selective property of the cell membrane. The cell membrane conductance was 1.38 ± 0.33 nS ($n=53$) in a Na-rich solution, and was effectively inhibited by 1mM Ba^{2+} (Fig. 1b). The effects of other K⁺ channel inhibitors were also examined (Fig. 1c-e). Quinine (1 mM) inhibited conductance as well as Ba^{2+}, whereas 2 mM TEA was without effect. Tolbutamide (3 mM), which is known to inhibit ATP-sensitive K⁺ channels at

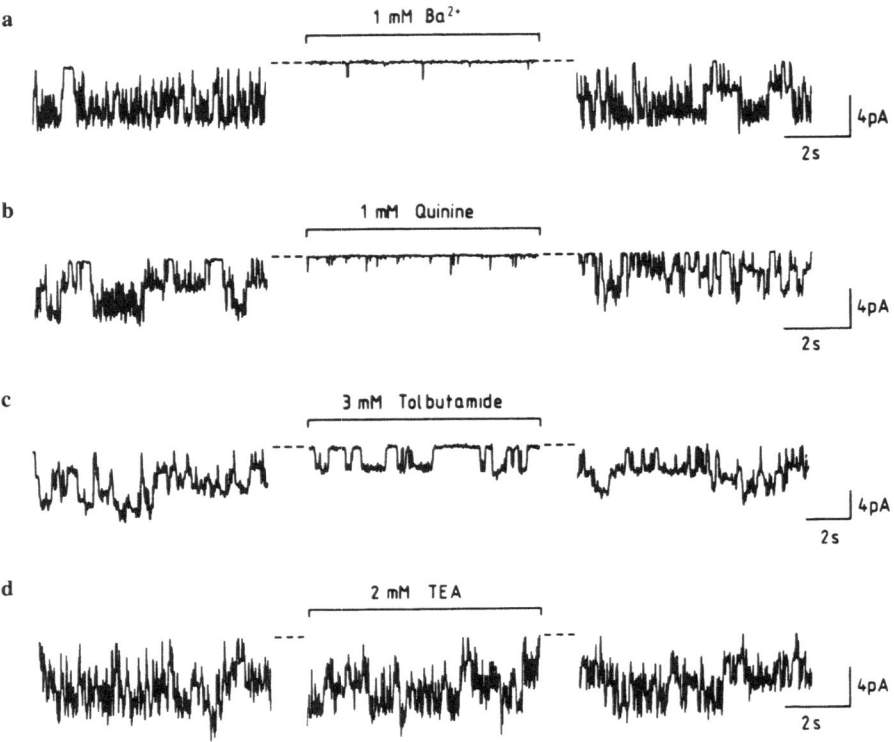

Fig. 2a-d. Effects of K$^+$ channel inhibitors on K$_{in}$ channels. These records were obtained from inside-out patches. The patch membrane potential was clamped throughout at -50 mV. The bath contained a 3 mM ATP solution with or without K$^+$ channel inhibitor

micromolar levels, inhibited the conductance only partially. These results indicate that the membranes of OK cells are K$^+$-selective and have a large K$^+$ conductance, which is inhibited by Ba^{2+} and quinine, but not by TEA.

Single-Channel Recordings

In order to find the K$^+$ channels responsible for membrane K$^+$ conductance, single-channel recordings were carried out. In cell-attached patches, an inwardly rectifying K$^+$ (K$_{in}$) channel [7] was most frequently observed. Since the other K$^+$ channels were rarely observed in cell-attached patches, we concluded that the K$_{in}$ channel contributed most to the membrane K$^+$ conductance in OK cells. This conclusion was further supported by other experiments, in which the effects of K$^+$ channel inhibitors were tested with outside-out patches. As shown in Fig. 2, the K$_{in}$ channel was inhibited strongly by Ba^{2+} and quinine, partially by tolbutamide, and was not inhibited by TEA. The sensitivities to these inhibitors were the same as those of the K$^+$ conductance of the cell membranes.

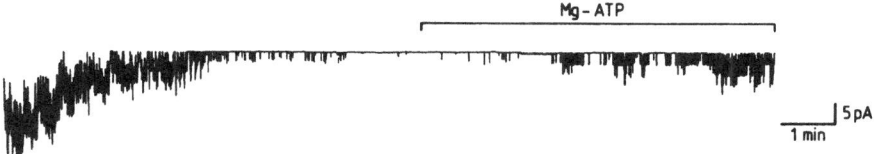

Fig. 3. Effects of intracellular Mg^{2+} and ATP on K_{in} channels. This record was obtained from an inside-out patch. The patch membrane was excised from the cell (at the left margin of the trace) in an ATP-free solution containing 1 mM Mg^{2+}, and then the internal surface of the patch membrane was exposed to 1 mM ATP solution. The patch membrane potential was clamped throughout at −50 mV

Effects of Mg^{2+} and ATP

The activity of K_{in} channels was stable in cell-attached patches. After excision of membrane patches from the cells (inside-out patches), however, channel activity declined with time ("run-down") in the absence of ATP (Fig. 3). This run-down was prevented by removal of Mg^{2+} from the bath solution, indicating that the run-down was due to a Mg^{2+}-induced inactivation of the channel. The channels inactivated by Mg^{2+} were reactivated by addition of ATP to the bath solution containing Mg^{2+}. The channel could not be reactivated by ATP in the absence of Mg^{2+}, or by AMPPNP, a nonhydrolyzable ATP analog, even in the presence of Mg^{2+}. Thus, the activity of K_{in} channels may be controlled by intracellular Mg^{2+} and ATP, probably via a dephosphorylation/phosphorylation process of the channel protein.

Effects of pH

The effects of pH on the K_{in} channel were examined, using excised patches. Changes in extracellular pH did not significantly affect the activity of the channel (Fig. 4a).

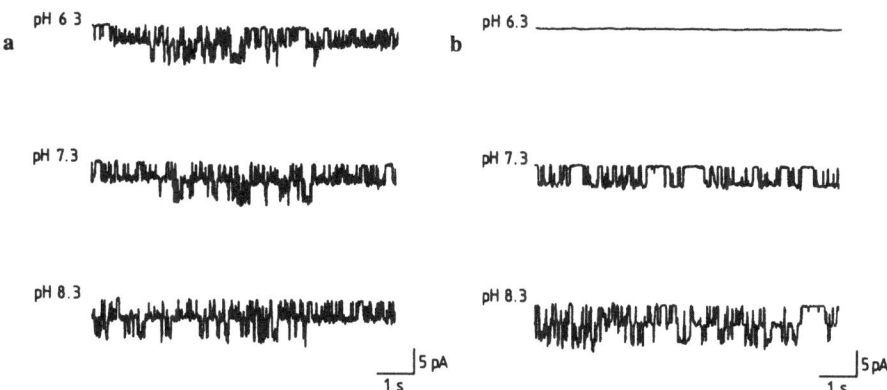

Fig. 4a,b. Effects of extracellular and intracellular pH on K_{in} channels. These traces were obtained from an outside-out (**a**) or an inside-out (**b**) patch. The patch membrane potential was clamped throughout at −50 mV. The bath contained a K-rich (**a**) or an ATP-free (**b**) solution adjusted to the indicated pH level

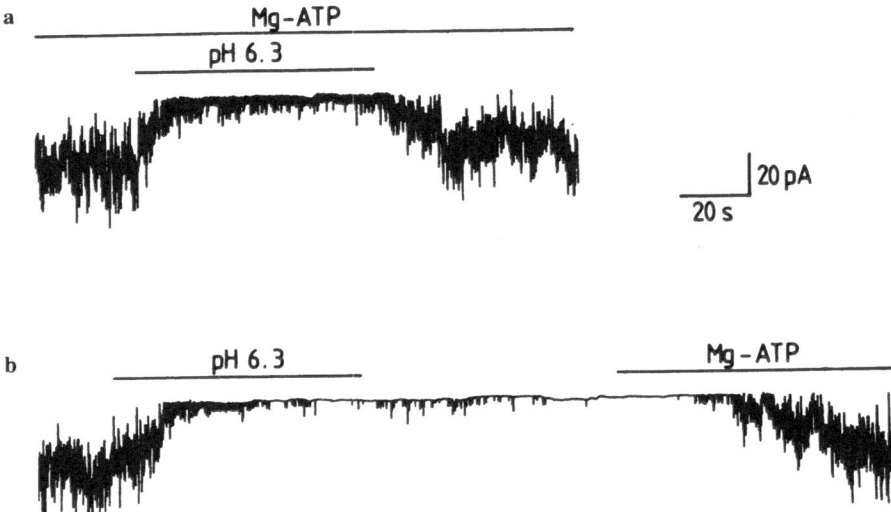

Fig. 5a,b. Effects of acid pH on K_{in} channels in the presence (**a**) or absence (**b**) of Mg-ATP. These records were obtained from an inside-out patch. **a**, the bath pH was changed from 7.3 to 6.3 by bath perfusion with 3mM ATP solutions for a given period of time. **b**, the bath pH was changed from 7.3 to 6.3 by bath perfusion with ATP-free solutions. After returning the pH to 7.3, ATP and Mg^{2+} were applied by perfusion with a 3mM ATP solution (pH 7.3)

On the other hand, changes in intracellular pH influenced channel activity remarkably (Fig. 4b). The channel was inhibited by acid pH and activated by alkaline pH.

The activating effects of alkaline pH were fully reversible, irrespective of the presence or absence of Mg-ATP. However, the inhibitory effects of acid pH were reversible only in the presence of Mg-ATP (Fig. 5a). In the absence of Mg-ATP, channel activity was not restored after returning the pH to 7.3 (Fig. 5b). This result indicates that H^+ inactivates the channels. The inactivated channels could be reactivated by adding Mg-ATP to the bath solution (Fig. 5b). All these findings would suggest that two different processes may be involved in the pH-effects: one, a protonation/deprotonation of the channel protein, and the other, a H^+-induced inactivation of the channel, which is probably caused by a dephosphorylation of the channel protein.

A Model of Channel Regulation

Figure 6 illustrates our model of channel regulation. According to this model, the K_{in} channel can be in four different states: one open state, where the channel protein is phosphorylated and deprotonated, and three closed states which are dependent on protonation and dephosphorylation of the protein. The transition from the open state to a closed state is considered to occur via dephosphorylation or protonation of the channel protein. The dephosphorylation process is promoted by Mg^{2+} and H^+, and the phosphorylation requires Mg-ATP. The observation that the channels inactivated by Mg^{2+} and H^+ in the absence of ATP were reactivated by Mg-ATP is consistent with this

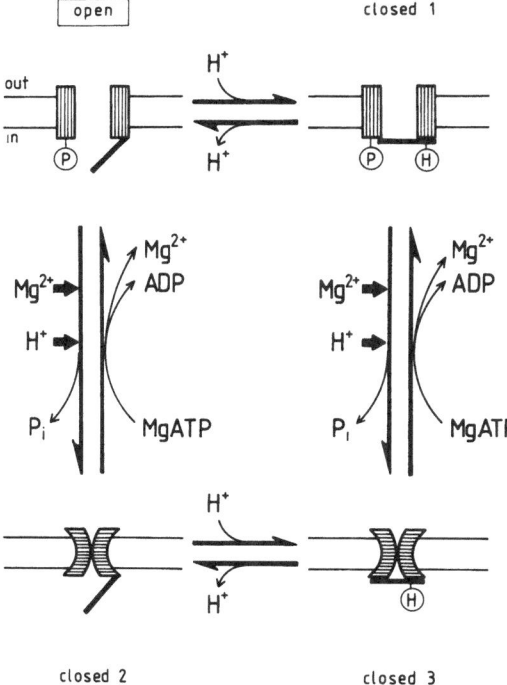

Fig. 6. A schematic model of regulation of the K_{in} channel

model. In the presence of Mg-ATP, the channel protein remains phosphorylated, because of continuous phosphorylation by Mg-ATP. Thus, this model can also explain the results which show that the pH-effects were fully reversible in the presence of ATP.

Acknowledgments. The authors are grateful to Dr. M. Fukase (Kobe Univ.) for providing us with OK cells, and to Drs. K. Kotera, N. Hagiwara and M. Kubokawa in our laboratory for their help, advice and encouragement in carrying out these experiments.

This work was supported by Grants-in-Aid for Scientific Research from the Ministry of Education, Science and Culture, Japan, and by a grant from The Salt Science Foundation to Prof. Mamoru Fujimoto (390B-4, 1990).

References

1. Giebisch G, Aronson PS (1986) The proximal nephron. In: Andreoli TE, Hoffman JF, Fanestil DD, Schults SG (eds) Physiology of membrane disorders. Plenum, New York, pp 669–700
2. Koyama H, Goodpasture C, Miller MM, Teplitz RL, Riggs AD (1978) Establishment and characterization of a cell line from the American opossum (*Didelphys virginiana*). In Vitro 14:239–246

3. Miller RT, Pollock AS (1987) Modification of the internal pH sensitivity of the Na$^+$/H$^+$ antiporter by parathyroid hormone in a cultured renal cell line. J Biol Chem 262:9115–9120

4. Ubl J, Murer H, Kolb H-A (1988) Ion channels activated by osmotic and mechanical stress in membranes of opossum kidney cells. J Membr Biol 104:223–232

5. Cole JA, Eber SL, Poelling RE, Thorne PK, Forte LR (1987) A dual mechanism for regulation of kidney phosphate transport by parathyroid hormone. Am J Physiol 253:E221–E227

6. Malmström K, Stange G, Murer H (1987) Identification of proximal tubular transport functions in the established kidney cell line, OK. Biochim Biophys Acta 902:269–277

7. Ohno-Shosaku T, Kubota T, Yamaguchi J, Fukase M, Fujita T, Fujimoto M (1989) Reciprocal effects of Ca^{2+} and Mg-ATP on the 'run-down' of the K$^+$ channels in opossum kidney cells. Pflügers Arch 413:562–564

8. Ohno-Shosaku T, Kubota T, Yamaguchi J, Fujimoto M (1990) Regulation of inwardly rectifying K$^+$ channels by intracellular pH in opossum kidney cells. Pflügers Arch 416:138–143

9. Hamill OP, Marty A, Neher E, Sakmann B, Sigworth FJ (1981) Improved patch-clamp technique for high-resolution current recording from cells and cell-free membrane patches. Pflügers Arch 391:85–100

10. Martell AE, Smith R (1977) Critical stability constants, vol 1. Other organic ligands. Plenum, New York

Regulation of K$^+$ Channels in the Thick Ascending Limb

WILLIAM B. GUGGINO[1]

SUMMARY. The apical K$^+$ conductance in the thick ascending limb (TAL) is important in the recycling of the K$^+$ which enters via the apical Na/K/Cl cotransport; in generating the positive transepithelial potential; and in the reabsorption of Na$^+$ across the paracellular pathway. Two types of K$^+$ channels have been identified in the apical membrane of the TAL. One group of K$^+$ channels is inhibited by ATP [1–3]; these are referred to as the ATP-sensitive channels. A second group is Ca^{2+}-activated [4–12]; because of their relatively large single channel conductance, they have been called Ca^{+2}-activated, maxi-K$^+$ channels. In this review, the properties and modulators of these groups of channels and their physiological role in TAL function are discussed.

Introduction

The TAL of the kidney reabsorbs NaCl, preferentially to water diluting tubular fluid [14]. The reabsorption of NaCl by this segment occurs via a combination of transcellular and paracellular routes. NaCl is taken into the cell across the apical cell membrane via a triple Na/K/2Cl cotransporter which is present in parallel with an apical K$^+$ conductance. This apical K$^+$ conductance functions to recycle the K$^+$ out of the cell across the apical cell membrane. Several transporters are present in the basolateral cell membrane, including the Na/K pump, a K$^+$ conductance, a K/Cl cotransporter, and a Cl$^-$ conductance. These basolateral transporters function to move Na$^+$ and Cl$^-$ out of the cell and to recycle the K$^+$ which moves into the cell via the Na/K pump (see Fig. 1).

The arrangement of an apical cell membrane, which is almost exclusively K$^+$ conductive and a basolateral cell membrane, which is conductive to both Cl$^-$ and K$^+$ is an important feature of the thick ascending limb. This arrangement of conductances

[1]Department of Physiology, the John Hopkins University, Baltimore, MD 21205, USA

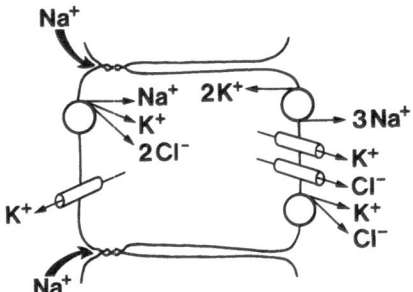

Fig. 1. A model of transcellular and paracellular ion transport in the thick ascending limb and the amphibian diluting segments. (Adapted from [14])

generates a lumen positive transepithelial potential, which, combined with a highly Na^+ conductive paracellular shunt pathway, allows about half of the Na^+ reabsorbed by the thick ascending limb to cross the paracellular pathway. This is an efficient mechanism, because for every Na^+ that is reabsorbed via a transcellular route an additional Na^+ is reabsorbed via a paracellular pathway. Because the Na/K pump is the major source of energy for the reabsorption of solutes by the thick ascending limb, this increased efficiency doubles the amount of Na^+ which is reabsorbed per turnover of the pump (see [14] for a review).

Several investigators have focussed attention on the biophysics and regulation of ion channels in the apical cell membrane of the thick ascending limb [1–12]. Most have utilized the path clamp technique, whereas others have isolated apical membrane vesicles to study the properties of the apical K^+ conductance, using radiolabelled K^+ or Rb^+ fluxes. These studies have been performed on rat or rabbit TAL cells, purified apical membranes, cultured medullary thick ascending limb (MTAL) cells, and amphibian diluting segments. The diluting segment is the amphibian homologue of the mammalian thick ascending limb.

Types of Potassium Channels in the Thick Ascending Limb

There are two classes of K^+ channels present in the apical cell membrane of the TAL and the diluting segment. The first group contains the ATP-sensitive K^+ channels (Fig. 2a). These channels have been observed primarily in both cell attached and excised patches of the apical cell membranes of freshly isolated TAL cells. The open probability of the channels is high in unstimulated cells (Fig. 2a). ATP-sensitive K^+ channels display inward rectification and a higher single channel conductance when current is carried into the cell than when current moves in the outward direction (Fig. 2b). The ATP-sensitive channels in the rat medullary thick ascending limb [1] have a higher single channel conductance (60 pS for inward current; 31 pS for outward current) than those in the rabbit [3] cortical thick ascending limb (22 pS for inward current; 10 pS for outward current). There are additional differences. The rabbit channel is not sensitive to either pH or Ca^{2+}, whereas the open channel probability of the rat channel is reduced by increasing H^+ or Ca^{2+} concentrations on the intra-

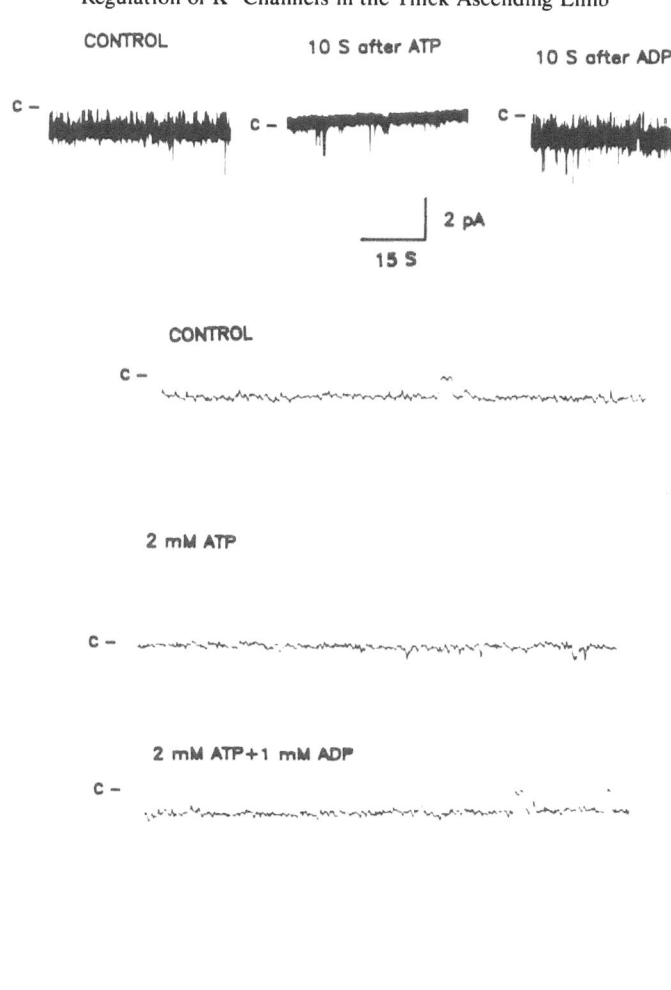

Fig. 2a. Inside-out patch at 33–37°C of the apical cell membrane of the rabbit TAL. Note that in control the channel is mostly in the open state; 1 mM ATP blocks the channel and 2 mM ADP reverses the effect. Recorded at 25 mV transmembrane potential (with respect to a bath ground). (Adapted from [3] with permission)

cellular face of the channel. The reason for these differences between the channels is not understood.

When exposed to millimolar amounts of ATP on the cytoplasmic face of the membrane in an excised patch configuration, channel open probability decreases dramatically, suggesting that ATP blocks these channels (Fig. 2a). The blocking effect of ATP can be reversed by addition of millimolar amounts of ADP. Thus, hormonal control of these channels depends heavily upon the metabolic state of the thick ascending

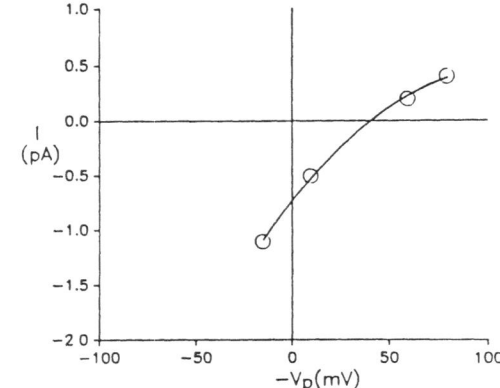

Fig. 2b. Current versus voltage relationship of ATP-dependent K⁺ channel in a cell attached patch of the rabbit TAL. (Adapted from [3] with permission)

limb cell. At high transport rates it is expected that Na/K pump activity is high and ATP concentrations are low. In this transport state, the channel will spend most of the time in the open configuration. If these channels are present in the apical cell membrane in large numbers, at lower levels of ATP, the channels would be expected to contribute significantly to apical K⁺ recycling.

A second group of channels found in the thick ascending limb and diluting segments includes the Ca²⁺-activated K⁺ channels (see Fig. 3a). These channels are activated by increasing concentrations of Ca²⁺ on the intracellular face of the membrane (Fig. 3b). In contrast to the ATP-sensitive channels, the Ca²⁺-dependent channels have a linear conductance over a wide range of voltages. They usually have a large single channel conductance of 100–200 pS.

Ca²⁺-activated K⁺ channel activity is voltage dependent, with positive voltages increasing and negative voltages decreasing, open probability. However, voltage does not directly affect the channel gating mechanism. Instead, voltage affects gating by influencing Ca²⁺ binding [4]. Ca²⁺-activated K⁺ channel activity is also decreased at acid pH (see Fig. 3b). Again, the effect of increased hydrogen ion concentration is not direct, instead it decreases Ca²⁺ binding to the gating mechanism. Finally, in one study, ATP has been shown to inhibit Ca²⁺-activated K⁺ channel activity in the diluting segment [9].

Two factors are thought to increase Ca²⁺-activated K⁺ channel activity in physiological conditions: antidiuretic hormone and membrane stretch induced by cell swelling. In the next two sections, I will focus specifically on these two mechanisms.

Hormonal Stimulation of Calcium-Activated Potassium Channels

An increase in net NaCl reabsorption by the thick ascending limb must involve increases in rates of transport through both the cotransporter and the apical K⁺ conductance (see Fig. 1). One factor which is known to increase NaCl reabsorption in

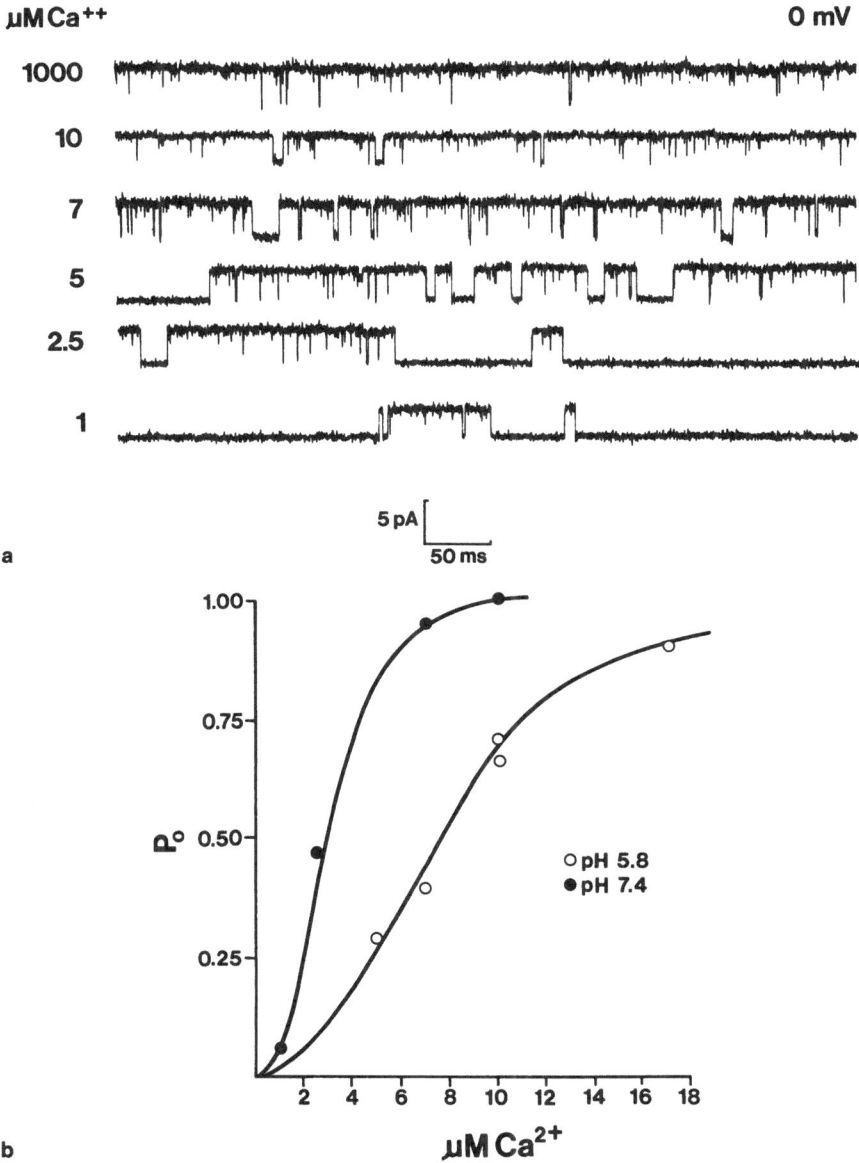

Fig. 3a. Ca²⁺ dependence of a K⁺ channel in the apical cell membrane of cultured thick ascending limb cells. The tracing is from an excised patch clamped at 0 mV. Ca²⁺ was varied on the intracellular face of the channel. **b.** Open probability versus Ca²⁺ of channels in an excised patch clamped at 0 mV. The channel spends about half of the time in the open state at 3 μM Ca²⁺ at pH 7.4 but is at almost 10 μM Ca²⁺ at pH 5.8. (Reproduced from [4])

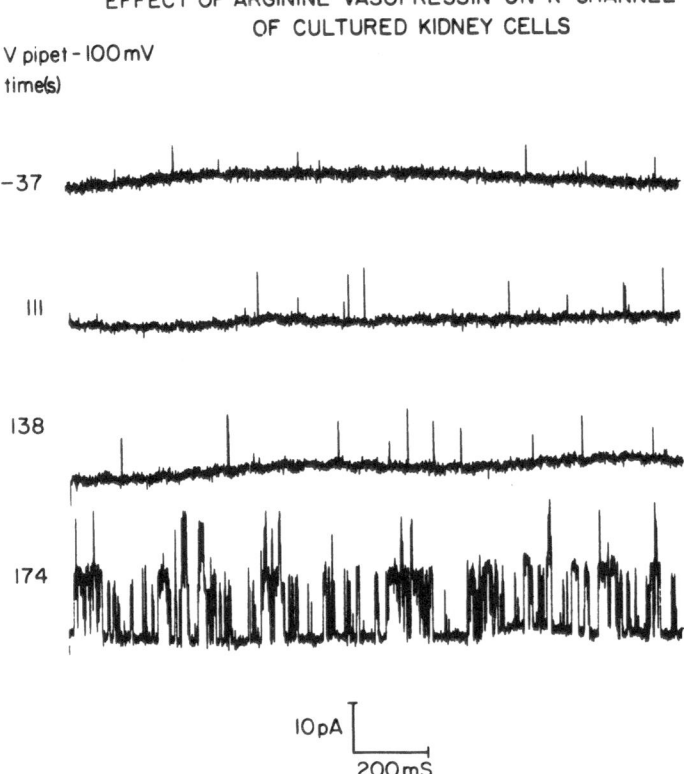

Fig. 4. The effect of arginine vasopressin (*ADH*) on a cell-attached patch held at 100 mV. *Top trace* shows that channel activity is low before ADH. *Lower traces* show the times for maximal increase in open probability to occur. (Reproduced from [8])

the mouse medullary TAL is arginine vasopressin ADH (see [15]). In cell attached patches of primary cultures of chick kidney cells, application of ADH increases Ca^{2+}-activated, maxi K^+ channel activity several-fold (see Fig. 4). Forskolin also activates maxi-K^+ channels in these cells. Since the major action of forskolin is to increase adenylate cyclase activity, the activation of Ca^{2+}-activated K^+ channels is probably via an increase in cAMP. Since ADH produces its effect through an increase in cAMP [16], it is safe to conclude that the ADH-induced increase in Ca^{2+}-activated K^+ channel activity occurs via an increase in cAMP levels. Although the final steps in the cascade by which ADH leads to an increase in channel activity are not known, experiments in isolated and purified apical cell membranes suggest that cAMP-dependent phosphorylation of the channel may play a role in activating Ca^{2+}-activated K^+ channels in this segment [11,24].

For example, Ca^{+2}activated K^+ channels can be purified from apical membranes of the mammalian thick ascending limb, using a calmodulin-affinity column [11]. These

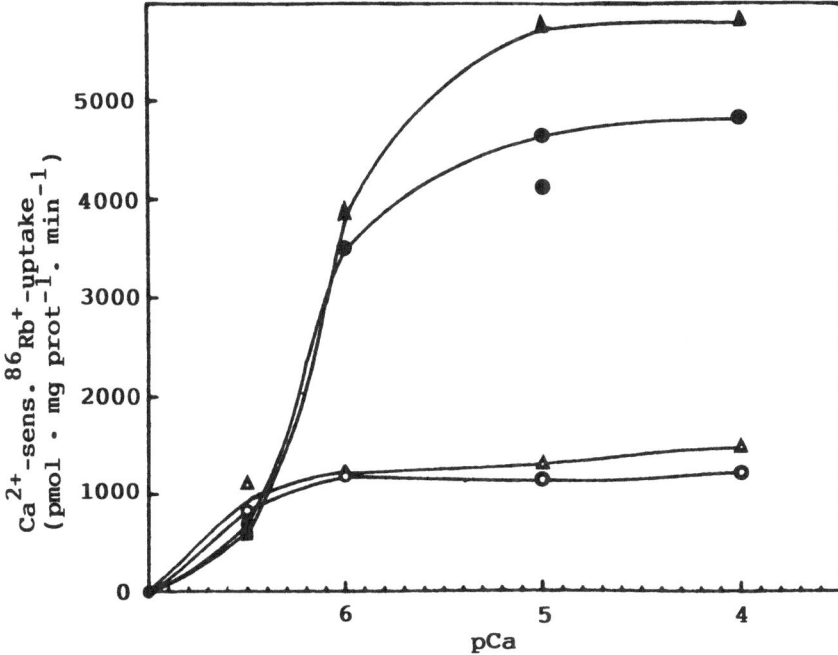

Fig. 5. ⁸⁶Rb⁺ uptake after phosphorylation of purified K⁺ channel protein in reconstituted vesicles (▲, ●) compared to uptake without phosphorylation (△, ○). K⁺ channel was purified on a calmodulin affinity column and reconstituted into phospholipid vesicles. Uptake was measured at different Ca²⁺ concentration. Uptake was also measured in the presence (▲, △) and absence (●, ○) of 0.1 μM calmodulin. (Reproduced from [11] with permission)

channels can also be reconstituted into phospholipid vesicles. Phosphorylation in this configuration by cAMP-dependent kinase stimulates by several-fold the maximum activity of Ca²⁺-activated K⁺ channels (Fig. 5). Interestingly, calmodulin by itself stimulates channel activity and is required for the phosphorylation-induced activation to occur. Since the activity of calmodulin is Ca²⁺-dependent andADH is known to cause an increase in intracellular Ca²⁺ in cultured cells, stimulation of Ca²⁺-activated K⁺ channels by ADH may involve the actions of Ca²⁺, both through calmodulin and cAMP-dependent phosphorylation.

Stimulation of Calcium-Activated Potassium Channels in Hyposmotic Solutions

Epithelial cells in the kidney medulla must maintain their volume despite large changes in extracellular osmolalities which occur during the diuretic versus antidiuretic state [see 13]. Thick ascending limb cells in isolated and perfused mouse tubules and in a cloned MTAL rabbit cell line regulate volume when exposed to hypotonic solutions [20]. In most kidney cells, K^+ efflux during volume regulation occurs via K^+ channels. There is evidence that Ca^{+2}-activated K^+ channels participate in regulatory volume decrease in hyposmotic solutions [12,18–21].

For example, in a cell attached patch configuration, stretching the cell membrane of cultured MTAL cells, by applying negative pressure to the patch pipette, causes a large increase in Ca^{+2}-activated K^+ channel open probability (see Fig. 6a). This effect is dependent upon extracellular Ca^{2+}, because removal of Ca^{2+} from only the pipette solution eliminates this effect of membrane stretch. Ca^{+2}-activated K^+ channels are not intrinsically stretch sensitive. For example, Ca^{+2}-activated K^+ channels are activated by membrane stretch only in the intact cell but not in excised patches.

Membrane stretch is expected to occur when cells swell following exposure to hyposmotic solutions. Figure 6b shows that exposing cultured medullary thick ascending limb cells to hyposmotic solutions causes a large increase in Ca^{+2}-activated K^+ channel open probability recorded in cell attached patches. This increase in open probability does not occur in the absence of extracellular Ca^{2+}.

These observations following membrane stretch or exposure to hyposmotic solutions suggest that membrane stretch acts to increase the influx of Ca^{2+} via stretch-sensitive Ca^{2+} channels. This influx of Ca^{2+} either raises intracellular Ca^{2+} directly or stimulates internal release. It is the increased intracellular Ca^{2+} which increases the open probability of Ca^{+2}activated K^+ channels in the apical cell membrane. The increase in Ca^{+2}activated K^+ channel open probability would result in enhanced K^+ loss from the cell. An enhanced K^+ loss, accompanied by anion, would be important for the volume regulatory processes of the thick ascending limb cell to occur. Similar activation of Ca^{2+}-activated K^+ channels by stretch has also been demonstrated in opossum kidney cells [21], in choroid plexus [18], and in *Necturus* proximal tubule cells [19]. In choroid plexus and *Necturus* proximal tubule, stretch is thought to act directly to increase Ca^{2+} influx, while in opossum kidney, Ca^{2+} is released from intracellular stores. The widespread occurrence of this Ca^{2+}-dependent stretch mechanism in different cell types suggests that maxi-K^+ channels may play an important role in volume regulation in hyposmotic solutions.

A rise in intracellular Ca^{2+} has been observed in cultured MTAL cells exposed to hyposmotic solutions (Figs. 7a and b). For example, exposure of cultured MTAL cells to hyposmotic solutions causes a maximal increase in intracellular Ca^{2+} in 40–60 seconds, followed by a decline toward baseline values (Fig. 7a). In hyposmotic solutions (42% decrease of osmolality), intracellular Ca^{2+} concentration increases from 163.5 ± 11.6nM (n=22) to a peak value of 738.6 ± 65.8 nM (n=22) at a rate of 12.5 ± 1.4nM/s (n=20). Intracellular Ca^{2+} concentration then decreases and reaches a value of 479.9 ± 43.4nM (n=21) at 200 seconds. Verapamil and nifedipine in the hyposmotic solution inhibit the increase of intracellular Ca^{2+} in a dose dependent manner (Fig. 7b). This sensitivity of Ca^{2+} influx to Ca^{2+} channel inhibitors such as verapamil and nifedipine [22] suggests that Ca^{2+} channels in either the apical or basolateral cell membrane of cultured MTAL cells are activated by stretch in hyposmotic solutions.

Thus, the simplest model of volume regulation in MTAL cells involves swelling which activates a nifedipine- and verapamil-sensitive Ca^{2+} channel. Increased entry through Ca^{2+} channels increases intracellular Ca^{2+} and thereby stimulates apical Ca^{2+}-activated K^+ channels to release cellular K^+. However, several pieces of information taken together show that the mechanism of activation of Ca^{2+}-activated K^+

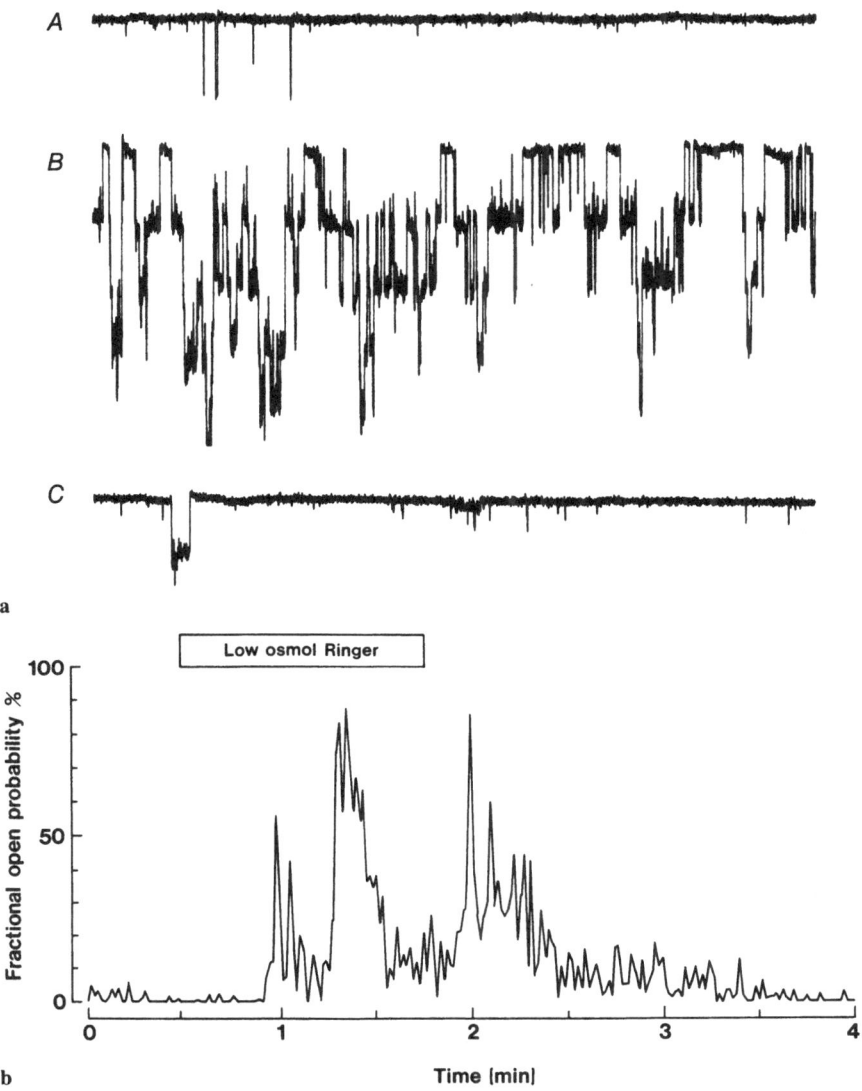

Fig. 6a. Negative pressure activation of K+ channels in apical cell membrane of an MTAL cell. Tracing from a cell attached patch clamped at 0 mV. *A* was recorded before, *B* during, and *C* following application of −40 cm water of negative pressure. Suction increased the open probability from 0.1 to 89%. **b** Time course of low osmotic pressure activation. Osmolalities of the control and low osmotic Ringer were 293 and 219, respectively. Data were obtained from a cell attached patch at 0 mV. (Reproduced from [12])

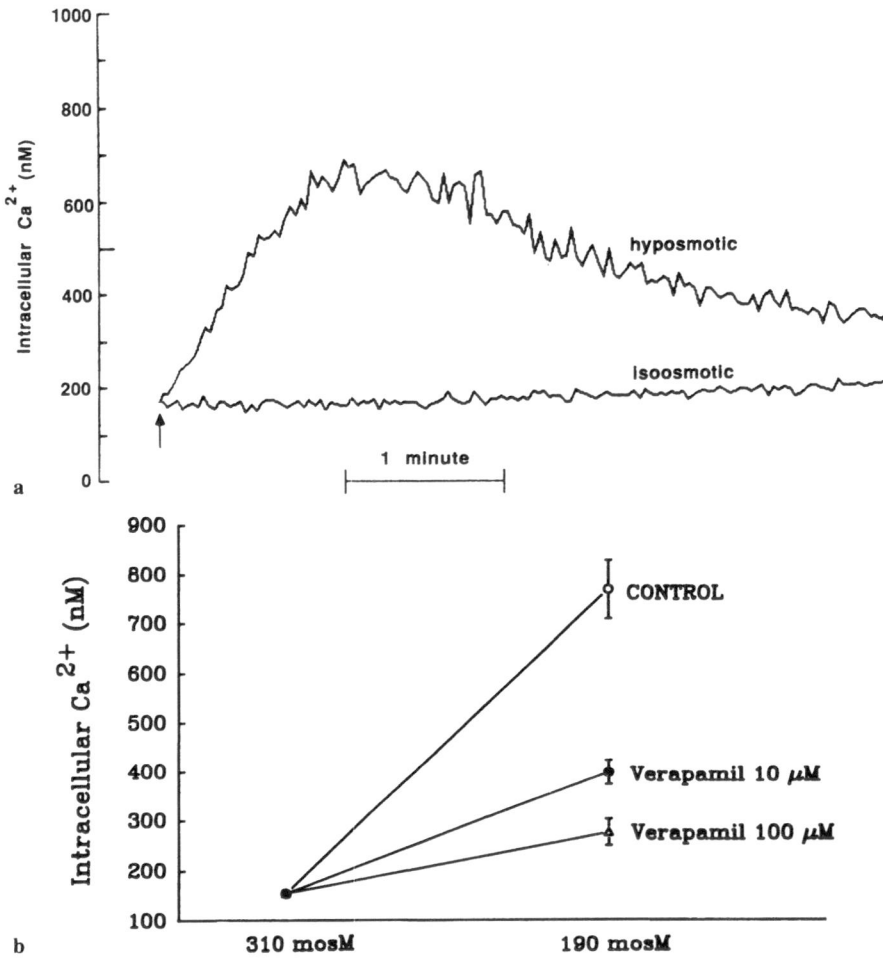

Fig. 7a. Measurements of intracellular Ca^{2+} in hyposmotic and isosmotic solutions. Aliquots of suspended MTAL cells were loaded with Fura-2 and fluorescence measured in an SLM-500C fluorometer. At the *arrow*, cells were exposed to either control isosmotic (315 mosmol/kg H_2O, *lower tracing*) or hyposmotic (180 mosmol/kg H_2O, *upper tracing*) medium. **b** Effect of verapamil on the hyposmotic-induced increase in intracellular Ca^{2+}. Peak increases of intracellular Ca^{2+} concentration in hyposmotic media were measured. The cells were exposed to hyposmotic medium (180 mosmol/kg H_2O) in the presence or the absence of two different concentrations of verapamil. The maximum increase of intracellular Ca^{2+} in these different conditions was measured. (Reproduced from [20])

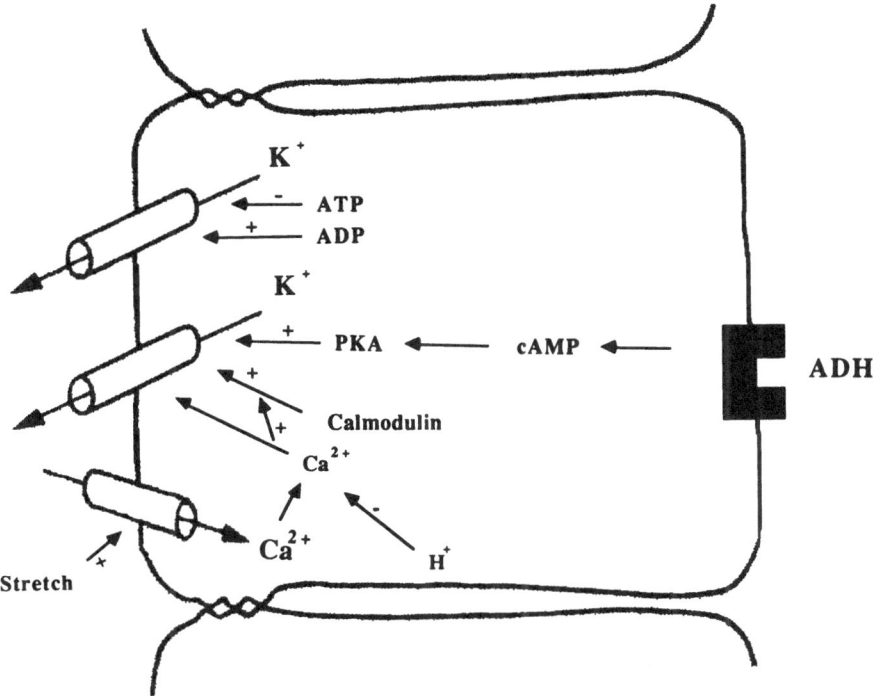

Fig. 8. Model of K⁺ channel regulation in the thick ascending limb. Three channels are depicted, *from upper to lower*: an ATP sensitive K⁺ channel; a Ca^{+2}-activated K⁺ channel; and a Ca^{2+} channel. For convenience the Ca^{2+} channel is located in the apical cell membrane, but direct evidence is not available for the exact location of the verapamil-sensitive Ca^{2+} entry pathway. (Model is a summary of data from [1–12] and [20–25]) ADH, arginine vasopressin

channels may be more complex. For example, in MTAL cells, one limitation of this hypothesis is an apparent discrepancy in the amount of Ca^{2+} released by hypotonicity versus the amount required to activate K⁺ channels. Open probability curves for Ca^{2+}-activated K⁺ channels in excised patches from MTAL cells show that these channels require 3uM Ca^{2+} to spend about half of the time in the open state (see Fig. 3b). However, exposure of cells to a change in osmolality that is known to stimulate Ca^{2+}-activated K⁺ channels in cell attached patches increases intracellular Ca^{2+} to only 400 nM. The channels would be expected to be mostly closed at 400 nM Ca^{2+}. As described below, at least two possible explanations could account for this apparent discrepancy.

First, stimulation of Ca^{+2}-activated K⁺ channels in hyposmotic solutions may not be driven directly via an increase in intracellular Ca^{2+}. For example, as mentioned above, Ca^{+2}-activated K⁺ channels purified from the apical cell membrane of thick ascending limb are stimulated by calmodulin and protein kinase A (see Fig. 5). It is possible that an increase in intracellular Ca^{2+} in hyposmotic solutions activates calmodulin, which in turn stimulates Ca^{+2}-activated K⁺ channels. Alternatively, hyposmotic solutions could cause a phosphorylation of the channel or an associated regulatory protein (perhaps via a Ca^{2+}-dependent kinase) which may cause activation of the channel.

Second, it is possible that the increase in intracellular Ca^{2+} in MTAL cells exposed to hyposmotic solutions is not uniform throughout the cell. The local Ca^{2+} concentration near the plasma membrane could be high enough to activate Ca^{2+}-activated K^+ channels. Recently, a restricted volume in cardiac cells, of only 0.3% of the total volume of the cell, has been hypothesized to exist near the plasma membrane [23]. If such a restricted volume of even 10% exists in intact MTAL cells, then the apparent rise of 400 nM could represent a 4uM increase in a local area near the plasma membrane.

Review

Two classes of K^+ channels have been identified in the apical cell membrane of the thick ascending limb. One class is inwardly rectifying and inhibited by ATP. ATP-sensitive channels have a high open probability in resting thick ascending limb cells and are probably involved in generating the resting apical K^+ conductance. A second class contains the large conductance, maxi K^+ channels. These channels have a very low open probability at resting levels of cell Ca^{2+}, but are stimulated by ADH and by hyposmotic solutions. Ca^{+2}-activated K^+ channels in the TAL are mediated by intracellular Ca^{2+}, pH, calmodulin, and PKA-mediated phosphorylation (Fig. 8). Clearly, K^+ channels in the apical cell membrane are highly regulated, which is important both for net transepithelial NaCl reabsorption and for volume regulation.

Acknowledgments. This work was supported by NIH grant DK 32753. Thanks to Dr. C. Montrose-Rafizadeh and Zeitlin for editorial comments on the manuscript.

References

1. Bleich M, Schlatter E, Greger R (1990) The luminal potassium channel of the thick ascending limb of Henle's loop. Pflugers Arch 415:449–460
2. Greger R, Bleich M, Schlatter E (1990) Ion channels in the thick ascending limb of Henle's loop. Renal Physiol Biochem 13:37–50
3. Wang W, White S, Geibel J, Giebisch G (1990) A potassium channel in the apical membrane of rabbit thick ascending limb of Henle's loop. Am J Physiol 258:F244–F253
4. Cornejo M, Guggino SE, Guggino WB (1989) Calcium-activated potassium channels from cultured renal medullary thick ascending limb cells:effects of pH. J Membr Biol 110:49–55
5. Cornejo M, Guggino SE, Guggino WB (1989) Calcium-activated potassium channels from cultured renal medullary thick ascending limb cells: effects of pH. J Membr Biol 110:49–55
6. Guggino SE, Guggino WB, Green N, Sacktor B (1987) Blocking agents of calcium activated potassium channels in cultured medullary thick ascending limb cells. Am J Physiol 252:C128–C137
7. Guggino SE, Guggino WB, Green W, Sacktor B (1987) Calcium-activated potassium channels in cultured medullary thick ascending limb cells. Am J Physiol 252:C121–C127

8. Guggino SE, Suarez-Isla BA, Guggino WB, Sacktor B (1985) Forskolin and antidiuretic hormone stimulate a calcium-activated potassium channel in cultured kidney cells. Am J Physiol 249:F448–F455

9. Hunter M, Giebisch G (1988) Calcium-activated potassium channels of Amphiuma early distal tubule: inhibition by ATP. Pflugers Arch 412:331–333

10. Hunter M, Kawahara K, Giebisch G (1988) Calcium-activated epithelial potassium channels. Min Electrol Metab 14:48–57

11. Klaerle DA, Jorgensen PL (1988) Role of calcium-activated potassium channel in regulation of NaCl reabsorption in thick ascending limb of Henle's loop. Comp Biochem Physiol [A] 90:757–765

12. Taniguchi T, Guggino WB (1989) Membrane stretch: a physiological stimulator of calcium-activated potassium channels in thick ascending limb. Am J Physiol 257:F347–F352

13. Montrose-Rafizadeh C, Guggino WB (1990) Cell volume regulation in the nephron. Annu Rev Physiol 52:761–72

14. Guggino WB, Oberleithner H, Giebisch G (1988) The amphibian diluting segment. Am J Physiol 254:F615–F627

15. Hebert SC, Andreoli TE (1984) Control of NaCl reabsorption in the thick ascending limb. Am J Physiol 246:F745–F756

16. Handler JS, Orloff J (1981) Antidiuretic hormone. Annu Rev Physiol 43:611–624

17. Hebert SC, Sun A (1988) Hypotonic cell volume regulation in mouse medullary thick ascending limb: effects of ADH. Am J Physiol 255:F962–F969

18. Christensen O (1987) Mediation of cell volume regulation by Ca^{2+} influx through stretch-activated channels. Nature 330:66–68

19. Filipovic D, Sackin H (to be published) Stretch-activated calcium currents in renal proximal tubule. Am J Physiol

20. Montrose-Rafizadeh C, Guggino WB (to be published) Role of potassium and calcium channels in volume regulation by rabbit medullary thick ascending limb vesicles. Am J Physiol

21. Ubl J, Murer H, Kolb H-A (1988) Hypotonic shock evokes opening of Ca^{2+}activated K channels in opossum kidney cells. Pflugers Arch 412:551–553

22. Hosey MM, Lazdunski M (1988) Calcium channels: molecular pharmacology, structure and regulation. J Membr Biol 104:81–105

23. Lederer WJ, Niggli E, Hadley RW (1990) Sodium-calcium exchange in excitable cells: fuzzy space. Science 248:283

24. Reeves WB, McDonald GA, Mehta P, Andreoli TE (1989) Activation of potassium channels in renal medullary vesicles by cAMP-dependent protein kinase. J Membr Biol 109:65–72

25. Hunter M, Oberleithner H (1988) Whole-cell potassium currents in single early distal tubule cells. Am J Physiol 255:F699–F703

Ion Channels in the Distal Convoluted Tubule in Primary Culture

Jean Merot, Michel Tauc, Michel Bidet, and Philippe Poujeol[1]

Summary. Cortical distal bright convoluted tubules (DCTb) were microdissected from rabbit kidneys and cultured in a hormonally-defined medium. The cultured cells grew as a monolayer and retained the morphological and biochemical characteristics of the original tubule. The cultured epithelia developed a transepithelial potential of 3.11 ± 0.53 mV that was oriented negatively towards the apical compartment. The apical membrane of the cells exhibited a sodium conductance sensitive to 10^{-6} M amiloride and 10^{-7} M phenamil and a small K^+ conductance which was blocked by 5 mM Ba^{2+}. The basolateral membrane was highly permeable to K^+. Patch clamp analysis conducted on the apical membrane of the cells revealed the presence of three types of ionic channel. The first was a small conductance cation channel (3 pS), sensitive to phenamil, which resembled the Na^+ channel, but the specificity of which seemed to be altered in excised configuration. The second was a non selective cation channel, it did not discriminate between Na^+ and K^+ and had a conductance of 20.5 pS. It was strongly voltage-dependent and required a high calcium concentration (1 mM) to its cytoplasmic face. The last channel was a small conductance highly selective K^+ channel (8 pS). These three channels could account for the macroscopic Na^+ and K^+ conductances found in the apical membrane of rabbit DCTb in primary culture.

Introduction

The study of the physiological properties of distal nephron segments is difficult owing to the presence of different cell types along this structure. In the rabbit, the very early distal tubule (bright part DCTb) contains only one cell type and the transi-

[1]Département de Biologie, Service de Biolgie Cellulaire, Centre d'Etudes Nucléaires de Saclay, 91191 Gif sur Yvette Cedex, France

tion to the following segment is sharp. However, probably due to the difficulties of gaining access to this segment in vivo and of microdissecting it without collagenase, little is known about the ionic channels present in the apical membrane. Cell culture technique provides a potential means of overcoming some of these problems. Thus, to investigate the properties of DCTb, we developed primary cultures of a well-defined nephron segment. The monolayers exhibited a transepithelial voltage, oriented negatively toward the apical membrane, which was inhibited by amiloride, phenamil, and 5 mM Ba^{2+} applied on the apical side. This confirms the results reported in DCTb perfused in vitro [1] and indicates that both Na^+ and K^+ conductances exist in the apical membrane. Patch clamp analysis reveals the existence of several types of channels which could well account for the macroscopic conductance of the apical membrane.

Materials and Methods

Primary Cultures

The primary cell culture technique has been described in detail in previous papers [2–4]. The cortical fragments of early distal convoluted tubule (bright part) of 4–5 week-old New Zealand rabbit kidneys were carefully dissected under sterile conditions. The kidneys were cut into small pyramids which were incubated in a dissection medium containing 0.1 mg/ml collagenase (Cooper, USA). The tubules were seeded in collagen-coated culture wells filled with primary culture medium composed of equal mixtures of Dulbecco's modified Eagle medium (DMEM) and HAM F12 (Gibco) containing 15 mM $NaHCO_3$, 20 mM HEPES (pH 7.5), 2 mM glutamine, 5 µg/ml insulin, 5.10^{-8} M dexamethasone, 10 ng/ml EGF, 5 µg/ml transferrin, 3.10^{-8} M sodium selenite, 10^{-8} M triiodothyronine, 100 U/ml penicillin, and 100 µg/ml streptomycin. Cultures were maintained at 37°C in 5% CO_2 − 95% air water saturated atmosphere. The medium was changed 4 days after seeding and every 2 days thereafter. The antibiotics were definitively removed from the medium after the first rinsing. The culture chamber was custom made. A polycarbonate filter formed the bottom of the cylinder and was coated with rat tail collagen. The surface available for tubular growth was 0.2 cm^2.

Electrophysiological Study

Vt was measured on 15–20-day-old cultures grown on permeable chambers by recording the difference between two calomel electrodes connected to the bathing solution by KCl-saturated Agar bridges (Keitley 601 electrometer). The basal side was grounded. The transepithelial resistance (Rt) was estimated by applying square-current pulses (1.5 µA, 2 sec duration) through Ag-AgCl electrodes and measuring Vt changes with electrodes placed as near as possible to the epithelium surface. Vt was measured with RPMI medium (Gibco) bathing apical and basolateral compartments. Rt measurements were corrected for series resistances measured after removing the cells from the support at the end of the experiment. All the experiments were performed at room temperature.

Patch Clamp Experiments

The single channel recordings were made on the apical membrane of 15–20-day-old cultured cells grown on a permeable support. Patch pipettes were made in two steps from hematocrit capillaries, using a vertical puller, coated with Sylgard 184 and fire polished immediately before using. Pipettes filled with NaCl solution had a resistance of 5–10 MΩ. Seals between 10 and 50 gigaΩ were achieved by applying a slight suction when the pipette was lowered onto the cell. Channel currents were recorded with RK 300 patch clamp amplifier (Biologic, France), stored on digital audio tapes using a DTR 1200 recorder (Biologic, France), and visualized on a digital oscilloscope (Nicolet Instruments, Madison, Wis., USA). For consistency throughout the paper the potential is defined as the potential on the cytoplasmic face of the membrane relative to the pipette. In cell-attached experiments, the intracellular potential that contributes to the actual membrane potential was assumed to be -60 mV. On the recordings given in the Figures, upward deflections represent currents of positive charge moving from the cell interior to the pipette. All experiments were performed at room temperature.

Data Analysis

Channel current amplitudes were measured by replaying the tape onto a digital oscilloscope (Nicolet Instruments, Madison, Wis., USA). The current-voltage (I/V) relations of the channels were constructed from the average amplitude of 10–20 well defined transitions between closed and open current levels at each applied potential.

Solutions

In patch clamp experiments the NaCl solution contained (in mM): 140 NaCl, 5 KCl, 1 $CaCl_2$, 1 $MgCl_2$, 5 glucose, and 10 HEPES, at pH 7.4. The KCl solution contained (in mM): 140 KCl, 5 NaCl, 1 $MgCl_2$, and 10 HEPES, at pH 7.2. The calcium concentration, (10^{-5} or 10^{-3} M), was adjusted by the addition of $CaCl_2$. In Cl^- free solution 140 mM NaCl was replaced by 70 mM Na_2SO_4. In Na^+ free solution 140 mM NaCl was replaced by 140 mM choline chloride.

Calculations

The values are presented as means $\pm$ SE. Student's t test was employed to determine statistical significances of differences.

Results

Electrophysiological Studies

The cultures growing on permeable chambers reached the edges of the culture wells (0.63 cm²) 15–20 days after seeding. They had a transepithelial potential that was oriented negatively towards the apical surface of the monolayer (Vt = -3.11 ± 0.53 mV, $n=9$). The apical and basolateral ionic membrane conductances of the cells were assessed by examining the effects of different ionic channel blockers and solutions on Vt. When applied on the apical side of the monolayer the diuretic amiloride (10^{-6} M) induced, within 1 second, a sharp depolarization (Vt = -0.43 ± 0.08 mV, $n=9$). Vt returned to its control value when amiloride was rinsed out. Phenamil (10^{-7} M), a specific epithelial sodium channel blocker, inhibited the Vt (-0.22 ± 0.11 mV, $n=8$) when applied on the apical side of the culture. As for amiloride, the effect was completely reversible. Addition of both drugs on the basolateral side of the cultured DCTb remained without significant effect on Vt. On the apical membrane, the application of 5 mM Ba^{2+} hyperpolarized the Vt (Vt = -6.9 ± 2.3 mV, $n=7$), whereas 10 mM tetraethylammonium (TEA) did not modify Vt. At the basolateral face of the monolayer, KCl solution or 1 mM Ba^{2+} induced a strong depolarization of Vt.

Patch Clamp Experiments

Gigaseals were obtained in 50% of the trials. In the cell attached mode only 10% of the patches contained channel activity. At least three different channels were characterized during the experimental series.

Poorly Selective Na⁺ Channel

Cell Attached Configuration

The predominant ion channel recorded in the cell attached mode had a low conductance and a slow open kinetic. An example of this, when pipette and bath contained the NaCl solution, is given in Fig. 1a. At resting membrane potential (Vm = -60 mV or Vp = 0) channel currents were directed from the pipette to the cell interior. The current amplitude was small (0.15 pA) and increased when the membrane potential was hyperpolarized from -80 to -120 mV. The current voltage relation for these experiments is shown in Fig. 1b. For membrane potentials between -140 and -40 mV, the relation was linear and the mean channel conductance was 3.0 ± 0.1 pS, ($n=5$). Due to the very low current flowing through the channel, it was impossible to detect a significant activity above -40 mV. Moreover, at high positive membrane potential, channel openings were never recorded. Similar data were obtained when the NaCl solution in the pipette was replaced by Na_2SO_4 solution (Fig. 1b). In a series of experiments we perfused both sides of the culture while the patch was in the cell-attached configuration with the tetramethylammonium (TMA)Cl solution, keeping the NaCl solution in the pipette. This maneuver induced, in some cases, an increase of channel activity. Figure 2b is an example of single channel records showing the appearance of inward current events after 3 minutes TMACl exposure. Histograms of currents amplitude shown in Fig. 2b demonstrate the increase in the channel openings at resting membrane potential (Vm = -60 mV, Vp = 0 mV). In this typical experiment the open probability increased from 0.03 to 0.6. From the I/V relationship after exposure to TMACl, the mean conductance was 6.70 ± 1.7 pS ($n=3$).

Excised Patch Configuration

In order to investigate the ionic selectivity of the channel, experiments were performed on excised patches. Inside-out patches were made from cell attached configurations. At first, the patch was studied with NaCl solution in the pipette and in the

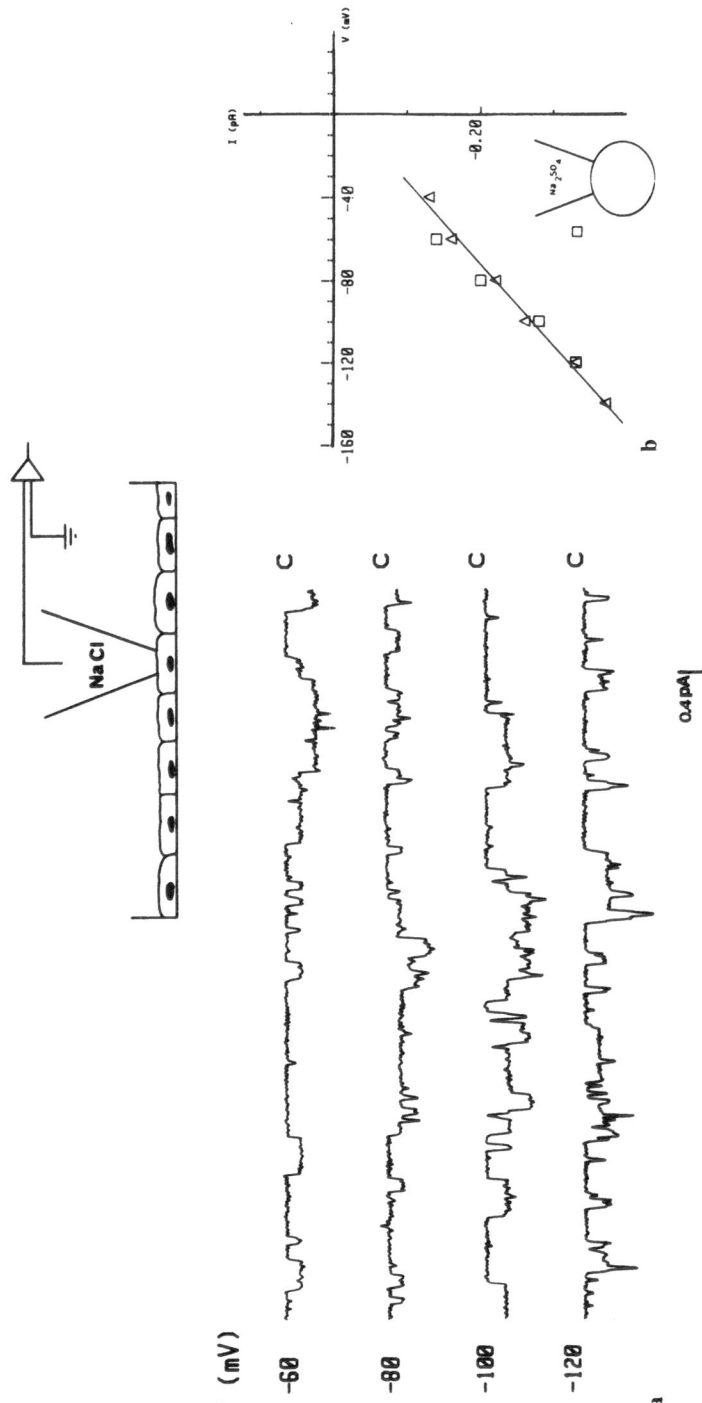

Fig. 1a. Single channel current recordings in a cell-attached patch. Channel openings are *downward*. The pipette and the bath contained NaCl solution. The membrane holding potentials are indicated on the *left of each recording*. *C* on the *right* of the *recordings* indicates the closed state of the chan- nel. **b** current-voltage (I/V) relationships of the channel in the cell-attached condition ($n=5$). The pipette and the bath contained the same solution as in **a** ($\triangle$) or contained 70 mM Na_2SO_4 ($\square$)

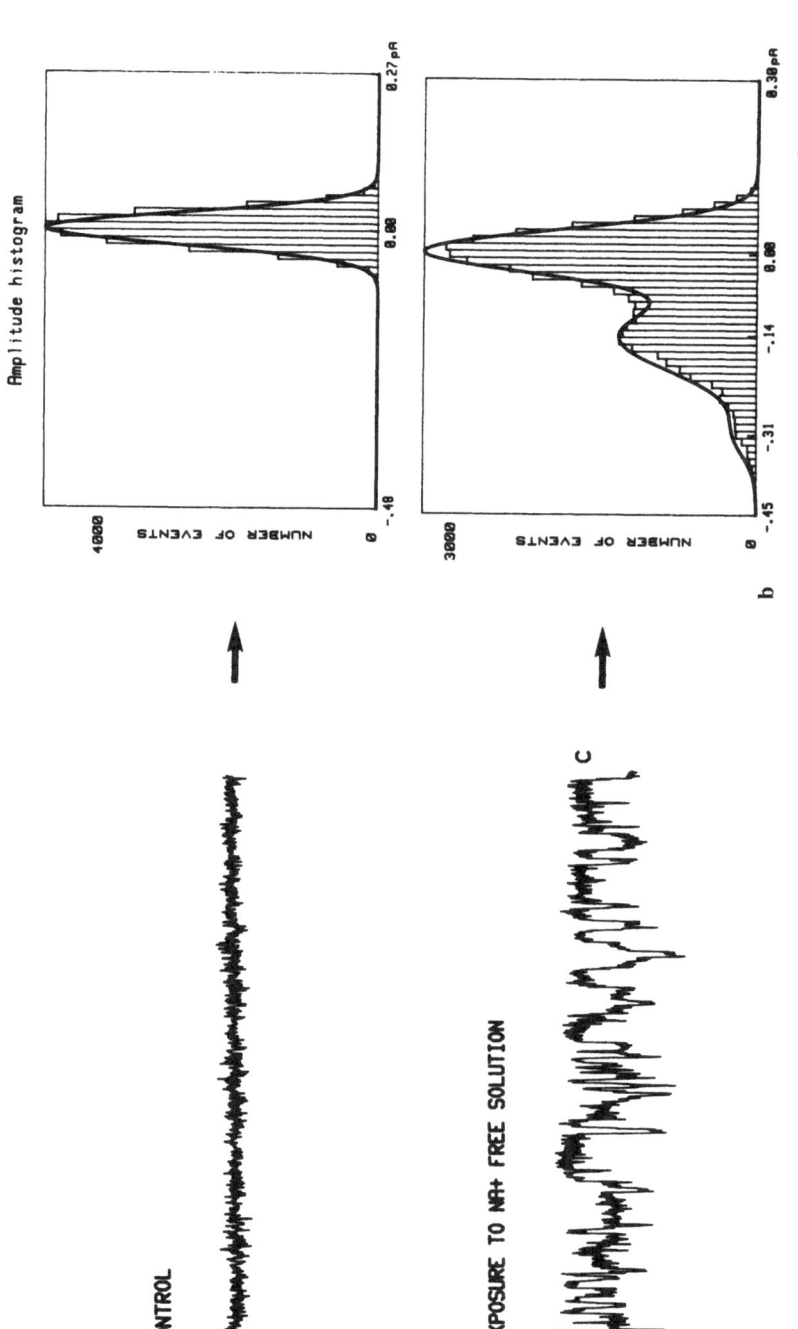

Fig. 2a,b. Effect of external sodium removal on the activity of poorly selective sodium channel, recorded in cell attached configuration. **a** The membrane potential was −60 mV (Vp = 0 mV) and the channel openings were *downward deflections*. **b** Current amplitude histograms plot channel events frequency versus amplitude (*pA*). Control histogram (*upper*) with the sodium solution in the bath shows that the channel was in closed state (0 pA). After replacing the tetramethylammonium sodium bath by (TMA)⁺, channel activity appeared in the patch membrane (*lower*)

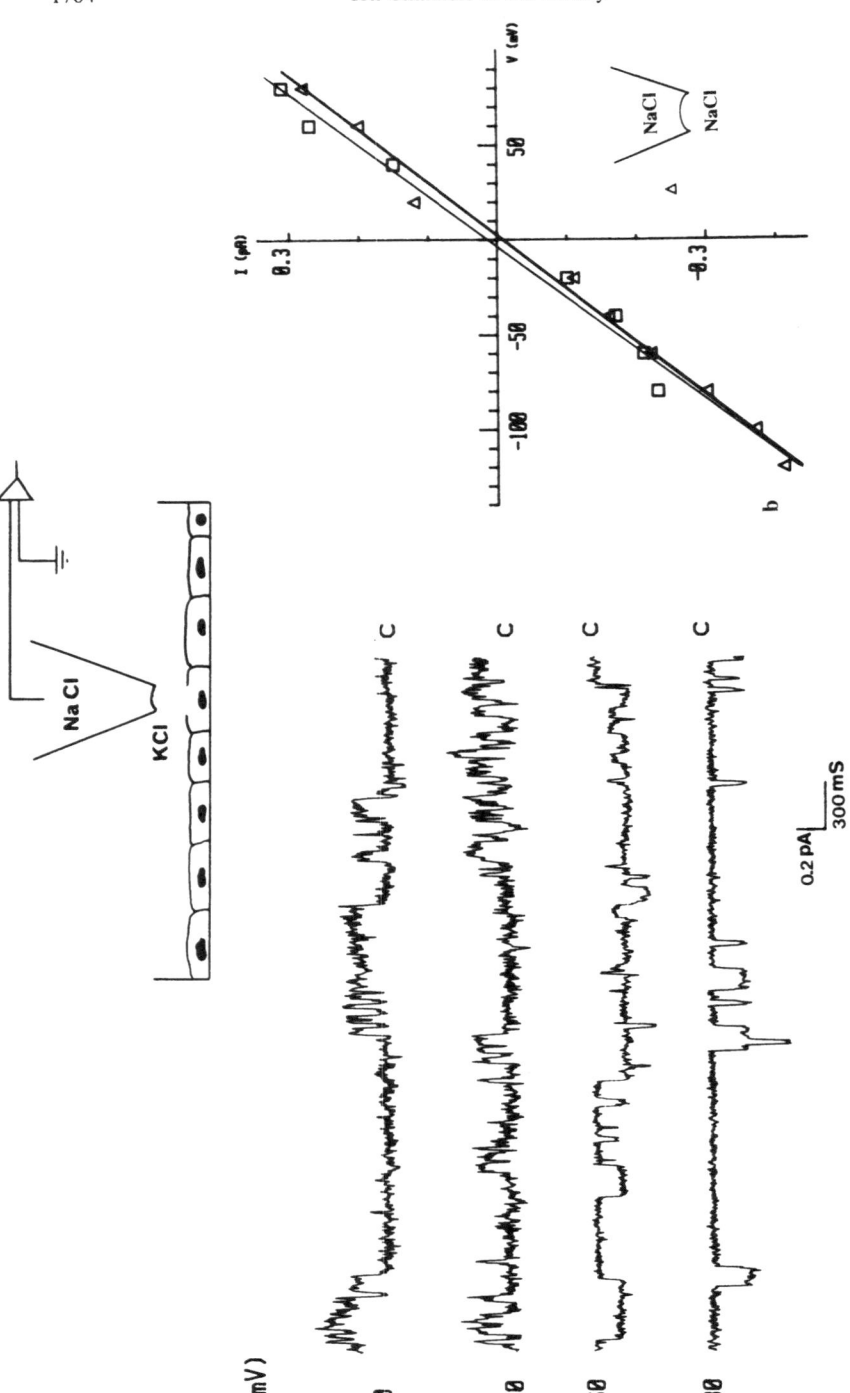

Fig. 3a. Single channel current recordings of the poorly selective sodium channel in an inside-out patch. The pipette contained NaCl solution and the bath contained KCl solution. Membrane holding potentials are given on the *left* of the recordings. C indicates the closed state of the channel. **b** current-voltage (I/V) relationships of the channel in the excised patch. The pipette and the bath contained NaCl solution (Δ, n=5). The bath solution was replaced by KCl solution (□, n=5)

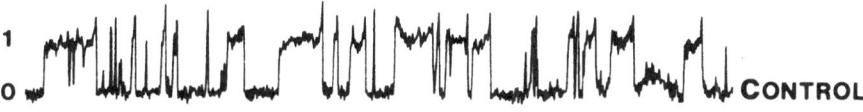

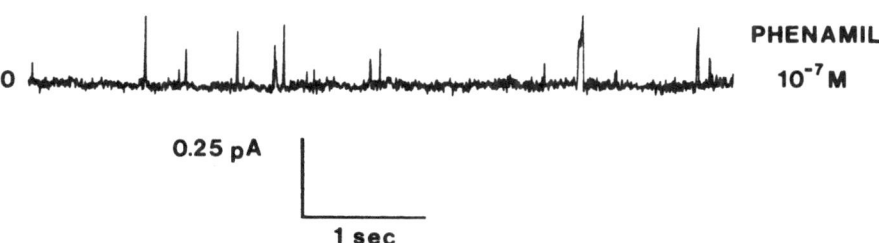

Fig. 4. Effect of 10^{-7} M phenamil applied on the cytosolic side of an inside-out excised patch. The membrane holding potential was $+80$ mV. The pipette contained NaCl solution and the bath contained KCl solution. The recordings represented three different experiments

bath and the I/V curves were constructed, then the cytoplasmic NaCl solution was replaced by KCl solution. Figure 3a illustrates the single channel currents recorded in KCl solution. At -60 and -80 mV holding potentials, the channel openings were downward deflections. Positive membrane potentials increased the noise of the recording and often broke the seal. The channel openings were upward directed and the current amplitude was near that measured at negative potentials. The I/V relationship was linear with a 0 mV reversal potential, and the channel conductance was 3.8 ± 0.2 pS ($n=5$). These values were not significantly different from those obtained when the bath contained the NaCl solution (Fig. 3b). The data indicate a low selectivity for Na$^+$ over K$^+$ ions.

The effect of phenamil on channel activity was tested from the cytosolic side of the inside-out patches (Fig. 4). Addition of 10^{-7} M phenamil almost completely inhibited the channel openings.

Non Selective Cationic Channel

Another type of ionic channel was observed in excised inside-out patches, although no channel activity was recorded in the cell attached condition. Typical channel current recordings are presented in Fig. 5a, where the pipette contained the NaCl solution and the bath the KCl solution. The channel openings are upward at negative holding membrane potentials (-40, -80 mV), and downward at positive potentials. The I/V relationship of the channel in these experiments was linear (Fig. 5b) and a channel conductance of 22.9 ± 1.2 pS ($n=5$) was calculated from the slope of the straight line. The current reversal potential was not different from 0 mV. Since the equilibrium potentials for Na$^+$, K$^+$, and Cl$^-$ were $+84$, -84, and 0 mV respectively,

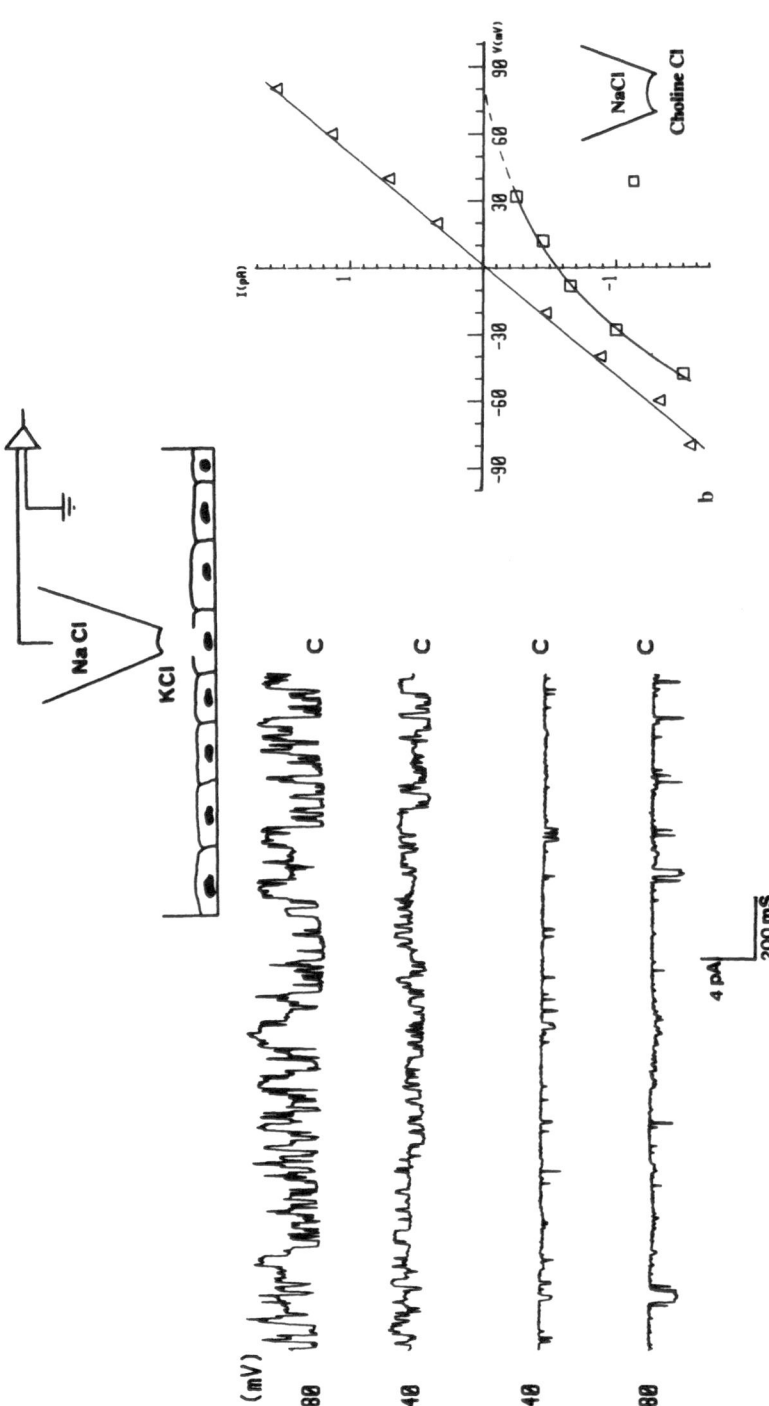

Fig. 5.a. Single channel current recordings of the non-selective cationic channel in an excised inside-out patch. The pipette contained NaCl solution and the bath contained KCl solution. The different membrane holding potentials are indicated on the *left* of each recording. *C* indicates the closed state of the channel. **b** current-voltage (I/V) relationships of the channel in different conditions. (△) corresponds to experiments in which pipette and bath contained the same solutions as in **a** (□) represents experiments in which the bath contained a choline chloride solution

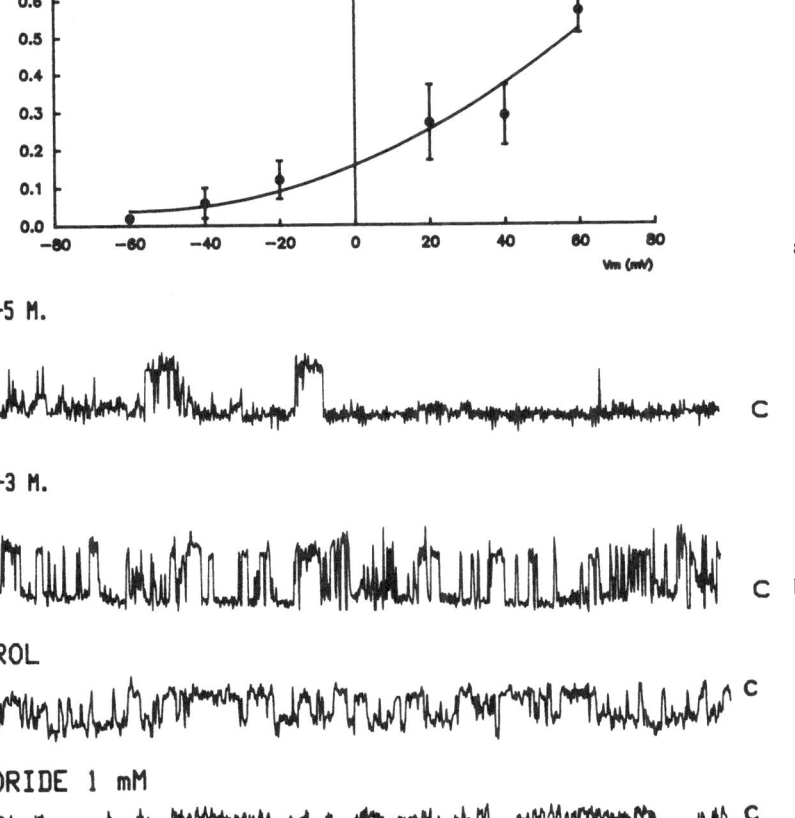

Ca++ 10-5 M.

C

Ca++ 10-3 M.

C   b

CONTROL

C

AMILORIDE 1 mM

C

PHENAMIL 10⁻⁶ M

C

1 pA

100 mS

c

Fig. 6.a. Open probability of the non-selective cationic channel versus membrane holding potentials. The data were fitted according to exponential function. **b** Effect of cytosolic calcium concentration on non-selective cationic channel activity. The pipette contained NaCl solution and the bath contained KCl solution with two different Ca^{2+} concentrations. The membrane holding potential was +60 mV and the channel openings were *upward* deflections. **c** Effects of amiloride and phenamil on non-selective cationic channel recorded on an inside-out excised patch. The pipette contained NaCl solution and the bath contained KCl solution. The membrane holding potential was −60 mV and the channel openings were *downward* deflections. C indicates the closed state of the channel

the channel must either not have discriminated between Na$^+$ and K$^+$ or must have been Cl$^-$ selective. To investigate these possibilities, the KCl in the bath was replaced by 140 mM Na gluconate. Because this maneuver did not significantly modify the reversal potential (data not given) we concluded that the channel was cationic and did not discriminate between Na$^+$ and K$^+$. In contrast, replacement of bath NaCl solution by choline chloride modified the I/V relationship, since a Goldman type rectification for Na$^+$ ions was observed. In this condition, the maximal channel conductance was 22.4 pS and the reversal potential obtained by extrapolation of the I/V curve was 80 mV.

The channel activity was clearly voltage-dependent. As illustrated in Fig. 6a, the opening probability was an exponential function of the membrane potential. Another characteristic of the channel is the high calcium concentration needed on the cytoplasmic side for its activation. Figure 6b illustrates an experiment in which a patch was excised in a KCl solution containing 10 μM calcium. Only one channel of low activity was observed: increasing the calcium concentration to 1 mM enhanced the channel activity. To test whether the non selective cation channels might correspond to the poorly selective Na$^+$ channel described above, we applied high amiloride concentration or 10^{-7} M phenamil on the cytoplasmic face of an inside-out excised patch. Neither drugs inhibited the channel (Fig. 6c).

K$^+$ Channels

In excised patch experiments, we recorded a K$^+$ channel, although no activity was found in the cell attached configuration. Figure 7a shows the single channel currents when the pipette contained the NaCl solution and the bath contained KCl solution. At 0 mV holding potential, the channel openings were upwardly directed and might have corresponded to K$^+$ currents, since Na$^+$ currents would have produced downward deflections and Cl$^-$ was at the electrochemical equilibrium. The I/V relationship was linear (Fig. 7b) and the extrapolated reversal potential was -76 ± 9 mV ($n=3$) (Fig. 7b), indicating a high selectivity for K$^+$ over Na$^+$ ions (pK/pNa = 65). Figure 7c shows that the addition of 1 mM barium to the cytosolic side of the patch completely blocked the channel activity recorded at 0 mV.

Discussion

In an attempt to further understand the function of DCTb, we undertook primary cultures of microdissected nephron segments. Most of the morphological, biochemical and antigenic properties of DCTb in primary culture have been described in detail in a previous paper [4]. Monitoring the transepithelial voltage and resistance showed that Vt was inhibited by the diuretic drug amiloride at low concentration. This effect was rapid and completely reversible. It indicates the existence of a Na$^+$ channel in the apical membrane of DCTb in culture [5], a hypothesis confirmed by experiments using phenamil. Phenamil is a derivative of amiloride, which is the most potent known inhibitor of the epithelial Na$^+$ channel [6,7]. With regard to the K$^+$ movements, barium applied apically hyperpolarized the Vt, showing a small K$^+$ conductance at this level. In contrast, barium applied to the basolateral side of the monolayer strongly depolarized the Vt, as did KCl perfusion. Thus our data are quite in agree-

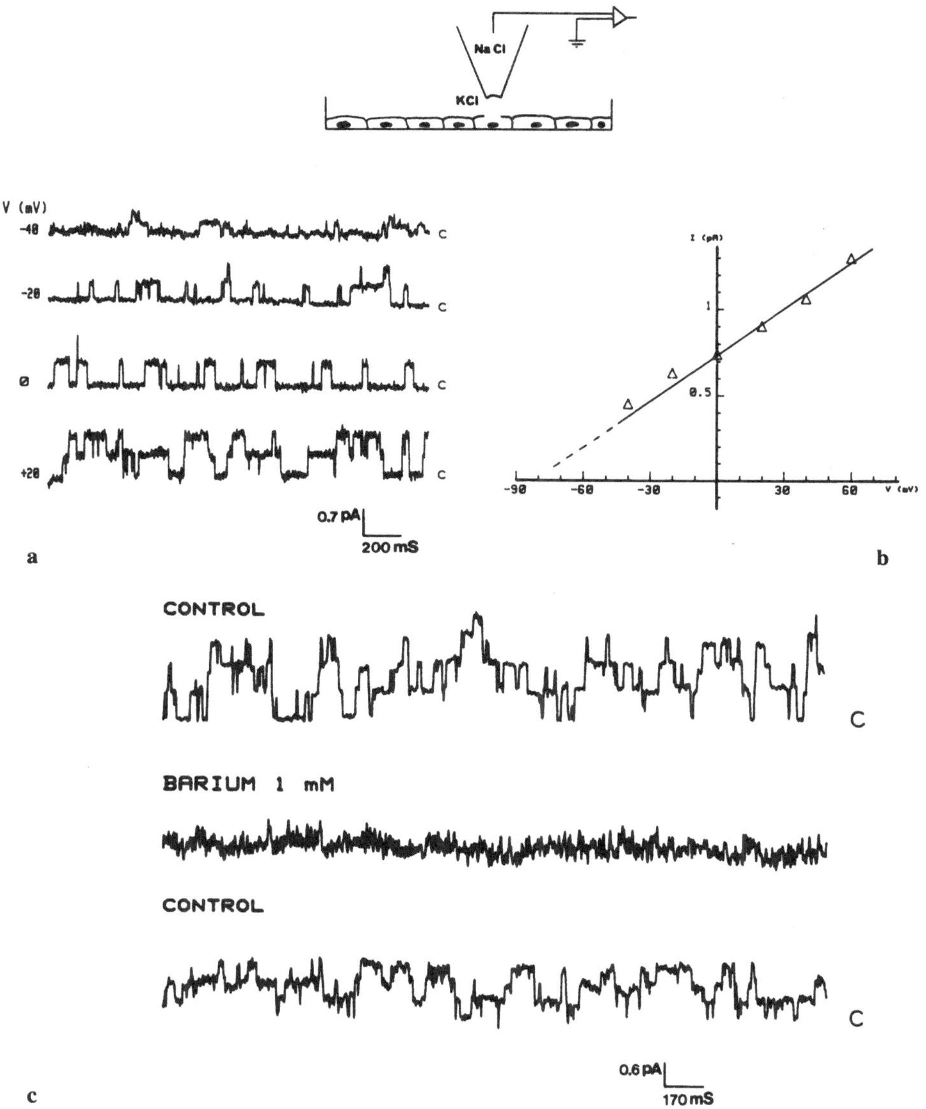

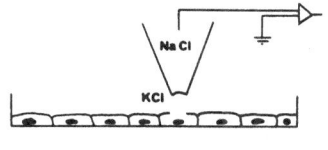

Fig. 7.a. Single K⁺ channel currents recorded in an inside-out excised patch. The pipette contained NaCl solution and the bath contained KCl solution. Membrane holding potentials are given on the *left* of the *recordings*. *C* indicates the closed state of the channel. **b** current-voltage (I/V) relationship of the channel in excised patches (*n*=3). The pipette and the bath contained the same solution as in **a**. **c** Effect of barium on K⁺ channel currents recorded in an inside-out patch. The pipette contained NaCl solution and the bath contained KCl solution with or without 1 mM barium. The membrane holding potential was 0 mV and the channel openings were *upward* deflections

ment with those reported by Yoshitomi et al. [8] on in vitro microperfused rabbit DCT. Single channel analysis performed on the apical membrane revealed the existence of various ionic channels, one of which was recorded in the cell attached configuration. It was a small conductance channel (3 pS) and the data lead us to conclude that in this configuration the current was probably carried by Na$^+$ ions. However, when the patches were excised from the membrane, the channel also allowed K$^+$ to pass. The gating properties (data not shown) and the conductance of this channel were not modified by the excision process. Moreover, phenamil (10^{-7} M) completely inhibited the channel openings, although the current flowing through the channel was K$^+$ current (Fig. 4). According to Palmer and Frindt [9], in the rat collecting duct, Na$^+$ channels have a low conductance but have a very high Na$^+$ selectivity. However, conditions could exist where this selectivity may be impaired. Thus, it appears that the ionic selectivity of Na$^+$ channels could depend on the culture conditions [10] and/or on the lipidic environment of the channel itself [11]. Moreover, a process of degradation by proteolytic enzymes could also explain the loss of selectivity of some Na$^+$ channels [12]. In cell attached experiments we have observed that the replacement of external Na$^+$ by TMA induced the appearance of channel activity. For the moment we have no further indication regarding the ionic selectivity of this channel. However, in the light of experiments performed by Ling and Eaton [131], this channel could correspond to a Na$^+$ channel which was masked by the Na$^+$ self-inhibition phenomenon. In addition to this channel species, the apical membrane contained another channel which did not discriminate between Na$^+$ and K$^+$. Its gating behavior, conductance, and low Ca^{2+} sensitivity were very similar to those reported for the Ca^{2+} sensitive cation channel in various tissues [3,14,15]. In the cultured DCTb we, unfortunately, never demonstrated the channel in the cell-attached configuration. Paulais et al. [16] have recently shown that a Ca^{2+} activated non specific cation channel is present in the basolateral membrane of the mouse cortical thick ascending limb (cTAL). Moreover, another type of non selective cation channel was recorded in the basolateral membrane of the rabbit proximal tubule [17], so the channel could exist in the intact structure. We have already found a non selective cation channel in the apical membrane of each of the nephron segments that we have cultured, i.e., proximal convoluted tubule [3], cortical thin ascending limb [18], and cortical collecting tubule [19]. As in the present study, this channel was never sensitive to amiloride or phenamil. Light et al. [20], on the other hand, observed an amiloride sensitive non specific cation channel in the apical membrane of inner medullary collecting duct in primary culture. Thus the question arises whether there are several kinds of non-specific cation epithelial channels. In the excised configuration we also found a low conductance high selective K$^+$ channel, which showed some analogies with that described in the apical membrane of rabbit [21] and rat [22] cortical collecting tubule.

In conclusion, the present study demonstrates that the electrophysiological properties of DCTb can profitably be investigated in primary culture. The action of amiloride and phenamil in depolarizing the Vt indicates the presence of a Na$^+$ conductance in the apical membrane of DCTb in culture. By using the patch clamp technique we identified a channel which could account for the Na$^+$ conductance, although we were not able to establish its selectivity with certainty. We also recorded a non selective cation channel, the exact role of which remains to be determined. Nevertheless, since we have shown that 10^{-6} M amiloride blocked 85% of the Vt, it is possible that the remaining 13% would be due to sodium transport via the non-selective channel which is insensitive to amiloride. On the other hand, the low conductance K⁺ channel that we have demonstrated in the apical membrane could mediate K⁺ secretion in DCTb. Such a secretion has now been demonstrated by Shimizu et al. in microperfused DCTb [1].

References

1. Shimizu T, Yoshitomi K, Taniguchi J, Imai M (1989) Effect of high NaCl intake on Na⁺ and K⁺ transport in the rabbit distal convoluted tubule. Pflugers Arch 414:500–508
2. Tauc M, Merot J, Bidet M, Koechlin N, Gastineau M, Othmani L, Poujeol P (1989) Antigenic expression of aminopeptidase M, dipeptidyl-peptidase IV and endopeptidase by primary cultures from rabbit kidney proximal tubule. Histochemistry 91:17–30
3. Merot J, Bidet M, Gachot B, Le Maout S, Tauc M, Poujeol P (1988) Patch clamp study on primary culture of isolated proximal convoluted tubules. Pflugers Arch 413:51–61
4. Merot J, Bidet M, Gachot B, Le Maout S, Koechlin N, Tauc M, Poujeol P (1989) Electrical properties of rabbit early distal convoluted tubule in primary culture. Am J Physiol 257:F288–F299
5. Garty H, Benos DJ (1988) Characteristics and regulatory mechanisms of the amiloride-blockable Na⁺ channel. Physiol Rev 68:309–373
6. Barbry P, Frelin C, Vigne P, Cragoe ED, Lazdunski M (1988) ³[H]Phenamil, a radio-labelled diuretic for the analysis of amiloride-sensitive Na⁺ channels in kidney membranes. Biochem Biophys Res Commun 135:25–32
7. Garvin JL, Simon SA, Cragoe EJ, Mandel LJ (1985) Phenamyl: an irreversible inhibitor of sodium channels in the toad urinary bladder. J Membr Biol 87:45–54
8. Yoshitomi K, Shimizu T, Taniguchi J, Imai M (1989) Electrophysiological characterization of rabbit distal convoluted tubule cell. Pflugers Arch 414:457–463
9. Palmer LG, Frindt G (1986) Amiloride sensitive Na channels from the apical membrane of the rat collecting tubule. Proc Natl Acad Sci USA 83:2767–2770
10. Hamilton KL, Eaton DC (1986) Regulation of single sodium channels in renal tissue: a role in sodium homeostasis. Fed Proc 45(12):2713–2717
11. Sariban-Sohraby S, Latorre R, Burg M, Olans L, Benos D (1984) Amiloride-sensitive Na channels reconstructed into planar lipid bilayer membranes. Nature 308:80–82
12. Kolb HA, Brown CDA, Murer H (1986) Characterization of a Ca-dependent maxi K channel in the apical membrane of a cultured renal epithelium (JTC-12 P3). J Membr Biol 92:207–215
13. Ling BN, Eaton DC (1989) Effects of luminal Na⁺ on single Na⁺ channels in A6 cells, a regulatory role for protein kinase C. Am J Physiol 256:F1094–F1103
14. Fichtner H, Frobe U, Busse R, Kolhardt M (1987) Single non selective cation channels and Ca²⁺-activated K⁺ channels in aortic endothelial cells. J Membr Biol 98:125–133
15. Yellen G (1982) Single Ca²⁺-activated nonselective cation channels in neuroblastoma. Nature 296:357–359
16. Paulais M, Teulon J (1989) A cation channel in the thick ascending limb of Henle's loop of the mouse kidney: inhibition by adenine neucleotides. J Physiol 413:315–327
17. Gögelein H, Greger R (1986) A voltage dependent ionic channel in the basolateral membrane of late proximal tubules of the rabbit kidney. Pflugers Arch 407:S142–S148
18. Merot J, Bidet M, Gachot B, Tauc M, Poujeol P (1988) Patch clamp characterization of K⁺ and non selective channels in the apical membrane of rabbit early distal convoluted tubule in primary culture. Act Physiol Pharmacol Bulg 14:102(A)
19. Merot J, Bidet M, Tauc M, Poujeol P (1987) Etude des canaux ioniques dans des cultures primaires de différents segments de néphron de lapin. J Physiol (Paris) 82(3):63(A)

20. Light DB, McCann FV, Keller TM, Stanton BA (1988) Amiloride-sensitive cation channel in apical membrane of inner medullary collecting duct. Am J Physiol 255:F278–F286

21. Koeppen BM, Beyenbach KW, Helman SI (1984) Single channel currents in renal tubules. Am J Physiol 247:F380–F384

22. Frindt G, Palmer LG (1989) Low-conductance K channels in apical membrane of rat cortical collecting tubule. Am J Physiol 256:F143–F151

Index